Handbook of Sensory Physiology

Volume VI/1

Vestibular System Part 1: Basic Mechanisms

By

D. Bagger-Sjöbäck · A. Brodal · B. Cohen · G.F. Dohlman · J.M. Fredrickson
R.R. Gacek · B.E. Gernandt · H.H. Kornhuber · O.E. Lowenstein · H. Markl
G. Melvill Jones · O. Pompeiano · W. Precht · D.W.F. Schwarz · J. Wersäll

Edited by

H.H. Kornhuber

With 251 Figures

Springer-Verlag Berlin · Heidelberg · New York 1974

ISBN 3-540-06889-9 Springer-Verlag Berlin · Heidelberg · New York
ISBN 0-387-06889-9 Springer-Verlag New York · Heidelberg · Berlin

Library of Congress Cataloging in Publication Data. Kornhuber, Hans. Vestibular System. (Handbook of Sensory Physiology, v. 6/1-2). Contents: pt. 1. Basic Mechanisms — pt. 2. Psychophysics, Applied Aspects and General Interpretations. 1. Vestibular Apparatus. I. Bagger-Sjöbäck. II. Title. III. Series. [DNLM: 1. Vestibular Apparatus. 2. Vestibular Nuclei. WL700 H236 v. 6] QP351.H34 vol. 6/1-2 [QP471] 591.1'82'08s [591.1'82]. 74-14870.

Typesetting and printing: Roth sel. Ww., München; Binding: Brühlsche Universitätsdruckerei, Gießen

Preface

The details of the receptor mechanism are not yet fully understood for any sensory system. However, sufficient data are available (for the vestibular system and for other systems) to permit meaningful tracking of the sensory messages through the nervous system and via conscious experience. The reception, processing, storage and output of information in man and other animals, as done by means of receptors, neurons, secretory cells and muscle fibers, are collectively referred to as mind. Sensory physiologists tend to disbelieve in extrasensory perception.

Sensory physiology in general is an area upon which different sciences and methods converge. Anatomists, physiologists, psychologists, physicists, chemists, and engineers have made important contributions to sensory physiology. What is special about vestibular physiology is the fact that many research workers are clinicians, living under the constant pressure of their patient's demands. This is a disadvantage when it comes to writing handbooks, but an advantage for the patient, since research is guided by clinical practice and can be quickly applied. Modern methods, such as recording from single nerve units and the correlation of electrophysiological and psychophysical data, have greatly contributed to our knowledge, yet the study of lesions is still important, especially in the vestibular field.

Part 1 of the vestibular volume of the Handbook of Sensory Physiology is devoted to basic anatomic and physiologic data; Part 2 deals with psychophysics, clinical and other applied aspects, and general interpretations. This division is rather artificial. Anatomists and physiologists will need to read the general interpretations of Part 2 if they are to acquire a coherent understanding of the system. Conversely, otologists, neurologists, psychologists, engineers, and aviation specialists will require the data in Part 1 as well as those in Part 2. Some general sensory physiology, namely a comparison of the vestibular system with other sensory systems, is given in the Introduction (Part 1).

Ulm, June 1974 HANS HELMUT KORNHUBER

List of Contributors

BAGGER-SJÖBÄCK, D., Department of Otolaryngology, B 53, Huddinge Sjukhus, S-14186 Huddinge, Sweden

BRODAL, A., Anatomisk Institutt Universitetet i. Oslo, Karl Johans gate 47, (Domus Media), Oslo 1, Norwegen

COHEN, B., Department of Neurology, Atran 710, Mount Sinai School of Medicine, 100 th Street and Fifth Avenue, New York, N.Y. 10029, USA

DOHLMAN, G.F., Bretton Place, Apt. 1811, 44 Jackes Avenue, Toronto 7, Canada

FREDRICKSON, J.M., Dept. of Otolaryngology, University of Toronto, Medical Sciences Building, Room 7310, 1 Kings College Circle Toronto, Ontario M5 S1 A8 Canada

GACEK, R.R., Private Offices, Dept. of Otolaryngology, Massachusetts Eye and Ear Infirmary, 243 Charles Street, Boston, Mass. 02114, USA

GERNANDT, B.E., Grev Turegatan 82 IV, S-11438 Stockholm, Sweden

KORNHUBER, H.H., Abt. f. Neurologie der Universität, D-7900 Ulm, Steinhövelstraße 9, Germany

LOWENSTEIN, O.E., Dept. of Zoology and Comparative Physiology, University of Birmingham, Neurocommunications Research Unit, Medical School, Birmingham B15 ZTJ, England

MARKL, H., Fachbereich Biologie der Universität, D-7750 Konstanz, Postfach 733, Germany

MELVILL JONES, G., Aviation Medical Research, McGill University, McIntyre Sciences Bldg., 3655 Drummond Street, Montreal, P. Q., Canada

POMPEIANO, O., Istituto di Fisiologia della Universita di Pisa, Via S. Zeno N. 29–31, Pisa, Italia

PRECHT, W., Max-Planck-Institut für Hirnforschung, Neurobiologische Abt., D-6000 Frankfurt-Niederrad, Deutschordenstraße 40, Germany

SCHWARZ, D.W.F., Dept. of Otolaryngology, University of Toronto, Toronto, Canada

WERSÄLL, J., Department of Otolaryngology, B 53, Huddinge Sjukhus, S-14186 Huddinge, Sweden

Vestibular System

Part 1: Basic Mechanisms

Contents

Part 2: Psychophysics, Applied Aspects and General Interpretations

Contents

A. Introduction

A. Introduction

By

H. H. KORNHUBER, Ulm

With 5 Figures

Contents

I. History of Vestibular Research

The history of vestibular research begins early in the nineteenth century. Against a background of the known anatomical structure of the labyrinth in different animals, the work of PURKINJE (1820), FLOURENS (1824), MENIÈRE (1861), GOLTZ (1870), BREUER (1874), MACH (1874), and EWALD (1892) led to the conclusion that the vestibular end-organs have a different function from hearing, and that they regulate body and eye positions and if disturbed, give rise to vertigo. BÁRÁNY in 1906 introduced the caloric test for clinical use.

After the torsion-pendulum motion of the cupula had been demonstrated by STEINHAUSEN in 1931, VAN EGMOND, GROEN and JONGKEES (1949) gave a quantitative description of the mechanics of the torsion pendulum. The quantitative functional analysis of the otoliths was the work of VON HOLST (1950). The interpretation that the kinocilium determines the directional sensitivity of the cupula was given by LOWENSTEIN and WERSÄLL in 1959.

Central vestibular reflex mechanisms in the brainstem and cerebellum were investigated by HÖGYES (1913), MAGNUS (1924), LORENTE DE NÓ (1928), RADEMAKER (1931), and recently by HASSLER (1956), FERNÁNDEZ (1960), BENDER (1964), PASIK (1964), ASCHAN et al. (1964) and COHEN (1971). The neural basis of optokinetic nystagmus was studied by TER BRAAK (1936). The functional morphology of the central vestibular connections was investigated by LORENTE DE NÓ (1928), SZENTÁGOTHAI (1943), BRODAL, POMPEIANO and WALBERG (1962) and CARPENTER (1964). Electrophysiological recordings of the activity of single vestibular nerve fibers and cells were made by LOWENSTEIN and SAND (1940), ADRIAN (1943), DUENSING and SCHAEFER (1957), ITO et al. (1964), TRINCKER (1965), and recently by PRECHT, LLINÁS, SHIMAZU, FERNÁNDEZ and GOLDBERG, and others. The neuronal background of saccadic and pursuit eye movements was elucidated by ROBINSON, FUCHS, SCHILLER and others. The cortical projection of the vestibular nerve was discovered in the cat by WALZL and MOUNTCASTLE (1949), and its location in the postcentral gyrus of the monkey was found by KORNHUBER and FREDRICKSON (1965). DEECKE et al. (1974) investigated the thalamic vestibular representation. Vestibulo-spinal relations were studied by GERNANDT (1959), POMPEIANO (1972) and WILSON (1972). The convergence of deep somatic and vestibular afferents was found by KORNHUBER and ASCHOFF (1964) in the motor cortex and by FREDRICKSON et al. (1965) in the vestibular nuclei. A theory of vestibular function in connection with the general motor system was given by KORNHUBER (1970, 1971).

The clinical characteristics of lesions at different levels of the vestibulo-oculomotor system have been collected and interpreted by BÁRÁNY (1907), DE KLEIJN and VERSTEEGH (1924), NYLEN (1931), JUNG (1953), FRENZEL (1955), BENDER (1962), KORNHUBER (1966), and others. The basis of clinical findings with the galvanic test was investigated by DOHLMAN. Vestibular problems in aerospace medicine were studied by GRAYBIEL (1964).

In contrast to the rapid progress made in the neurophysiology of the vestibular system, research on the metabolism of the vestibular endorgans and on secretion and absorption of the endolymph has advanced more slowly for several reasons. The flow of endolymph to the endolymphatic sac was demonstrated by GUILD in 1927, yet no basis has been found for preventive or conservative treatment of Menière's disease.

II. The Vestibular System in Relation to Other Sensorimotor Systems

Vestibular receptors are located within the labyrinth together with auditory receptors, and both are hair-cell mechanoreceptors. Nevertheless, the vestibular system has very little to do with the auditory system. Throughout the brain, the vestibular system joins deep somatic afferents but not auditory afferents.

On the one hand, the vestibular system is a sensory system with access to the cerebral cortex, conscious perception, and memory. On the other hand, it is a motor system that regulates body posture and eye position. In both respects it is helpful to compare the vestibular system with other sensory systems and to consider it within the framework of the general motor system.

The sensory sisters of vestibular sense are somatic proprioception and visual motion perception in the peripheral field. The motor brothers of the vestibular nuclei are the cerebellar nuclei. As described in more detail elsewhere in this volume, the vestibular nuclei stabilize body and eye positions (in the same way as a gun platform is stabilized on a battleship) in order to ensure safe, goal-directed movements and clear vision. However, if there were nothing but this holding regulation, we would not be able to change our body or eye positions. For active movement something more than holding regulation is necessary, e.g. function generators and programs for movements. The simplest active movement is a small step of standard size. Steps of this kind occur frequently in the motion of invertebrates; often in these animals a single neuron can generate bursts of action potentials that underlie the standard step movements. Vertebrates have developed more complex neuronal machinery for this purpose: first, the reticular nuclei of the brainstem tegmentum, which generate the quick phases of nystagmus, and second, for more complex tasks, the cerebellar cortex, which has a direct connection with the vestibular nuclei. After this system had proved its usefulness, another set of holding regulators evolved, analogous in function to the vestibular nuclei, i.e. the cerebellar nuclei. They do not, as the vestibular system does, regulate the position of the entire body but only of special parts, such as limbs or the eyes, and they obey, not labyrinthine inputs, but the commands of the forebrain.

Let us for a moment consider the stabilization of the eye position in greater detail. The retina is a slow device. It is slow, not only because it operates by photochemistry, but because it is a little brain in itself, a distally located part of the bigger brain, adjacent to the photoreceptors because it has to solve the intensity problem created by earth's rotation. Vision must work over a broad range of intensity, which is why neural mechanisms are necessary in addition to photochemical mechanisms of adaptation (automatic gain control of the response). If the reader moves his index finger back and forth in front of his eyes in a horizontal plane through an angle of about 15° at a frequency of about 4 Hz, his vision will be blurred because of the slowness of retinal information processing. However, if he keeps his finger still and moves his head through the same angle at the same

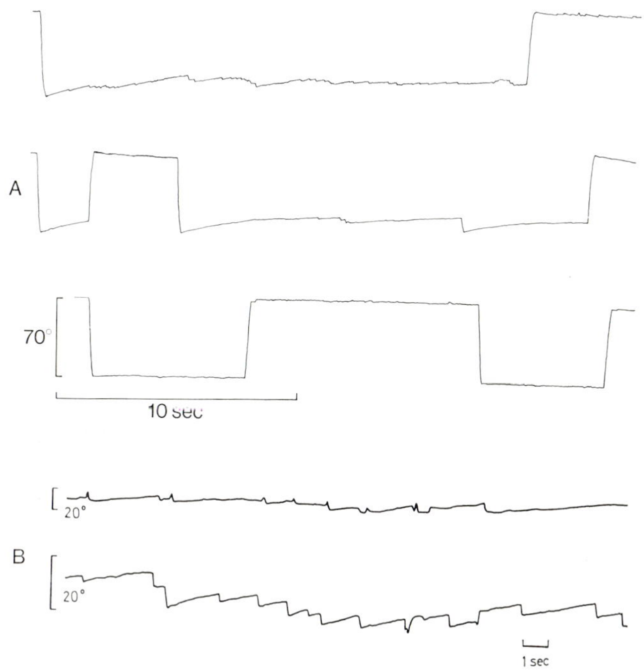

Fig. 1. A: Inability of the normal human oculomotor-vestibular system to maintain eccentric eye positions after exclusion of vision. Lower record: steady maintenance of eye position (35° right and left of midline) with visual fixation. Upper two records: In the same normal person the eyes drift toward midposition in darkness. This drift is partially compensated by saccades, forming a gaze nystagmus. Horizontal leads (FROM BECKER and KLEIN, 1973). B: Inability of the normal human vestibular system to maintain a steady eye position after lid closure. Spontaneous nystagmus in a normal young lady towards left-down with both eyes closed. Upper curve vertical, lower curve horizontal leads; DC recording (From KAMEI and KORNHUBER, 1974)

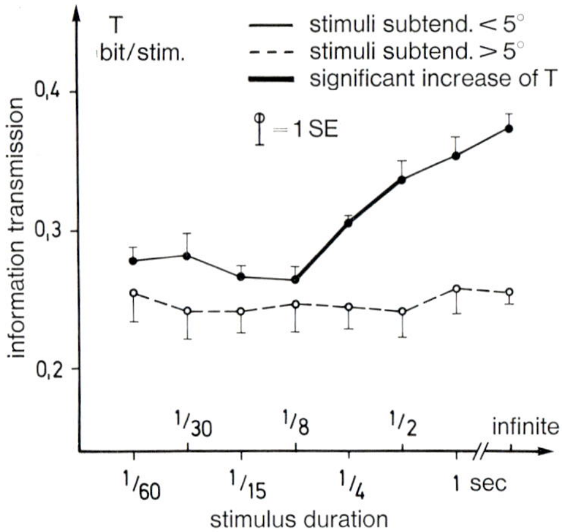

Fig. 2. Information transmission in human visual perception of size (length of horizontal lines presented in random order, method of "absolute judgement") is constant for stimulus durations up to $^1/_8$ sec, but increases significantly at stimulus durations which allow eye movements (250 and 500 msec). This increase occurs, however, only with stimuli of short length subtending visual angles of foveal extension (up to 5°). There is no increase in transmission of length information with long lines subtending visual angles of more than 5°, even up to infinitely long stimulus durations that allow many eye movements. A nonlinear distribution of stimuli of different lengths was used so as to saturate equally well both foveal and peripheral vision; there were 24 stimuli subtending visual angles from 10 min of arc to 5°, and 33 stimuli for angles from 5° to 44° (From BECHINGER, KONGEHL, KORNHUBER and WALTHER, 1974)

frequency, his vision will be clear because vestibular stabilization of eye position works faster. The advantage vestibular regulation has over visual is that its frequency response is better. If vestibular regulation is abolished, vision is still good so long as the head is not moved. A typical complaint of patients with bilateral damage of peripheral vestibular function is that they have to stand still to read a clock on the wall. It is the same with body position: vestibular deficit is most obvious when one is walking on uneven ground in darkness.

Vestibular regulation of eye position is better than visual at the higher frequencies, but worse in the low frequency range. The vestibular apparatus cannot accurately maintain an eccentric eye position if vision is excluded, and the eyes drift back to midposition (BECKER and KLEIN, 1973). Even in midposition there is spontaneous nystagmus in many normal persons when vision is excluded (KAMEI and KORNHUBER, 1974). Thus, continuous visual regulation is necessary in order to hold the eyes constant in a definite position.

The function of the saccadic eye movements which commence from the platform of stabilized eye position is, of course, to direct the fovea with its high visual acuity towards objects of interest. Is there any additional function of the saccades; for instance, do they contribute to the perception of size? At first glance it may seem that they do, because transmission of information about the visual perception of length increases when the stimulus lasts long enough to allow for eye movements, whereas below that stimulus duration information transmission is constant. However, if information transmission is considered separately for small stimuli (subtending visual angles of foveal size up to 5°) and for larger stimuli, only the small stimuli yield an increase in information transmission with eye movements; with larger stimuli there is no increase up to an infinite presentation duration which allows many eye movements (BECHINGER et al., 1974). Thus, the increase with small stimuli is due to better working conditions for the foveal visual channel: many eye movements per se do not result in length information transmission that is better than the visual sensory information transmission at very short presentations.

This lack of feedback from the oculomotor system, with its spindle afferents from eye muscles, to visual size perception, corresponds to a lack of feedback from eye movements as such to conscious perception, and to the suppression of visual motion perception during the saccadic eye movements and fast phases of nystagmus that provides visual space constancy. The reader may do the following simple experiment: let him observe the visual objects in front of him in a field about 5° in diameter. He will always know the position of his eyes but will be barely conscious of his eye movements. Let him now close one eye, put the tips of his index and middle fingers on the lid and look at the objects again with the other eye, moving the eye through the same angle: he will be surprised by the strong tactile sensation evoked by his eye movements. Most naive subjects are unaware of any eye movements taking place during vestibular nystagmus with the eyes open in darkness, or with the eyes closed. A very few report some unilateral tension in the eyes during nystagmus or rhythmic eye movements, but without knowing to which side. After anesthesia of the conjunctival sac (without anesthesia of the eye muscles, of course) none of the subjects feels any eye movements during vestibular nystagmus (LANGE and KORNHUBER, 1964).

Most eye movements occur unconsciously, or half-consciously at most. This is true for vestibular eye movements and also for most saccades. The brain is not interested in knowing about eye movements, but it knows the position of the eyes, and this is what it needs to know for all other visually guided movements, e.g. hand movements. The knowledge of eye position is represented in the cortex in the frontal eye field (BIZZI, 1968).

Fast phases of nystagmus and saccades are helpful if additional information can be gained by foveal inspection. However, in situations where this is not the case, saccades may "mask" visual information processing. Therefore, in such situations (e.g. with stimuli lasting 250 msec or less) eye movements are inhibited for about 200 msec following the end of the stimulus. This inhibition does not occur if stimuli are presented long enough to allow for two or more eye movements (cf. Fig. 3).

Vision and audition are tele-senses, receiving information from distant events. Vestibular sensation belongs to proprioception; it tells us about the position and motion of our body. Touch tells us about changes on our skin, and explores the surface and shape of tactile objects. While the cochlea uses location to represent frequency, touch preserves location as such but carries out a rough local frequency analysis of events, using three sets of receptors of different adaptive behavior (KORNHUBER, 1972). Vision is interested in location, in motion within the visual field, and in the orientation of lines and the pattern of figures. The vestibular system is less sophisticated, but in one respect it is more basic: it tells vision what is up and down. A subject wearing reversing spectacles finds on the first day that

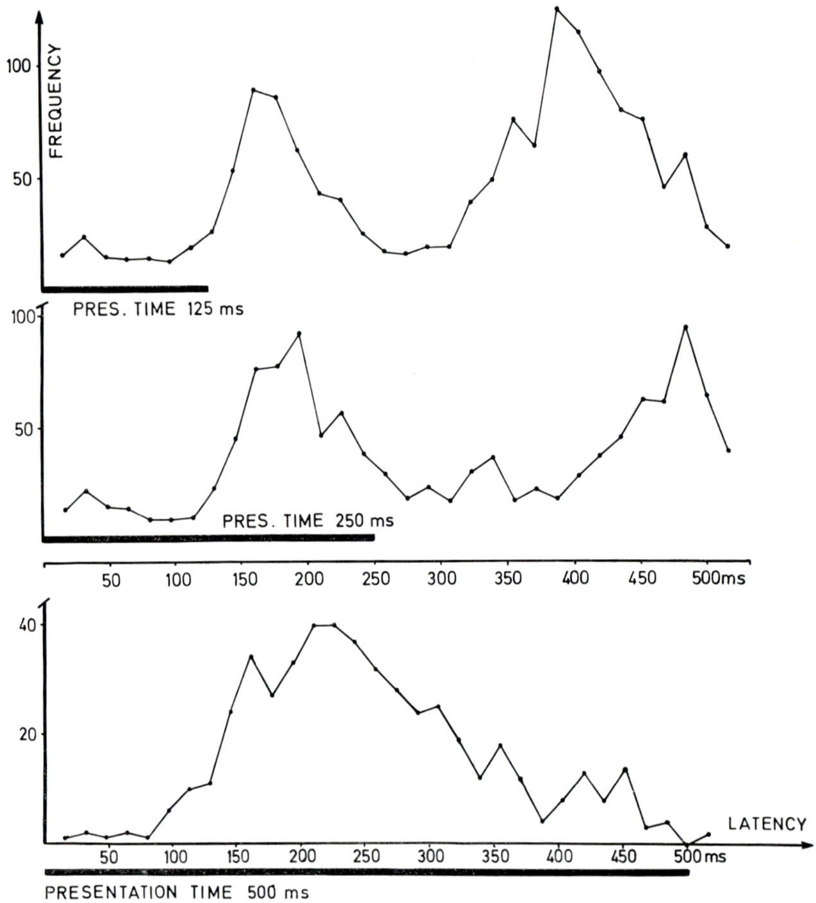

Fig. 3. Analysis of eye movements during the experiments shown in Fig. 2 reveals that the sudden increase of foveal information transmission between stimulus durations of 125 and 250 msec is due to the first saccadic eye movement, which occurs with a latency of about 150 to 250 msec. Furthermore, the frequency distribution of saccades is bimodal with stimuli of 125 and 250 msec, but unimodal with 500 msec stimuli. With stimulus durations of 125 and 250 msec, the first peak of saccades is followed by an inhibition of saccadic eye movements, which lasts about 200 msec after the end of the stimulus. The function of this inhibition is to ensure undisturbed visual information processing in a situation in which more saccades cannot obtain additional information. This inhibition does not occur with stimuli of 500 msec duration. Average of 2 subjects (From BECHINGER, KONGEHL, KORNHUBER and WALTHER, 1973)

everything is upside down; gradually, however, the richer visual system gives way and lets the vestibular and proprioceptive systems determine what is up and what is down. When the spectacles are removed after several days, there is a transient after-effect of the newly established sensory coordination (STRATTON, 1897; KOHLER, 1951).

Vestibular (and other proprioceptive) orientation within the field of gravity does not work equally well in all directions; it refers mainly to the upright position. Therefore, it signals small deviations from the vertical most sensitively

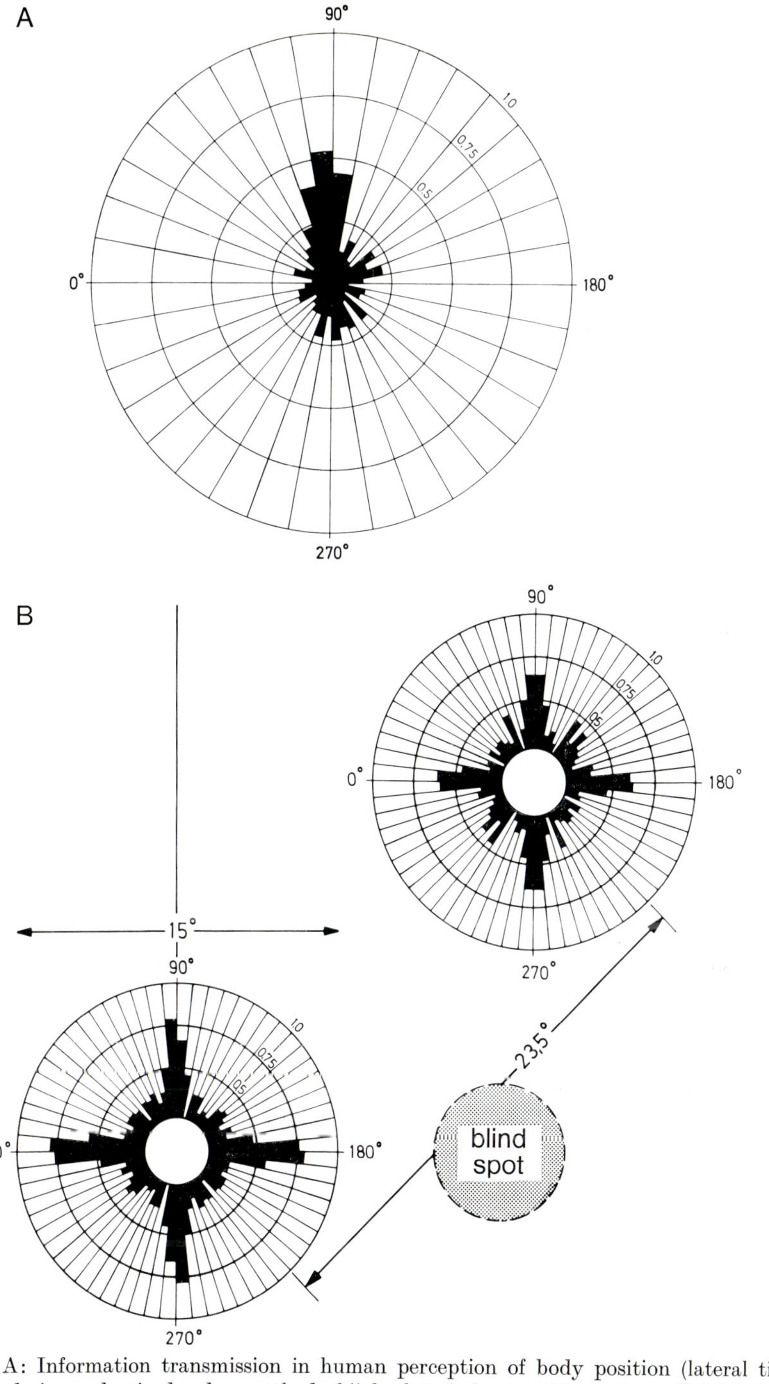

Fig. 4. A: Information transmission in human perception of body position (lateral tilt of whole body in randomized order, method of "absolute judgement") is not equally distributed over the different positions. Vestibular perception of body position is most sensitive near the upright position. In this plot on polar coordinates, the extension of the radial length of the vector is partial information transmission (From BRÜGEL, GIEDKE, KONGEHL and KORNHUBER, 1972). B: In visual perception of angular orientation, information transmission shows maxima around the vertical and horizontal positions in the central (lower left graph) as well as the peripheral visual field (upper right graph); plot similar to A. Stimulus duration $^1/_{60}$ sec, 11 normal subjects (From BECHINGER, KONGEHL and KORNHUBER, Pflügers Arch. **319**, 1970)

(BRÜGEL et al., 1972; see Fig. 4). Deviations from the vertical in the head down position or deviations from the horizontal are much less well perceived. On the other hand, visual perception of the orientation of lines has maxima in both vertical and horizontal directions (BECHINGER et al., 1970; see Fig. 4).

The threshold of vestibular acceleration perception is very low and the effects are alarming, but vestibular sensation disappears during rotation of constant velocity because of the mechanical construction of the receptor organs. In this situation, visual motion perception takes over. As long as visual motion occurs within a steady field of objects, we know that the object is moving. But as soon as the whole visual environment moves, as signalled by the peripheral visual field, we have the impression that we ourselves are moving (circular vection) while the environment is still (BRANDT et al., 1971). Active head movements under conditions of circular vection induced by visual motion even result in Coriolis-like effects and motion sickness similar to those experienced during real rotations of the body (see DICHGANS, Vol. VIII of this handbook). The effect of visual stimuly in the peripheral field is even stronger on linear than on circular vection (BERTHOZ et al. 1974).In other words, vision in the peripheral field acts like the vestibular system and supplements it at constant velocity motions. Convergence of visual motion and vestibular afferents occurs not only at higher levels of the nervous system but also in the vestibular nuclei, and the visually evoked activity is even projected along the efferent pathway to the labyrinth (SCHMIDT et al., 1972).

Vision in the peripheral field has generally been underrated. Though it is weak in differentiating details, peripheral vision overall is strong in detecting changes in motion and brightness, in static and dynamic spatial orientation, and even in transmission of information about size, line orientation, and figures. For example, the maximum flow of information (channel capacity) of size perception, expressed in bits per stimulus, is about six times higher in peripheral than central vision (BECHINGER et al., 1973).

Another case where the cooperation of the vestibular system is important is somatic proprioception. The location of the labyrinths in the head is correct for regulating eye position. Therefore, the contribution of neck proprioception to eye stabilization is very small and in the same direction as the labyrinthine contribution. For the regulation of body position, this location is useful only in fishes. In higher vertebrates with a freely moving head, the labyrinths indicate body position only in conjunction with afferents from neck receptors. Neck receptor activity must be subtracted from vestibular messages in order to give the correct signal for maintaining equilibrium in the tilting situation (VON HOLST and MITTELSTAEDT, 1950). For this reason, the neck reflexes are exactly opposite to the labyrinthine tilting reflexes, which depend on the vertical channels and otoliths. Because of the importance of deep somatic afferents for the vestibular regulation of body position, there are certain regions of the vestibular nuclei where most neurons respond to vestibular and deep somatic afferents, mainly from the neck and the proximal joints of the limbs (FREDRICKSON et al., 1965). This coordination of vestibular and deep somatic afferents occurs throughout the vestibular system, from the vestibular nuclei via the thalamus up to the vestibular sensory and motor cortical areas (KORNHUBER and ASCHOFF, 1964; see also Chap. D. VI., this volume). In

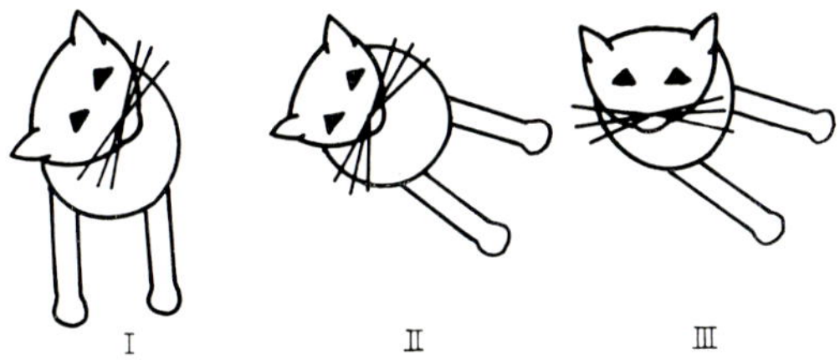

Fig. 5. The labyrinths sense the position of the head but not of the body. Therefore, neck receptor messages must be taken into account to enable the labyrinths to regulate body position. In position I body posture is normal yet the labyrinths sense oblique position. In III this cat is falling, although for the labyrinths everything is in order; the neck receptors signal in this case that postural reflexes must be activated to prevent falling. Only in case II, when labyrinth messages are not abolished by contradictory neck afferents, will the labyrinths give rise to tilting reflexes (From KORNHUBER, Hals-Nasen-Ohrenheilkunde, Handbook, Stuttgart: Thieme Verlag, 1966)

contrast to the poor sensory representation of eye movements, vestibular sensation of head or body movements is strongly represented in conscious experience and has access to long-term memory. The location of the vestibular cortical sensory area in a field juxtaposed and analogous in function to area 2 (in which deep somatic sensation and kinesthesia is represented) ensures strong access not only to the motor cortex but also to the posterior parietal regions (area 7) in which messages from all senses converge to form a unified image of the spatial situation.

References

ADRIAN, E.D.: Discharges from vestibular receptors in the cat. J. Physiol. (Lond.) **101**, 389–407 (1943).

ASCHAN, G., EKVALL, L., GRANT, G.: Nystagmus following stimulation in the central vestibular pathways using permanently implanted electrodes. Acta oto-laryng. (Stockh.) Suppl. **192**, 63–77 (1964).

BÁRÁNY, R.: Untersuchungen über den vom Vestibularapparat des Ohres reflektorisch ausgelösten rhythmischen Nystagmus und seine Begleiterscheinungen. Mschr. Ohrenheilk. **40**, 191–297 (1906).

BÁRÁNY, R.: Physiologie und Pathologie des Bogengangsapparates beim Menschen. Wien: Deuticke 1907.

BECHINGER, D., KONGEHL, G., KORNHUBER, H.H.: Visuelle Informationsübertragung beim Menschen: Richtungsanisotropie im peripheren wie zentralen Sehfeld. Pflügers Arch. **319**, R 157 (1970).

BECHINGER, D., KONGEHL, G., KORNHUBER, H.H.: Glanz und Elend des peripheren Sehens (The virtues of peripheral vision). Pflügers Arch. **339**, R 89 (1973).

BECHINGER, D., KONGEHL, G., KORNHUBER, H.H., WALTHER ,C.: What do the eye movements contribute to the visual perception of length? Pflügers Arch. Physiol. **347**, R 63 (1974).

BECKER, W., KLEIN, H.M.: Accuracy of saccadic eye movements and maintenance of excentric eye positions in the dark. Vision Res. **13**, 1021–1034 (1973).

BENDER, M.B.: Neuroophthalmology. In: A.B. BAKER, Ed. Clinical neurology. New York: Hoeber 1962.

BENDER, M.B., SHANZER, S.: Oculomotor pathways defined by electric stimulation and lesions in the brainstem of the monkey. In: BENDER, Ed. The oculomotor system. New York: Hoeber 1964.

BERTOZ, A., PAVARD, B., YOUNG, L.: Rôle de la vision périphérique et interaction visuo-vestibulaires dans la perception exo-centrique du mouvement linéaire chez l'homme. C.R. Acad. Sci. (Paris) **278**, 1605–1608 (1974).

BIZZI, E.: Discharge of frontal eye field neurons during saccadic and following eye movements in unanesthetized monkeys. Exp. Brain Res. **6**, 69–80 (1968).

BRAAK, J.W.G. TER: Untersuchungen über optokinetischen Nystagmus. Arch. néerl. Physiol. **21**, 309 (1936).

BRANDT, T., WIST, E., DICHGANS, J.: Optisch induzierte Pseudocoriolis-Effecte und Circularvection. Ein Beitrag zur optisch-vestibulären Interaktion. Arch. Psychiat. Nervenkr. **214**, 365–389 (1971).

BREUER, J.: Über die Funktion der Bogengänge des Ohrlabyrinthes. Wien. med. Jahrb. **4**, 72 (1874).

BREUER, J.: Neue Versuche an den Ohrbogengängen. Pflügers Arch. ges. Physiol. **44**, 135–152 (1889).

BRODAL, A., POMPEIANO, O., WALBERG, F.: The vestibular nuclei and their connections. Anatomy and functional correlations. Springfield/Ill.: C.C. Thomas; Edinburgh: Oliver and Boyd 1962.

BRÜGEL, R., GIEDKE, H., KONGEHL, G., KORNHUBER, H.H.: Information transmission in the human perception of angular orientation. Pflügers Arch. **335**, R 79 (1972).

CARPENTER, M.B.: Ascending vestibular projections and conjugate horizontal eye movements. p. 150–189. In: FIELDS and ALFORD, Eds. Neurological aspects of auditory and vestibular disorders. Springfield/Ill.: C.C. Thomas 1964.

COHEN, B.: Vestibulo-ocular relations. p. 105–148. In: BACH-Y-RITA and COLLINS, Eds. The control of eye movements. New York and London: Academic Press 1971.

DEECKE, L., SCHWARZ, D.W.F., FREDRICKSON, J.M.: Nucleus ventroposterior inferior (VPI) as the vestibular thalamic relay in the rhesus monkey. Exp. Brain Res. **20**, 88–100 (1974).

DOHLMAN, G.: Experimentelle Untersuchungen über die galvanische Vestibularisreaktion. Acta oto-laryng. (Stockh.) SUPPL. **8**, (1929).

DUENSING, F., SCHAEFER, K.P.: Die Neuronenaktivität in der Formatio reticularis des Rhombencephalons beim vestibulären Nystagmus. Arch. Psychiat. Nervenkr. **196**, 265–290 (1957).

DUENSING, F., SCHAEFER, K.P.: Die Aktivität einzelner Neurone im Bereich der Vestibulariskerne bei Horizontalbeschleunigungen unter besonderer Berücksichtigung des vestibulären Nystagmus. Arch. Psychiat. Nervenkr. **198**, 225–252 (1958).

EGMOND, A.J., VAN, GROEN, J.J., JONGKEES, L.B.W.: The mechanics of the semicircular canal. J. Physiol. (Lond.) **110**, 1–17 (1949).

EWALD, J.R.: Physiologische Untersuchung des Endorgans des N. octavus. Wiesbaden: Bergmann 1892.

FERNÁNDEZ, C.: Interrelations between flocculonodular lobe and vestibular system. pp. 285–296. In: G.L. RASMUSSEN and W.F. WINDLE, Eds. Neural mechanisms of the auditory and vestibular systems. Springfield/Ill.: C.C. Thomas 1960.

FERNÁNDEZ, C., GOLDBERG, J.M.: Physiology of peripheral neurons innervating semicircular canals of the squirrel monkey. II. Responses to sinusoidal stimulation and dynamics of peripheral vestibular system. J. Neurophysiol. **34**, 661–675 (1971).

FLOURENS, P.: Recherches experimentales sur les propriétés et les fonctions du système nerveux dans les animaux vertébrés. Paris: Crevot 1824.

FREDRICKSON, J.M., SCHWARZ, D., KORNHUBER, H.H.: Convergence and interaction of vestibular and deep somatic afferents upon neurons in the vestibular nuclei of the cat. Acta oto-laryng. (Stockh.) **61**, 168–188 (1965).

FRENZEL, H.: Spontan- und Provokationsnystagmus als Krankheitssymptom. Berlin-Göttingen-Heidelberg: Springer 1955.

FUCHS, A.F., LUSCHEI, E.S.: Unit activity in the brainstem related to eye movement. Bibl. ophthal. (Basel) **82**, 17–27 (1872).

GERNANDT, B.: Vestibular mechanisms. In: Handbook of physiology, section I Neurophysiology, Vol. I, p. 549–564. Washington, D.C.: Amer. Physiolog. Soc. 1959.

GOLTZ, F.: Über die physiologische Bedeutung der Bogengänge des Ohrlabyrinthes. Pflügers Arch. ges. Physiol. **3**, 172–192 (1870).

GRAYBIEL, A.: Vestibular sickness and some of its implications for space flight. p. 248–270. In: FIELDS and ALFORD, Eds. Neurological aspects of auditory and vestibular disorders. Springfield/Ill.: C.C. Thomas 1964.

GUILD, S.R.: The circulation of the endolymphe. Amer. J. Anat. **39**, 57–81 (1927).

HASSLER, R.: Die zentralen Apparate der Wendebewegungen. Arch. Psychiat. Nervenkr. **194**, 456–480 und 481–516 (1956).

HÖGYES, A.: Der Nervenmechanismus der assoziierten Augenbewegungen. Wien: Urban & Schwarzenberg 1913.

VON HOLST, E.: Die Arbeitsweise des Statolithenapparates bei Fischen. Z. vergl. Physiol. **32**, 60–120 (1950).

VON HOLST, E., MITTELSTAEDT, H.: Das Reafferenzprinzip (Wechselwirkungen zwischen Zentralnervensystem und Peripherie). Naturwissenschaften **37**, 464–475 (1950).

ITO, M.: Cerebellar control of the vestibular neurones: Physiology and Pharmacology. Progr. Brain Res. **37**, 377–390 (1972).

ITO, M., YOSHIDA, M.: The cerebellar-evoked monosynaptic inhibition of Deiters' neurons. Experientia (Basel) **20**, 515–516 (1964).

JUNG, R.: Nystagmographie: Zur Physiologie und Pathologie des optisch-vestibulären Systems beim Menschen. In: G. v. BERGMANN et al., Eds. Handbuch der inneren Medizin, 4. Ed., Vol. V/1, p. 1325. Berlin-Göttingen-Heidelberg: Springer 1953.

JUNG, R., KORNHUBER, H.H.: Results of electronystagmography in man: the value of optokinetic, vestibular and spontaneous nystagmus for neurologic diagnosis and research. p. 428–482. In: M.B. BENDER, Ed. The oculomotor system. New York: Hoeber 1964.

KAMEI, T., KORNHUBER, H.H.: Spontaneous and head-shaking nystagmus in normal and in patients with central lesions. Canad. J. Otolaryng. **3** (1974).

DE KLEYN, A., VERSTEEGH, C.: Schwindelanfälle und Nystagmus bei einer bestimmten Lage des Kopfes. Acta oto-laryng. (Stockh.) **6**, 99–105 (1924).

KOHLER, J.: Über Aufbau und Wandlung der Wahrnehmungswelt. Sitz. Ber. österr. Akad. Wiss. phil. hist. Kl. 227, 1, 1951.

KORNHUBER, H.H.: Physiologie und Klinik des zentralvestibulären Systems (Blick- und Stützmotorik). In: BERENDES, LINK und ZÖLLNER, Eds. Hals-Nasen-Ohrenheilkunde, Handbuch, Vol. III, part. 3, p. 2150–2351. Stuttgart: Thieme 1966.

KORNHUBER, H.H.: Das vestibuläre System, mit Exkursen über die motorischen Funktionen der Formatio reticularis, des Kleinhirns, der Stammganglien und des motorischen Cortex sowie über die Raumkonstanz der Sehdinge. In: W.D. KEIDEL and K.H. PLATTIG, Hrsg. Vorträge der Erlanger Physiologentagung 1970, S. 173–203. Berlin-Heidelberg-New York: Springer 1971.

KORNHUBER, H.H.: Motor functions of the cerebellum and basal ganglia: the cerebello-cortical saccadic (ballistic) clock, the cerebello-nuclear hold regulator, and the basal ganglia ramp (voluntary speed smooth movement) generator. Kybernetik 8, 157–162 (1971).

KORNHUBER, H.H.: Tastsinn und Lagesinn. In: Somatische Sensibilität, Geruch und Geschmack (Sinnesphysiologie I), Band 11 aus GAUER, KRAMER und JUNG, Hrsg. Physiologie des Menschen. München, Berlin, Wien: Urban & Schwarzenberg 1972.

KORNHUBER, H.H., ASCHOFF, J.C.: Somatisch-vestibuläre Integration an Neuronen des motorischen Cortex. Naturwissenschaften **51**, 62–63 (1964).

KORNHUBER, H.H., FREDRICKSON, J.M., FIGGE, U.: Die cortikale Projection der vestibulären Afferenz beim Rhesus-Affen. Pflügers Arch. ges. Physiol. **283**, R 20 (1965).

LANGE, G., KORNHUBER, H.H.: Nichtwahrnehmung der Augenbewegungen und corneoconjunctivale Entstehung des subjectiven Augenzuges beim vestibulären Nystagmus. Acta oto-laryng. (Stockh.) **58**, 503–509 (1964).

LORENTE DE NÓ, R.: Die Labyrinthreflexe auf die Augenmuskeln nach einseitiger Labyrinthexstirpation nebst einer kurzen Angabe über den Nervenmechanismus der vestibulären Augenbewegungen. Berlin, Wien: Urban & Schwarzenberg 1928.

LORENTE DE NÓ, R.: Vestibulo-ocular reflex arc. Arch. Neurol. (Chic.) **30**, 245–291 (1933).

LOWENSTEIN, O., SAND, A.: The individual and integrated activity of the semicircular canals of the elasmobranch labyrinth. J. Physiol. (Lond.) **99**, 89–101 (1940).

LOWENSTEIN, O., WERSÄLL, J.: A functional interpretation of the electron-microscopic structure of the sensory hairs in the cristae of the elasmobranch Raja clavata in terms of directional sensitivity. Nature (Lond.) **184**, 1807–1810 (1959).

MACH, E.: Über den Gleichgewichtssinn. Sitzungsber. kaiserl. Akad. Wissensch. Wien, Math. Nat. Kl. 69, III, 44 (1874).

MACH, E.: Grundlinien der Lehre von den Bewegungsempfindungen. Leipzig: Engelmann 1875.

MAGNUS, R.: Körperstellung. Berlin: Springer 1924.

MENIÈRE, P.: Sur une forme de surdité grave dépandant d'une lésion de l'oreille interne. Bull. d'Otol. etc. **26**, 241 (1861).

NYLEN, C.O.: A clinical study on positional nystagmus in cases of brain tumour. Acta otolaryng. (Stockh.) Suppl. **15** (1931).

PASIK, P., PASIK, T.: Oculomotor functions in monkeys with lesions of the cerebrum and the superior colliculi. In: M.B. BENDER, Ed. The oculomotor system. New York: Hoeber 1964.

POMPEIANO, O.: Spinovestibular relations: anatomical and physiological aspects. Progr. Brain Res. **37**, 263–296 (1972).

PRECHT, W., LLINÁS, R.: Responses of vestibular nuclear neurons to ampullar input. Progr. Brain Res. **37**, 89–107 (1972).

PURKINJE, J.E.: Beiträge zur näheren Kenntnis des Schwindels aus heautognostischen Daten. Med. Jb. (Wien) **6**, 79–125 (1820).

RADEMAKER, G.J.: Das Stehen. Berlin: Springer 1931.

ROBINSON, D.A.: Models of oculomotor neural organization, p. 519–538. In: BACH-Y-RITA and COLLINS, Eds. The control of eye movements. New York, London: Academic Press 1971.

ROBINSON, D.A., KELLER, E.L.: The behavior of eye movement motoneurons in the alert monkey. Bibl. ophthal. (Basel) **82**, 7–16 (1972).

SCHILLER, P.H.: Some functional characteristics of the superior colliculus in the rhesus monkey. Bibl. ophthal. (Basel) **82**, 130–138 (1972).

SCHMIDT, C.L., WIST, E.R., DICHGANS, J.: Efferent frequency modulation in the vestibular nerve of goldfish correlated with saccadic eye movements. Exp. Brain Res. **15**, 1–14 (1972).

SHIMAZU, H.: Organization of the comissural connections: physiology. Progr. Brain Res. **37**, 177–190 (1972).

STEINHAUSEN, W.: Über den Nachweis der Bewegung der Cupula in der intakten Bogengangsampulle des Labyrinthes bei der natürlichen rotatorischen und calorischen Reizung. Pflügers Arch. ges. Physiol. **228**, 322–328 (1931).

STRATTON, G.M.: Vision without inversion of the retinal image. Psychol. Rev. **4**, 341, 463 (1897).

SZENTÁGOTHAI, J.: Die zentrale Innervation der Augenbewegungen. Arch. Psychiat. Nervenkr. **116**, 721–760 (1943).

TRINCKER, D.: Physiologie des Gleichgewichtsorgans, p. 310–361. In: BERENDES, LINK und ZÖLLNER, Eds. Hals-Nasen-Ohrenheilkunde, Handbuch, Vol. III, part 1. Stuttgart: Thieme 1965.

WALZL, E.M., MOUNTCASTLE, V.B.: Projection of vestibular nerve to cerebral cortex of the cat. Amer. J. Physiol. **159**, 595 (1949).

WILSON, V.J.: Vestibular influences on alpha motoneurons in the cervical and thoracic cord. Progr. Brain Res. **37**, 233–242 (1972).

B. Comparative Morphology and Physiology

Chapter I.

The Perception of Gravity and of Angular Acceleration in Invertebrates

By

H. Markl*, Konstanz

With 27 Figures

Contents

I. Introduction

It is not just scientific curiosity which makes physiologists turn to lower animals for subjects of their experiments; often enough they have supplied excellent preparations for the analysis of mechanisms which could only be dealt with with difficulties, if at all, in Vertebrates. Furthermore, most biologists feel that they do not understand a particular organ and its function completely unless they have learned how it has developed in evolution.

* Fachbereich Biologie der Universität Konstanz.

There are two approaches to the question of how "lower" forms achieve what a vertebrate achieves with the aid of its vestibular apparatus. A sensory physiologist is likely to inquire how — if at all — invertebrates perceive the stimuli a vertebrate perceives by means of its vestibular organs, or more specifically, since the adequate stimulus for vestibular sense organs is mechanical energy in the form of acceleration (linear, angular, sometimes sinusoidal), which sense organs of lower animals respond to these stimuli. On the other hand, someone more interested in understanding how sense organs are used by an animal, might reason that vestibular sense organs are used in vertebrates to control the body's position in space and to monitor intended changes or compensate for imposed changes in this position, and ask whether invertebrates can do the same and which sense organs they apply.

Both approaches are valid. The second, behavioral line of reasoning includes such mechanisms as optical means of posture control, which are not closely related to vestibular senses in vertebrates (though these very mechanisms may replace vestibular ones in some invertebrates). Thus it seemed preferable to limit the scope of this review to mechanoreceptor mechanisms in invertebrates, which are involved in posture control. In addition, attention will be drawn to tonus-controlling effects of such organs as well as to their possible role in vibration reception. However, though statocysts were regarded as hearing organs for a long time, surprisingly few investigators have studied their sensivity to vibration in lower animals.

A phylogenetic approach has been chosen, since it is for taxonomic rather than functional reasons that "lower forms" are contrasted to vertebrates in this volume. The appropriate way to deal with them is therefore phylum by phylum.

Definitions: The terms "longitudinal, dorsoventral and transverse axes" are usually self-explanatory in bilaterals. Rotations about these axes are called respectively rolling, yawing and pitching.

Gravireception will be used as a short term for "perception of gravity".

Bibliography: Most of the earlier literature is collected in MANGOLD (1913), PLATE (1924), KOLMER (1926) and VON BUDDENBROCK (1952). The handbooks by GRASSÉ, HYMAN and BULLOCK and HORRIDGE are valuable sources of references. SCHÖNE (1959) gives a review of some modern concepts for the behavioral analysis of the maintenance of equilibrium. The most recent reviews of the subject matter can be found in GORDON and COHEN (1971) and Fortschritte der Zoologie **22**, (1973). Only the more important publications used in the preparation of this paper are cited in the bibliography. They give access to additional material.

II. General Remarks

A capacity to orient the body's axes with respect to gravity during rest or during locomotion has been reported in most or all invertebrate phyla. Responsiveness to angular acceleration is only well known in arthropods and mollusks. Sense organs presumably used for gravireception have also been described in most groups, though experimental proof of their function is often poor or unavailable. Only a few crustaceans, insects and mollusks have been studied more thoroughly, and analysis at the level of the receptor cell has rarely been undertaken even in these groups.

Methods used in the study of gravireception and angular acceleration perception in invertebrates have generally been of the following types:

A. Gravireception:

I. Responses to gravity.

1. An animal upon which a change of position of a body axis relative to gravity has been forced reacts with sustained compensatory movements directed at regaining the former, undisturbed position in space. The experiment can be performed in stationary animals, which respond by *righting* themselves, or during locomotion, for instance on a seesaw. Response to gravity is assumed if the reaction persists after elimination of all other possible sources of orienting stimuli and if essentially similar manipulations, which do not change the angle between a body-axis and gravity — e.g. a change of position in the horizontal plane — do not evoke compensatory movements.

2. An animal keeps the position of its eyes in space as constant as possible if its body's spatial orientation is changed, thus stabilizing retinal images (compensatory eye movements).

II. Localization of gravireceptors.

1. Elimination experiments. Reactions of type I1 or I2 are no longer observed after destruction of a suspected gravireceptor. Quite often in behavioral experiments it is extremely difficult to decide whether an operation has eliminated the relevant receptor or only damaged some other link in the chain between receptor and effector.

2. Recording of the electrical activity of a suspected gravireceptor, when defined gravitational stimuli are applied. A gravireceptor should be capable of indicating a sustained position by having a tonic or phasictonic response characteristic. Whether a receptor thus shown to be able to perceive gravity is actually used for that purpose by the animal should always be confirmed by behavioral experiments.

3. By way of analogy or by inferring homology, organs are frequently described as gravireceptors if similarly constructed organs have been demonstrated to respond to gravity in other, preferably closely related, animals. This can obviously not be regarded as more than a working hypothesis.

The most common type of gravireceptor is the *statocyst*, a fluid-filled sac containing particles (one *statolith* or numerous *statoconia*) of higher density than the fluid. The cyst wall contains sensory cells that register the position of these particles, which depends on the direction of the gravitational force. Occasionally, a statolith is located inside a cell (*lithocyte*) which often together with others, may give weight to a pendulumlike projection of the surface, the *lithostyle*. The direction in which this pendulum hangs down is monitored by receptors. In insects, two entirely different types of gravireceptors have been described (cf. p. 41, 42); for still another type see also p. 40.

III. Further characteristics of orientation with respect to gravity.

Gravity orientation during locomotion can also be classified by the sign of the reaction (positive: parallel to the gravitational field; negative: antiparallel to it), the capacity to orient at an any angle varying between 0° and 360° to gravity (menotaxis, compass orientation), or the way paired receptors are used (independently or not).

For a discussion of the classification of orientation mechanisms, see FRAENKEL and GUNN (1961), JANDER (1963, 1966), SCHÖNE (1973). FRAENKEL and GUNN also discuss the investigations by CROZIER and others on peculiarities of geotactic orientation of animals with and without statocysts on inclined surfaces (see also CLARKE, 1970).

For many animals, light is as important a factor as gravity for the conservation of equilibrium. A close connection between orientation by these two stimuli is therefore frequently noticed. Commonly, a positive (negative) phototactic tendency goes with a negative (positive) geotactic one. In insects, the capacity to switch from light orientation to a corresponding angle of gravity orientation is very common ("transposition", cf. von FRISCH (1965) and LINSENMAIR-ZIEGLER (1970) for references). Many swimming, and probably many flying animals also, control their equilibrium by stabilizing their dorsoventral axis in the direction of light and of gravity. If the two stimuli are given under different angles, a resultant orientation is often assumed. This fact has been profitably used for the analysis of gravireception since it was noted by von BUDDENBROCK (1914).

B. The perception of angular acceleration.

Compensatory turns opposing an accelerated rotation imposed upon the animal are recorded in tests analogous to those described under AI and AII. Receptors are localized by finding out which organs have to be eliminated to upset this reaction. Eye movements that compensate for rotations are called *nystagmus*.

III. Protozoa

A considerable number of publications have appeared on geotactic responses in ciliates, mostly in *Paramecium*, though most of the work was done more than thirty years ago. Unquestionably, these protozoa migrate upward when exposed to a variety of stimuli, most noticeably when exposed to increased concentrations of carbon dioxide. This movement is said to be oriented by gravity. The mechanism of this orientation is far from being understood (JAHN and BOVEE, 1967). Whereas KOEHLER (1922, 1930) concludes from his experiments with iron-fed *Paramecium* that cell inclusions of higher density act as statoliths and thus make the cell sensitive to gravity, DEMBOWSKI (1931) maintains that orientation depends on the fact that the posterior half of the body is heavier than the anterior half. MERTON (1935) was unable to confirm this experimentally. However, ROBERTS (1970) concludes from experiments on *Paramecium* and on small-scale models that the cause of geotaxis in Protozoa is a body shape-dependent, gravity-induced hydrodynamic torque. ANDERSON and DUMONT (1966) describe the ultrastructure of an organelle found only in ciliates of the families *Bütschliidae* and *Paraisotrichidae* which would fit nicely into KOEHLER's scheme of gravireception. These ciliates possess vacuoles containing concrements of a calcium compound which come into close contact with ciliary rootlets. Little is known about responses to gravity in these endocommensals.

It should be emphasized in this connection that statoliths are generally intracellular in the simplest metazoans (coelenterates).

Porifera

No responses to gravity are on record.

IV. Coelenterata

A. Cnidaria

Coelenterates are the simplest animals equipped with true gravireceptors. The HERTWIG brothers (1878) gave a classic anatomical account of what they regarded as hearing organs in medusae. They concluded that in Coelenterata these organs evolved independently two or three times, from club-like projections of the body surface, some of whose entodermal or ectodermal cells are loaded with *intracellular* calcareous particles. These lithostyles hang openly from the body surface, or become enclosed in capsules. Sensory cells are arranged around the pendulum so as to monitor its position. HORRIDGE (1969, 1971) has reexamined some of these organs with the electron microscope. The sensory cells bear non-motile cilia of the (9+2) filament pattern, the line connecting the two central filaments at right angles to the line of the expected deflexion by the statolith. These cilia emerge from a craterlike membrane ring or a ring of fingerlike microvilli without fibrillar structure. HORRIDGE hypothesizes that gravity receptors in coelenterates may have developed from groups of cells bearing non-motile cilia which are sensitive to underwater vibration. When the bases of these receptors were loaded with a calcareous secretion the vibration receptors were further perfected and a way was opened for the evolution of a loaded pendulum which could be displaced by gravity when the animal changed its position in space.

Considering how much detail we know about the morphology of these organs, experimental evidence to support the assumption that they are gravireceptive is often far from being impressive. Few organisms have been studied with any care, most of them scyphomedusae.

Polyps:

Statocysts or comparable organs have only very rarely been found in the polyps of Hydrozoa or Anthozoa. However, remarkably clear geotropic reactions occur in *Aglaophenia* (LOEB, 1891), while *Cerianthus* (LOEB, 1891) and *Pennatula* (FRAENKEL and GUNN, 1961) burrow geotactically. The *Aglaophenia* colony grows straight up even in the dark; change of position is corrected for in subsequently grown portions. *Corymorpha palma* rights itself when placed in a horizontal posture as long as the neuromuscular system is intact (PARKER, 1917). CAMPBELL (1972) described a remarkable statocyst with no cilia or nerve cells in this hydroid polyp: a spherical cavity between terminal entodermal cells of the stolons of *Corymorpha* contains a statolith presumably originating from an entodermal cell, which seems to affect ectodermal contractile cell processes directly, so that the stolon is directed straight downward.

Medusae:

Hydrozoa:

"Static organs" have been described in Lepto-, Limno-, Trachy- and Narcomedusae.

Leptomedusae: Depending on age and species, 8 to several hundred "statocysts" are developed on the underside of the velum. The organ is an open pit (*Mitrocoma*) or, more frequently, a closed vesicle (Fig. 1). Ectodermal litho-

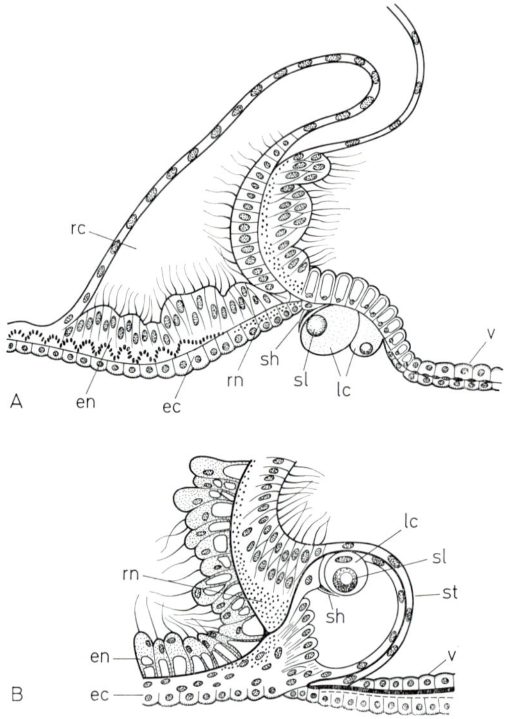

Fig. 1. A: Lithostyles in the open subvelar crypt of *Mitrocoma annae* (Leptomedusae) in a radial section through the margin of the bell. The larger lithocyte is flanked by a sensory hair. B: Lithostyle as a closed vesicle in *Aequorea forskali* (Leptomedusae). *ec*: ectoderm; *en*: entoderm; *lc*: lithocyte; *rc*: ring canal; *rn*: ring nerve; *sh*: sensory hair; *sl*: statolith; *st*: statocyst; *v*: velum (From Bütschli, 1925, after O. and R. Hertwig, 1878)

cytes project clublike into the cavity. They are surrounded by one to several sensory haircells.

Trachymedusae and *Narcomedusae* possess from 4 to 80 lithostyles on the underside of the exumbrellar margin (only in *Hydroctena* are they in aboral position: Dawydoff, 1953). Lithostyles hang openly (*Cunina* (Fig. 2), *Aeginopsis*) or enclosed in a cyst (*Rhopalonema*, *Geryonia* (Fig. 3)). Lithocytes are generally entodermal, though Horridge finds they are extracellular in *Cunina*. Epithelial cells surrounding the lithocytes carry cilia which touch the body wall around the lithostyle. Some or all of these are thought to be sensory. In *Geryonia*, which has the most complex "static organ" found in medusae (Fig. 3), each sensory cell carries one non-motile (9+2) cilium amidst approximately 200 microvilli which have no fibrillar organization (Horridge, 1969).

There is no experimental proof for the static function of the organs in hydromedusae hitherto mentioned. Fraenkel (1925) and Bozler (1926) describe equilibrating movements in *Aequorea*, *Tima* and *Geryonia*, but have not located the sense organs responsible for this reaction.

In the *Limnomedusa Gonionemus*, removal of the "static organs" did not affect orientation in space at all during locomotion (Murbach, 1903, 1905).

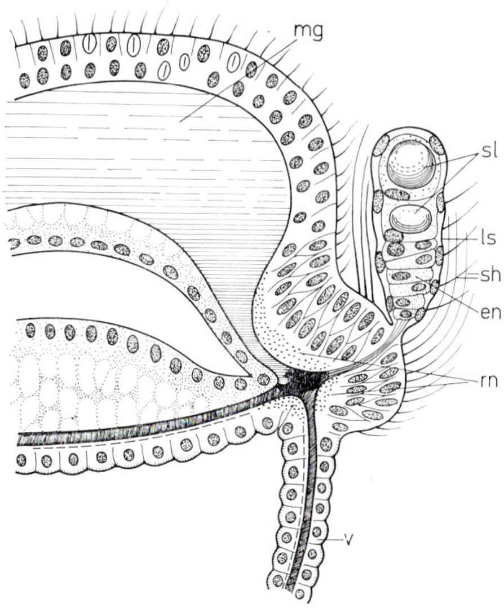

Fig. 2. Lithostyle of *Cunina lativentris* (Narcomedusae) in a radial section through the margin of the bell. *en*: entoderm; *ls*: lithostyle; *mg*: mesogloea; *rn*: ring nerve; *sh*: sensory hair; *sl*: statolith; *v*: velum (From Bütschli, 1925, after O. and R. Hertwig, 1878)

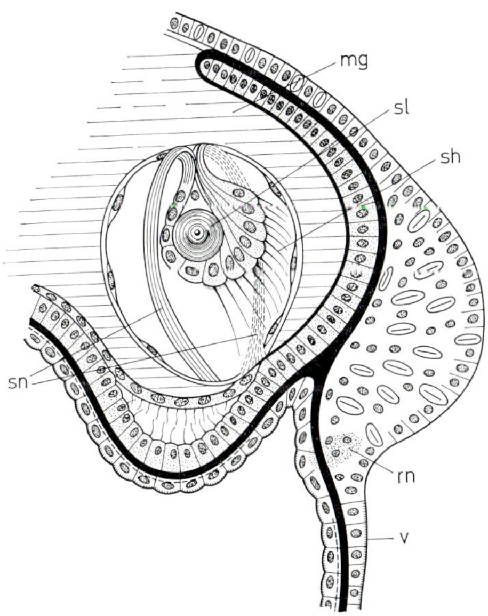

Fig. 3. Statocyst of *Carmarina hastata* (= *Geryonia*) (Trachymedusae) in a radial section through the margin of the bell. Horridge finds the sensory hairs surrounded by numerous microvilli. *mg*: mesogloea; *rn*: ring nerve; *sh*: sensory hair; *sl*: statolith; *sn*: statocyst nerve; *v*: velum (From Bütschli, 1925, after O. and R. Hertwig, 1878)

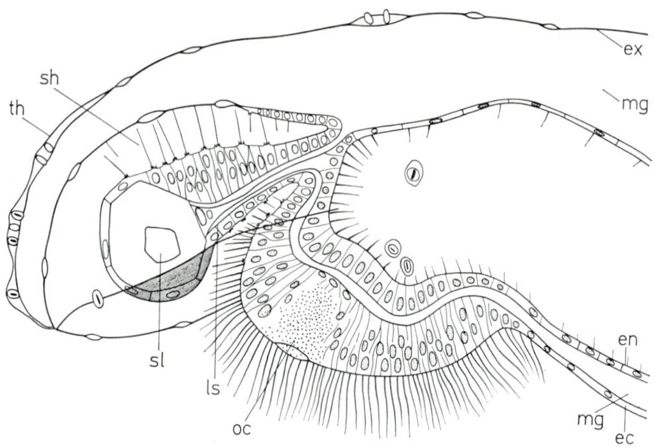

Fig. 4. Longitudinal section through the marginal sense organ of *Nausithoe albida* (Coronata). At the base of some of the sensory hairs, the craterlike membrane ring is shown, from which these hairs originate in HORRIDGE's description. *ec*: ectoderm; *en*: entoderm; *ex*: exumbrella; *ls*: lithostyle; *mg*: mesogloea; *oc*: ocellus; *sh*: sensory hair; *sl*: statolith; *th*: tectorial hood (Redrawn from O. and R. HERTWIG, 1878)

Scyphozoa:

The marginal body (rhopale) of scyphomedusae plays a part in the conservation of equilibrium. It is a transformed tentacle, hanging from the margin of the bell and more or less protected by surrounding tissue (Fig. 4). The typical number is 8, though in *Polyclonidae* there are 12 and in *Sthenonidae* 16 rhopalia, and in some forms (e.g. *Tessera*) there are none. In the distal part of the rhopale, entodermal cells produce statoliths, which contain calcium sulfate, carbonate, and phosphate (SPEK, 1914; YAMASHITA, 1957). Non-motile cilia project from sensory cells at the base of the tentacle towards the surrounding wall. They are bent differently according to the direction in which the rhopale dangles. The function of these organs has been studied experimentally by LEHMANN (1923), FRAENKEL (1925), BOZLER (1926a, b, c) and HORSTMANN (1934). LEHMANN concludes the marginal bodies are unimportant in orientation, since the animals (*Chrysaora* and *Cyanea*) are swimming in a mechanically stable equilibrium but influence the tonus and contraction frequency of the bell musculature. The other authors have accumulated convincing evidence for a gravireceptive role of these sense organs in *Cotylorhiza*, *Rhizostoma*, *Pelagia*, *Aurelia* and *Cyanea*. These medusae can maintain a defined position in space independently of mechanical stability, be it exumbrella down or up or at any angle to the vertical. Thus oriented, they can move on a straight course. They compensate for passive rotations by contracting the bell asymmetrically. This depends on the presence of marginal bodies, which, in addition, enhance the frequency of contraction (general stimulating effect). If only one rhopale is left intact, its deflexion in opposite directions triggers opposite effects on bell contractions.

It is remarkable that even in these low animals, the equilibrating system is not set invariably at one particular position in space, but can stabilize quite a variety of positions relative to gravity. Even here a servo-mechanism seems to be at work in which some higher center sets the control variable.

B. Ctenophora

Since the first detailed anatomical descriptions by Chun (1880) and Hertwig (1880), the *apical organ* of ctenophores has often attracted the interest of physiologists. Its structure is unique (Fig. 5) (ultrastructural details from Horridge, 1965a, 1966, 1971; and Krisch, 1973). Balanced upon four groups of cilia, the statolith stands in the center of the organ. It is composed of numerous cells stemming from the statocyst floor which contain calcareous particles. The balancers consist of 100–200 cilia of the (9+2) pattern. Balancers and lith are roofed over by a translucid dome of interwoven cells and cilia, which leaves only four small openings at its base. Through these, ciliated grooves lead from the base of the balancer cilia to the apical end of the comb-plate rows, each groove bifurcating and serving two rows. The comb-plates are the organs of locomotion and consist

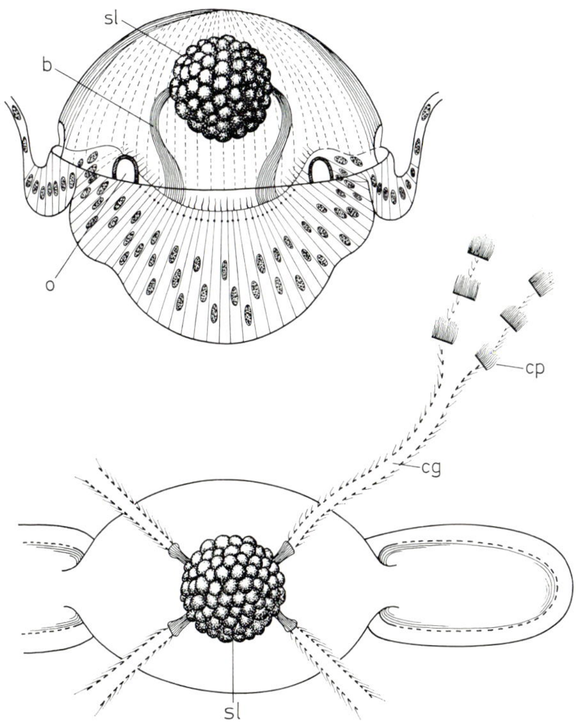

Fig. 5. Diagram of the apical sense organ of the ctenophore *Callianira*. A: seen laterally; epithelim in optical section; B: apical view. *b*: balancer cilia; *cg*: ciliated groove; *cp*: comb plate; *o*: opening of the translucid roof; *sl*: statolith (Redrawn from Bütschli, 1925). For correcting details according to electron microscopic studies see text p. 25

of thousands of cilia adhering together and moving as one. In a slowly swimming ctenophore, waves of ciliary beats run along the comb-plate rows from their apical to their oral ends, all 8 rows beating with approximately the same frequency.

Verworn (1891) and Bauer (1910) were the first to study maintenance of equilibrium in Ctenophora, especially in *Beröe*, and the role the apical organ plays in it. The normal position of these animals is mouth up or down, though they are able to assume any other angle to gravity during locomotion. Passive rotations from any of these positions are compensated for by a change of beating frequency in some of the comb-plate rows. If, for instance, an upward-swimming *Beröe* is tilted, comb-plates beat more frequently on the lower side and less frequently on the upper side: this brings the animal back into its former position; in animals swimming downward the opposite occurs. This righting reaction is dependent on an intact apical organ. Control of equilibrium can also be upset by cutting across the apical ends of the 8 comb-plate rows: after this operation the rows beat at independent frequencies. This demonstrates a coordinating function of the apical organ, which was confirmed in *Mnemiopsis* by Coonfield (1934, 1936). Horridge (1965, 1966) added further details. In *Bolinopsis*, *Pleurobrachia* and *Vexillum*, the balancer cilia are normally stiff and straight. At regular intervals one of them gives a rapid beat towards the center of the organ. This beat triggers a wave of activity along the ciliated groove down to the corresponding pair of comb-plate rows. The cilia of the groove and of the comb-plates beat only when activated by the balancers in this way. The frequency of the balancers' beat depends on their loading by the statolith. Whether the frequency decreases or increases when a balancer is deflected in a given direction depends on the animal's orientational "tendency." Coonfield (1934), Horridge (1965) and Sleigh (1968) conclude from their experiments that conduction of excitation from the balancer cells through the ciliated groove and along the plate rows is not nervous but "neuroid", i.e. from epithelial cell to epithelial cell. Velocity of conduction is 4.1 cm/sec in *Beröe* and 7.3 cm/sec in *Pleurobrachia*. In *Cestus*, Horridge recorded from ciliated cells with a microelectrode: coincident with the power stroke of the cilia, the cell is depolarized; depolarizations are graded and not followed by a refractory period. Presumably this depolarization is conducted from cell to cell, thereby coupling the beat of different cells, since it has been demonstrated that depolarization of a cell makes its cilia beat rapidly. In spite of convincing evidence for neuroid ciliary co-ordination in ctenophores, there are other experiments (Verworn, 1891; Tamm, 1973) which seem to force us to conclude that the co-ordination depends entirely on mechanical interaction between adjacent comb-plates. Tamm (1973) may have resolved this controversy by demonstrating the existence of both mechanisms, the neuroid one in lobate ctenophores with a continuation of the ciliated grooves between the comb-plates, and the mechanical one in cydippids and beroids in which the grooves end at the first aboral plates of the comb-rows. It has been suggested that motile cilia account for the extreme vibration sensitivity of ctenophores. If this is true, the cells act simultaneously as receptors and effectors. Thurm (1968) has shown that this could well be so in cells bearing motile cilia. However, Krisch (1973) describes specialized cilia with a modified root on the floor of the apical organ of *Pleurobrachia*, which she assumes to be vibration-sensitive. A common role as gravireceptor and vibration detector is thus possible for the apical organ of Ctenophora. It should be noted that the inclusion of photoreceptive cells into the apical organ has also been suggested.

V. Plathelminthes

Statocysts have been reported only in *Turbellaria*. Among the *Archoophora* they are generally found in *Acoela* and they are common in *Nematodermatida*, *Catenulida*, and, among *Neoophora*, in *Proseriata* (AX, 1961). Loss of statocysts can be regarded as secondary. Typically, there is one, rarely two cysts on the surface of or embedded in the cerebral ganglion. The ultrastructure of the organ has still to be examined; its sensory supply is not at all clear. The justification for calling it a gravireceptor is based on the scanty evidence described below. *Convoluta* (FRAENKEL, 1929) and *Otoplana* (JÄGER, 1932) show a positive geotactic response when disturbed, and a negative one when not irritated. They compensate for imposed rotations by muscular reactions, though locomotion is achieved by means of cilia. When centrifuged, the animals orient by the resultant mechanical force. If *Convoluta* is cut across, leaving the cerebral ganglion with the statocyst in a piece of only one tenth the length of the rest, only the head part will orient by gravity. Headless pieces of *Polychoerus* have great difficulty in righting themselves until ganglion and statocyst have been regenerated (KEIL, 1929).

Most cercariae of *Trematoda* display negative geotactic responses when freshly released from their hosts. This phenomenon has been studied in detail in *Opisthioglyphe* (STYCZYNSKA-JUREWICZ, 1961).

VI. Nemertini

Statocysts are occasionally found, for instance one to two pairs in the dorsal rind of the ventral lobe of the cerebral ganglion in *Ototyphlonemertidae* (HYMAN). Neither fine structure nor function of these organs seem to have been investigated.

VII. Nemathelminthes

"Statocysts" have been suggested in some *Nematodes*, *Rotatoria* and *Gastrotricha*, though on equivocal grounds (BULLOCK and HORRIDGE, 1965). No analysis of gravity reactions has come to my attention, except for that by BOLIN (1926), who reports negative geotactic orientation in several rotatorians under the influence of increased concentrations of CO_2 and H_2S.

No gravity reactions seem to be on record in *Kamptozoa* or *Priapulida*.

VIII. Annelida

No statocysts were discovered in *Myzostomatida* or *Clitellata*, though VERWEY (cited by DIJKGRAAF, 1961a) found *Lumbricus* sensitive to gravity.

Polychaeta: Most of the morphological data on "statocysts" in Polychaeta come from EHLERS (1892) and FAUVEL (1907), who found them in *Ariciidae*, *Arenicolidae*, *Terebellidae* and *Sabellidae*. MERKER and VAUPEL-von HARNACK (1967) report unicellular cysts in the cerebral ganglion of the archiannelid *Protodrilus*. In none of these families is every species equipped with cysts; only in

Arenicolidae do they seem to be fairly typical. A pair of statocysts may be developed in the first (*Arenicolidae*) or second (*Terebellidae*, *Sabellidae*) segment. In *Ariciidae* up to six pairs are found, the first of which is located several segments behind the prostomium. *Orbiniidae* possess up to 20 pairs of cysts (BULLOCK and HORRIDGE, 1965). The organs can always be derived from dorsolateral invaginations of the body surface. These can remain open crypts (e.g. in the ariciid *Scoloplos*), or become closed vesicles communicating with the surface by a duct (most species), which may be almost closed in older specimens. In all these cases statoliths are small particles taken from the outside and cysts are ciliated. Finally there are species with completely closed statocysts, which secrete their own calcareous statolith (e.g. *Arenicola cristata*, *Myxicola*) or statoconia (*Arenicola grubei*, *A. ecaudata*). Only in those with one lith was a ciliated epithelium encountered, though our knowledge of the fine structure of these organs hardly justifies such a statement. LAVERACK (1968) has made a beginning in studying the ultrastructure of the cyst in *Arenicola marina*. He found two different types of cilia; some had the (9+2) pattern, and others had bladderlike blown-up distal parts, with a frame of branched and divergent central fibrils.

Responses to gravity, and the participation of statocysts in these responses, were studied by von BUDDENBROCK (1912) in *Arenicola grubei* and *A. claparedei* and by the same author (1913) in *Arenicola marina*, *Myxicola infundibulum* and *Branchiomma vesiculosum*.

When *A. grubei* is put on the surface of the sand, it burrows exactly vertically downward and compensates for rotations. Deafferentiation of one statocyst does not prevent orientation with respect to gravity, while deafferentiation of both does. *A. marina* prefers a different angle (40–50°) downward and its burrowing directions are more variable (JÄGER, 1932). *A. claparedei* — a species with no statocysts — appears at first glance to behave similarly. However, its front end is not directed by gravity but by another mechanism: it is always bent to the ventral side in the exposed worm and begins to burrow when it finds contact with the substrate.

Branchiomma and *Myxicola* are interesting in that they dig in the sand with their rear ends first, so that the position of the leading segments cannot be directed by bringing the statocysts into the intended position. One cyst is sufficient for correct orientation and for compensation of imposed rotations. *Branchiomma* will still dig in the sand after elimination of both cysts, though with no defined orientation. Orientation of burrowing is further complicated in this worm by proprioceptive reflexes, which enable it to proceed downward even if the rear end has been bent passively upward while the front end with the statocysts remained unmoved. The basic principle seems to be a tendency to keep head and tail parallel as long as statocyst reflexes are not involved.

Polychaetes equipped with statocysts are typically sessile. It is, however, curious that some closely related forms with apparently very similar ecology may have the cysts (e.g. *Branchiomma*, *Myxicola*) and others (e.g. *Sabella*, *Spirographis*) do not. Clearly, these sense organs cannot be of crucial biological importance, though species without cysts have been found to burrow more slowly and less precisely downward.

Neither statocysts nor gravireceptive reactions seem to have been reported in *Sipunculida*, *Echiurida*, *Onychophora*, *Tardigrada* or *Pentastomida*.

IX. Arthropoda. Crustacea

Crustacea are the classic subjects for the study of gravireception in lower animals. It was primarily through experiments with them that DELAGE (1887) came to realize that "otocysts" of invertebrates were not, or not only, hearing organs, but primarily sense organs for the maintenance of equilibrium. It was again in Crustacea that KREIDL (1893) proved this beyond all doubt by his iron-filing experiment. Compensatory eye movements, first described in crabs by CLARK (1896) have been widely used to test equilibrium receptors in Crustacea. They stabilize the visual field against displacements of the head or body. HORRIDGE (1965b) draws attention to the biological significance they may have for sun orientation in these animals. Processing of sensory input from the eyes together with information from statoreceptors has been studied in the crayfish with the aid of neurophysiological methods by WIERSMA and YAMAGUCHI (1967). In addition to, or instead of conservation of equilibrium with respect to gravity, Crustacea make ample use of optical means of postural control (for a summary see SCHÖNE, 1959). It was in *Hemimysis* that BUDDENBROCK (1914) discovered the "dorsal light orientation." In addition to its sensitivity to gravity, the statocyst of some Crustacea has been shown to respond to angular acceleration and to vibration. A review is given by COHEN and DIJKGRAAF (1961).

A. Gravireception

No static organs have been reported in *Entomostraca*, nor have reactions to gravity been described in them (PLATE, 1924, mentions statocysts in copepods; I was unable to trace his source). Among the *Malacostraca*, statocysts have been described in some species of *Anaspidacea*, *Isopoda*, *Cumacea*, *Amphipoda* and in most *Mysidacea* and *Decapoda*. The organs are located in the head (Amphipoda, Cumacca), the basal segment of the first antenna (Anaspidacea, Decapoda), the telson (Isopoda) or in the endopodit of the last abdominal pair of legs (Mysidacea).

Again it ought to be emphasized that the lack of a statocyst does not mean that a species does not have statoreactions. Adult *Squilla* (Stomatopoda), for example, have been shown to control their posture with reference to gravity; the mechanism of perception is not understood (von BUDDENBROCK, 1914).

Neither the morphological nor the experimental evidence (LANGENBUCH, 1928) can be regarded as firm enough to allow the inference of a gravireceptive role for the head organs of Amphipoda. The statocyst of *Cyathura* (Isopoda) has interesting structural peculiarities (only three sensory hairs; a muscle between cyst and body wall); its extirpation abolishes the animal's capacity for positively geotactic burrowing in the mud, as well as its ability to compensate for rotations (LANGENBUCH, 1928). *Anaspides* has a statocyst which can be regarded as homologous to the organ in Decapoda. It is remarkable in that it has no statoliths; instead, the sensory hairs are distally swollen like clubs. It has been suggested that every sensory hair acts as a "statolith" and receptor in one. A similar disposition was encountered in the decapod *Typhlocaris* (SIEWING, 1957)[1]. Detailed anatomical and experimental investigations are very necessary in all these forms.

Only mysids and decapods have been the objects of thorough studies.

Mysidacea:

The anatomy of the cyst has been described by HENSEN (1863) and BETHE (1895). It is found in the base of the medial tail appendages and communicates with the exterior by an almost closed duct. Its floor is tilted outward by 45°. About 60 sensory hairs carry a single statolith, which is secreted by the wall of the cyst and consists of calcium fluoride. DELAGE (1887) was the first to find that blinded mysids also deprived of their statocysts were unable to maintain their equilibrium during swimming. Von BUDDENBROCK (1914) reviews experiments by BETHE (1895) and BAUER (1908) critically and confirms DELAGE's results, while he also emphasizes the role of the eyes in postural orientation. He finds unilateral extirpation of a statocyst has no effect upon orientation in blinded animals.

All authors agree that the statocyst makes mysids highly sensitive to water-borne vibration.

Decapoda:

The anatomy of the decapod statocyst was described by HENSEN (1863), PRENTISS (1900), KINZIG (1921), PANNING (1924), COHEN (1955, 1960) and SANDEMAN and OKAJIMA (1972). The ultrastructure of the sensory hairs was studied by SCHÖNE and STEINBRECHT (1968) in *Astacus fluviatilis* (Fig. 6). Surprisingly, a single hair is supplied by three sensory cells inserting at the joint of the hair through a common cuticular chorda up to 200 μm in length; thus, the same mechanical stimulus seems to be transmitted to all three cells. PATTON (1969) was able to drive up to three units by movements of a single hair in the lobster statocyst; one was phasically, the other tonically excited, the last one tonically inhibited by deflection of the hair.

The statocyst develops as an invagination, generally from the dorsal wall of the basal antennular segment. The fluid-filled, ectodermal sac is never anatomically closed, though it is often functionally closed. Its cuticular lining is cast off and renewed during each molting together with the contents of the cyst. The statolith typically consists of sand grains, which are actively introduced by the animal after molting. They are usually cemented together by a secretion of cyst wall glands. Occasionally the lith is secreted completely (e.g. *Sergestes*, *Leucifer*, *Hippolyte*, all of which are Natantia). Reports, mainly of crabs, that statoliths are absent altogether, cannot be regarded as conclusive since careful inspection revealed small heaps of particles of external origin in the species which were reinvestigated (*Carcinus* and *Maja*: DIJKGRAAF, 1956a; *Scylla*: SANDEMAN and OKAJIMA, 1972).

Due to protuberances from the wall, the form of the brachyuran statocyst is very complicated; in some species there is almost a division into two canals shaped like two toroids and joined approximately at right angles to each other.

1 NICKLAUS (1968) suggested a gravireceptive function for club-shaped mechanoreceptor hairs on the cerci of the orthopteran insect *Acheta*. For a possibly comparable mechanism in tunicates see p. 64.

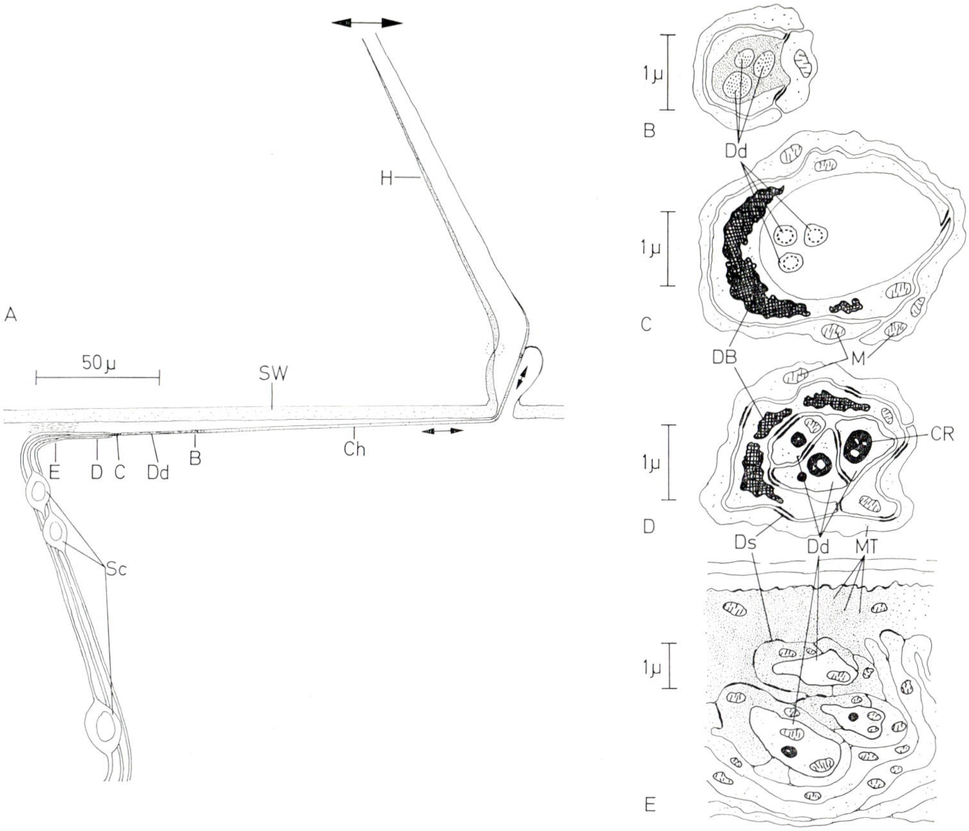

Fig. 6. A: Structure of a statocyst receptor hair in *Astacus fluviatilis*. Only the basal part of the hair is drawn, sectioned along its plane of symmetry. Hypodermis and sheath cells are omitted. Double arrows indicate stimulus-transferring movements. Arrows B, C, D, E refer to the sites of the transverse sections. B–E: Semi-diagrammatic transverse sections through the dendrites at different levels, together with part of their sheath cells. B: at the point of dendrite insertion in the chorda. C: ciliary segment of the dendrites. D: inner segment of dendrites; note connecting desmosomes. E: dendrites separated by sheath cells. *Ch*: Chorda; *CR*: Ciliary rootlet; *DB*: Dense body; *Dd*: Dendrite; *Ds*: Desmosome; *H*: Hair shaft; *M*: Mitochondrion; *MT*: Microtubuli; *Sc*: Sensory cell; *SW*: Statocyst wal (Courtesy of SCHÖNE and STEINBRECHT)

Sensory hairs vary in number (*Crangon*: 26 (PRENTISS, 1900); *Homarus*: about 500 (COHEN, 1955)), length, and arrangement. Functional importance is attached to the fact that quite often not all hairs have contact with the statoliths, different groups of hairs are differentiated in structure, and the spatial arrangement of some receptors suggests specialization with respect to rotation about the three body axes. Crabs and lobster have been studied best in this respect. In *Carcinus*, the following types are found: 1) hooklike hairs approximately 50 μm in length; some of them are loosely connected to the minuscule lith, others are free. 2) thread hairs, over 300 μm long, very thin and never in contact with the lith. Both types are partly plumed. 3) Irregularly grouped hairs of intermediate length, again not

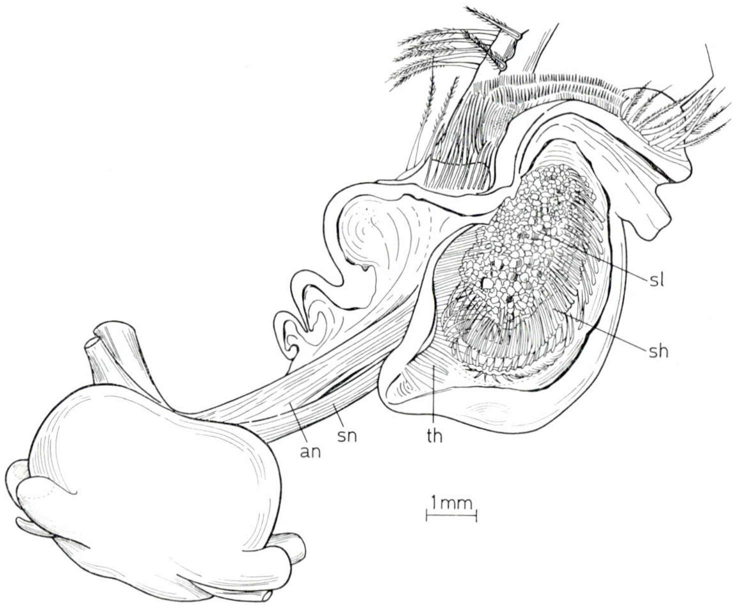

Fig. 7. The right statocyst and its nervous connection to the supra-esophageal ganglion in *Homarus americanus* seen in dorsal view. The statocyst nerve (sn) lies on the dorsolateral aspect of the antennular nerve (an) and is seen as a distinct bundle. The wall of the basal antennular segment has been removed to expose the cyst lying in the lumen of the segment. The dorsal wall of the cyst has been taken off and the compact statolith (sl) composed of sand grains cemented together is seen on the floor of the cyst. The sensory hairs on the cyst floor (sh) are arranged in a crescent shape with the inner three rows contacting the lith, while the irregular outer row projects freely into the fluid. The fine thread hairs (th) are seen projecting horizontally into the cyst fluid from the medial cyst wall (From COHEN, 1960)

in contact with the lith. There is some doubt as to whether the latter are sensory at all (HENSEN, 1863; PRENTISS, 1900; DIJKGRAAF, 1955, 1956a, b). Similar types of hairs are found in *Scylla*, the statolith hairs being 3–4 μm long, less than 1 μm in diameter and unfeathered (SANDEMAN and OKAJIMA, 1972). In the lobster the sensory hairs are arranged in two main groups (Fig. 7): about 400 hairs are stationed in four rows in a crescent pattern on the floor of the cyst adjacent to the lith, though only three of the rows have contact with it, not all of them equally close. Their average length is about 540 μm at a basal diameter of 25 μm; hairs up to 850 μm in length occur. In addition there are about 70 thread hairs in a row along the posterior medial wall. They project horizontally into the cyst and are about 600 μm long, their base being approximately 5 μm thick (COHEN, 1955). Three groups of hairs have been described in crayfish (*Cambarus* and *Astacus*: PRENTISS, 1900; PANNING, 1924).

Development of the statocyst has been followed by PRENTISS (1900) in *Homarus* and *Carcinus*. In *Homarus* it appears gradually; the third instar has a shallow sac without sensory hairs or lith, the fourth is equipped with a functional statocyst. In *Carcinus*, the cyst is suddenly present in the Megalopa (4th instar).

Up to the end of the last century, crustacean "otocysts" were generally regarded as hearing organs. Analysis of their equilibrating function began with DELAGE (1887), who showed that the shrimp *Palaemon* is unable to swim on an even keel when deprived of its statocysts. Consequently, EXNER proposed the crucial experiment performed by KREIDL (1893): after letting a molted shrimp introduce iron filings into its statocysts and then exposing it to a strong magnetic field, he was able to induce the animal to assume a posture which brought its dorsoventral axis in line with the resultant of gravitational and magnetic forces. Since the mechanical force exerted by the lith upon the receptors depends on the animal's position in space, this demonstrated that gravity was an adequate stimulus for the organ. PRENTISS (1900) confirmed DELAGE's and KREIDL's experiments and added further evidence: *Virbius*, a shrimp without statocysts, cannot keep its equilibrium when forced to swim after blinding. Larvae of crab and lobster cannot orient by gravity up to the third instar. From the fourth on, when statocysts have developed, blinding no longer affects spatial orientation.

CLARK (1896) and BETHE (1897) independently discovered compensatory static eyestalk reflexes in crabs, which only occur when the statocysts are intact. DIJKGRAAF (1955, 1956a, b) later proved that the hooklike sensory hairs are responsible for the perception of gravity. A stretch-sensitive proprioceptor at the base of the antennula monitors its position in *Panulirus*, and enables the animal to discriminate between afferences from the statocysts which are due to a change of the body's position in space, and those which are due to the active movement of the antennula (SCHÖNE and SCHÖNE, 1967; SCHÖNE, 1971). Since the positions of eyestalks can readily be measured in many decapods, this was the method of choice to probe more deeply into the function of statocysts by means of behavioral experiments.

One of the questions that aroused interest was the functional coordination of the two statocysts. Unilateral extirpation was found to have no or only temporary effects on orientation in *Palaemon* (DELAGE, 1887), *Penaeus* (BEER, 1899) and *Leander* (ALVERDES, 1926). On the other hand, BETHE (1897) found compensatory eyestalk movements of the contralateral eye diminished in *Carcinus*, whereas BURROWS and HORRIDGE (1968) maintain that each statocyst affects the movements of both eyestalks in the same way. From experiments in *Astacus*, KÜHN (1914) concluded that each statocyst controls only compensatory movements against rolling in an ipsilateral direction. In addition, he maintained that even in the untilted resting position each statocyst is continuously excited and would induce postural-control reflexes, were it not for the fact that the effects elicited by the two cysts cancel each other. That the assumption of unilateral positional control by each statocyst was incorrect, was elegantly proved by SCHÖNE (1954). Stimulating the exposed sensory hairs directly by bending them laterally, he evoked the same compensatory reflexes as by rotation of the intact animal. Bending the hairs in opposite directions produced reciprocal reactions. Each cyst can thus exert bidirectional control of position and initiate the appropriate righting reactions of both sides (DAVIS, 1968).

From reliable quantitative experimentation on *Astacus*, *Homarus*, *Palaemonetes*, *Crangon* and *Carcinus*, SCHÖNE drew the following conclusions on statocyst function in decapods. The sensory hairs are stimulated by a lateral shearing force

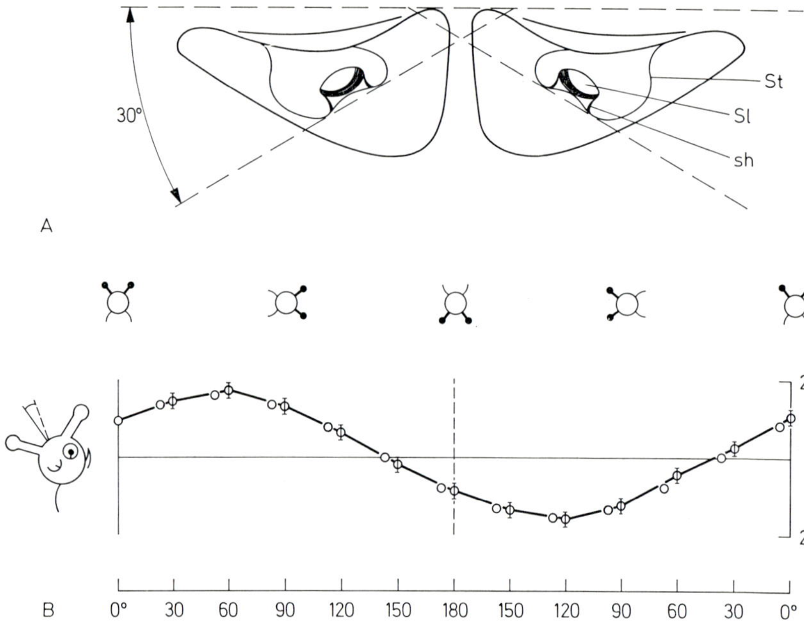

Fig. 8. A: Section through the antennules of *Palaemonetes varians* at the level of the statocysts. Note that the floor of the cyst is tilted by about 30°. *sh*: sensory hair; *St*: statolith; *St*: statocyst. B: Compensatory eyestalk positions of *Palaemonetes varians* in various degrees of rotation about the longitudinal axis after unilateral elimination of a statocyst. Ordinate: deviation of the bisector of the angle between the two eyestalks from the dorsoventral axis (see inset on left); abscissa: angle between the dorsoventral axis and gravity see insets at top). Vertical lines: threefold standard deviation; small circles give the best-fitting sine curve. The maximum of reaction is shifted by 30° to the left, since it is at this position that the floor of the intact statocyst stands vertical (see A) and shear is maximal on the sensory hairs (Redrawn from Schöne, 1954)

which the statolith exerts upon them. Since the floor of the statocyst is generally not exactly horizontal, receptors are excited when the animal is in its normal resting position (Fig. 8); compensatory reactions are not apparent because the effects of both sides are in balance. They become apparent after unilateral removal of the statolith. The animal then assumes a position in which lateral shear of the lith upon the hairs is minimal. In *Palaemonetes*, compensatory eyestalk movements were measured to $\pm 2°$ accuracy while the animal was rotated by 360° around its longitudinal axis. There is a sinusoidal relation between the angle of rotation and the compensatory position of the eyestalks (Fig. 8). This proves a linear dependance of eyestalk movement on receptor excitation, since the shearing force depends also on the sine of the rotation angle. Since the curve of eyestalk positions after removal of the left lith and the one after removal of the right lith add to the curve of the intact animal (Fig. 9), afferences of both statocysts seem to be simply added centrally.

There is a remarkable difference between the effect of taking away the statolith and that of extirpating the cyst: if one first empties both cysts, the animal

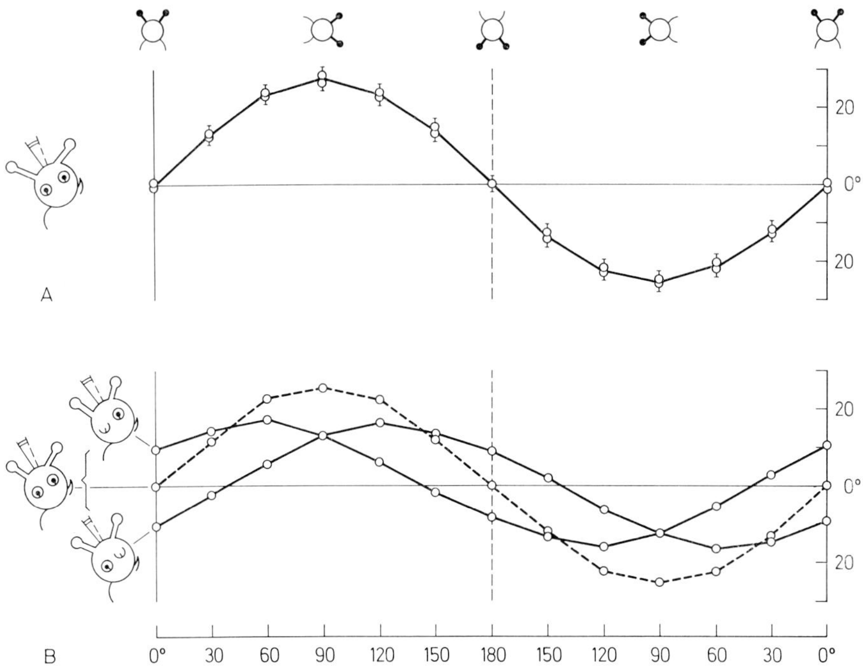

Fig. 9. Compensatory eyestalk reflexes of *Palaemonetes varians* in various positions during rotation about the longitudinal axis. Abscissae and ordinates as in Fig. 7. A: normal animals; B: continuous curves from unilaterally statocystless animals. Broken curve derived from addition of the two continuous curves. Note the agreement between this curve and the curve in A (From SCHÖNE, 1954)

is unable to compensate for imposed tilt but shows no asymmetry of movements; if one of the two empty cysts is then removed, dramatic compensatory movements in the direction of the operated side occur. This demonstrates a continuous spontaneous activity of the sensory epithelium, the activity of both cysts normally being in balance. Unilateral loss of this spontaneous discharge as well as unilateral loss of excitation by the statolith is compensated for by a central nervous process. This enables a crayfish to assume a normal posture after recovery from unilateral damage. The central nature of the mechanism can be nicely demonstrated by first letting a crayfish compensate for unilateral loss of a cyst and then taking away the other one, too: a strong tendency to turn in the opposite direction of the turns after removal of the first cyst is the result. Central balancing of unequal afferent influx is of great biological importance, since unequal filling of the cysts thus cannot affect the behavior of the animal permanently.

By centrifuging freely swimming *Crangon* and *Palaemonetes* heading obliquely downward or upward, and by recording their swimming angles under 1, 1.3, and 2.2 g acceleration, SCHÖNE (1957) demonstrated that the statocysts control position in the pitching plane as well as in the rolling plane. The animals always swam at an angle to the horizontal such that the product of the sine of the angle between the plane of the sensory epithelium and the horizontal multiplied by the force of acceleration remained constant. This proves that statocysts are not only used to control a basic resting posture, but also to steer a course with respect to gravity. The control mechanism is a feedback system which keeps a set level of stimulation constant at the receptors. The setting of the loop depends on many factors, customarily subsumed as the animal's "mood".

Fortunately these inferences from the results of behavioral experiments in decapods are backed up by neurophysiological recordings from afferent sensory neurons in the statocyst nerve (COHEN, KATSUKI and BULLOCK, 1953: *Panulirus* and *Loxorhynchus*; COHEN, 1955, 1960; KNOX, 1970: *Homarus*). In the normal resting position most receptors discharge continously and arhythmically (KNOX, 1970). After removal of the lith, hairs which had been in contact with it assume an angle of approximately 40° from the cyst floor and their sensory neurons keep discharging spontaneously. Bending a hair towards the vertical increases the frequency of discharge through the first 15°; further displacement in this direction makes the frequency decrease, so that at about 40° upward deflexion the activity drops below the level of spontaneous discharge in the resting position. Bending the hair down from the resting position also causes the discharge frequency to decrease. Accordingly, the single hair has a bell-shaped response curve. Different receptor hairs are set at different points within their response range by their relation to the statolith mass, and peak response therefore occurs in different receptors at different positions of the animal in space. This provides a means of resolving the ambiguity inherent in this type of response characteristic. Even

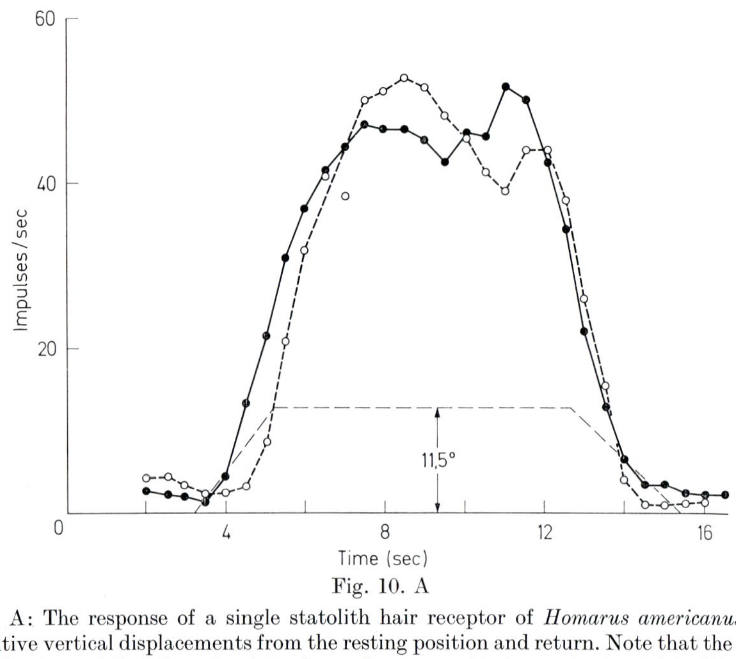

Fig. 10. A

Fig. 10. A: The response of a single statolith hair receptor of *Homarus americanus* to two consecutive vertical displacements from the resting position and return. Note that the response is nonadapting and that there is relatively good agreement between the two trials. B (see p. 38): Response of a single thread hair receptor from the statocyst of *Homarus americanus* when bent backward by 83° 34′ and held there and then returned to its resting position. Note initial rapid adaptation and subsequent gradual fall in frequency. -----: stimulus (From COHEN, 1960)

though a single receptor fires with the same frequency at two different levels of stimulation, it is possible to distinguish between the two levels by differences in the composite sensory input pattern from many receptor channels. Receptor threshold — difficult to define in a spontaneously active system — was measured as less than 6° displacement optimally; this fits in with SCHÖNE's data on the behavioral threshold of reaction.

By recording from the nerve while rotating the isolated anterior cephalothorax of *Homarus* about longitudinal and transverse axes, COHEN (1955) was able to characterize two types of position receptors. Their response to rotation is abolished by removal of the lith.

Type I discharges with a specific frequency adapting slightly only initially for each position maintained within a certain range about the transverse axis (Fig. 10A). Beyond the sensitive range, the receptor remains spontaneously active at a relatively low, constant frequency. The tonic discharge at a given position is independent of the direction from which the position was approached. This type was only found to be responsive to rotation about the transverse axis and it reaches a certain frequency earlier during a fast rotation than during a slow one.

Type II receptors are responsive to rotations either about the transverse or about the longitudinal axis. Their response is phasic-tonic: in addition to a static response which again is independent of the direction of approach, there is a distinct sensitivity to the direction and velocity of movement. During movement toward the region of maximal static response, the frequency increases, while during movement away from it the receptors stop firing; only after an interval do the responses come up to a stationary level. Units responsive to rotation about the longitudinal axis usually have their maximal response when rotation is 45–90°. Units responsive to rotation about the transverse axis can reach the maximum rostrum up or rostrum down.

Single statolith hairs in the crab *Scylla* are unidirectionally sensitive, there being hairs with maximal sensitivity for different directions; the response to deflection has a high impulse-frequency initial phase and a long-term tonic level. When the stimulus is removed, units stop firing abruptly (SANDEMAN and OKAJIMA, 1972).

B. Perception of Angular Acceleration

Compensatory locomotor or eyestalk reactions evoked in blinded *Carcinus* by rotation about the vertical axis and abolished by removal of the statocysts were described by BETHE (1897) and have been confirmed by von BUDDENBROCK and FRIEDRICH (1933), SCHÖNE (1954) and DIJKGRAAF (1955, 1956a, b). The phenomenon has also been reported in *Palaemon* (KREIDL, 1893), *Astacus* (LYON, 1900), *Maja* (DIJKGRAAF, 1955, 1956a, b) and *Scylla* (SANDEMAN and OKAJIMA, 1972, 1973a, b), whereas in *Pagurus* (COHEN and DIJKGRAAF, 1961), *Uca* (LYON, 1900) and *Palinurus* (DIJKGRAAF, 1956c) statocysts were not found to be involved in rotation perception. Detailed behavioral evidence concerning the receptors involved in *Carcinus*, *Maja* and *Eriocheir* has been presented by DIJKGRAAF (1955, 1956a, b) and COHEN and DIJKGRAAF (1961). These crabs respond to angular acceleration about all three axes. During continuous, constant-velocity

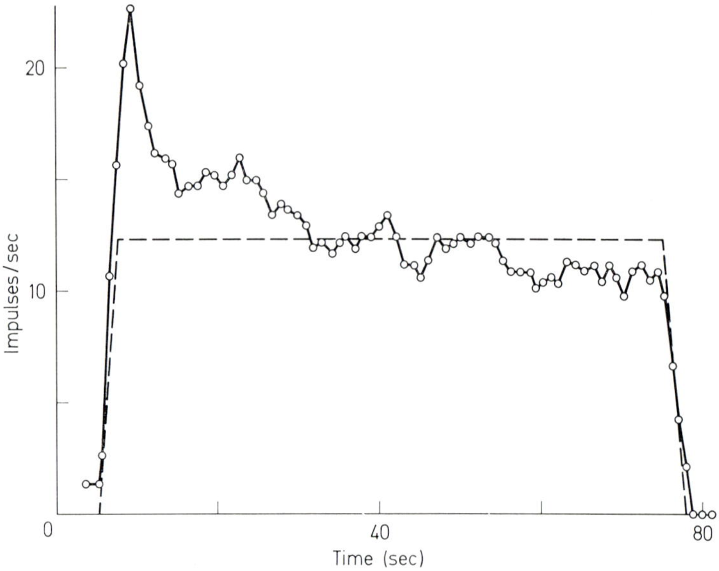

Fig. 10. B

rotation about the vertical axis, the eyestalks return slowly to their symmetrical position. A sudden arrest of rotation causes after-nystagmus in the opposite direction, as opposed to nystagmic movements at the onset of rotation. All reflexes due to angular acceleration are abolished in blinded crabs, if the thread hairs of the statocysts are denervated or destroyed. This operation does not affect static reflexes. It can therefore be concluded that thread hairs are stimulated by fluid movement within the statocyst, caused by angular acceleration and deceleration. In *Scylla* electrical recordings from all types of receptor hairs show that the thread hairs are most probably responsive to rotation about the vertical axis, free hook hairs to rotation about the horizontal axes (Sandeman and Okajima, 1972, 1973a, b).

In *Homarus*, Cohen (1955, 1960) recorded the response to angular acceleration from the statocyst nerve. Again it was shown that thread hairs perceive this stimulus. The single unit apparently responds to rotation about all three axes. The sensory cells are spontaneously active and increase their discharge rate with posterior and/or ventral deflexion, while they decrease it during either anterior or dorsal deflexion. Response is not purely phasic (Fig. 10B), but it is completely independent of the animal's static position in space. Thread hairs have little stiffness: it takes them about 20 sec to return to their resting position after maximal bending. In recordings from the whole statocyst nerve, acceleration receptors respond to rotation with either a burst or a depression of discharge, depending on the direction of movement. These patterns can be reconciled with response characteristics of single units, by taking into account how the fluid moves in the cyst during rotation about any of the three axes. The threshold for rostrum-up rotation was found to be between 5–15°/sec². A threshold for rotation of 6°/sec was reported for thread hairs in *Scylla* by Sandeman and Okajima (1972).

Since thread hairs are sensitive to rotation in all three planes, a given response must be highly ambiguous. It could be assumed that the animal could easily overcome this ambiguity by correlating the response with corresponding positional information from the statolith hairs. However, behavioral experiments on crabs showed that even after elimination of the position receptors rotation about all three axes still evokes appropriate compensatory reactions. So the acceleration system alone must be able to resolve the direction of rotation (COHEN and DIJKGRAAF, 1961). SANDEMAN and OKAJIMA (1972) demonstrated that due to the directions of fluid flow in the vertical and horizontal canals of the statocyst in *Scylla*, rotation about any body axis can be unambiguously coded by thread hairs and free hook hairs of both statocysts, though not in the receptors of only one side. These authors (1973a, b) have also traced the physiological and morphological bases of statocyst-controlled compensatory eye movements (nystagmus) in this crab and found the system to function in remarkable convergence to the one in vertebrates.

Additional properties of the decapod statocyst

Vibration sensitivity of the statocyst has been inferred from behavioral experiments (e.g. in *Palaemon* and *Palaemonetes*: BEER, 1898) and was proved by recording from the statocyst of *Panulirus* (COHEN, KATSUKI and BULLOCK, 1953) and *Homarus* (COHEN, 1955). In the latter, type I and II positional receptors are generally sensitive to vibration, while acceleration receptors are little affected. In addition, there are specific vibration-sensitive units, presumably long hairs in the anterolateral part of the sensory cushion. They only respond to solid-borne vibration, and not to waterborne or airborne sound.

Furthermore, statocyst removal has been reported to have a pronounced effect on the muscular tonus either of the whole animal or of one side after unilateral operation (see BETHE, 1897; and FRÖHLICH, 1904b, for examples).

X. Chelicerata

Very little is known about gravireception in this class. JÄGER (1932) found the pseudoscorpion *Obisium* oriented positively or negatively on a seesaw. PETERS (1932) and HOLZAPFEL (1934) demonstrated that orb-weaving spiders make use of gravity orientation for finding their way in their webs. Nothing is known about the receptors involved.

No responses to gravity have been recorded in *Myriapoda*. It is doubtful whether the matter has ever been investigated with care.

XI. Insecta

A. Gravireception

Orientation with respect to gravity is common, and may even be general in insects (BÜCKMANN, 1962; JANDER, 1963; MARKL, 1963; MARKL, 1974). Almost any insect tested shows positive or negative geotactic orientation (according to the conditions) when put on a vertical or inclined surface if optical orientation is made impossible. When put on a board which is tipped end over end while the insect is running upward or downward, it will immediately turn through 180° to regain its former position relative to the vertical (e.g. BAUNACKE, 1912; JÄGER, 1932; MARKL, 1962). Compass orientation relative to gravity, i.e. a straight course that keeps up a constant angle relative to the direction of gravity is found in many if not most adult insects. For the mechanisms of orientation, see MARKL (1974). *Bledius* and *Dyschirius* (Coleoptera) dig burrows within a few degrees of vertical into the beach sand, and continue to find the steepest direction when forced to dig along an inclination of only 3° above the horizontal (BÜCKMANN, 1954, 1955). Even in larvae, orientation by gravity is not missing (caterpillars: LAMMERT, 1925; TABOURET-KELLER, 1957; dipteran larvae: von STUDNITZ, 1932; beetle larvae: QUEINNEC, 1967).

Gravity orientation is not only widespread in insects; it is probably developed to a more perfect degree and serves more important biological functions than in most other groups of invertebrates. JANDER (1963), and JANDER, HORN and HOFFMANN (1970) have demonstrated that many insects (e.g. *Carausius morosus*, *Apis mellifica* (JANDER and JANDER, 1970), *Formica polyctena*), can keep the same angle relative to the steepest direction on an inclined surface regardless of the angle of inclination of the surface (as long as it is above threshold). During their tail-wagging dances on a vertical comb, honeybees indicate the angle between the sun azimuth and the direction from hive to foodsource by orienting the straight part of their dance relative to gravity: the vertical upward direction is equivalent to the direction towards the sun; any deviation from this direction is translated into an equally large angle between the vertical and the tail-wagging run (VON FRISCH, 1965). This ability to switch from light- to gravity-orientation under conservation, or at least under lawful translation, of the compass angle, has been called *transposition* by its discoverer, VON FRISCH (1948), and has been found to be ubiquitous in insects. That indicates how widespread their ability to perceive gravity is. (Examples: dungbeetles: BIRUKOW, 1954; ants: VOWLES, 1954; JANDER, 1957; caddisflies: JANDER, 1960; many others: TENCKHOFF-EIKMANNS, 1959; LINSENMAIR-ZIEGLER, 1970). It has even been shown that social hymenopterans can learn specific compass angles relative to gravity in order to find their way out to a foodsource and back home again (MARKL, 1964, 1966a, b).

Considering these abilities for gravity orientation the fact that sense organs used for gravireception in insects have escaped discovery for a long time is surprising. Improved understanding of how land insects perceive gravity has only been achieved a decade ago.

The only case where a statocystlike receptor may be at work, is an aquatic dipteran larva (*Limnobiidae*). A pair of open ventral invaginations in the last abdominal segment is said to contain particles. These are whirled around by rhythmical pulsations. The direction in which they settle down might be monitored by two sensory hairs. However, not all gravity responses are abolished after removal of these organs (VON STUDNITZ, 1932).

Apart from this, two fundamentally different principles of gravity perception are known in insects.[2]

2 A third type was suggested by NICKLAUS (1968) in the gryllid *Acheta*: club-shaped cercal hairs change their impulse-discharge frequency depending on their position in space. No behavioral test has proved whether these receptors are actually used to control gravity-oriented reactions in these animals.

Buoyancy receptors of aquatic Hemiptera.

In *Nepa rubra* and *Ranatra linearis (Nepidae)*, BAUNACKE (1912) described static organs which depend for their function on the animal's air supply. When the bug changes its position in space, the air store distributes unevenly over the animal, due to its buoyancy. Sensory hairs on several spots along the abdomen, which move with the air-water boundary, indicate this change of distribution and thus provide the animal with information about the direction of the gravitational force. The organs are different in larvae and adults.

Larvae possess two ventral abdominal grooves in which an air supply is held by a thick fence of bristles. In the 3rd, 4th, 5th and 6th segments there is a spot on each side, where there are no bristles; at these points the air has broad contact with the water and sensory hairs monitor the position of the air-water boundary. If the animal heads upward, the air will push out the receptor hairs in the anterior sites and pull them in at the posterior ones. In adults, there are no ventral air grooves; air is stored under the elytra. Static sense organs are retained only in the 4th, 5th and 6th segments (Fig. 11). Receptor hairs have differentiated into

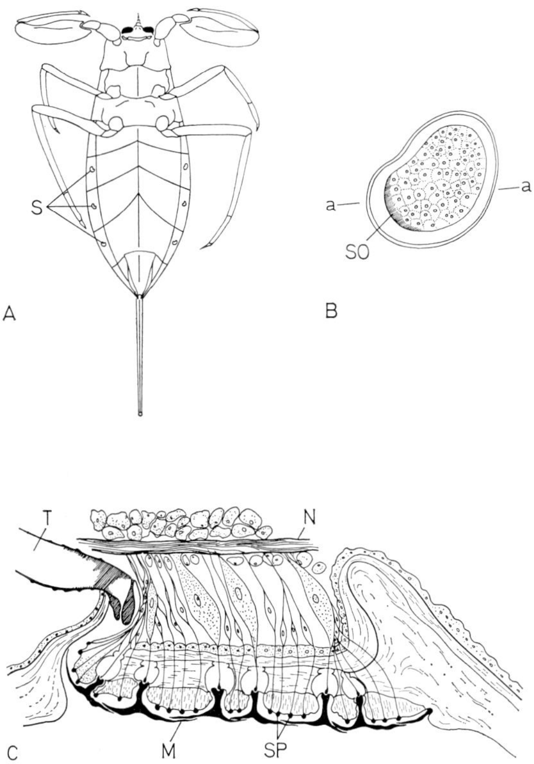

Fig. 11. A: Imago of *Nepa rubra* from the ventral side. S: Spiracular sense organs of equilibrium. B: Enlarged sense organ. *SO*: Spiracular opening. *a–a*: line of section of Fig. C (A and B from MARKL, 1963). C: Section through the sense organ, ventral side down. *M*: Membrane of overlapping expanded margins of the umbrellatype sensilla; *SP*: sensory papillae; *N*: Nerve; *T*: Trachea (Redrawn from THORPE and CRISP, 1947)

two types (THORPE and CRISP, 1947) and are located next to the segmental spiracles. One type of hair holds air under its umbrellalike, overlapping distal end, while the other — for which the sensory nature remains to be proved — has only a small external papilla between the stalks of the umbrellae. When air is pushed out of or sucked into the spiracle due to the animal's position in space, the umbrellas move with the air-water interface and respond to these displacements in a phasic-tonic manner (D. Bonke, results of single-unit recordings, pers. comm.). Exstirpation experiments by BAUNACKE and by THORPE and CRISP leave no doubt that these organs act as gravireceptors. Selective exstirpation of different combinations of the six receptor sites (MARKL and BONKE, in preparation) show that the system works as a pressure-difference measuring device, which compares right-left differences in hydrostatic pressure as well as those in anterior-posterior direction. Females, which are larger and therefore more sensitive to pressure-differences than males, find the upward leading direction even on a surface which is tilted by only 2°; they must therefore perceive pressure differences which are not larger than 0.24 mm H_2O.

Nepa is not sensitive to the absolute hydrostatic pressure. However, perception of the absolute hydrostatic pressure seems to be the main function of a pair of similarly constructed organs at the spiracles of the 2nd abdominal segment of *Aphelocheirus aestivalis (Naucoridae)* (THORPE and CRISP, 1947). Though these may, in addition, have a stabilizing function against rotations about the longitudinal axis, they cannot indicate turn about the transverse axis as the three sets of organs in *Nepa* can. *Aphelocheirus* perceives hydrostatic pressure with them, and upward or downward swimming is triggered according to the pressure level, and is then oriented by other means than gravity.

Other waterbugs (*Corixidae, Naucoridae, Notonectidae*) are thought to perceive gravity in the following way: the buoyancy of an air-bubble between head and prothorax deflects the antennae (RABE, 1953). This is at variance with results of BOTH (1935) and OEVERMANN (1936), so that the decision is up to further experimentation.

Proprioceptive gravity perception in land insects.

A new type of insect gravireceptor was described by LINDAUER and NEDEL (1959) in the honeybee and further investigated by MARKL (1962, 1964, 1966a, b, 1971) in ants and bees, by HORN (1973) in honeybees and bumblebees, by BÄSSLER (1965) and WENDLER (1964, 1965) in *Carausius* and by HORN (1970) and JANDER, HORN and HOFFMANN (1970) in a variety of insects. It is based on the following mechanism: Proprioceptors monitor the relative positions of body parts or measure the strain exerted by one upon the other due to its weight. The position of these body parts and the distribution of strains depends to an extent on the animal's position in space, since the weight of appendages will always pull downward. By processing proprioceptive afferences with respect to the effect produced by gravity, the insect can obtain information about the direction of this force. This mechanism must discriminate against proprioceptive afferences deriving from joint displacements or strains set up by mechanical forces other than gravity, e.g. action of the insect's own muscles. It can be surmised that it is by comparing the input from several sets of receptors that the tonic action of gravity — with equal direction and intensity upon all receptors — is selected against background noise. *Apis*, *Formica* and *Carausius* are the best understood with respect to this mechanism. In bees and ants the predominant proprioceptors used are groups of hair sensilla at several joints (hairplates). They are found on antennal joints, the neck, the petiole joint and at basal joints of the legs; in ants, one more joint — between petiole and gaster — is equipped with them (Fig. 12). By selectively

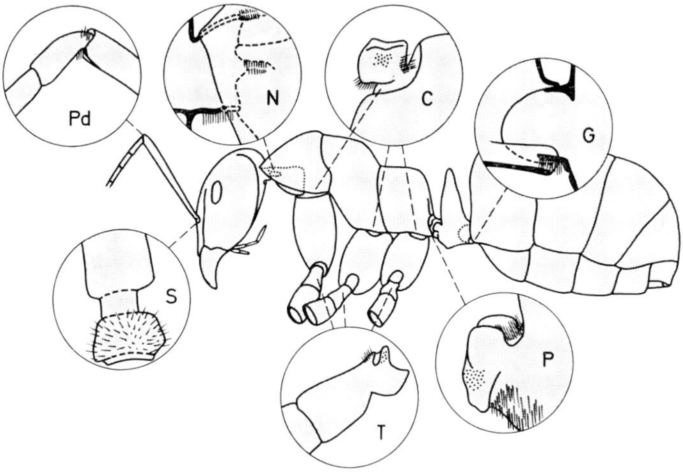

Fig. 12. Worker of *Formica polyctena*. The circles give enlarged views of the different joints bearing hair plates. The lines indicate, where the respective joints are located. *C*: coxal joint; *G*: gaster joint; *N*: neck joint; *P*: petiole joint; *Pd*: joint between 1st and 2nd antennal segments; *S*: joint between antenna and head; *T*: joint between coxa and trochanter (Redrawn from MARKL, 1965)

blocking joints, severing appendages, singeing off hairplates or deafferentiating them, LINDAUER and NEDEL, and MARKL found the following joints involved in gravity perception: neck and petiole in the bee, and antennal, neck, petiole, gaster and coxal joints in ants. Little importance could be attributed to antennal joints and coxal joints in bees; they are also of minor importance for gravireception in ants. These conclusions were derived from experiments designed to test whether the insects could compensate for imposed rotations when they were walking on a vertical or inclined surface after a joint or a combination of joints had been incapacitated. The insects were blinded or under dim red light. All the joints able to mediate gravity orientation were also supplied with hairplates. Though these thus seem to be the most important source of proprioceptive information for gravireception in these insects, this does not mean that the animals would not take advantage of additional proprioceptive input for the same purpose. In fact, there is evidence to support the assumption that they do (MARKL, 1966b). According to HORN (1973), in the honeybee the petiolar hairplates and leg proprioceptors control predominantly negatively and positively geotactic reactions, while the neck hairplates are of major importance in lateral or diagonal geotactic orientation.

Petiolar and leg organs must be left intact and unimpeded for the honeybee's independence of a gravity-oriented course from the angle of inclination of the substrate.

THURM (1963, 1964a, b, 1965) undertook a neurophysiological and ultrastructural analysis of the receptor unit in the major neck hairplate of the honeybee. The base of the sensory hair is asymmetrical due to the eccentric position of the dendritic ending at the joint membrane and to the construction of the hair joint, which does not allow the hair to be bent in all directions equally easy (Fig. 13). In different hairs of the same hairplate these preferential directions are

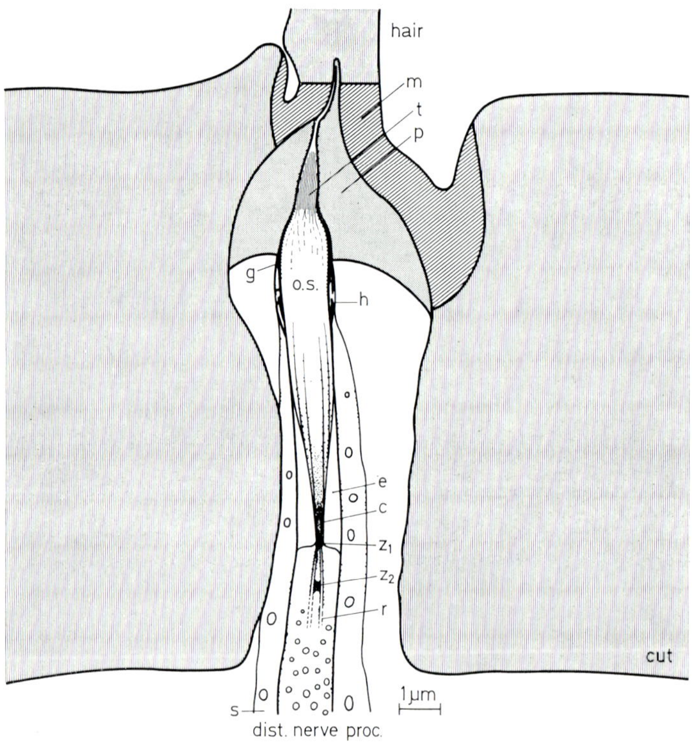

Fig. 13. Diagram of the basal structure of a sensillum from the major hair plate in the neck of the honeybee *Apis mellifera* as derived from electron micrographs. Note the asymmetrical structure of the joint. *c*: ciliary structure; *e*: extracellular space; *g*: granules; *h*: cuticular sheath; *m*: joint membrane; *o.s.*: outer segment; *p*: cap; *s*: Schwann cell; *r*: root fiber; *t*: tubular body; *cut*: cuticle; z_1 and z_2: centrosome-like structure (From THURM, 1964b)

distributed to coincide best with the expected direction of load. Each hair has one sensory cell. Its response to bending is phasic-tonic: after an initial peak of discharge, activity levels out in two phases of adaptation to a constant tonic discharge rate (Fig. 14). All response components depend on the angle of deflexion of the hair and the direction into which it is bent (Fig. 15). Response latency can be less than 1 msec under optimal conditions.

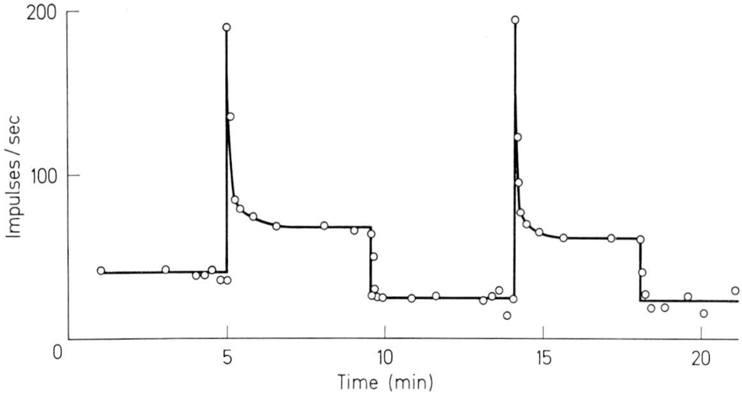

Fig. 14. Phasic-tonic response of a single hair sensillum from the hair plate in the neck of the honeybee to two consecutive deflexions. The maximum of the deflexion was reached in 10 msec (From THURM, 1963)

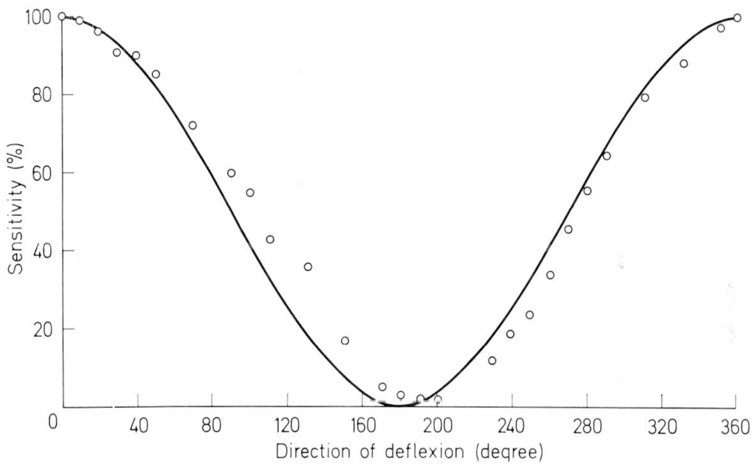

Fig. 15. Average sensitivity of five hair-plate receptors of the honeybee to deflexion into different directions as measured when the hair was fully bent. The direction of maximal sensitivity was set equal to 0°. Angles are measured from caudad to laterad. The continuous line gives a fitting cosine curve, lifted to cos 180° = 0 (From THURM, 1963)

BÄSSLER (1965) postulates that in *Carausius* gravity orientation is attributable to hair receptors which monitor the position of the basal leg joint and femoral chordotonal organs which measure the angle between femur and tibia. After a great variety of experimental manipulations, he proposed a mathematical model which accounts for all gravity reactions he has found in *Carausius*. It assumes that a central mechanism sets proprioceptive afferences indicating the load along the transverse axis or the longitudinal axis in relation, so that it corresponds formally to a division of the transverse-load afference by the longitudinal-load afference. WENDLER (1965) demonstrates that antennal proprioreceptors are also involved. From theoretical considerations and experimental evidence he concludes (WENDLER, 1971a, b) that still more proprioreceptors contribute to the gravireceptive mechanism, of which he thinks strain-receptors (e.g. campaniform sensilla) to be of decisive importance.

A similar means of gravireception was proposed by BÄSSLER (1958, 1961) for the mosquito *Aedes*, in which he names antennal and leg receptors, and for the beetle *Tenebrio*, where antennal and pro-mesothoracal joint receptors are mentioned as the proprioceptors involved, while HORN (1970) maintains that in *Tenebrio* only leg receptors are responsible for gravireception. JANDER et al. (1970) report leg receptors in all hemimetabolic neopterous insects and also in Megaloptera, Mecoptera and Coleoptera as the main sources of positional information. In *Osmylus* and *Calliphora*, leg receptors cooperate with other, still unknown proprioceptors, while in those Odonata, Lepidoptera and Hymenoptera tested, leg receptors are of little or no importance for gravity perception, other joints of the body being supplied with position-controlling devices (MARKL, 1962, 1971).

Interaction between the orientation by gravity and the influence of the earth's magnetic field was demonstrated by LINDAUER and MARTIN (1968) in the honeybee (see also MARTIN and LINDAUER, 1973). It explains hitherto poorly understood deviations from the expected course of gravity-orientation in Hymenoptera (VON FRISCH, 1965; MARKL, 1964, 1966a, b).

Little is known about the role of gravity perception in the maintenance of equilibrium in flight, though SCHNEIDER (1953) recorded well-defined compensatory reactions to positional changes in the rolling and pitching plane in *Calliphora* during stationary flight. The pertinent receptors were not localized. This problem deserves further study in insects (see also WILSON, 1971; WEIS-FOGH, 1971).

B. Perception of Angular Acceleration

Information on the perception of angular acceleration in walking insects is scanty. Blindfolded honeybees (KUWABARA, 1952) and ants compensate for rotation about their dorsoventral axis; proprioceptors at the basal joints of the legs respond to the stimulus (personal observations).

Insects in flight provide fine examples for the perception of rotation. Generally, many of them probably sense rotations in the yawing plane by means of antennal receptors, as has been shown in *Calliphora* by SCHNEIDER (1953) and in *Apis* by HERAN (1959).

Dragonflies (*Anax*) possess rotation receptors at the neck (MITTELSTAEDT, 1950). The head is large and heavy and is hung up rather loosely on the prothorax, so that inertial forces set up by rotation of the head are great, compared to friction in the joint and to elastic resistance. The position of the head is monitored by several hairplates. Any imposed rotation, whether around the longitudinal or around the transverse axis, is compensated for by the dragonfly in flight as long as these neck receptors are intact. They do not however, mediate any static positional reflexes. Optical mechanisms of posture control are very important in dragonflies, as well as this mechanoreceptive stabilizing system. The most significant role of the neck organs may be to make the dragonfly always fly in the direction where its eyes look, since the neck organs are the sensory device in the feedback system which always keeps head and trunk in line.

The most complicated organs for the perception of angular acceleration in insects are the halteres, the transformed hind wings of Diptera. This is not the place to review all the functions ascribed to them. They may have a general stimulatory effect on the animal (von Buddenbrock, 1919; Brauns, 1939; Faust, 1952) and serve as important mechanical stabilizers (Schneider, 1953). In addition, Fraenkel (1939), and Pringle (1948) proved that halteres are also used as gyroscopes in not too slowly flying diptera. Faust (1952) and Schneider (1953) added evidence in favor of this role from behavioral experiments.

Halteres are dumbell-shaped organs (Fig. 16) which oscillate rapidly in the vertical plane during flight, the frequency of oscillation being dependent on the

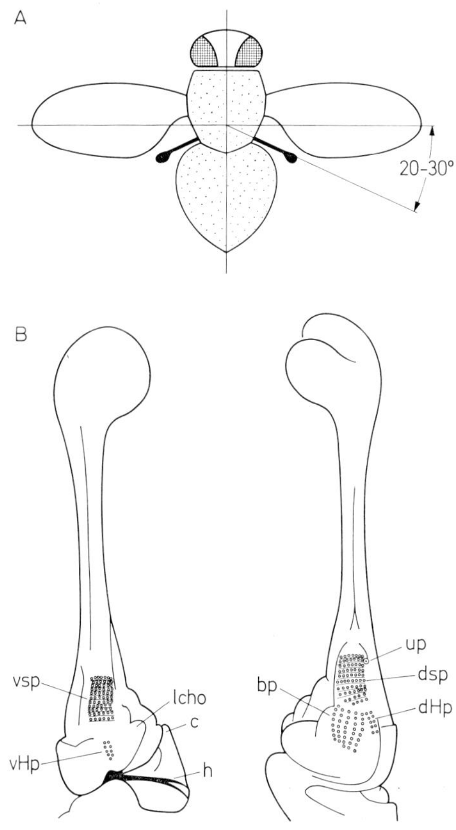

Fig. 16. A: Diagram of *Calliphora*, showing the position of the halteres. They oscillate at right angles to the paper plane (from Schneider, 1953). B: Ventral (left) and dorsal (right) view of the left haltere of *Lucilia sericata*. *c*: condyle of the secondary articulation; *h*: main hinge line; *bp*: basal plate; *dsp*: dorsal scapal plate; *dHp*: dorsal Hicks papillae; *lcho*: large chordotonal organ; *up*: undifferentiated papilla; *vsp*: ventral scapal plate; *vHp*: ventral Hicks papillae (From Pringle, 1948)

mechanical resonance of the system. They are articulated about a horizontal hinge; further distally, a secondary articulation allows a slight, damped movement about a vertical axis. Rotation of the fly sets up torques at the base of each haltere, which act about an axis at right angles to the moving stalk in the plane of oscillation. Magnitude and periodicity of torques differ for different planes of rotation. The base of the haltere is lavishly supplied with sense organs (Fig. 16) (in *Calliphora* about 400). A dorsal and a ventral group of various campaniform sensilla and a small chordotonal organ respond to strains set up by the primary oscillation of the haltere, whereas another group of dorsal campaniforms (the basal plate) and a large chordotonal organ respond to the gyroscopic torques set up during rotations. Though the receptors of both halteres together would enable the fly to discriminate between the torques produced by rotations about all three axes, PRINGLE concluded that it only uses these sense organs for the perception of rotation in the yawing plane. FAUST (1952), however obtained behavioral data, which do support the view that they monitor rotation in all three planes. Electrophysiological recordings from the haltere nerve (PRINGLE, 1948) and behavioral experiments (SCHNEIDER, 1953) in which compensatory reactions of the wings after imposed rotation about the dorsoventral axis were measured verified the derivations from the morphology and the mechanics of the system.

XII. Mollusca

Statocysts are part of the typical sensory equipment of a mollusc, except in Amphineura, which have none. They arise as ectodermal invaginations which are usually closed off as cysts, though occasionally an open communicatory duct to the exterior exists. The cyst is often found near the pedal ganglion, but its innervation derives generally from the cerebral ganglion. BARBER (1968) and VINNIKOV (1971) have reviewed gross and fine structure of molluscan statocysts, and CHARLES (1966), WELLS (1966) and WOLFF (1973) have also reviewed their functions.

Monoplacophora

A pair of statocysts with ducts to the surface is found in *Neopilina* (LEMCHE and WINGSTRAND, 1959).

A. Pelycopoda

The pair of statocysts is absent only in a few forms (e.g. in *Vermetus*, *Pinna*, *Janthina* and in adult *Tridacnidae*, which possess them as larvae). It is usually found close to the pedal ganglia, though sometimes (for instance in *Arca* and *Modiolus*) it is located near the cerebral ganglia, which always provide the innervation. Protobranchs, *Mytilidae*, some species of *Pecten* and some others have an open duct from the statocyst to the body surface; in these groups external particles are introduced as statoliths. In all others, the liths are secreted by the cyst; sessile *Ostreidae* have none at all.

BARBER (1968) and BARBER and DILLY (1969) find supporting cells with microvilli and haircells in the sensory epithelium of *Pecten*, the latter bearing (9+2) type cilia and a few microvilli; in some cells the cilia are arranged in a ring, while in others they stand in rows, the direction of the cilia — and presumably also their physiological polarization — being given by the position of their basal feet, which stand perpendicular to the line connecting the two central ciliary filaments. The cilia are fastened to the lith. VON BUDDENBROCK (1915) found the left (upper) cyst better developed in nine species of *Pecten*; it contains a large, granular statolith and its epithelium has two types of haircells, one with long and one with short cilia, whereas the right cyst is smaller and has only one type of cilia and its small statolith is a loose mass of particles.

Studies on responses to gravity in bivalves are scarce and need reexamination. *Pecten opercularis* usually swims with its dorsoventral axis at an angle of about 45° to the vertical, ventral side up, and compensates for rotations about the longitudinal axis. Deafferentiation of the left statocyst upsets orientation. No influence from the right cyst has been detected. However, not all static reactions are abolished after section of both statocyst nerves, even when light-orientation is excluded. The animals are, for instance, still able to right themselves when turned over. It is not known where positional information comes from in this case (VON BUDDENBROCK, 1915).

Solenidae burrow positively geotactically in the sand. FRAENKEL (1927) centrifuged them in a rotating trough filled with wet sand. Their burrows were then directed along the mechanical resultant. There is no proof that the statocysts are responsible for this behavior.

Scaphopoda

Statocysts are similar to those of bivalves. They do not seem to have been investigated experimentally.

B. Gastropoda

Statocyst morphology has been described in various gastropods by ILYIN (1900), TSCHACHOTIN (1908), SCHMIDT (1912), PFEIL (1921), BAECKER (1932), DIJKGRAAF and HESSELS (1969), QUATTRINI (1967), GEUZE (1968), LAVERACK (1968), BARBER and DILLY (1969), COGGESHALL (1969), WOLFF (1969), VINNIKOV (1971) and STAHLSCHMIDT and WOLFF (1972); the last eight investigations made use of the electron microscope. The cyst, surrounded by connective tissue, is usually close to the pedal ganglion, but is innervated from the cerebral ganglion in all cases but one (*Australorbis*: PAN, 1958).

Two types of epithelial cells are generally found in the cyst of pulmonates (*Lymnaea*: GEUZE; *Planorbis*: VINNIKOV; *Limax* and *Arion* (Fig. 17): WOLFF; *Helix*: LAVERACK), prosobranchs (*Pomacea*: STAHLSCHMIDT and WOLFF) and opisthobranchs (*Aplysia*: COGGESHALL; DIJKGRAAF and HESSELS; *Pterotrachea*: BARBER and DILLY). Small "supporting" cells carry microvilli and occasionally modified cilia, and separate the sensory haircells, called "giant" cells in pulmonates and opisthobranchs, which in addition to microvilli or stereocilia bear (9+2)-type kinocilia. In *Lymnaea*, two kinds of sensory cells are distinguished (high and low cells), the low ones being found mainly at the dorso-latero-rostral side, the high ones at the opposite cyst wall. The kinocilia are rooted in a basal apparatus (Fig. 18) which usually has a striated root to one side and a basal foot to the other, the latter being absent in *Pterotrachea*. The basal feet of all cilia of

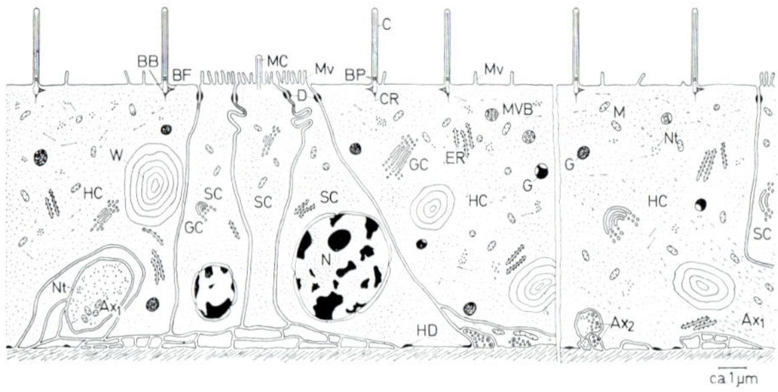

Fig. 17. Diagram of the statocyst wall of *Limax* and *Arion* with hair cells (HC) and small supporting cells (SC). Ax_1: afferent axons; Ax_2: endings of presumably efferent axons containing numerous vesicles; *BF*: basal foot; *BB*: basal body; *BP*: basal plate; *C*: cilium; *MC*: modified cilium; *CR*: ciliary root; *D*: desmosomes; *ER*: endoplasmic reticulum; *G*: granulum; *GC*: Golgi complex; *HD*: hemidesmosomes; *M*: mitochondrium; *Mv*: microvilli; *MVB*: multivesicular body; *N*: nucleus; *Nt*: neurotubuli; *W*: whorl. The basal membrane and the connective tissue envelope of the cyst are indicated by the striated zone beneath the cells (From Wolff, 1969)

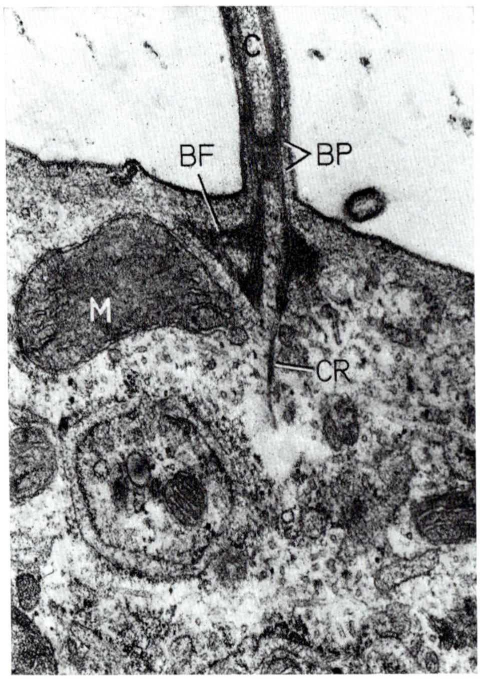

Fig. 18. Sagittal section through a kinocilium of a hair cell of *Limax*. For abbreviations see Fig. 17 (From Wolff, 1969)

a given hair cell can point in the same direction (*Pomacea*) or are directed centrifugally or centripetally. In the latter cases, each cell is sensitive to stimulation tangential to its surface from any direction (Wolff, 1968, 1970a, 1973b; Wood and von Baumgarten, 1972). The number of sensory cells is very small in the cyst of pulmonates and opisthobranchs, usually between 10 and 15; in two species of *Aplysia*, regardless of the animal's body size, there are always 13 sense cells per cyst, as there are in *Pleurobranchaea* (Wood and von Baumgarten, 1972). In prosobranchs there are more hair cells, e.g. 2500–3000 in *Pomacea*, though the diameter of the cyst is only about 400–450 μm, as compared to 100–200 μm in pulmonates (Wolff, 1973a). The statocysts are usually filled with numerous calcareous statoconia, which in the intact cyst are seen in dancing motion, when they come close to the beating cilia of the wall. They seem to be secretory products of the supporting cells. In the haircells of pulmonates large whorls of endoplasmic reticulum are typically found. Efferent innervation of the cyst has been demonstrated in pulmonates (Wolff, 1968, 1969, 1970b) and has been shown to be very probable also in *Pomacea* (Stahlschmidt and Wolff, 1972).

The structure and function of the heteropod statocyst are excitingly complicated (Ilyin, 1900; Tschachotin, 1908; Polimanti, 1911; Friedrich, 1932; Barber and Dilly, 1969). In *Pterotrachea* (Fig. 19) the cyst has a sensory macula on its lower side — which is dorsal, since the animals swim on their back. The macula contains the haircells, each of which bears 30–60 (9+2)-type cilia lacking basal feet but nevertheless arranged in centripetally oriented rings, judging by the positions of the central ciliary filaments. The rest of the cyst is covered by ciliated cells of a different type: their long cilia adhere together as pointed tufts. Axons are said to originate from all these cells. Numerous supporting cells are interspersed between the ciliary ones, so that the latter are completely separated from each other. A group of multipolar cells sits externally on the cyst and is connected with the cerebral ganglion. Tschachotin describes these as contractile, but this is equivocal.

Each cyst contains a large calcareous statolith. Normally the lith is floating in the middle of the cyst with no contact with the wall, presumably due to fluid currents set up by the beat of the ciliary tufts. Every once in a while, all the tufts erect stiffly and push the lith onto the macula. The rhythm of this activity continues in isolated cysts, though less regularly. This fascinating mechanism has been known since 1908 but is still awaiting thorough physiological analysis.

Part of the axon bundle entering the cerebral ganglion from the statocyst decussates to the other side and ends there together with the ipsilateral tract.

Experiments, most of which have been performed on *Pterotrachea mutica*, have revealed a double function of the statocysts. Firstly, they are organs of equilibrium; removal or deafferentiation of both cysts makes the animal unable to keep its normal position in space. It swims dorsal side up when at rest — this is the mechanically stable position — and rolls erratically when disturbed. Unilateral extirpation initially makes the animals roll. After recovery, one statocyst alone allows normal postural orientation (Friedrich, 1932).

Secondly, statocysts have an important influence on the general control of muscular tonus in *Pterotrachea*; in this, they cooperate with eyes and cerebral ganglia. Each cyst influences the muscular tonus of both sides. Tschachotin developed a rather detailed scheme of the tonus-controlling pathways originating from statocysts and cerebral ganglia, which should be accessible to neurophysiological verification.

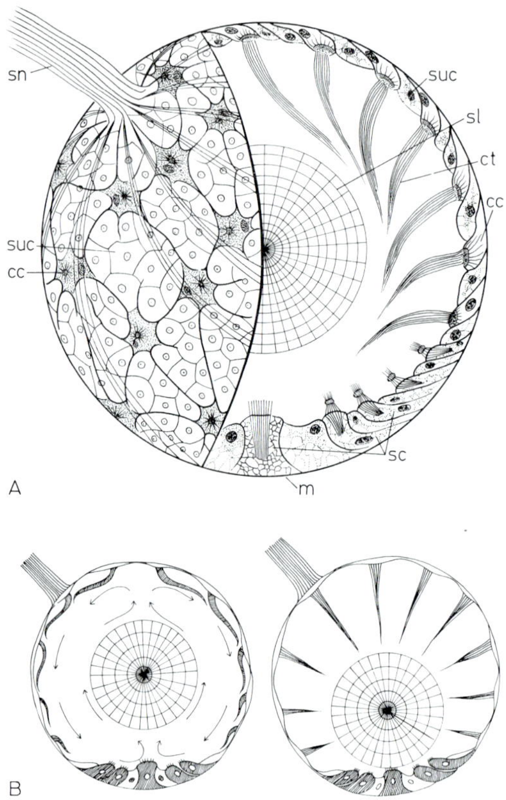

Fig. 19. Statocyst of *Pterotrachea*. A: Diagrammatic view. On the left side, the cyst is seen from outside. On the right side: section through the center. *cc*: ciliated cells; *ct*: ciliary tufts; *m*: macula; *sc*: sensory cell; *sl*: statolith; *sn*: statocyst nerve; *suc*: supporting cell. (From BÜTSCHLI, 1925, after TSCHACHOTIN, 1908). B: Two phases of ciliary activity in the statocyst of *Pterotrachea*. Left: ciliary tufts beating; the statolith floats in the middle of the cyst. Right: ciliary tufts erected; the statolith is pushed upon the macula (From TSCHACHOTIN, 1908)

Orientation by gravity during locomotion on inclined surfaces, as well as righting responses and static compensatory eye reflexes, have been studied in several Pulmonates, though no experimental evidence on the participation of the statocysts in these responses was obtained by BAUNACKE (1913), JÄGER (1932), PIÉRON (1927, 1928, 1929), VON BUDDENBROCK (1935), and WOLFF (1970a). The same is true of FRAENKEL's (1927b) investigation of gravity orientation in *Littorina*, where orientation by the resultant mechanical force was demonstrated in centrifuged snails. MCCLARY (1966) found no change in orientation behavior in *Pomacea* after removal of statocysts, though he may have checked the animals too late (4 days) after the operation, when compensation had occurred. Only LEVER and GEUZE (1965) and GEUZE (1968) were successful in extirpating the statocysts of *Lymnaea stagnalis* and proving their involvement in geotactic locomotion: animals with no statocysts at either side move erratically on an inclined surface; unilateral extirpation results in deviations to the intact side from the downward direction which is preferred in air, and to the treated side from the upward course chosen under water. To the same effect, DIJKGRAAF and HESSELS (1969) studied correction movements (head leading) against rotation around horizontal axes in free-swimming *Aplysia*. While unilateral section of the stato-nerve did not affect posture and postural reflexes, bilateral operation abolished compensatory movements and made the snails swim in somersaults. The cysts do not mediate responses to rotations about a dorsoventral axis. Reflectory pathways controlling turns in opposite directions originate from each statocyst. Both pathways controlling turn in the same direction run through the ipsilateral cerebropedal connective to the ipsilateral pedal ganglion. Similar correction movements were reported for *Helix* by WOLFF (1970a).

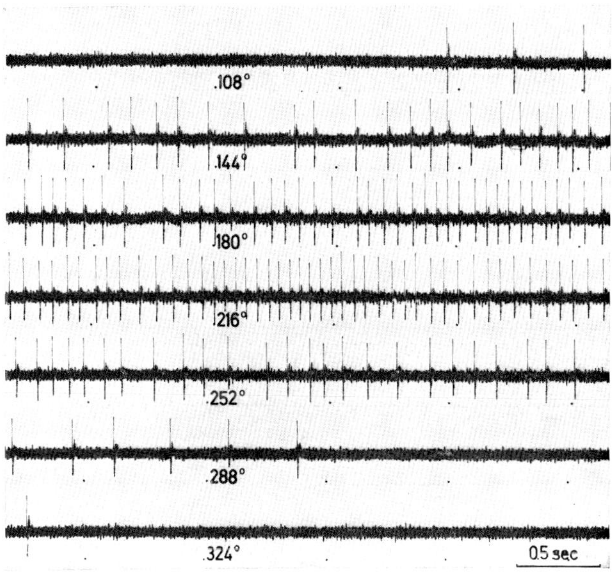

Fig. 20. Recording from a single sensory unit in the statocyst nerve of *Arion empiricorum* during rotation of the animal to the right around its longitudinal axis by 360° with 10°/sec angular velocity (From WOLFF, 1973a)

The electric activity from the statocyst nerve of gastropods (*Helix*, *Arion*: WOLFF, 1968, 1970a, b; *Pleurobranchaea*: WOOD and VON BAUMGARTEN, 1972; *Aplysia*: WOLFF, 1973b) has been recorded while the preparation was rotated about the longitudinal or transverse axes. A single unit can respond to rotations about both axes and is therefore multidirectionally sensitive, but responds only within a limited steric angular range. The response ranges of different cells can cover from 120°–220° and can overlap (Figs. 20, 21). Maximal response is at different angles in different receptor cells. All have a phasic-tonic response characteristic and show a low activity even in the resting position of the animal. They do not respond to rotations about the vertical axis or to angular acceleration.

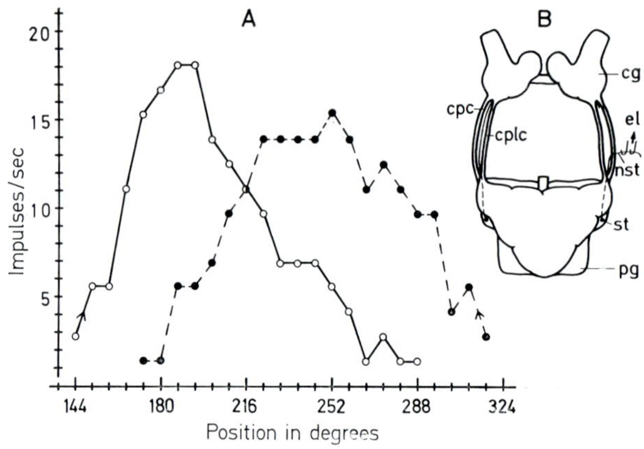

Fig. 21. A: Response of a single unit from the statocyst nerve of *Arion empiricorum* to rotation about the transverse axis with constant angular velocity (10°/sec) and in opposite directions (o——o: head down, to be read from left to right; ●----●: head up, to be read from right to left). For each point the frequency has been averaged over an interval of 7.2°. B: Diagram of the esophageal ganglion mass of *Arion*. *cg*: cerebral ganglion; *el*: recording electrodes; *cpc* and *cplc*: cerebropedal and cerebropleural connectives; *nst*: statocyst nerve; *pg*: pedal ganglion *st*: statocyst (From WOLFF, 1968)

DIJKGRAAF and HESSELS (1969) found no rotation sensitivity in *Aplysia* either in behavioral experiments. Thus, gastropod statocysts are gravireceptors only. The information about position in space is contained entirely in the pattern of stimulated sense cells, not in their individual discharge rates, which may be the same for widely different positions in the activity range of a cell. In addition to afferences, efferent activity was recorded from the nerve, which is dependent on contralateral statocyst excitation (WOLFF, 1970b). A bundle of thin axons was found running along the main statocyst nerve in *Limax and Arion*, and axon endings carrying numerous vesicles at the base of the sensory cells, which may carry the efferent activity (WOLFF, 1969)*.

C. Cephalopoda

All cephalopods have statocysts, which in higher forms are the most differentiated equilibrium organs in invertebrates.

In *Nautilus (Tetrabranchiata)*, the statocyst is rather simple and gastropodlike, connected by a duct to the outside and almost filled by a large, granular statolith. There are sensory cells throughout the cyst wall; there is no separation of a macula or crista from the rest of the cells (YOUNG, 1965).

The morphology of the statocyst of *Dibranchiata* has been carefully studied with conventional techniques by HAMLYN-HARRIS (1903), ISHIKAWA (1924),

* Note added in proof: ALKON and BAK (1973) and DETWILER and ALKON (1973) recorded intracellularly from haircells in the statocyst of the opisthobranch *Hermissenda*. The mechanically excited generator response is depolarizing. Haircells of the same and of the opposite statocysts have an inhibitory hyperpolarizing interaction by means of chemical and electrical synapses.

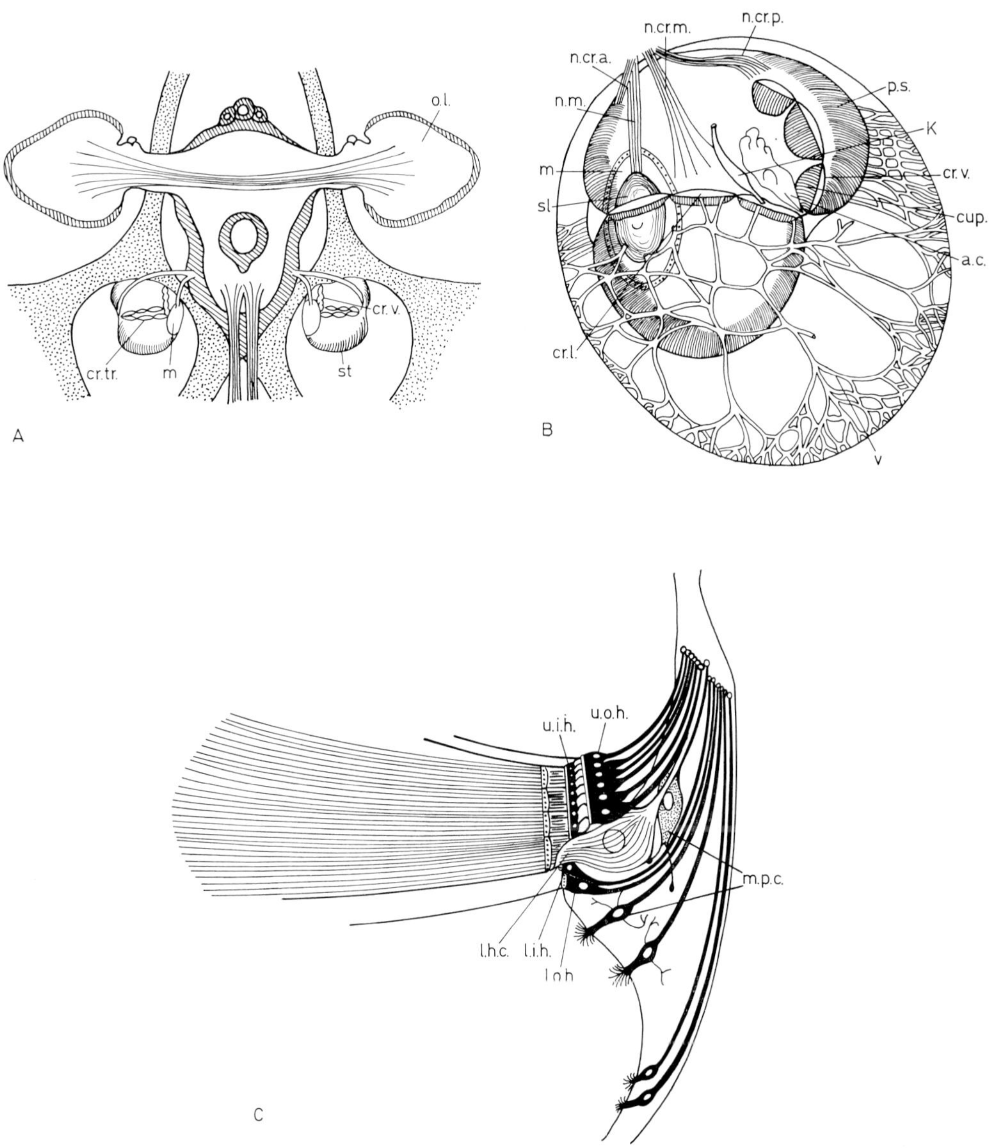

Fig. 22. A: Diagram showing the position of the statocysts in *Octopus vulgaris*. The figure represents a transverse section through the central ganglia as seen from the front. *cr. tr.*: transverse crista; *cr.v.*: vertical crista; *m*: macula; *o.l.*: optic lobe; *st*: statocyst. B: Left statocyst seen from the lateral side. "Cupulae" and statolith are drawn diagrammatically. *a.c.*: antecrista; *cr.l.*: longitudinal crista; *cup*: "cupula" (the flap of cilia of the crista haircells); *K*: Kölliker's canal; *n.cr.a*: anterior crista nerve; *n.cr.m.*: middle crista nerve; *n.cr.p.*: posterior crista nerve; *n.m.*: macular nerve; *p.s.*: posterior *sac*; *sl*: statolith; *v*: vessels. C: Diagram of the types of cells probably present in a portion of a single-row section of the crista. *l.h.c.*: large haircells; *l.i.h.*: lower inner haircells; *l.o.h.*: lower outer haircells; *m.p.c.*: multipolar cells; *u.i.h.*: upper inner haircells; *u.o.h.*: upper outer haircells. (Only one example of each hair type is drawn) (Redrawn from Young, 1960)

KLEIN (1932) and YOUNG (1960), and with the aid of transmission and scanning electron microscopes by BARBER (1966), VINNIKOV et al. (1967), BARBER and BOYDE (1968), BOYDE and BARBER (1969) and BUDELMANN et al. (1973). For a review see BUDELMANN (in press).

The statocyst of *Octopus* — a fluid-filled sac 4 mm in diameter in a 500 g specimen — hangs in a fluid-filled cavity enclosed in the cartilage surrounding the brain (Fig. 22A). Kölliker's canal, a ciliated duct lying in the wall of the cyst and opening at one end into its cavity, while the other ends blind, is regarded as a rudiment of the invagination duct and is thought to be involved in the control of the statocyst fluid.

Three concentrations of sensory cells — all bearing kinocilia — are found together with supporting cells: those of the macula, those of the crista, and others scattered in the rest of the wall of the sac, most densely in its posterior portion.

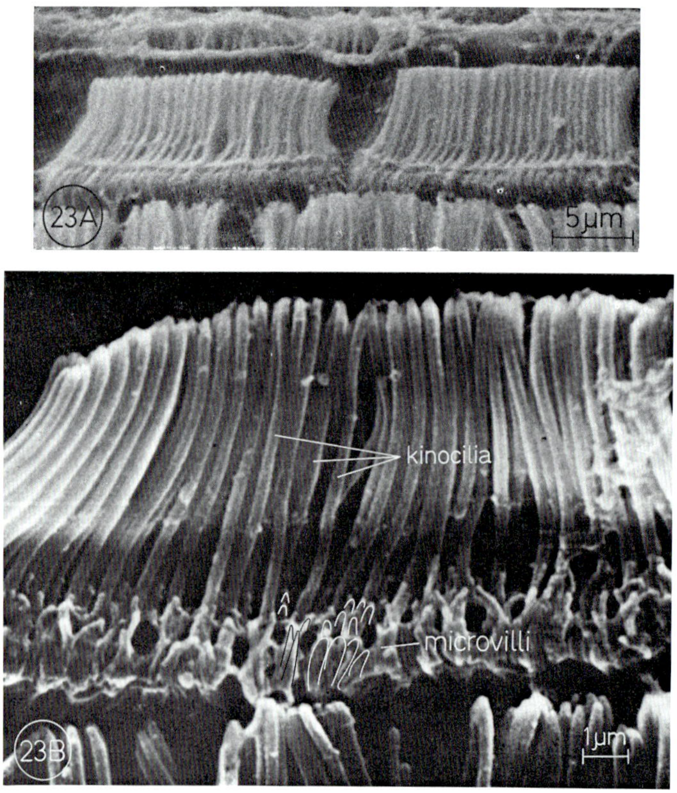

Fig. 23. A, B: Hair cell groups of the crista transversalis posterior of the left statocyst of *Sepia officinalis* as seen in the scanning electron microscope. C: Macula of the right statocyst of *Octopus vulgaris*. *D* dorsal, *V* ventral, *M* medial, *L* lateral. The arrow indicates the macula nerve. Some of the ciliary groups are partly covered by the remains of the mucus layer. D: Hair cell group of the macula statica princeps of the left statocyst of *Sepia officinalis* (A, C, D: from BUDELMANN et al., 1973; B: unpublished SEM-photograph by courtesy of Dr. B.-U. BUDELMANN)

The macula is a vertical oval area of haircells on the anteromedial wall, with a calcareous statolith hanging from it (Fig. 22 B). The planes of the right and left maculae subtend 90° open to the front. The crista is a greatly elongated ridge, with a course in each of the three planes, each section being innervated by a separate nerve. Each of the three parts is further divided into three subsections with their own flaps of massed hairs. In front of the vertical crista there is a rigid plate of cartilage, the anticrista, which may influence the movement of the fluid

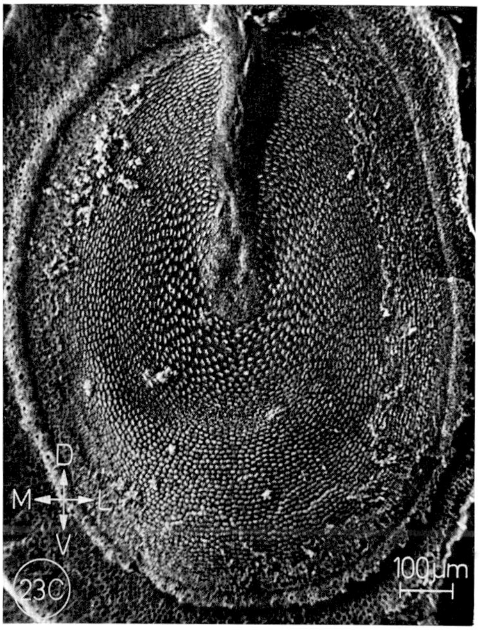

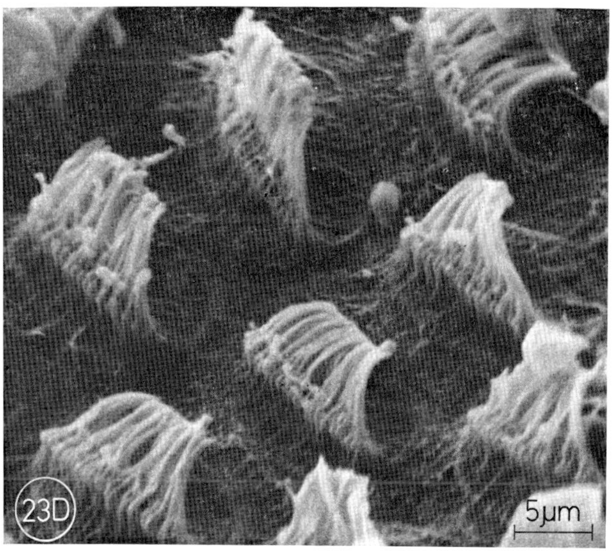

during rotation. The crista contains large haircells at its center, arranged in alternate sections with one row or two rows. Each row contains about 35 large hair cells per section. Flanking these, there are inner and outer rows of smaller hair cells; these show characteristic differences and are asymmetrical above and below (Fig. 22C).

The fine structure of the crista and of the macula are similar. All haircells are primary receptor cells. At their distal end, they bear elongated groups of up to 200 kinocilia of the (9+2) type, together with many short microvilli. The cilia measure about 10 μm. The two central filaments of each cilium are in line with the long axis of the ciliary group of the cell, whereas the basal feet of the cilia are at right angles to this axis. In the crista, the long axis of each group coincides with the long axis of the crista (Fig. 23A, B); both possible polarization directions of the hair cells are present in some crista segments. The connection of the cilia to the fragile cupula of amorphous and fibrous material is not yet quite clear.

In the macula (Fig. 23C, D) the long axes of the ciliary groups are oriented on concentric ellipses, all basal feet pointing away from the center. There are about 5100 hair cells in the *Octopus* macula, while the macula nerve contains about 9200 axons, the difference presumably being accounted for by efferent fibers (BUDELMANN et al., 1973).

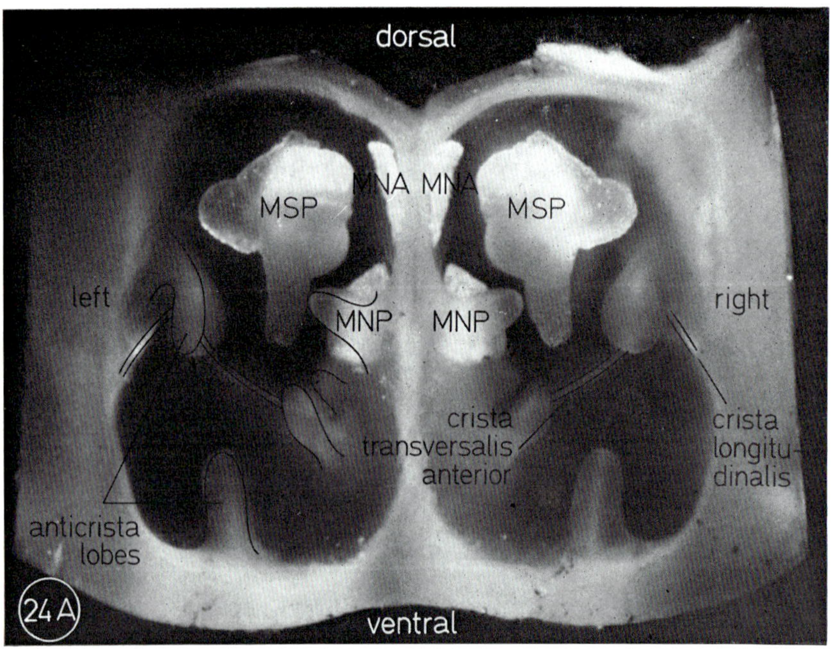

Fig. 24. A: Section through the statocysts of *Sepia officinalis*. MSP statolith on the macula statica princeps; MNA and MNP: statoconial layers on macula neglecta anterior and posterior, respectively (Unpublished photograph by courtesy of Dr. B.-U. BUDELMANN). B: Macula statica princeps of the left statocyst of *Sepia officinalis* (From BUDELMANN et al., 1973)

Desmosomes connect haircells and supporting cells. Below the macula and crista, there is a plexal nervous layer. In addition to cell bodies of the haircells, this contains multipolar cells, some of which also carry cilia. Others may be peripheral neurons, since their dendrites seem to come in contact with haircells, though ultrastructural evidence of synapses is not yet available. Furthermore, there are nerve endings assumed to be efferent around the apical part of the haircells.

The fluid contents of the cyst and the fluid surrounding the cyst have a very similar ionic composition. There is no high potassium concentration in the cyst (AMOORE et al., 1959).

In *Decabrachia*, there is almost no free space between cyst and cartilage, and instead of one, there are several anticristae (11–12 in Sepia, Fig. 24A), forming an elaborate system of loops around four sections of the crista. The macula (Fig. 24B) is divided into sections, often three; two of them stand vertical, at right angles to each other, the third horizontal. One vertical macula carries a statolith, the other two are covered by statoconia in *Sepia*. In *Sepia* the four sections of the crista contain ca. 700 hair cells each, the three maculae together 8600 hair cells; the respective numbers for *Loligo* are 600 and 4400 cells (BUDELMANN et al., 1973).

Vampyromorpha possess a fluid space around the cyst, have 9 anticristae, one macula, and a crista in three planes (BARBER, 1968).

Experimentation on the function of statocysts in Cephalopoda began with DELAGE (1887). He found blinded and statocystless *Octopus* were disoriented

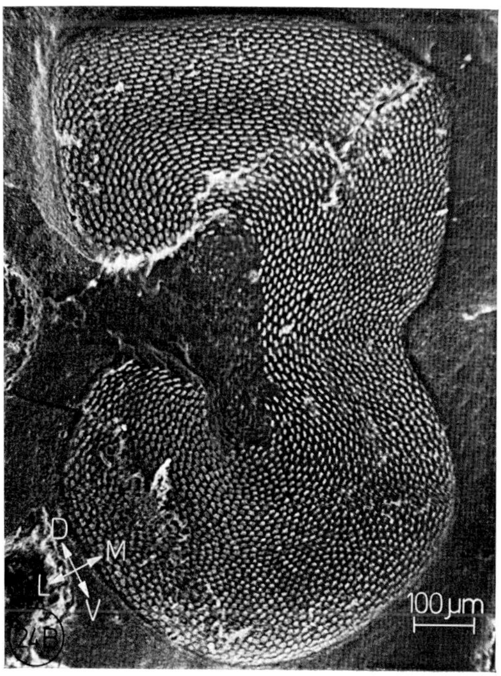

during swim, and even while walking they could not avoid swaying and rocking. These experiments were confirmed and expanded by von Uexküll (1895), Fröhlich (1904a), and Muskens (1904) in *Eledone*, and by Boycott (1960) and Wells (1960) in *Octopus*. After bilateral extirpation, *Octopus* rolls, somersaults, corkscrews and zigzags around when forced to swim, and lands any way up on the bottom of the tank. There is no apparent recovery even after several weeks. After unilateral extirpation, orientation is almost normal; only a slight tendency to circle around, with the intact side outward, is noticed. The capacity to right themselves, though with difficulty, is still present in blinded and bilaterally statocystless animals, probably due to tactile reflexes. In contrast to Fröhlich, Boycott and Wells found no notable influence of the statocyst on general muscular tonus; vibration sensitivity is also unaffected by statocyst removal.

The dependance of compensatory eye movements (counterrolling and vertical shift of the eye axis) on statocyst function in *Octopus* rotated around its transverse or longitudinal axes with two, one or no statocysts intact was carefully measured by Budelmann (1970). While intact animals counterroll with both eyes when rotated around the transverse axis and shift the axes of both eyes in opposite directions when rotated around the body's long axis, both kinds of eye movements

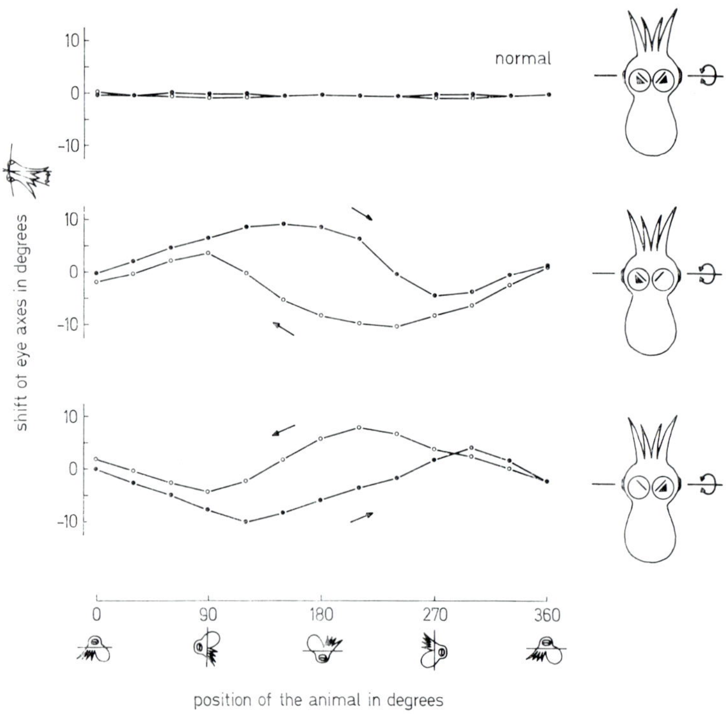

Fig. 25. Shift of eye axes (difference between shift angle of left and right eyes) of an intact *Octopus* (above) and after removal of the right (middle) or left (below) statolith during rotation in opposite directions (open and closed signs) around the transverse axis of the body (From Budelmann, 1970)

are found at the same time after rotation about one of both axes after unilateral exstirpation of a statocyst (Fig. 25). Reaction intensities in these animals are, however, only half of those in the intact state. Reactions reduced by 50% are also found in intact animals when they are rotated around a diagonal axis which stands so that one macular surface is at an exact right angle to this axis and the other parallel to it. All these reactions remain unchanged when the mechanical force acting on the statolith is increased up to 1.8 times by centrifugation of the animal. All compensatory eye reactions are abolished after extirpation of both statocysts or even after removal of the statoliths from the macular epithelia. From these experiments, BUDELMANN concludes that the effect of the two cysts on these reactions is additive, each organ affecting both eyes. Though shear of the statolith stimulates the sensory epithelium, it is only the direction, not the magnitude, of shearing forces that influences the eye movements. This differs remarkably from the gravireceptive mechanism in Crustacea and vertebrates, in which both magnitude and direction of the shearing force vector influence compensatory eye movements. The difference is not due to different properties at the level of the receptor cell, which are similar in cephalopods and vertebrates (BUDELMANN, in press).

BUDELMANN (in press) extended these behavioral investigations to compensatory eye and head movements in *Sepia* in order to elucidate the contribution of its three different maculae oriented in the three planes. Basically the gravireceptive function is similar to that in *Octopus*. Unilateral removal of statolith and statoconia leads to non-compensated eye-rolling and head-tilt, while the orientation of the whole body is unaffected. Only after destruction of the macular epithelia by extirpation of the cyst or by injection of Novocain into it, does rolling of the whole animal to the intact side result, an indication of spontaneous activity of the unloaded sense cells. The compensatory reactions are under the additive control of all 6 available maculae: any one of the six systems allows 20% of the normal reactions, any two 35–40%, three 65%, and four 80–85%, while 5 intact systems give reactions of normal intensity not different from those in the intact animal.

MUSKENS (1904) described an interesting connection between the presence of the equilibrium organs and eye position in *Eledone*. The slitlike pupil normally always remains horizontal, regardless of the body's position in space. After statocyst removal, the control of eye position is lost. WELLS (1960) confirmed this in *Octopus*, and found that completely statocystless animals are unable to discriminate between vertical and horizontal optical patterns. This shows that postural information from the statocysts is not centrally integrated with retinal input; on the contrary, the position of the retina relative to the external environment is kept constant, the statocyst information being used as reference. Both eyes are connected with both statocysts. Postural information from the statocysts seems not to be available for learning processes in *Octopus*.

Behavioral experiments on *Octopus* (DIJKGRAAF, 1961b) and on *Sepia* by DIJKGRAAF (1963), COLLEWIJN (1970) and MESSENGER (1970) have yielded data on the sensitivity to *angular acceleration* in cephalopods. Compensatory turning reactions of the eyes, the head, or the whole animal during and after rotation on a horizontal turntable in *Octopus* and upon rotation about all three axes in *Sepia* clearly depend on rotatory acceleration and deceleration. Postrotatory reflexes are not very pronounced in seeing animals, but are conspicuous in blinded ones. Unilateral extirpation of the statocyst does not affect reactions to rotations in either direction. Since compensatory reactions persist in blinded animals as long as at least the posterior crista has an intact innervation, there is little doubt that the cristae act as receptors for angular acceleration, which had already been inferred from anatomical studies.

Little has been published on electrophysiological recording from statocyst receptors in cephalopods, though more results are being prepared for publication by Wolff and Budelmann (pers. comm.). Maturana and Sperling (1963) recorded from single units in the horizontal crista nerve of *Octopus*. They found no spontaneous discharge but high sensitivity to low-frequency vibration. Budelmann and Wolff (1973), who recorded from all cristae nerves of the same species, report a resting discharge in all nerves. The longitudinal crista reacts to angular acceleration and deceleration around the longitudinal axis, the transversal crista around the transverse axis, and the vertical crista around the vertical axis. Rotation to one side inhibits the resting discharge during acceleration, while the activity is increased during deceleration; the response pattern reverses when rotation is in the opposite direction. The responses of crista units to angular acceleration and deceleration clearly change as a function of the orientation of the receptors with respect to gravity, which demonstrates that the cristae are also sensitive to linear gravitational acceleration.

XIII. Tentaculata

No gravity receptors have been described in *Bryozoa* and *Phoronidea*.

Lingulus (Brachiopoda) is equipped with one pair of cysts, though it is doubtful whether these are even innervated (Hyman). There is no experimental evidence on the subject.

XIV. Echinodermata

Control of posture in Echinodermata, their righting reactions, and their orientation during burrowing have been reviewed in great detail by Reese (1966). Only some of the salient features are therefore described here.

Among the *Holothuroidea*, statocysts are found in *Synaptida*, *Elasipoda* and *Molpadonia*. Gross morphological data have been published by Cuenot (1891), Clark (1898), Becher (1909), and Yamanouchi (1929a). *Synaptida* and *Molpadonia* have five pairs of statocysts close to the calcareous ring, each pair situated directly upon one of the 5 radial nerves (Fig. 26). Some *Elasipoda* have up to 100 cysts along their five radii. The epithelium of the cyst is ciliated. Statoliths are normally numerous, each lith being contained in a free lithocyte. According to Plate (1924), the lith material is not calcium carbonate.

Loeb (1891) was the first to describe gravity responses in a holothurian. *Cucumaria* crawls up an inclined surface and turns around when tilted. Clark (1899), Olmsted (1917) and Stier (1933) report similar, but not always negative, geotactic responses. Burrowing is gravity-oriented in *Synapta* (von Buddenbrock, 1912) and *Caudina* (Yamanouchi, 1927, 1929a, b).

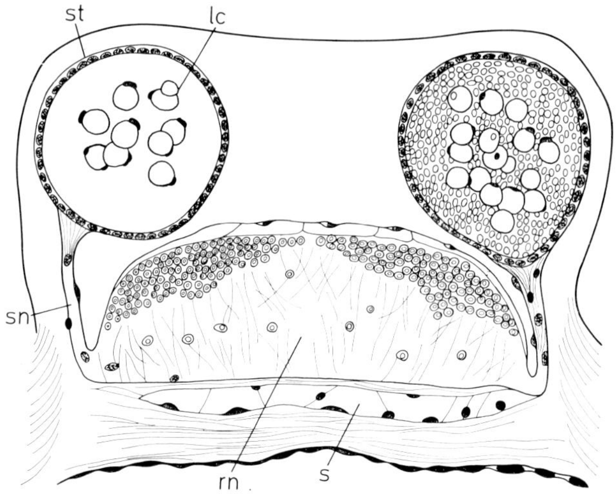

Fig. 26. A pair of statocysts of *Synapta inhaerens*. The right cyst is sectioned almost tangentially. *lc*: lithocyte (containing statolith); *rn*: radial nerve; *s*: sinus; *sn*: statocyst nerve; *st*: statocyst (From CUENOT, 1891)

It has not yet proved possible to extirpate the statocysts in these animals. The "best" evidence for their participation in gravity perception comes from OLMSTED (1917), who cut *Synaptula* across behind the calcareous ring: only the front part (with statocysts) continued to crawl upward. Data published by YAMANOUCHI (1929a, b) on *Caudina*, however, are not consistent with this result; an isolated anterior piece orients by gravity, but so does the rear part, where there are no statocysts. Not surprisingly, righting reactions are found in holothurians with cysts as well as in those without them (CROZIER, 1915).

No gravireceptors have been located in *Pelmatozoa*, *Echinoidea*, *Asteroidea* or *Ophiuroidea*. CUENOT suggested that sphaeridia of echinoids might function as gravireceptors (see also LEWIS, 1968). Indeed, their removal slows down righting reactions (DELAGE, 1902; PARKER, 1927); however, BOLIN (1926b) found *Psammechinus* just as well oriented with respect to gravity after removal of all sphaeridia as before. Therefore, present evidence does not justify calling these organs gravireceptive. Nevertheless, as in holothurians, responses to gravity have been frequently noticed in all these echinoderms.

Psammechinus persistently crawls up in aquaria and turns around when tilted end over end. All the spines and also the intestines can be removed without upsetting orientation; nor does filling of the coelom cavity with air change its sign (BOLIN, 1926b). In negative geotactic *Centrechinus* any radius can lead during oriented locomotion (PARKER, 1922). There are similar reports on geotactic locomotion in Asteroidea (LOEB, 1891; JÄGER, 1932; CROZIER, 1935a, b), where even single arms show the reaction (MANGOLD, 1909). KALMUS (1929) was able to change the sign of orientation by fixing a piece of cork to the body of *Asterina*. He concluded that this starfish perceives gravity from the body's pull on the podia. However, simply handling the animal can also change the sign of orientation (CROZIER, 1935b).

Righting reactions have been studied extensively in echinoderms (see Reese, 1966, for a summary). Even isolated arms of starfish can right. Wolf (1925) maintained that ophiuroids and asteroids with iron-filled intestines orient by a magnetic field. Fraenkel (1928) was unable to confirm this. His experimental animals righted nicely even after the intestines had been removed. He doubts whether righting reactions are oriented by gravity at all, and thinks stereotyped movements of appendages and tactile sensory reflexes may well be sufficient to explain all observed reactions, a view which is also supported by Tortonese (1950).

Pogonophora, Chaetognatha, Enteropneusta, Pterobranchia: neither equilibrium organs nor equilibrium reactions of these groups are mentioned in the literature.

XV. Tunicata

A "statocyst" is present in the third intermuscular space of the gonozoid of *Doliolum*. A duct opens to the surface (Plate, 1924; Bone, 1959). Adult ascidians do not have a static organ. However, their larvae as well as Appendicularia (Larvacea) possess an unpaired unicellular statocyst to the left at the base of the brain.

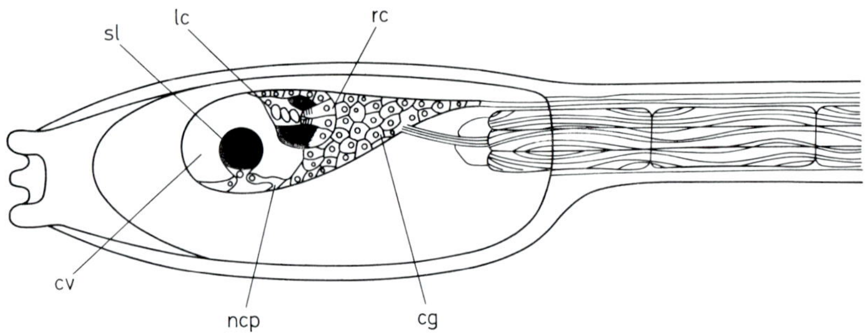

Fig. 27. Diagram of head region of the tadpole of *Ciona intestinalis*. *cg*: cerebral ganglion; *cv*: cavity of the cerebral vesicle; lc: lens cell; *ncp*: nerve cell process; *rc*: retinal cell; *sl*: statolith (From Dilly, 1962)

Dilly (1962) gives details of the structure in the tadpole of *Ciona intestinalis* (Fig. 27). The "lithocyte" has a free part, the "head", projecting into the cavity of the cerebral vesicle, and a "foot" contained within a mound of cells, among which neurons are suspected. The head is filled with pigment which is heavier than ordinary tadpole tissue. The neck connecting head and foot is only 0.75 μm across. The foot contains filaments, which may be derived from a ciliary apparatus. Tadpoles show negative geotactic reactions for two hours after hatching; two hours before settling down, the sign of the reaction is reversed. There is no proof of any gravireceptive function of the "statocyst".

Cephalochordata (Acrania)

Neither gravity receptors nor gravity responses are on record.

XVI. Concluding Remarks

Our knowledge of invertebrate receptors for gravity and for angular acceleration is far from complete. The fine structure and the response characteristics of the single sensory unit and the integration and processing of sensory afferences into motor commands and behavioral patterns of orientation will have to be carefully studied in many more forms before reliable generalizations can be ventured. There are good indications, however, even now that this search for basic mechanisms will not be in vain. To give one example: the use of sensory cells bearing kinocilia, the ultrastructure of which is intimately related to the cells' polarization of sensitivity, is now known to be common to groups as far apart as Coelenterata, Mollusca and Vertebrata. On the other hand, it must always be borne in mind that invertebrates, as opposed to vertebrates, are not an evolutionally homogeneous, monophyletic group. What we can often reasonably expect therefore are not general "invertebrate solutions" to gravireceptive problems, but rather solutions typical for all Metazoa or characteristic of a single phylum or of a few phyla of close relationship. The ever-present possibility of convergent evolution, especially in organs as much under the selective pressures of specific functions as sensory systems are, makes caution essential even when phylogenetic interpretations and generalizations seem all too self-evident.

As to the pattern of occurrence of specialized gravireceptors in invertebrates, there seems to be no general phylogenetic, ecological, or ethological explanation of why equilibrium organs are distributed among the taxonomic groups as they are. There can be little doubt that gravireceptors have evolved independently many times in different groups. It is true that these receptors are more often found in animals that move freely in all directions than in sedentary ones or those which move about slowly on the ground, but exceptions are far too numerous to be neglected. Orientation by light can replace orientation by gravity in many cases, but in yet other species both types of mechanisms have been perfected side by side.

It may be that gravireceptors have evolved from organs which formerly acted as vibration receptors in some cases or as generally stimulating organs in others. These functions could have been served in other groups by mechanisms which were not readily transformable into gravity-perceiving organs. Thus, it may have been more or less a matter of chance whether an ancestral form had or had not the type of material "at hand", which could easily develop into a gravireceptor. In that case, it would be useless to search for a common denominator as the causative factor in the evolution of gravireceptors in all groups of organisms which we now find equipped with them.

References

Alkon, D.L., Bak, A.: Hair cell generator potentials. J. gen. Physiol. **61**, 619–637 (1973).

Alverdes, F.: Stato-, Photo- und Tangoreaktionen bei zwei Garnelenarten. Z. vergl. Physiol. **4**, 699–765 (1926).

Amoore, J.E., Rodgers, K., Young, J.Z.: Sodium and potassium in the endolymph and perilymph of the statocyst and in the eye of *Octopus*. J. exp. Biol. **36**, 709–714 (1959).

Anderson, E., Dumont, J.N.: A comparative study of the concrement vacuole of certain endocommensal ciliates — a so-called mechanoreceptor. J. Ultrastruct. Res. **15**, 414–450 (1966).

Ax, P.: Verwandtschaftsbeziehungen und Phylogenie der Turbellarien. Ergebn. Biol. **24**, 1–68 (1961).

Bäcker, R.: Die Mikromorphologie von *Helix pomatia* und einigen anderen Stylommatophoren. Ergebn. Anat. Entwickl.-Gesch. **29**, 449–585 (1932).

Bässler, U.: Versuche zur Orientierung der Stechmücken: die Schwarmbildung und die Bedeutung des Johnstonschen Organs. Z. vergl. Physiol. **41**, 300–330 (1958).

Bässler, U.: Zum Schweresinn von Mehlkäfern und Stechmücken. Z. Naturforsch. **16b**, 264–267 (1961).

Bässler, U.: Proprioreceptoren am Subcoxal- und Femur-Tibia-Gelenk der Stabheuschrecke *Carausius morosus* und ihre Rolle bei der Wahrnehmung der Schwerkraftrichtung. Kybernetik **2**, 168–193 (1965).

Barber, V.C.: The fine structure of the statocyst of *Octopus vulgaris*. Z. Zellforsch. **70**, 91–107 (1966).

Barber, V.C.: The structure of mollusc statocysts, with particular reference to Cephalopods. Symp. Zool. Soc. (Lond.) **23**, 37–62 (1968).

Barber, V.C., Boyde, A.: Scanning electron microscopic studies of cilia. Z. Zellforsch. **84**, 269–284 (1968).

Barber, V.C., Dilly, P.N.: Some aspects of the fine structure of the statocysts of the molluscs *Pecten* and *Pterotrachea*. Z. Zellforsch. **94**, 462–478 (1969).

Bauer, V.: Über die reflektorische Regulierung der Schwimmbewegungen bei den Mysiden mit besonderer Berücksichtigung der doppelsinnigen Reizbarkeit der Augen. Z. allg. Physiol. **8**, 343–370 (1908).

Bauer, V.: Über die anscheinend nervöse Regulierung der Flimmerbewegung bei den Rippenquallen. Z. allg. Physiol. **10**, 231–248 (1910).

Baunacke, W.: Statische Sinnesorgane bei Nepiden. Zool. Jahrb. Anat. **34**, 179–342 (1912).

Baunacke, W.: Studien zur Frage nach der Statocystenfunktion. (Statische Reflexe bei Mollusken). Biol. Zbl. **33**, 427–452 (1913).

Becher, S.: Die Hörbläschen der *Leptosynapta bergensis*. Ein Beitrag zur Kenntnis der statischen Organe. Biol. Zbl. **29**, 413–424 (1909).

Beer, T.: Vergleichend-physiologische Studien zur Statocystenfunktion. I. Über den angeblichen Gehörsinn und das angebliche Gehörorgan der Crustaceen. Arch. ges. Physiol. **73**, 1–41 (1898).

Beer, T.: Vergleichend-physiologische Studien zur Statocystenfunktion. II. Versuche an Crustaceen (*Penaeus membranaceus*). Arch. ges. Physiol. **74**, 364–382 (1899).

Bethe, A.: Die Otocyste von *Mysis*. Zool. Jahrb. Anat. **8**, 544–564 (1895).

Bethe, A.: Das Nervensystem von *Carcinus maenas*. Ein anatomisch-physiologischer Versuch. I. Theil. I. Mittheilung und II. Mittheilung. Arch. mikroskop. Anat. Entwickl.-Gesch. **50**, 460–546; 589–639 (1897). II. Theil. 3. Mittheilung. ibid. **51**, 382–452 (1898).

Birukow, G.: Photo-Geomenotaxis bei *Geotrupes silvaticus* Panz. und ihre zentralnervöse Koordination. Z. vergl. Physiol. **36**, 176–211 (1954).

Bolin, L.: Einwirkung des Lichtes und der Schwere auf die Bewegungen der Rotatorien. Int. Rev. ges. Hydrobiol. **16**, 118–124 (1926).

Bolin, L.: Der Geotropismus von *Psammechinus miliaris* O.F.M. Int. Rev. ges. Hydrobiol. **16**, 125–129 (1926).

Bone, Qu.: Observations upon the nervous systems of pelagic Tunicates. Quart. J. micr. Sci. **100**, 167–181 (1959).

Both, M.P.: Die Regulation des Luftschöpfens bei *Notonecta glauca L.* Z. vergl. Physiol. **21**, 167–175 (1935).

Boycott, B.B.: The functioning of the statocysts of *Octopus vulgaris*. Proc. roy. Soc. B **152**, 78–87 (1960).

Boyde, A., Barber, V.C.: Freeze-drying methods for the scanning electron-microscopical study of the protozoon *Spirostomum ambiguum* and the statocyst of the cephalopod mollusc *Loligo vulgaris*. J. Cell Sci. **4**, 223–239 (1969).

Bozler, E.: Reizphysiologische Untersuchungen an *Paramaecium*. Verh. Dtsch. Zool. Ges. Kiel 1926, p. 124–129 (1926a).

Bozler, E.: Sinnes- und nervenphysiologische Untersuchungen an Scyphomedusen. Z. vergl. Physiol. **4**, 37–80 (1926b).

BOZLER, E.: Weitere Untersuchungen zur Sinnes- und Nervenphysiologie der Medusen: Erregungsleitung, Funktion der Randkörper, Nahrungsaufnahme. Z. vergl. Physiol. **4**, 797–817 (1926c).

BRAUNS, A.: Morphologische und physiologische Untersuchungen zum Halterenproblem unter besonderer Berücksichtigung brachypterer Arten. Zool. Jahrb. Physiol. **59**, 245–390 (1939).

BUDDENBROCK, W. VON: Über die Funktion der Statocysten im Sande grabender Meerestiere (*Arenicola* und *Synapta*). Biol. Zbl. **32**, 564–585 (1912).

BUDDENBROCK, W. VON: Über die Funktion der Statocysten im Sande grabender Meerestiere. II. Mitteilung. Zool. Jahrb. Physiol. **33**, 441–482 (1913).

BUDDENBROCK, W. VON: Über die Orientierung der Krebse im Raum. Zool. Jahrb. Physiol. **34**, 479–514 (1914).

BUDDENBROCK, W. VON: Die Statocyste von *Pecten*, ihre Histologie und Physiologie. Zool. Jahrb. Physiol. **35**, 301–356 (1915).

BUDDENBROCK, W. VON: Die vermutliche Lösung der Halterenfrage. Pflügers Arch. ges. Physiol. **175**, 125–164 (1919).

BUDDENBROCK, W. VON: Über unsere Kenntnis von der Funktion der Statocysten der Schnekken, mit besonderer Berücksichtigung der kompensatorischen Augenbewegungen. Biol. Zbl. **55**, 528—534 (1935).

BUDDENBROCK, W. VON: Vergleichende Physiologie. I. Sinnesphysiologie. Basel: Birkhäuser 1952.

BUDDENBROCK, W. VON, FRIEDRICH, H.: Neue Beobachtungen über die kompensatorischen Augenbewegungen und den Farbensinn der Taschenkrabben (*Carcinus maenas*). Z. vergl. Physiol. **19**, 747–761 (1933).

BUDELMANN, B.-U.: Die Arbeitsweise der Statolithenorgane von *Octopus vulgaris*. Z. vergl. Physiol. **70**, 278–312 (1970).

BUDELMANN, B.-U.: Gravity receptor function in Cephalopods with particular reference to *Sepia officinalis*. Fortschr. Zool. (in print).

BUDELMANN, B.-U., WOLFF, H.G.: Gravity response from angular acceleration receptors in *Octopus vulgaris*. J. comp. Physiol. **85**, 283–290 (1973).

BUDELMANN, B.-U., BARBER, V.C., WEST, S.: Scanning electron microscopical studies of the arrangements and numbers of hair cells in the statocysts of *Octopus vulgaris*, *Sepia officinalis* and *Loligo vulgaris*. Brain Res. **56**, 25–41 (1973).

BÜCKMANN, D.: Die Leistungen der Schwereorientierung bei dem im Meeressande grabenden Käfer *Bledius bicornis* Grm. (Staphylinidae) Z. vergl. Physiol. **36**, 488–507 (1954).

BÜCKMANN, D.: Zur Leistung des Schweresinnes bei Insekten. Naturwissenschaften **42**, 78–79 (1955).

BÜCKMANN, D.: Das Problem des Schweresinnes bei den Insekten. Naturwissenschaften **49**, 28–33 (1962).

BÜTSCHLI, O.: Vorlesungen über vergleichende Anatomie. 3. Lfg. Sinnesorgane und Leuchtorgane. Berlin: Springer 1925.

BULLOCK, T.H., HORRIDGE, G.A.: Structure and function in the nervous systems of Invertebrates. 2 vol. San Francisco: Freeman 1965.

BURROWS, M., HORRIDGE, G.A.: Motoneurone discharges to the eyecup muscles of the crab *Carcinus*. J. exp. Biol. **49**, 251–267 (1968).

CAMPBELL, R.D.: Statocyst lacking cilia in the coelenterate *Corymorpha palma*. Nature (Lond.) **238**, 49–51 (1972).

CHARLES, G.H.: Sense organs (less Cephalopods). In: Physiology of Mollusca. K.M. WILBUR and C.M. YONGE, Eds. Vol. 2, pp. 455–521. New York: Academic Press 1966.

CHUN, C.: Die Ctenophoren des Golfes von Neapel und der angrenzenden Meeresabschnitte. Leipzig: Engelmann 1880.

CLARK, G.P.: *Synapta vivipara*. A contribution to the morphology of Echinoderms. Mem. Bost. Soc. nat. Hist. **5**, 53–88 (1898).

CLARK, G.P.: The synaptas of the New England coast. Bull. U.S. Fish. Comm. **19**, 21–31 (1899).

CLARK, J.P.: On the relation of the otocysts to equilibrium phenomena in *Gelasimus pugilator* and *Platyonichus ocellatus*. J. Physiol. (Lond.) **19**, 327–343 (1896).

Clarke, A.M.: Geotactic responses in infra-human animals: a note on a new relationship between gravitational variables. Aust. J. Psychol. **22**, 67–70 (1970).

Coggeshall, R.E.: A fine structural analysis of the statocyst in *Aplysia californica*. J. Morph. **127**, 113–132 (1969).

Cohen, M.J.: The function of receptors in the statocyst of the lobster *Homarus americanus*. J. Physiol. (Lond.) **130**, 9–34 (1955).

Cohen, M.J.: The response patterns of single receptors in the crustacean statocyst. Proc. roy. Soc. B **152**, 30–49 (1960).

Cohen, M.J., Dijkgraaf, S.: Mechanoreception. In: The Physiology of Crustacea. T.H. Waterman, Ed. Vol. 2, pp. 65–108. New York: Academic Press 1961.

Cohen, M.J., Katsuki, Y., Bullock, T.H.: Oscillographic analysis of equilibrium receptors in Crustacea. Experientia (Basel) **9**, 434–435 (1953).

Collewijn, H.: Oculomotor reactions in the cuttlefish, *Sepia officinalis*. J. exp. Biol. **52**, 369–384 (1970).

Coonfield, B.R.: Coordination and movement of the swimming-plates of *Mnemiopsis leidyi* Agassiz. Biol. Bull. **66**, 10–21 (1934).

Coonfield, B.R.: Apical dominance and polarity in *Mnemiopsis leidyi* Agassiz. Biol. Bull. **70**, 460–471 (1936).

Crozier, W.J.: The sensory reactions of *Holothuria surinamensis* Ludwig. Zool. Jahrb. Physiol. **35**, 233–297 (1915).

Crozier, W.J.: The geotropic response in *Asterina*. J. gen. Physiol. **18**, 729–737 (1935a).

Crozier, W.J.: On reversal of geotropism in *Asterina*. J. gen. Physiol. **18**, 739–742 (1935b).

Cuenot, L.: Etudes morphologiques sur les Echinodermes. Arch. Biol. (Liège) **11**, 313–680 (1891).

Davis, W.J.: Lobster righting responses and their neural control. Proc. roy. Soc. B **70**, 435–456 (1968).

Dawydoff, C.: Contribution à nos connaissances de l'*Hydroctena*. C. R. Acad. Sci. (Paris) **237**, 1301–1302 (1953).

Delage, Y.: Sur une fonction nouvelle des otocystes comme organes d'orientation locomotrice. Arch. zool. exp. gén. 2. sér. **5**, 1–26 (1887).

Dembowski, J.: Die Vertikalbewegungen von *Paramaecium caudatum*. III. Polemisches und Experimentelles. Arch. Protistenk. **74**, 153–187 (1931).

Detwiler, P.B., Alkon, D.L.: Hair cell interactions in the statocysts of *Hermissenda*. J. gen. Physiol. **62**, 618–642 (1973).

Dijkgraaf, S.: Rotationssinn nach dem Bogengangsprinzip bei Crustaceen. Experientia (Basel) **11**, 407–409 (1955).

Dijkgraaf, S.: Structure and functions of the statocysts in crabs. Experientia (Basel) **12**, 394–396 (1956a).

Dijkgraaf, S.: Über die kompensatorischen Augenstielbewegungen bei Brachyuren. Pubbl. staz. zool. (Napoli) **28**, 341–358 (1956b).

Dijkgraaf, S.: Kompensatorische Augenstieldrehungen und ihre Auslösung bei der Languste (*Palinurus vulgaris*). Z. vergl. Physiol. **38**, 491–520 (1956c).

Dijkgraaf, S.: Wahrnehmung und Beantwortung des Erdschwerereizes bei Tieren. Stud. gen. **14**, 479–494 (1961a).

Dijkgraaf, S.: The statocyst of *Octopus vulgaris* as a rotation receptor. Pubbl. staz. zool. (Napoli) **32**, 64–87 (1961b).

Dijkgraaf, S.: Nystagmus and related phenomena in *Sepia officinalis*. Experientia (Basel) **19**, 29–30 (1963).

Dijkgraaf, S., Hessels, H.G.A.: Über Bau und Funktion der Statocyste bei der Schnecke *Aplysia limacina*. Z. vergl. Physiol. **62**, 38–60 (1969).

Dilly, P.N.: Studies on the receptors in the cerebral vesicle of the ascidian tadpole. I. The otolith. Quart. J. micr. Sci. **103**, 393–398 (1962).

Ehlers, E.: Die Gehörorgane der Arenicoliden. Z. wiss. Zool. **53**, Suppl. 217–285 (1892).

Faust, R.: Untersuchungen zum Halterenproblem. Zool. Jahrb. Physiol. **63**, 325–366 (1952).

Fauvel, P.: Recherches sur les otocystes des annélides polychètes. Ann. Sci. nat. zool. 9. Sér. **6**, 1–142 (1907).

Fraenkel, G.: Der statische Sinn der Medusen. Z. vergl. Physiol. **2**, 658–690 (1925).

FRAENKEL, G.: Die Grabbewegung der Soleniden. Z. vergl. Physiol. **6**, 167–220 (1927a).

FRAENKEL, G.: Beiträge zur Geotaxis und Phototaxis von *Littorina*. Z. vergl. Physiol. **5**, 585–597 (1927b).

FRAENKEL, G.: Über den Auslösungsreiz des Umdrehreflexes bei Seesternen und Schlangensternen. Z. vergl. Physiol. **7**, 365–378 (1928).

FRAENKEL, G.: Über die Geotaxis von *Convoluta roscoffensis*. Z. vergl. Physiol. **10**, 237–247 (1929).

FRAENKEL, G.: The function of the halteres of flies (Diptera). Proc. Zool. Soc. Lond. (A) **109**, 69–78 (1939).

FRAENKEL, G., GUNN, D.L.: The orientation of animals. New York: Dover 1961.

FRIEDRICH, H.: Studien über die Gleichgewichtserhaltung und Bewegungsphysiologie bei *Pterotrachea*. Z. vergl. Physiol. **16**, 345–361 (1932).

FRISCH, K. VON: Die Tänze der Bienen. Österr. Zool. Z. **1**, 1–48 (1946).

FRISCH, K. VON: Tanzsprache und Orientierung der Bienen. Berlin-Heidelberg-New York: Springer 1965.

FRÖHLICH, A.: Studien über Statocysten. I. Versuche an Cephalopoden. Pflügers Arch. ges. Physiol. **102**, 415–473 (1904a).

FRÖHLICH, A.: Studien über die Statocysten wirbelloser Tiere. II. Mitteilung. Versuche an Krebsen. Pflügers Arch. ges. Physiol. **103**, 149–168 (1904b).

GEUZE, J.J.: Observations on the function and the structure of the statocysts of *Lymnaea stagnalis* (L.). Neth. J. Zool. **18**, 155–204 (1968).

GORDON, S.A., COHEN, M.J.: Gravity and the Organism. 474 p. Chicago and London: University of Chicago Press 1971.

GRASSÉ, P.-P. (Ed.): Traité de Zoologie. Paris: Masson 1952.

HAMLYN-HARRIS, R.: Die Statocysten der Cephalopden. Zool. Jahrb. Anat. **18**, 327–358 (1903).

HENSEN, V.: Studien über das Gehörorgan der Decapoden. Z. wiss. Zool. **13**, 319–412 (1863).

HERAN, H.: Wahrnehmung und Regelung der Flugeigengeschwindigkeit bei *Apis mellifica L.* Z. vergl. Physiol. **42**, 103–163 (1959).

HERTWIG, O., HERTWIG, R.: Das Nervensystem und die Sinnesorgane der Medusen. Leipzig: Vogel 1878.

HERTWIG, R.: Über den Bau der Ctenophoren. Jena. Z. Med. Naturw. **14**, (N.F. **7**) 313–457 (1880).

HOLZAPFEL, M.: Die nicht-optische Orientierung der Trichterspinne *Agelena labyrinthica* (Cl.) Z. vergl. Physiol. **20**, 55–116 (1934).

HORN, E.: Die Schwerkraftrezeption bei der Geotaxis des laufenden Mehlkäfers (*Tenebrio molitor*). Z. vergl. Physiol. **66**, 343–354 (1970).

HORN, E.: Die Verarbeitung des Schwerereizes bei der Geotaxis der höheren Bienen (*Apidae*). J. comp. Physiol. **82**, 379–406 (1973).

HORRIDGE, G.A.: Relations between nerves and cilia in Ctenophores. Amer. Zool. **5**, 357–375 (1965a).

HORRIDGE, G.A.: The optomotor response of the crab *Carcinus*. Proc. Symp. on Information Processing in Sight Sensory Systems, Pasadena, 57–74 (1965b).

HORRIDGE, G.A.: Pathways of co-ordination in Ctenophores. Symp. Zool. Soc. (Lond.) **16**, 247–266 (1966).

HORRIDGE, G.A.: Statocysts of medusae and evolution of stereocilia. Tissue and Cell **1**, 341–353 (1969).

HORRIDGE, G.A.: Primitive examples of gravity receptors and their evolution. In: Gravity and the Organism. S. GORDON and M. COHEN, Eds. pp. 203–221. Chicago: University of Chicago Press 1971.

HORSTMANN, E.: Untersuchungen zur Physiologie der Schwimmbewegungen der Scyphomedusen. Pflügers Arch. ges. Physiol. **234**, 406–420 (1934).

HYMAN, L.H.: The Invertebrates. New York: McGraw Hill 1940.

ILYIN, P.: Das Gehörbläschen als Gleichgewichtsorgan bei den Pterotracheiden. Zbl. Physiol. **13**, 691–694 (1900).

ISHIKAWA, M.: On the phylogenetic position of the cephalopod genera of Japan based on the structure of statocysts. J. Coll. Agr. Imp. Univ. Tokyo **7**, 165–210 (1924).

JÄGER, H.: Untersuchungen über die geotaktischen Reaktionen verschiedener Evertebraten auf schiefer Ebene. Zool. Jahrb. Physiol. **51**, 289–320 (1932).

JAHN, T.L., BOVEE, E.C.: Motile behavior of Protozoa. In: Research in Protozool. **1**, 39–198. T.T. CHEN, Ed. Oxford: Pergamon Press 1967.

JANDER, R.: Die optische Richtungsorientierung der Roten Waldameise (*Formica rufa L.*) Z. vergl. Physiol. **40**, 162–238 (1957).

JANDER, R.: Menotaxis und Winkeltransponieren bei Köcherfliegen (*Trichoptera*). Z. vergl. Physiol. **43**, 680–686 (1960).

JANDER, R.: Grundleistungen der Licht- und Schwereorientierung von Insekten. Z. vergl. Physiol. **47**, 381–430 (1963a).

JANDER, R.: Insect orientation. Ann. Rev. Entomol. **8**, 95–114 (1963a).

JANDER, R.: Die Phylogenie von Orientierungsmechanismen der Arthropoden. Verh. Dtsch. zool. Ges. Jena 1965, 266–306 (1966).

JANDER, R., HORN, E., HOFFMANN, M.: Die Bedeutung von Gelenkrezeptoren in den Beinen für die Geotaxis der höheren Insekten (Pterygota). Z. vergl. Physiol. **66**, 326–342 (1970).

JANDER, R., JANDER, U.: Über die Phylogenie der Geotaxis innerhalb der Bienen (Apoidea). Z. vergl. Physiol. **66**, 355–368 (1970).

KALMUS, H.: Versuche über die Bewegungen der Seesterne, besonders von *Asterina gibbosa*. Z. vergl. Physiol. **9**, 703–733 (1929).

KEIL, E.M.: Regeneration in *Polychoerus caudatus Mark.* Biol. Bull. **57**, 225–244 (1929).

KINZIG, H.: Untersuchungen über den Bau der Statocysten einiger decapoder Crustaceen. Verh. naturhist.-med. Verein Heidelberg N.F. **14**, 1–90 (1921).

KLEIN, K.: Die Nervenendigungen in der Statocyste von *Sepia*. Z. Zellforsch. **14**, 481–516 (1932).

KNOX, CH.K.: Signal transmission in random spike trains with applications to the statocyst neurons of the lobster. Kybernetik **7**, 167–174 (1970).

KOEHLER, O.: Über die Geotaxis von *Paramaecium*. Arch. Protistenk. **45**, 1–94 (1922).

KOEHLER, O.: Über die Geotaxis von *Paramaecium* II. Arch. Protistenk. **70**, 279–306 (1930).

KOLMER, W.: Statoreceptoren. Bau der statischen Apparate. Handb. Norm. Pathol. Physiol. A. BETHE, G. VON BERGMANN, G. EMBDEN und A. ELLINGER, Eds. **1**, 769–790 (1926).

KREIDL, A.: Weitere Beiträge zur Physiologie des Ohrlabyrinthes (II. Mitt.). Versuche an Krebsen. S.-B. Akad. Wiss. Wien, math.-nat. Kl. **102**, 149–174 (1893).

KRISCH, B.: Über das Apikalorgan (Statocyste) der Ctenophore *Pleurobrachia pileus*. Z. Zellforsch. **142**, 241–262 (1973).

KÜHN, A.: Versuche über die reflektorische Erhaltung des Gleichgewichtes bei Krebsen. Verh. Dtsch. zool. Ges. Freiburg 1914, 262–277 (1914).

KUWABARA, M.: Über die Funktion der Antenne der Honigbiene in Bezug auf die Raumorientierung. Mem. Fac. Sic. Kyushu Univ. Ser. E. **1**, 13–55 (1952).

LAMMERT, A.: Über Pigmentwanderung im Punktauge der Insekten, sowie über Licht- und Schwerkraftreaktionen von Schmetterlingsraupen. Z. vergl. Physiol. **3**, 225–278 (1926).

LANGENBUCH, R.: Über die Statocysten einiger Crustaceen. Zool. Jahrb. Physiol. **44**, 575–622 (1928).

LAVERACK, M.S.: On superficial receptors. Symp. Zool. Soc. (Lond.) **23**, 299–326 (1968).

LEHMANN, C.: Untersuchungen über die Sinnesorgane der Medusen. Zool. Jahrb. Physiol. **39**, 321–394 (1923).

LEMCHE, H., WINGSTRAND, K.G.: The anatomy of *Neopilina galathea* LEMCHE 1957 (Mollusca, Tryblidiacea). Galathea Rep. **3**, 9–73 (1959).

LEVER, J., GEUZE, J.J.: Some effects of statocyst extirpations in *Lymnaea stagnalis*. Malacologia **2**, 275–280 (1965).

LEWIS, J.B.: The function of the sphaeridia of sea urchins. Canad. J. Zool. **46**, 1135–1138 (1968).

LINDAUER, M., NEDEL, J.O.: Ein Schweresinnesorgan der Honigbiene. Z. vergl. Physiol. **42**, 334–364 (1959).

LINDAUER, M., MARTIN, H.: Die Schwereorientierung der Bienen unter dem Einfluß des Erdmagnetfeldes. Z. vergl. Physiol. **60**, 219–243 (1968).

LINSENMAIR-ZIEGLER, CHR.: Vergleichende Untersuchungen zum photogeotaktischen Winkeltransponieren pterygoter Insekten. Z. vergl. Physiol. **68**, 229–262 (1970).

LOEB, J.: Über Geotropismus bei Thieren. Arch. Physiol. **49**, 175–189 (1891).

LYON, E. P.: A contribution to the comparative physiology of compensatory motions. Amer. J. Physiol. **3**, 86–114 (1900).

MANGOLD, E.: Sinnesphysiologische Studien an Echinodermen. Ihre Reaktionen auf Licht und Schatten und die negative Geotaxis bei *Asterina*. Z. allg. Physiol. **9**, 112–146 (1909).

MANGOLD, E.: Gehörssinn und statischer Sinn. In: Handb. vergl. Physiol. H. WINTERSTEIN, Ed. **4**, 841–976 (1913).

MARKL, H.: Borstenfelder an den Gelenken als Schweresinnesorgane bei Ameisen und anderen Hymenopteren. Z. vergl. Physiol. **45**, 475–569 (1962).

MARKL, H.: Geomenotaktische Fehlorientierung bei *Formica polyctena* Foerster. Z. vergl. Physiol. **48**, 552–586 (1964).

MARKL, H.: Schwerkraftdressuren an Honigbienen. I. Die geomenotaktische Fehlorientierung. Z. vergl. Physiol. **53**, 328–352 (1966a).

MARKL, H.: Schwerkraftdressuren an Honigbienen. II. Die Rolle der schwererezeptorischen Borstenfelder verschiedener Gelenke für die Schwerekompassorientierung. Z. vergl. Physiol. **53**, 353–371 (1966b).

MARKL, H.: Proprioceptive gravity perception in Hymenoptera. In: Gravity and the Organism. S. GORDON and M. COHEN, Eds. pp. 185–194. Chicago: University of Chicago Press 1971.

MARKL, H.: Insect Behavior: Functions and Mechanisms. Ch. 1, pp. 3–148. In: Physiology of Insecta, Vol. III, M. ROCKSTEIN, Ed. New York: Academic Press 1974.

MARTIN, H., LINDAUER, M.: Orientierung im Erdmagnetfeld. Fortschr. Zool. **21**, 211–228 (1973).

MATURANA, H. R., SPERLING, S.: Unidirectional response to angular acceleration recorded from the middle cristal nerve in the statocyst of *Octopus vulgaris*. Nature (Lond.) **197**, 815–816 (1963).

MCCLARY, A.: Statocyst function in *Pomacea paludosa*. Malacologia **3**, 419–431 (1966).

MERKER, G., VAUPEL-VON HARNACK, M.: Zur Feinstruktur des Gehirns und der Sinnesorgane von *Protodrilus rubropharyngeus* Jaegersten (Archiannelida). Z. Zellforsch. **81**, 221–239 (1967).

MERTON, H.: Versuche zur Geotaxis von *Paramaecium*. Arch. Prostistenk. **85**, 33–60 (1935).

MESSENGER, J. B.: Optomotor responses and nystagmus in intact, blinded and statocystless cuttlefish (*Sepia officinalis* L.). J. exp. Biol. **53**, 789–796 (1970).

MITTELSTAEDT, H.: Physiologie des Gleichgewichtssinnes bei fliegenden Libellen. Z. vergl. Physiol. **32**, 422–463 (1950).

MURBACH, L.: The static function in *Gonionemus*. Amer. J. Physiol. **10**, 201 (1903).

MURBACH, L.: Further experiments on static function. 7th. Ann. Rep. Michigan Acad. Soc. 1905, 86–88 (1905).

MUSKENS, L. J. J.: Über eine eigenthümliche compensatorische Augenbewegung der Octopoden mit Bemerkungen über deren Zwangsbewegungen. Arch. Physiol. (Leipzig) 1904, 49–56 (1904).

NICKLAUS, R.: Zur Funktion der keulenförmigen Sensillen auf den Cerci der Grillen. Verh. Dtsch. Zool. Ges. Innsbruck 1968, 393–398.

OEVERMANN, H.: Das statische Verhalten einiger Wasserwanzenarten. Z. wiss. Zool. **147**, 595–628 (1936).

OLMSTED, J. M. D.: The comparative physiology of *Synaptula hydriformis* (Lesueur). J. exp. Zool. **24**, 333–379 (1917–1918).

PAN, C.-T.: The general histology and topographic microanatomy of *Australorbis glabratus*. Bull. Mus. Comp. Zool. Harvard **119**, 237–299 (1958).

PANNING, A.: Die Statocyste von *Astacus fluviatilis* (*Potamobius astacus* Leach) und ihre Beziehungen zu dem sie umgebenden Gewebe. Z. wiss. Zool. **123**, 305–358 (1924).

PARKER, G. H.: The activities of *Corymorpha*. J. exp. Zool. **24**, 303–331 (1917–1918).

PARKER, G. H.: The geo-tropism of the sea-urchin *Centrechinus*. Biol. Bull. **43**, 374–383 (1922).

PATTON, M. L.: Physiological evidence indicating that decapod statocyst hairs drive three sensory neurons. Amer. Zool. **9**, 1097 (1969).

PETERS, H.: Experimente über die Orientierung der Kreuzspinne *Epeira diademata Cl.* im Netz. Zool. Jahrb. Physiol. **51**, 239–288 (1932).

PFEIL, E.: Die Statocyste von *Helix pomatia L.* Z. wiss. Zool. **119**, 79–113 (1921).

Piéron, H.: Le rôle des statocystes chez les mollusques et les donneés fournies par l'étude du géotropisme des limaces. C. R. Soc. Biol. (Paris) **97**, (1927).

Piéron, H.: Sens statique et géotropisme chez les limaces. Remarques sur la notion de tropisme. J. Psychol. **26**, (1929).

Piéron, H.: Réactions géotropiques chez les limaces. Ann. Physiol. Physicochim. Biol. **4**, 44–63 (1928).

Plate, L.: Allgemeine Zoologie und Abstammungslehre. 2. Teil. Jena: Fischer 1924.

Prentiss, C. W.: The otocyst of Decapod Crustacea, its structure, development and functions. Bull. Mus. Comp. Zool. Harvard **36**, 167–251 (1900–1901).

Pringle, J. W. S.: The gyroscopic mechanism of the halteres of Diptera. Phil. Trans. B **233**, 347–384 (1948).

Polimanti, O.: Contributi alle fisiologia del movimento e del sisteme nervoso degli animali inferiori. Z. allgem. Physiol. **12**, 379–406 (1911).

Quattrini, D.: Osservazioni preliminari sulla ultrastruttura della statocisti dei molluschi gasteropodi polmonati. Boll. ital. Biol. sper. **43**, 785–786 (1967).

Queinnec, Y.: Etude des facteurs psychophysiologiques permettant la découverte de la plante-hôte par les larves néonates de l'altise d'hiver du Colza (*Psylloides chrysocephala L.*). Ann. Epiphyties **18**, 27–74 (1967).

Rabe, W.: Beiträge zum Orientierungsproblem der Wasserwanzen. Z. vergl. Physiol. **35**, 300–325 (1953).

Reese, E. S.: The complex behavior of Echinoderms. In: Physiology of Echinodermata. R. A. Boolootian, Ed. pp. 157–218. New York: Interscience 1966.

Roberts, A. M.: Geotaxis in motile micro-organisms. J. exp. Biol. **53**, 687–699 (1970).

Sandeman, D. C., Okajima, A.: Statocyst-induced eye movements in the crab *Scylla serrata*. I. The sensory input from the statocyst. J. exp. Biol. **57**, 187–204 (1972).

Sandeman, D. C., Okajima, A.: II. The responses of the eye muscles. J. exp. Biol. **58**, 197–212 (1973).

Sandeman, D. C., Okajima, A.: III. The anatomical projections of sensory and motor neurones and the responses of the motor neurones. J. exp. Biol. **59**, 17–38 (1973).

Schmidt, W.: Untersuchungen über die Statocysten unserer einheimischen Schnecken. Jena. Z. Med. Naturw. **48**, 515–562 (1912).

Schneider, G.: Die Halteren der Schmeißfliege (*Calliphora*) als Sinnesorgane und als mechanische Flugstabilisatoren. Z. vergl. Physiol. **35**, 416–458 (1953).

Schöne, H.: Statocystenfunktion und statische Lageorientierung bei decapoden Krebsen. Z. vergl. Physiol. **36**, 241–260 (1954).

Schöne, H.: Kurssteuerung mittels der Statocysten (Messungen an Krebsen). Z. vergl. Physiol. **39**, 235–240 (1957).

Schöne, H.: Die Lageorientierung mit Statolithenorganen und Augen. Ergebn. Biol. **21**, 161–209 (1959).

Schöne, H.: Gravity receptors and gravity orientation in Crustacea. In: Gravity and the Organism. S. Gordon and M. Cohen, Eds. pp. 223–235. Chicago: University of Chicago Press 1971.

Schöne, H., Schöne, H.: Integrated function of statocyst and antennular proprioceptive organ in the spiny lobster. Naturwissenschaften **54**, 289 (1967).

Schöne, H.: Steinbrecht, R. A.: Fine structure of statocyst receptor of *Astacus fluviatilis*. Nature (Lond.) **220**, 184–186 (1968).

Siewing, R.: Untersuchungen zur Morphologie der Malacostraca (Crustacea). Zool. Jahrb. Anat. **75**, 39–176 (1957).

Sleigh, M. A.: Metachronal co-ordination of the comb plates of the ctenophore *Pleurobrachia*. J. exp. Biol. **48**, 111–125 (1968).

Spek, J.: Die chemische Natur der Statoconien in den Rhopalien von *Rhizostoma pulmo* Les. Zool. Anz. **44**, 406–411 (1914).

Stahlschmidt, V., Wolff, H. G.: The fine structure of the statocyst of the prosobranch mollusc *Pomacea paludosa*. Z. Zellforsch. **133**, 529–537 (1972).

Stier, T. J. B.: Diurnal changes in activities and geotropism in *Thyone briareus*. Biol. Bull. **64**, 326–332 (1933).

STUDNITZ, G. VON: Statische Funktion der sogenannten pelotaktischen Organe (Schlammsinnesorgane) der Limnobiidenlarven. Zool. Jahrbuch. Physiol. **50**, 419–446 (1932).

STYCZYNSKA-JUREWICZ, E.: On the geotaxis, invasivity and span of life of *Opisthioglyphe ranae* Duj. cercariae. Bull. Acad. Pol. Sci. Cl. II. Ser. Sci. Biol. **9**, 31–35 (1961).

TABOURET-KELLER, A.: L'analyse experimentale du géotropisme de la chenille d'un Saturniide, *Automeris illustris W.* Union Intern. Sci. Biol. Bruxelles. pp. 99–115 (1957).

TAMM, S.L.: Mechanisms of ciliary co-ordination in ctenophores. J. exp. Biol. **59**, 231–245 (1973).

TENCKHOFF-EICKMANNS, J.: Licht- und Erdschwereorientierung beim Mehlkäfer *Tenebrio molitor L.* und bei einigen anderen Insekten. Zool. Beitr. N.F. **4**, 307–341 (1959).

THORPE, W.H., CRISP, D.J.: The orientation responses of *Aphelocheirus* (Hemiptera, *Aphelocheiridae* (*Naucoridae*)) in relation to plastron respiration; together with an account of specialized pressure receptors in aquatic insects. J. exp. Biol. **24**, 310–328 (1947).

THURM, U.: Die Beziehungen zwischen mechanischen Reizgrößen und stationären Erregungszuständen bei Borstenfeldsensillen von Bienen. Z. vergl. Physiol. **46**, 351–382 (1963).

THURM, U.: Das Rezeptorpotential einzelner mechanorezeptorischer Zellen von Bienen. Z. vergl. Physiol. **48**, 131–156 (1964a).

THURM, U.: Mechanoreceptors in the cuticle of the honeybee: fine structure and stimulus mechanism. Science **145**, 1063–1065 (1964b).

THURM, U.: An insect mechanoreceptor. I. Fine structure and adequate stimulus. II. Receptor potentials. Cold Spr. Harb. Symp. quant. Biol. **30**, 75–82; 83–94 (1965).

THURM, U.: Die Empfindlichkeit motiler Cilien für mechanische Reize. Verh. Dtsch. Zool. Ges. Heidelberg 1967, 96–105 (1968).

TORTONESE, E.: Ricerche sperimentale e comparative sui movimenti degli asteroidi. Arch. zool. ital. Napoli **35**, 217–250 (1950).

TSCHACHOTIN, S.: Die Statocyste der Heteropoden. Z. wiss. Zool. **90**, 343–422 (1908).

UEXKÜLL, J. VON: Physiologische Untersuchungen an *Eledone moschata*. Z. Biol. **31**, (N.F. **13**) 584–609 (1895).

VERWORN, M.: Gleichgewicht und Otolithenorgan. Pflügers Arch. ges. Physiol. **50**, 423–472 (1891).

VINNIKOV, Y.A.: Rezeptor gravitazii. Evoluzia strukturnoj, zitochimitscheskoj i funktionalnoj organisazii. In: "Problemy kosmitscheskoj biologii" Bd. XII. Hrsg. W.I. Tschernigovskij. Isdatelstvo Nauka Leningradskoje Otdelenije, Leningrad 1971.

VINNIKOV, Y.A., GASENKO, O.G., BRONSTEIN, A.A., TSIRULIS, T.P., IVANOV, V.P., PYATKINA, G.A.: Structural, cytochemical and functional organization of statocysts of Cephalopoda. Symp. on Neurobiology of Invertebrates, Akadémiai Kiadó, Budapest, pp. 29–48 (1967).

VOWLES, D.M.: The orientation of ants. I. Substitution of stimuli. II. Orientation to light, gravity and polarized light. J. exp. Biol. **31**, 341–355; 356–375 (1954).

WEIS-FOGH, T.: Flying insects and gravity. In: Gravity and the Organism. S. GORDON and M. COHEN, Eds. pp. 177–184. Chicago: University of Chicago Press 1971.

WELLS, M.J.: Proprioception and visual discrimination of orientation in *Octopus*. J. exp. Biol. **37**, 489–499 (1960).

WELLS, M.J.: Cephalopod sense organs. In: Physiology of Mollusca. K.M. WILBUR and C.M YONGE, Eds. Vol. 2, pp. 523–545. New York: Academic Press 1966.

WENDLER, G.: Laufen und Stehen der Stabheuschrecke *Carausius morosus*: Sinnesborstenfelder in den Beingelenken als Glieder von Regelkreisen. Z. vergl. Physiol. **48**, 198–250 (1964).

WENDLER, G.: Über den Anteil der Antennen an der Schwererezeption der Stabheuschrecke *Carausius morosus Br.* Z. vergl. Physiol. **51**, 60–66 (1965).

WENDLER, G.: Gravity orientation in insects: the role of different mechanoreceptors. In: Gravity and the Organism. S. GORDON and M. COHEN, Eds. pp. 195–199. Chicago: University of Chicago Press 1971.

WENDLER, G.: Körperhaltung bei der Stabheuschrecke: ihre Beziehung zur Schwereorientierung und Mechanismen ihrer Regelung. Verh. Dtsch. Zool. Ges. 65. Jahresvers. Helgoland 1971, pp. 214–219 (1971b).

WIERSMA, C.A.G., YAMAGUCHI, T.: Integration of visual stimuli by the crayfish central nervous system. J. exp. Biol. **47**, 409–431 (1967).

Wilson, D.M.: Stabilizing mechanisms in insect flight. In: Gravity and the Organism. S. Gordon and M. Cohen, Eds. pp. 169–176. Chicago: University of Chicago Press 1971.

Wolf, E.: Physiologische Untersuchungen über das Umdrehen der Seesterne und Schlangensterne. Z. vergl. Physiol. **3**, 209–224 (1925).

Wolff, H.G.: Elektrische Antworten der Statonerven der Schnecken (*Arion empiricorum* und *Helix pomatia*) auf Drehreizung. Experientia (Basel) **24**, 848–849 (1968).

Wolff, H.G.: Einige Ergebnisse zur Ultrastruktur der Statocysten von *Limax maximus*, *Limax flavus* und *Arion empiricorum* (Pulmonata). Z. Zellforsch. **100**, 251–270 (1969).

Wolff, H.G.: Statocystenfunktion bei einigen Landpulmonaten (Gastropoda). Z. vergl. Physiol. **69**, 326–366 (1970a).

Wolff, H.G.: Efferente Aktivität in den Statonerven einiger Landpulmonaten (Gastropoda). Z. vergl. Physiol. **70**, 401–409 (1970b).

Wolff, H.G.: Statische Orientierung bei Mollusken. Fortschr. Zool. **21**, 80–99 (1973a).

Wolff, H.G.: Multi-directional sensitivity of statocyst receptor cells of the opisthobranch gastropod *Aplysia limacina*. Mar. Behav. Physiol. **1**, 361–373 (1973b).

Wood, J., von Baumgarten, R.J.: Activity recorded from the statocyst nerve of *Pleurobranchaea californica* during rotation and at different tilts. Comp. Biochem. Physiol. **43A**, 495–502 (1972).

Yamanouchi, T.: Some preliminary notes on the behaviour of the Holothurian *Caudina chilensis* (J. Müller). Sci. Rep. Tohoku Imp. Univ. Sendai Ser. 4 (Biol.) **2**, 85–91 (1927).

Yamanouchi, T.: Notes on the behaviour of the Holothurian *Caudina chilensis* (J. Müller). Sci. Rep. Tohoku Imp. Univ. Sendai, Ser. 4 (Biol.) **4**, 73–115 (1929a).

Yamanouchi, T.: Reactions to centrifugal force in the Holothurian *Caudina chilensis* (J. Müller). Sci. Rep. Tohoku Imp. Univ. Sendai, Ser. 4 (Biol.) **4**, 521–532 (1929b).

Yamashita, T.: Über den Statolithen in den Sinneskörpern der Meduse *Aurelia aurita*. Z. Biol. **109**, 111–115 (1957).

Young, J.Z.: The statocysts of *Octopus vulgaris*. Proc. roy. Soc. B **152**, 3–29 (1960).

Young, J.Z.: The central nervous system of *Nautilus*. Phil. Trans. B **249**, 1–25 (1965).

Chapter II.

Comparative Morphology and Physiology

By

O.E. LOWENSTEIN, Birmingham

With 20 Figures

Contents

I. Introduction

The emergence of the vertebrates during organic evolution is still obscure. Zoologists find it impossible to single out any specific invertebrate type as the direct ancestor of one or the other of the earliest fish-like vertebrates. The protochordates point the way but there is rather a wide gap between them and the Agnatha or jawless fishes. These include the ostracoderms, the earliest known fossil chordates, and the living cyclostomes, hagfishes and lampreys. In both the ostracoderms and the cyclostomes the labyrinth has reached almost the extent of organization characteristic throughout the vertebrates. Its subdivision into semicircular canals and otolith organs is phylogenetically fundamental and is found in the labyrinth of the fossil ostracoderm *Kieraspis* (STENSIÖ, 1927) and in the cyclostomes.

Obviously the otolith organs have their analogues in the various types of statocysts found in the invertebrates, including the protochordates (see Chapter 2/1 by MARKL). Whether any of these statocysts, for instance the otolith-bearing sense ending in the tunicate larva, can be considered homologous with the chordate otolith organs will have to remain an open question. They are definitely functional analogues (VINNIKOV, 1974).

The semicircular canals have no such obvious analogues among sensory systems of the invertebrates. However, the principle of cupula-ensheathed hair processes of sensory cells monitoring fluid displacement is foreshadowed by the syphonal current sensors in tunicates such as *Ciona intestinalis*. Patches of primary sensory cells with apical sensory processes are distributed on the inside of the atrial or exhalant syphon. The hair processes are covered by flag-like sheaths of tunicin floating freely in the syphonal channel, and it is reasonable to suggest that they gauge the strength and direction of the syphonal current, though this has not yet been experimentally demonstrated (MILLAR, 1953). The homologous forerunners of the semicircular canals of the labyrinth are of course the lateral-line organs. The design and composition of their sense endings closely resemble those of the endings of the cristae in the semicircular canal ampullae. In fact, it is assumed that the whole labyrinth may represent the final stage in the submergence of originally superficial and free-standing neuromast organs of the lateral-line system below the body surface which have now become almost completely isolated from the outside medium and encapsulated in the brain case (PUMPHREY, 1950). The so-called ductus endolymphaticus maintains a tenuous connection with the outside world in the elasmobranch fishes only. Elsewhere it ends blindly, widening into a saccus endolymphaticus, whose function is discussed in Chapter C.III. by DOHLMAN.

II. Morphology

The membraneous labyrinth is surrounded by a cartilaginous or bony capsule filled with perilymphatic fluid and suspensory connective tissue acting as shock absorbers. The chemical composition of the perilymph is very similar to that of cerebrospinal fluid or haemolymph. The sensory nerves leave this capsule through foramina. Loss of perilymph is prevented in some cases by a jelly-like packing surrounding the nerve distal to the foramen. In vertebrates with a bony skull the labyrinth is enclosed in a bony labyrinth capsule replicating the general shape of the labyrinth, especially that of the semicircular canals. Bony tubes filled with perilymph surround the membraneous endolymph-filled canals.

Figure 1 shows the general appearance of the membraneous labyrinths in cyclostomes and fishes. The labyrinth consists of a membraneous sac filled with endolymph. This fluid has a completely different composition from other body fluids, which is regulated by complex mechanisms associated with glandular tissues forming part of the labyrinthine wall (see DOHLMAN, C.III.). It probably plays an important role in stimulus transduction.

The canals and their ampullae and the various recesses containing the otolith-bearing maculae are moulded from the initial spherical labyrinth vesicle. The semicircular canals are curved membraneous tubes continuous with the general labyrinth cavity at both ends. At one end, each canal widens into a near-spherical

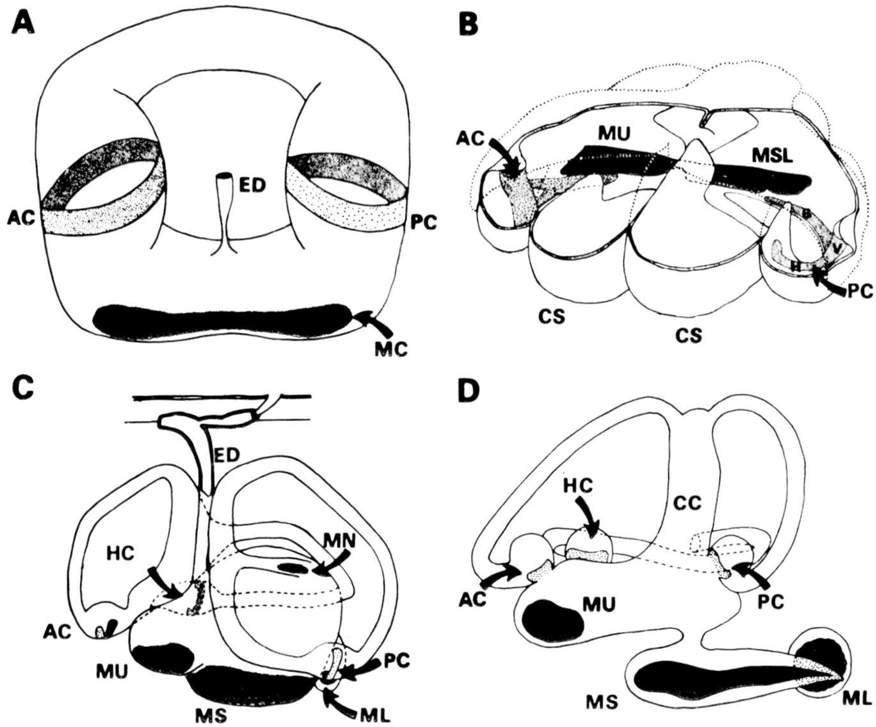

Fig. 1. The four chief morphological types of labyrinth in the agnathous and gnathostome fishes. A. Myxine; B. Lampetra; C. Elasmobranch; D. Cyprinoid. *AC* anterior crista; *B* basal arm of crista; *CC* crus commune; CS ciliated sac; *ED* endolymphatic duct (omitted in B and D); *H* horizontal arm of crista; *HC* crista of horizontal canal; *MC* macula communis; *ML* macula lagenae; *MN* macula neglecta; *MS* macula sacculi; *MSL* macula sacculi and macula lagenae; *MU* macula utriculi; *PC* posterior crista; *V* vertical arm of crista. A. unpublished original; B. after LOWENSTEIN, OSBORNE and THORNHILL, 1968; C. after RETZIUS; D. after v. FRISCH, 1936

space or ampulla containing the sensory apparatus. This consists of a crest-like ridge in the wall of the ampulla, the crista ampullaris, which carries a sensory epithelium made up of sensory cells and supporting cells (see WERSÄLL, C.I.). The sensory cells are secondary sensory cells of epithelial origin. They are ciliated at the apical end. The ciliary processes project into the ampullary lumen where they do not float freely in the endolymph, but are ensheathed in a jelly-like cupula. This forms a flexible but elastic superstructure to the crista and extends right through the lumen of the ampulla to the opposite ampullary wall, making close and probably fluid-tight contact with it (Fig. 3). The existence and mode of function of the cupula in living animals were first demonstrated by STEINHAUSEN (1931) and DOHLMAN (1935). The endolymph and cupula constitute a coupled movable system within the canal and ampulla, and in fact within the whole labyrinthine space with which the semicircular canals are in open communication. Rotary acceleration of the head creates cupula-endolymph inertia movements and these in turn lead to mechanical deformation of the hair processes of the sensory cells. The mechanical changes are finally transduced into changes in the electrical activity of the dendritic processes of sensory neurons which make synaptic contact with the bases of the sensory cells (*vide infra*). The canals are thus designed to monitor angular accelerations of the head in space (see MAYNE, 3/2). Vector analysis of the directions of such rotations is achieved by the spatial dispositions of the canals.

III. The Semicircular Canals

Typically the vertebrate labyrinth has three semi-circular canals, whose planes are almost at right angles to each other. There are two so-called vertical canals, the canalis verticalis anterior and canalis verticalis posterior, and one horizontal or lateral one, the canalis horizontalis or externus. The cyclostome labyrinth does not have the horizontal canal, and its vertical canals are represented by their ampullae, the canal parts forming relatively wide recesses in the labyrinthine space, especially in the Myxinoids, in which the name canal seems hardly appropriate (LOWENSTEIN et al., 1968; LOWENSTEIN and THORNHILL, 1970). The

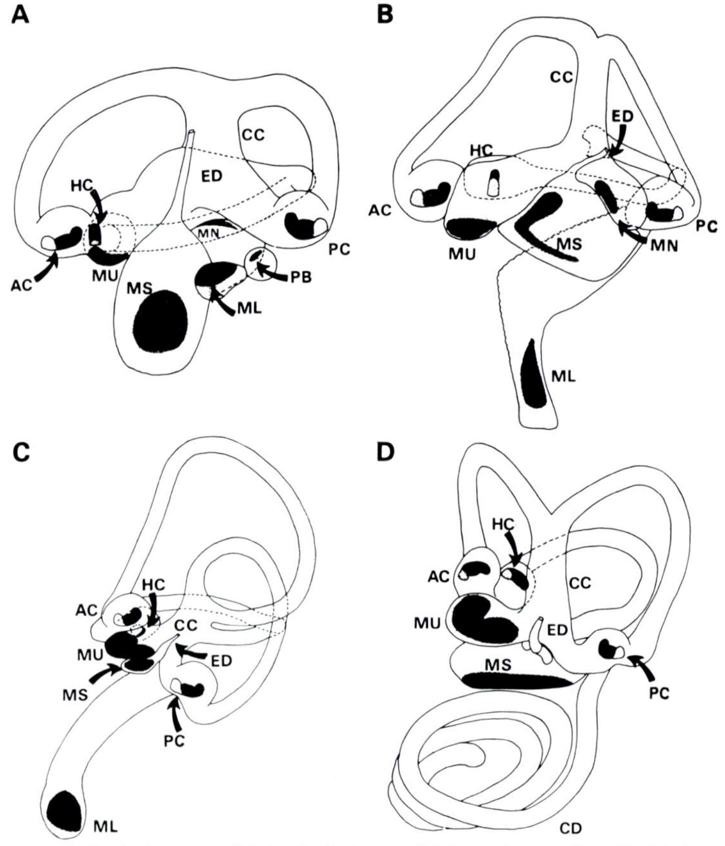

Fig. 2. Four morphological types of labyrinth in amphibians A; reptiles, B; birds, C; and mammals, D. Other symbols as in Fig. 1 (After RETZIUS, 1881)

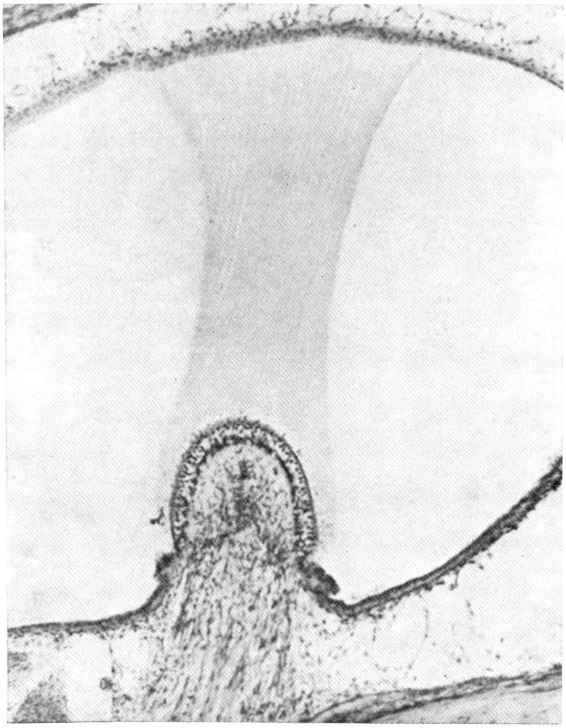

Fig. 3. Crista-cupula system of the horizontal semicircular canal of a squirrel monkey (From IGARASHI, 1966)

relative length, diameter and shape of the canals varies widely from species to species throughout the vertebrates (Fig. 2). The functional significance of these variations has not been minutely analyzed. It is, however, fairly safe to say that in free-swimming and flying animals and in animals with lively off the-ground activity the canals tend to be longer and of smaller diameter than in animals moving near the ground in relatively stable equilibrium. Generally the horizontal canal lies in a truly horizontal plane when the head of the animal is oriented in a position of active attention (GIRARD, 1930; DE BEER, 1947). This head posture is reflexly guaranteed by means of the gravitational responses based on otolith function.

IV. The Otolith Organs

Otolith organs are differential-density gravity sensors. A relatively specifically heavy mass of calcareous material lies anchored to and partially embedded in a jelly-like otolith "membrane" which in turn overlies a sensory epithelium, the so-called "macula statica". This is composed of sensory and supporting cells resembling those in the cristae of the canal ampullae. The hair processes of the sensory cells project into the otolith membrane and are mechanically deformed by displacement of the otolithic mass relative to the sensory epithelium. Such displacement occurs when the otolith organ changes its spatial disposition relative to the vertical as the head is tilted. The minute mechanism of stimulus transduction will be discussed later. There are typically three such otolith organs in the vertebrate labyrinth, the utriculus, the sacculus and the lagena, which are situated in the recessus utriculi, recessus sacculi, and recessus lagenae respectively.

The shape and consistency of otoliths varies throughout the vertebrates. In the majority of vertebrates the otoliths consist of conglomerates of crystals of calcium salts. A number of calcium salts are involved but the otoliths consist mainly of calcium carbonate (Carlström, 1963). The consistency of these conglomerates embedded in the ground substance of the otolith "membrane" is that of a stiff paste probably with a certain freedom of plastic flow (Figs. 4 and 5). However, in

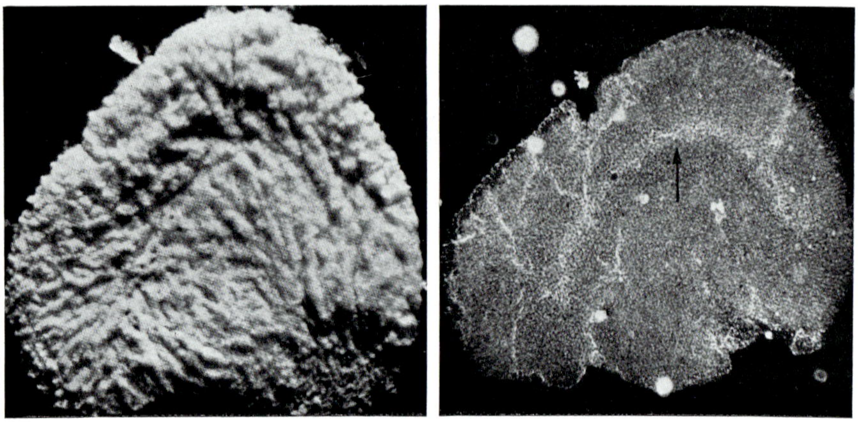

Fig. 4. Two photomicrographs of the same macula utriculi of the guinea pig with and without statoconia (From Engström, Lindeman and Ades, 1966)

the bony fishes the otoliths are solid objects of specific and constant shape. This shape is characteristic of the species, and the otoliths show growth in rings which can be used to determine the age of the fish. The utriculus otolith is called lapillus, that of the sacculus sagitta, and the otolith of the lagena is the asteriscus. In the cyprinoid minnow, for instance, the lapillus is almost spherical and the sagitta arrow-shaped with a fluted wing, while the astericus is a star-shaped disc with marginal flutings and a horseshoe-shaped ridge around the centre of the macula (Wohlfahrt, 1932) (Fig. 6). Mammals, with the exception of the monotremes, have only two otolith organs, utriculus and sacculus. The lagena, which in the Sauropsida has been displaced from the vestibular part of the labyrinth to the tip of the papilla basilaris or cochlea, has disappeared in the marsupials and eutherian mammals.

The maculae, like the semicircular canals, are arranged in different planes of space. The utriculus macula usually lies almost horizontally and the maculae of sacculus and lagena lie in two different, approximately vertical planes. It is therefore not surprising that different directional functions used to be attributed to the

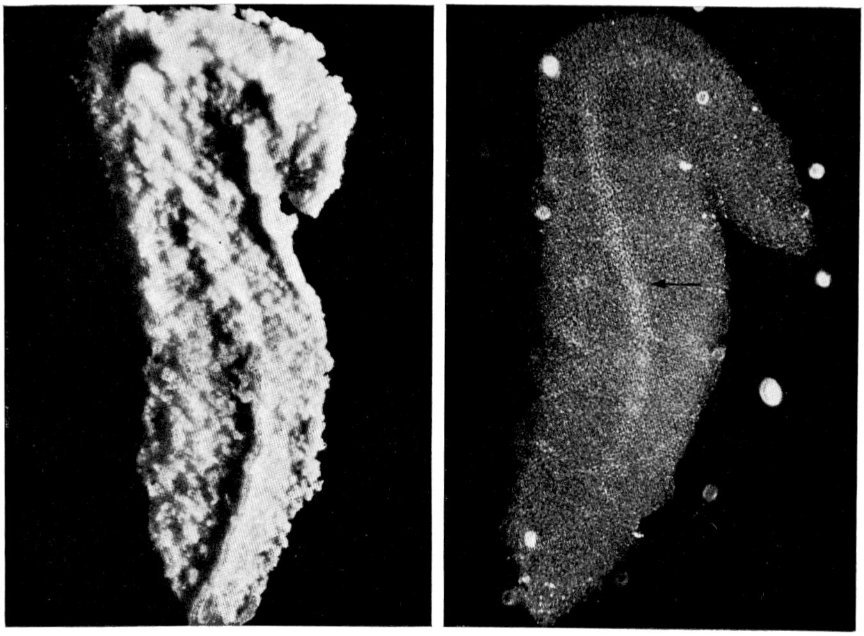

Fig. 5. Macula sacculi of the guinea pig. Right: the statoconia are in position over the macula surface. Left: the crystals have been removed from the macula and the figure shows the crystal layer only (From ENGSTRÖM, LINDEMAN and ADES, 1966)

three otolith organs (MAGNUS, 1924). As will be seen below, this analogy proved to be somewhat misleading. A further end organ, the so-called macula neglecta, is found associated with the median wall of the utriculus recess. It is not covered by an otolith and was called the crista quarta by some early investigators (EWALD, 1892).

V. General Survey of Range of Functions

The labyrinth has four main functions. It is an organ concerned with the maintenance and regulation of the tonus of the body musculature, including muscles not concerned with posture and locomotion, such as those involved in mastication. It is a receptor for angular accelerations, a receptor for gravitational and other linear accelerations and, finally, a receptor for vibrations over a wide range of frequencies. This applies not only to animals in which a cochlea or corresponding appendage is associated with the labyrinth, but also to the lower vertebrates in which only the "vestibular" parts of the labyrinth, i.e. semicircular canals and otolith organs, are present.

As organs controlling posture and movement, the labyrinthine end organs elicit reflexes of trunk, neck, limb, and eyemuscles. The study of these and their localization in the various endorgans was the first step in the comparative physiology of the vertebrate labyrinth.

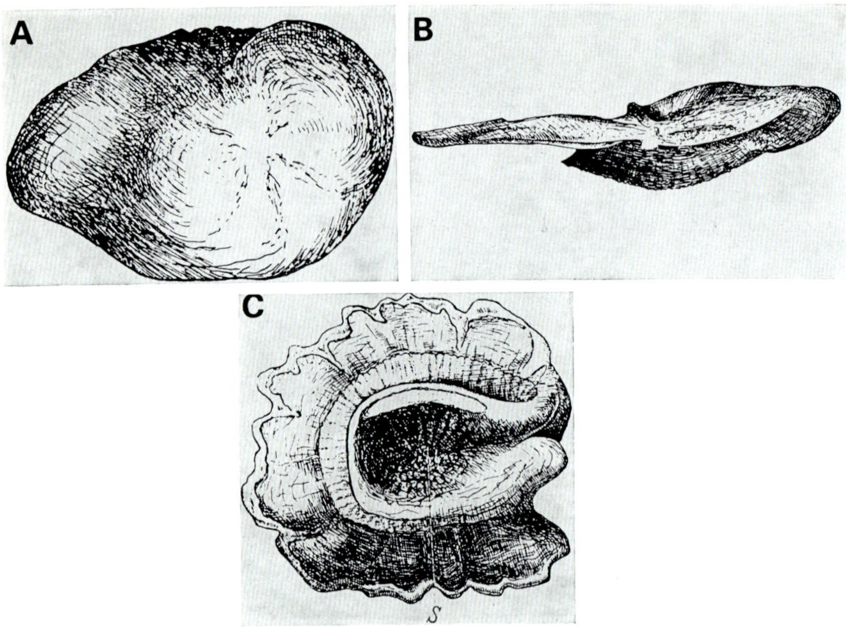

Fig. 6. The three otoliths in the labyrinth of the minnow (*Phoxinus laevis, L.*) *A* lapillus; *B sagitta*; *C* asteriscus (After WOHLFAHRT, 1932)

These studies, originating with the classic work of FLOURENS (1824), GOLTZ (1870), MACH (1875), CRUM-BROWN (1873/74), BREUER (1889, 1891) and EWALD (1892), were based on the results of two main experimental approaches, *viz.* analysis of the consequences of operative elimination of the labyrinth as a whole or in part, unilaterally or bilaterally, and study of the effects of mechanical, thermal, and electrical stimulation of the exposed organ. This has been thoroughly reviewed by MAXWELL (1923), MAGNUS (1924), FISCHER (1926), MAGNUS and DE KLEIJN (1926), GRAHE (1926), CAMIS and CREED (1930) and LOWENSTEIN (1936, 1950). Apart from a short summary, only the data which are still the focal points of present-day experimentation or theorizing will be mentioned here.

EWALD (1892) was the first to show the effect of operative elimination of parts of the labyrinth on muscle tonus, and in his theory of the "tonus labyrinth" he stressed the wide compass of tonic influence emanating from the labyrinth. This "stimulatory" function of the labyrinth (WOLSKY, 1933) is supplementary to that of control of postural reflexes, although in many cases these reflexes consist in an adjustment in the tonic state of effector muscles rather than rapid tetanic contractions. Postural reflexes are restorative, in cases of passive displacement of the head or body from their normal or zero position (compensatory reflexes), or contribute to intricate networks of servo-mechanisms controlling the postural changes of head, body, and limbs during active movement (see JONES, Chapter 7). These mechanisms function in close collaboration with sensory inputs from other receptor systems such as integumental, tactile, and pressure receptors, stretch receptors in muscles and tendons, and not least from the eyes.

Vision plays an important part in the control of posture and movement and it is therefore not surprising that the eye muscles rank high amongst the effectors jointly controlled by sensory inputs from the retina and the semicircular canals and otolith organs. Eye movements and eye postures are in fact the main indicators used by vestibular physiologists in the quantitative study of functional parameters.

Eye nystagmus consists of a slow compensatory deviation and a jerk-like return to the central resting position of the eye, and takes place roughly in the spatial plane in which the head is subjected to angular acceleration. This involves all six extrinsic eye muscles, the appropriate pair carrying out the nystagmic movement while the remaining four are responsible for adjusting the position of the eyeball in the orbit in accordance with the spatial orientation of the head. In animals with little capacity for conjugated eye movements, such as the amphibians, reptiles, and birds, the whole head shows nystagmic responses to angular accelerations executed by the neck muscles.

The gravitational responses of the eyes consist of lasting deviations of the eyeballs from their normal position in the orbit. The eyeball either deviates upwards and downwards or carries out a conjugated counter-rolling movement about the axis running through the centre of the pupil. Under certain circumstances positional nystagmus of the eyes is observed in the stationary head. Together with the per-rotatory nystagmus the postural eye deviations ensure that the field of vision existing before the passive or active postural change is preserved unaltered until the extent of the movement makes this impossible.

During active movement and in prolonged "voluntary" deviation from the normal resting position of the head in space the compensatory responses of eyes, neck, and limbs can of course be modified or entirely overruled by other servo-mechanisms. If this were not so it would be impossible for an animal to lie on its side without being automatically pulled-up by the labyrinthine righting reflexes in which compensatory responses of eye, neck and limb muscles all participate. A detailed account of vestibular reflexes is beyond the scope of this chapter. They have been mentioned because their observation before and after operative interference with the labyrinth was the only basis for the analysis of vestibular function before the advent of Adrian's oscillographic technique of impulse recording from sensory nerves made it possible to investigate the mode of functioning of the various end organs in the labyrinth directly (Adrian, 1947).

The data obtained by the neurophysiological approach are described below. Besides allowing the solution of a number of outstanding problems in vestibular physiology it posed a number of questions that were not answered until the electron microscope made it possible to study of the ultrastructure and innervation of the labyrinthine sensory cells.

VI. The Hair Cell and its Role in Mechano-Electric Transduction

The mechano-electric transducer element which is vital to all functional properties of vestibular end organs is the hair cell (see also Wersäll, C.I.) (Fig. 7). This type of sensory cell is found exclusively in vertebrate animals and has been

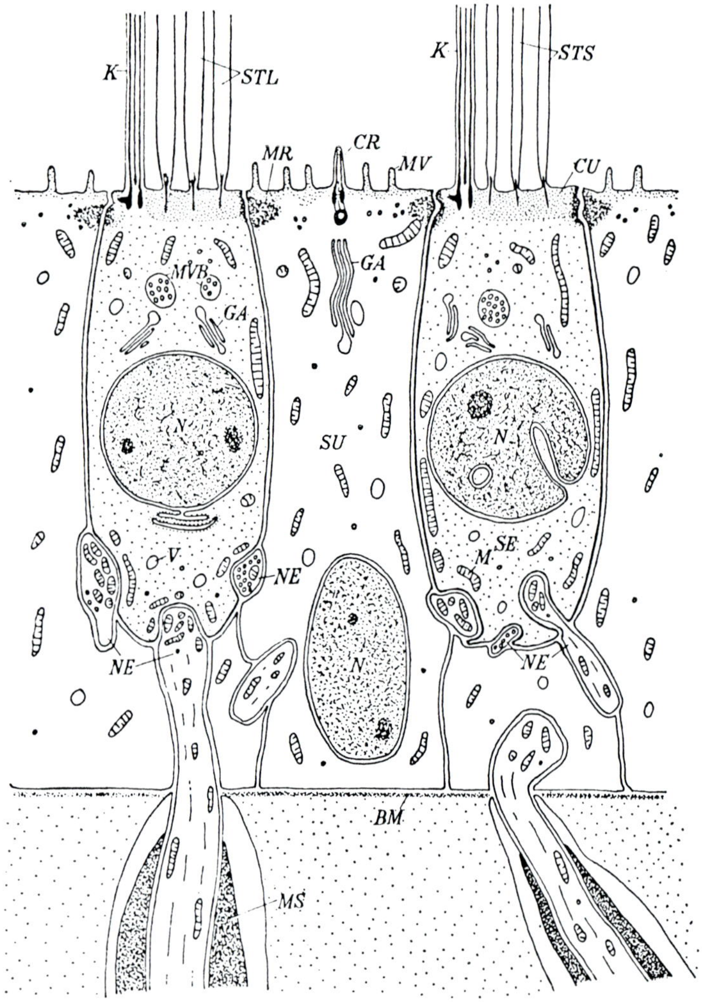

Fig. 7. Schematic drawing of the general structure of the sensory epithelia in the ray (*Raja clavata*). Two sensory cells are shown. One has a hair process composed of 'large'-and the other a hair process composed of 'small'-diameter stereocilia. Nerve endings make contact with the base of the sensory cells. The supporting cells bear numerous microvilli and a short ciliary rod on their free apical surfaces. *BM* basement membrane; *CR* ciliary rod; *CU* cuticle; *GA* Golgi apparatus; *K* kinocilium; *M* mitochondrion; *MS* myelin sheath; *MR* membrana reticularis; *MV* microvillus; *MVB* multivesicular body; *N* nucleus; *NE* nerve endings; *SE* sensory cell; *STL* 'large'L-diameter sterocilia; *STS* 'small'-diameter sterocilia; *SU* supporting cell; *V* vesicle (From Lowenstein, Osborne and Wersäll, 1964)

described as a secondary sensory cell of epithelial origin. It is usually described as ciliated. It is now known that only one of the apical processes, the so-called kinocilium, is morphologically a true cilium. All the other processes, the "stereocilia" are perhaps best described as villi. They are arranged in intersecting rows. The number varies but fields of more than 50 sterocilia are quite common. They are usually shorter than the kinocilium, their length decreasing with increasing distance from the kinocilium. Hair cells of this kind are found in all organs belonging to the acoustico-lateralis system, i.e. in the ear and in the lateral-line organs of fishes and aquatic amphibians. All the hair bundles are ensheathed either in jelly-like cupulae or in membranes of similar consistency. In these cases the hair bundles are lodged in cylindrical canals spaced out in the substance of the covering structures. In the case of the membrana tectoria of the mammalian cochlea the

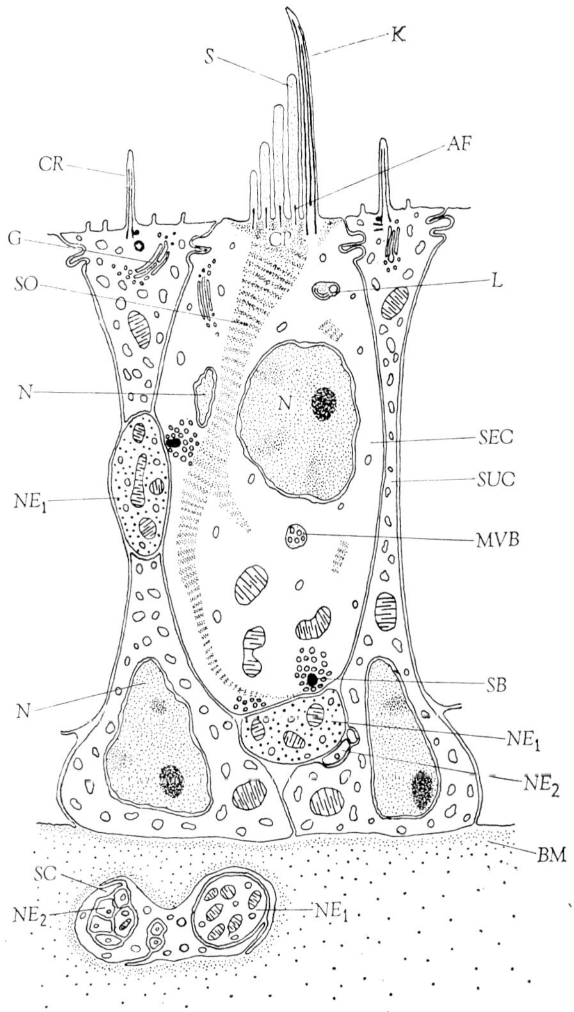

Fig. 8. Schematic drawing of a single sensory cell from a crista of the ammocoete labyrinth. Note the striated organelle which originates from the cuticular plate and runs to the base of the cell where it terminates in close proximity with a synapse. *AF* axial fibre; *BM* basement membrane; *CR* ciliary rod; *CP* cuticular plate; *G* golgi apparatus; *K* kinocilium; *L* lysosome; *MVB* multivesicular body; *N* nucleus; NE_1 large nerve endings; NE_2 small nerve endings *S* stereocilia; *SB* synaptic bar; *SC* Schwann cell; *SEC* sensory cell; *SO* striated organelle; *SUC* supporting cell (From LOWENSTEIN and OSBORNE, 1964)

hairs, which are all stereocilia, reach the membrane with their tips but do not penetrate. The kinocilium is represented by its basal body only in the hair cells of the cochlea. This must be taken into account when the role of the kinocilium in the mechano-electric transduction process is discussed.

The stereocilia are rooted by simple filamentous processes in what is known as the cuticular plate, an electron-dense part of the apical cytoplasm of the cell. The root of the kinocilium stands in a niche in this cuticular plate and does not seem to be in physical contact with it. The apical end of the hair cell must play a part in mechano-electric transduction; mechanical deformation of the hair processes is generally thought to be the first step in transduction. This immediately raises the question as to whether the deformation of the kinocilium or that of the stereocilia is the operative factor. There is a hypothesis that the kinocilium operates as a mobile cilium in reverse (GRAY and PUMPHREY, 1958) and that the active mechanical deformation of a motile cilium is initiated by an electric event at the basal structure. Conversely, passive deformation of the kinocilium of the hair cell could be thought to give rise to an electric charge in the cytoplasm surrounding the basal body of the organelle, which might in turn set the modulation of the activity of the cell in motion as described below. This presupposes a pathway between the kinocilial root or its immediate cytoplasmic environment and the cell membrane involved in the formation of the synaptic sites near the base of the cell (see WERSÄLL, C.I.). In the cyclostome 'fish', the lamprey, the soma of the hair cell contains an intriguing structure; the cuticular plate gives rise to a "striated organelle" with an average periodicity of 130 μm (Figure 8). This electron-dense structure extends towards the base of the cell, passing the nucleus and ending near the cell wall, often but not always near synaptic sites (LOWENSTEIN et al., 1968). A search for similar structures in other vertebrates has so far not been successful. It has not been reported in the hair cells of the lateral line and does not appear to be present in hair cells of *Myxine* (LOWENSTEIN and THORNHILL, 1970). A similar structure has been found in diseased hair cells of the human macula utriculi (FRIEDMAN et al., 1965) and in hair cells of rats (OSBORNE, pers. comm.). If this structure were more common it would be tempting to assign to it the role of a pathway of excitation from the top to the bottom of the sensory cell.

The possibility that the stereocilia act as part of the transducer system cannot be ruled out. They form a bulky projection of the cytoplasm into or towards the covering structures (cupulae, otolith membranes, membrana tectoria), and are surrounded by cell membranes continuous with that of the hair-cell soma. Thus their surface area is 20 times that of the rest of the cell (DOHLMAN, 1960; TRINCKER, 1965). The stereocilia are very probably coated with a layer of mucopolysaccharide (a hyalouronate of potassium) intervening between their surface and the wall of the cylindrical tubes spaced out in the cupula and otolith membrane. There has been some speculation on the possible part played by displacement potentials generated by the mechanical deformation of such a mucopolysaccharide. This may rest on the possibility that such potentials might directly affect the resting potentials of the hair cell membrane (CHRISTIANSEN, 1964; TRINCKER, 1965). Even if this controversial point is disregarded, the fact remains that the mass of stereocilia firmly anchored in the cuticular plate might propagate a mechanical effect from cupula to cytoplasm, e.g. that tilting or twisting of the cuticular plate could affect the cytoplasm directly or via the basal body of the kinocilium. If this were so, the absence of the kinocilium in the hair cells of the cochlea would be of no functional consequence. The significance of the stereocilia might also lie in their possible contribution to the restoring force which brings the cupula back to its normal position after deviations. TRINCKER (1965) reports that the hair bundles carry an electrostatic surface charge of up to 80 mv and believes that this is instrumental in spacing the hair processes and thus giving them rigidity and resilience. If this is true, the stereocilia are an integral and important component of the mechanical system.

At least in mammals, the potassium concentration in the endolymph is the same as that in the interior of the hair cell. TRINCKER argues that the apical surface of the hair cell can thus hardly be involved in a transduction mechanism based upon a potassium battery. The fact that the hair bundle carries an electrostatic charge points accordingly to its non-impermeability and to condenser-like behaviour which may by associated with microphonics obtained from semicircular canals up to a frequency of mechanical charge of 120 kHz.

The high potassium concentration in the endolymph may play a part in the control of the gelatinous mechanical properties of the cupula jelly with its high content of acid mucopolysaccharide. It should not be overlooked, however, that the potassium concentration in the endolymph is not equally high in all vertebrates (MURRAY and POTTS, 1961) and that generalizations based on the concentration in mammals may be dangerous. The chemical composition of the endolymph is of fundamental importance to the function of the system (Tables 1 and 2). It will be dealt with in a different context elsewhere (DOHLMAN, C.5.).

Table 1.

	Content (meq/liter) Perilymph	Endolymph (Utriculus)	Authors
Potassium			
Guinea pig	4,8	144,4	SMITH, LOWRY and WU (1954)
	5,0	142,0	CITRON, EXLEY and HALLPIKE (1956)
Man	7–8	140–160	RAUCH and KÖSTLIN (1958)
Sodium			
Guinea pig	150,3	15,8	SMITH, LOWRY and WU (1954)
	148	26	CITRON, EXLEY and HALLPIKE (1956)
Man	135–150	13–16	RAUCH and KÖSTLIN (1958)
Chloride			
Guinea pig	121,5	107,1	SMITH, LOWRY and WU (1954)
	120	110	CITRON, EXLEY and HALLPIKE (1956)
Man	135	120–130	RAUCH and KÖSTLIN (1958)

After TRINCKER (1965).

Table 2. *Concentrations of sodium, potassium chloride and urea in mM/kg in the perilymph, endolymph and Lorenzini jelly of Raja clavata*

	Na	K	Cl	Urea
Perilymph	281	3.54	321	447
Endolymph	295	63.4	391	381
Lorenzini jelly	443	12.5	581	74.8

From MURRAY and POTTS (1961).

Synaptic Structures

The nature of the link-up between hair cell and the associated nerve endings deserves comment from a functional point of view. The fact that the hair cell soma contains synaptic structures typical for chemical transmission from the hair cell to the dendritic ending of the terminal branches of the eighth nerve raises its status from that of a simple ciliated epithelial cell to that of a true neuronal element. The vesicles associated with the cytoplasm in these synapses very probably contain a neurotransmitter whose nature is not yet known. The presence of synaptic endings filled with vesicles at the base of a type II hair cell (and outside the calix of the type I hair cell of higher vertebrates) strongly suggests that the hair cell is under efferent control (see GACEK, C.IV.). It is not yet known whether or not close-junction electric synapses are also associated with the hair cell (SPOENDLIN, 1965).

Functionally, all this means that the hair cell, the most peripheral element in this mechanoreceptive system, may be deeply involved in the processing of the information received at the input end.

VII. The Resting Discharge

A low-frequency resting discharge has consistently been reported ever since the first successful recording of the electrical activity of the lateralis system (HOAGLAND, 1933a, b, c, d; SAND, 1937) and of the labyrinth (ROSS, 1936; LOWENSTEIN and SAND, 1936). HOAGLAND and ROSS failed to assign a functional role to this "spontaneous" activity, describing it either as "noise" or as an artefact caused by operative interference with the system. The functional significance of this resting discharge became clear, however, during an analysis of the responses of the semicircular canals of the dogfish by LOWENSTEIN and SAND (1936). The main point of this analysis was to find out of whether a semicircular canal responds to and provides information to the central nervous system on rotational stimuli in one direction only (MCNALLY and TAIT, 1932; LOWENSTEIN, 1936) or in two opposite directions (EWALD, 1892, and other authors, especially those working on mammals). LOWENSTEIN and SAND (1940b) found that in a considerable proportion of the single-unit preparations the unit showed a low-frequency resting discharge. This discharge was often astonishingly regular — much more regular than that recorded from nerves of the lateralis system; the frequency was increased by angular acceleration of the canal in one direction and decreased or abolished by acceleration in the opposite direction. In the right horizontal canal rotated in its own plane, acceleration to the right (ipsilateral acceleration) increased, acceleration to the left (contralateral acceleration) decreased the impulse frequency. As a unit of the left horizontal canal simultaneously increases its activity on acceleration to the left and decreases it on acceleration to the right, the central nervous system receives oppositely changing signals from the two sides (Fig. 9). These results were confirmed by LEDOUX (1947) in electrophysiological experiments on the frog. If the signals are relayed to antagonistic effector muscles such as the rectus externus and internus of the left eye, the compensatory phase of the eye response to horizontal rotation to the left will be achieved by an increase in tonus in the rectus internus under the influence of the increased discharge activity of the

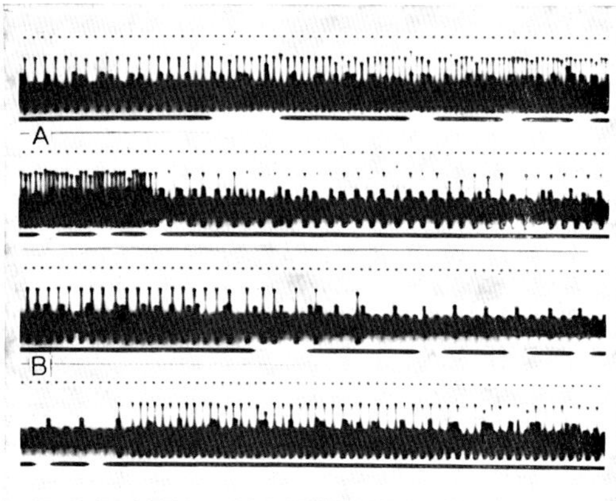

Fig. 9. Oscillograph records from the nerve branch to the left horizontal ampulla of the ray (*Raja clavata*) showing the response of a single unit to angular acceleration to the left (A) and to the right (B). The lower strip of each pair is the continuation of the upper. Time in 0.05 sec is marked at the top of the record, and the acceleration is recorded by the signal line at the bottom. Successive gaps in the line mark the revolution of the turntable. The acceleration in record A is 15° per sec^2; in record B, 20° per sec^2 (From LOWENSTEIN and SAND, 1940b)

left horizontal canal and a simultaneous relaxation of the rectus externus governed by the decrease in tonic influx from the right horizontal canal. Of course, it can be argued that the coordination of the activity of a pair of antagonistic muscles need not be controlled jointly by two antagonistic peripheral receptors. An intrinsic Sherringtonian mechanism would do equally well, as was shown by experiments on the pike (*Esox lucius*) in which LOWENSTEIN (1937) severed the nerve to the horizontal ampulla on one side. This operation leaves the fish with a permanent tonic deviation of the eyes towards the treated side (as if it were rotated towards the intact side). This asymmetry is obviously due to the asymmetric influx of resting discharge from the intact semicircular canal; it acts only on the rectus externus of the eye on the treated side and on the rectus internus of the eye on the intact side. The antagonists follow suit in a Sherringtonian manner. The experiment is instructive, showing clearly that the resting discharge is a source of vestibular tonus. This, then, is its primary function.

If a fish is subjected to angular acceleration in the plane of the horizontal canals after this operation, compensatory eye movements and nystagmus are superimposed on the basic eye deviation. Responses are shown both to ipsi- and to contralateral acceleration with respect to the intact semicircular canal, and owing to the existence of the lasting eye deviation, the contralateral eye response elicited by the diminution of the discharge activity in the intact canal is the more clearly observable of the two but does not take the form of a full nystagmus. This demonstrates the second function of the resting discharge. It makes the semicircular canal a bidirectional receptor by allowing upwards and downwards modulation of the basic activity by oppositely directed stimuli. The above results of unilateral canal elimination show clearly that the central nervous system does in fact utilize both directional types of information.

Of course, this is not necessarily so in all vertebrate classes. McNALLY and TAIT performed an extensive series of experiments on frogs and claimed emphatically that the semicircular canals are unidirectional (McNALLY and TAIT, 1925). Similarly, TENDELENBURG and KÜHN (1908) found that labyrinthine responses to rotation in reptiles were unidirectional, i.e. to rotation towards the side of the intact labyrinth only. In contrast to this, GRIBENSKI (1963) showed that after unilateral elimination of a horizontal semicircular canal by nerve sectioning and central compensation of the consequent tonus asymmetry, there were reflex responses to horizontal rotations to both the intact and the operated side. GRIBENSKI attributes this result to a fundamental bi-directionality of the amphibian semicircular canal. On the other hand, bidirectionality has consistently been reported in fishes, birds, and mammals, although there is a significant degree of ipsilateral preponderance (BREUER, 1889; EWALD, 1892). Indeed there are claims of equal sensitivity to rotation in opposite directions in man (HALLPIKE, 1960), but this may be due to the mode of the central utilization of peripheral signals, as suggested by the fact that the overall voltage influx on upward and downward modulation of the resting activity is likely to be unequal; increase in discharge activity from a moderate resting frequency is unlimited, in contrast to its inhibition to the point of total abolition.

The parameter of input used by the central nervous system is obviously of crucial importance. An increase of the discharge rate in a semicircular canal unit from 10 impulses/sec to 50 impulses/sec on ipsilateral acceleration can only correspond to a maximum decrease of 10 impulses/sec in the discharge rate on contralateral acceleration of the same intensity. Unfortunately, we do not know the calculus used by the 2nd or 3rd order neurons. Nevertheless the possibility has to be envisaged that in squatting animals, for example, the unilateral preponderance of responses to oppositely directed canal stimulations may be maximal or complete.

The Hair-Cell Map

Returning to the hair cell, we can now ask how the bidirectionality of the semicircular canal is based on a similar bidirectionality of the sensory cell. For purely heuristic reasons we can assume that the kinocilium is the first level in the transduction process. In free-living ciliated animals and in ciliary epithelia the stroke of the cilium is usually directionally polarized. The working stroke takes place in a plane perpendicular to the plane of the two central filaments in the (9+2) arrangement. Moreover, one of the peripheral filaments has a basal excrescence, the so-called basal foot (LOWENSTEIN et al., 1964). In mobile cilia this electron-dense structure lies in the plane of the working stroke and points in its direction (GIBBONS, 1961).

If we accept the electrophysiological findings on the mode of functioning of the horizontal canal as our starting point, we note that cupula-endolymph action in one direction increases and in the opposite direction decreases the frequency of the resting discharge. Let us assume that in a single-unit preparation we have in fact one hair cell only under observation. It would be interesting to know how this cell is oriented on the crista ampullaris with reference to the direction of the cupula-endolymph action. We know that ipsilateral angular acceleration is

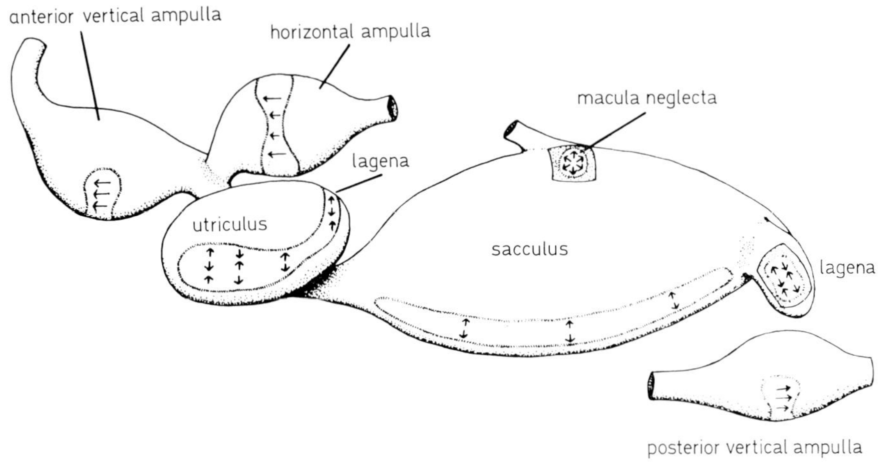

Fig. 10. Diagram of the polarity of sensory hair bundles found in the cristae and maculae of the left labyrinth of the ray (*Raja clavata*). Part of the dorsal wall of the sacculus above the macula neglecta and of the posterior wall of the lagena have been cut away to show their two sensory areas. In this schematic rendering of the sensory hairs the orientation of the hair bundle is symbolized by an arrow, the arrow-head indicating the position of the kinocilium (After LOWENSTEIN, OSBORNE and WERSÄLL, 1964)

excitatory. From the data of STEINHAUSEN (1931) and DOHLMAN (1936) on cupula movements during rotatory stimulation of the horizontal semicircular canal, we know that ipsilateral acceleration causes the cupula to move away from the canal towards the ampullo-utricular opening (utriculo-petal cupula movement). And that conversely, contralateral acceleration leads to utriculo-fugal cupula deflexion. Ultrastructural mapping of the hair cells and their orientation on the crista has shown that all hair cells point in the same direction. Figures 10 and 11 show that their kinocilia are on the side of the hair bundle facing the utriculus and that the basal feet of all kinocilia point towards the utriculus and away from the canal end of the ampulla. It seems reasonable to assume that this uniform arrangement of the kinocilia is functionally significant, and that deflexion of the kinocilium towards the utriculus initiates the excitatory increase in the discharge rate in an ampullary nerve fibre and deflexion away from the utriculus leads to a decrease in or complete inhibition of the impulse discharge. The observed behaviour of the freely beating cilium adds credence to our conclusions. Equating the working stroke of the mobile cilium with an excitatory and its oppositely directed recovery stroke with an inhibitory state, we postulate that the captive kinocilium has a corresponding functional polarization. Deflexion of the whole hair bundle in the plane of and towards the basal foot leads to an increase, deflexion in the opposite direction to a decrease or abolition of impulse activity in the associated afferent nerve. Experiments on the lateral-line organs have confirmed that experimentally imposed deflexion of the hair bundle in the direction of the basal foot of the kinocilium is excitatory and deflexion away from it inhibitory (GÖRNER, 1963; FLOCK, 1967).

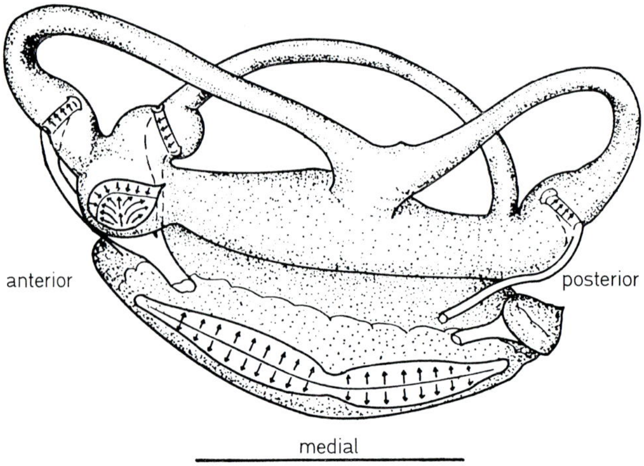

Fig. 11. Schematic drawing of the fish labyrinth (*Lota vulgaris*) illustrating the orientation of the sensory cells in the sensory areas with regards to the kinocilia in the hair bundles. The arrow-head denotes the position of the kinocilium (From Wersäll, Gleisner and Lundquist, 1967)

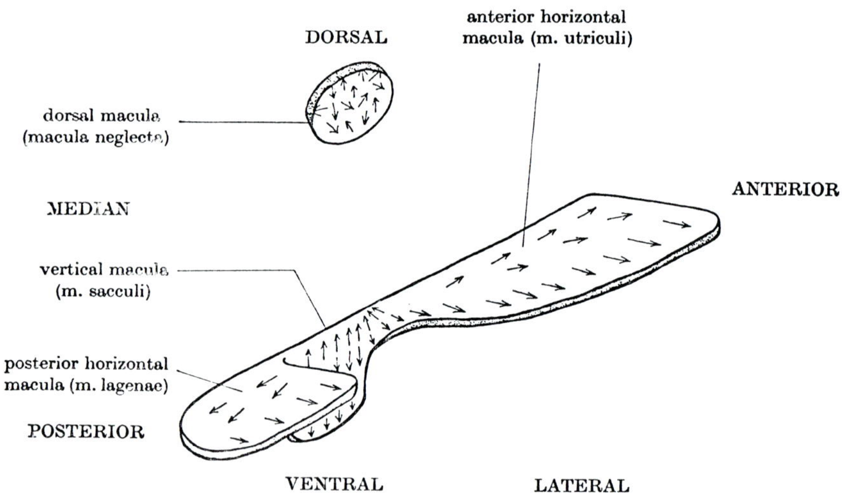

Fig. 12. Diagram to illustrate the general orientation of the sensory cells of the maculae of the right labyrinth of the lamprey (*Lampetra vulgaris*) as seen from dorso-laterally and posterior to the lagena (From Lowenstein, Osborne and Thornhill, 1968)

The vertical canals offer an interesting test case. It has long been known that angular acceleration in or near the plane of a vertical canal leads to effector responses which suggest that in this situation utriculo-fugal deflexion of the cupula is the preponderant stimulus. This was borne out by the electrophysiological analysis of the impulse discharge both in elasmobranch fishes (Lowenstein and Sand, 1940a) and in the frog (Ledoux, 1949). If our hypothesis concerning the functional significance of the polarization and topographic arrangement of the hair cells

Response of canals to	Reaction of right eye	*Contracting* muscle, mainly responsible for reaction
A. Tilting right 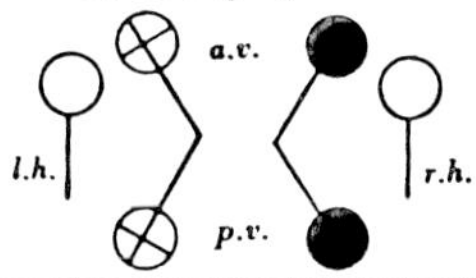	Vertical deviation upwards	Superior rectus
B. Tilting left 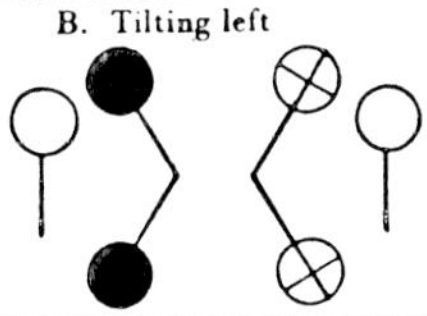	Vertical deviation downwards	Inferior rectus
C. Tilting forwards 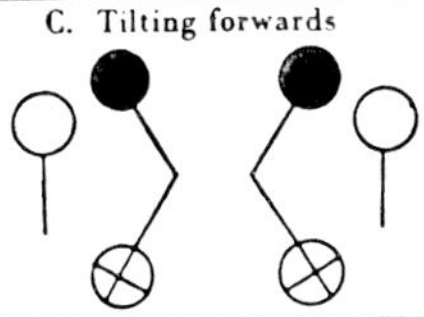	Rolling upwards	Inferior obliquus
D. Tilting backwards 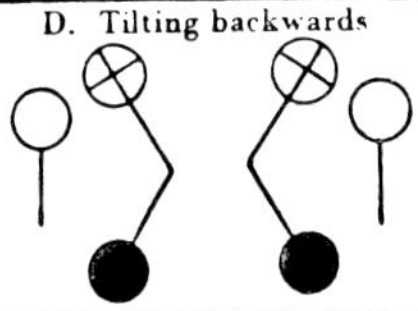	Rolling downwards	Superior obliquus
E. Clockwise rotation 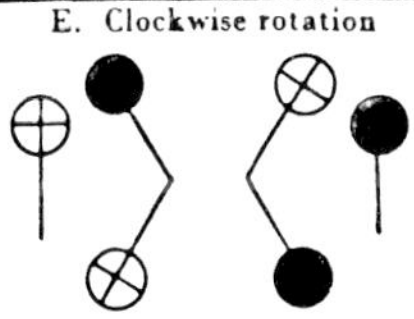	Horizontal deviation forwards	Internal rectus

F. Correlation between excitation of the vertical canals and contraction of the superior and inferior recti and obliqui

Inferior rectus
Inferior obliquus

Superior rectus
Inferior obliquus

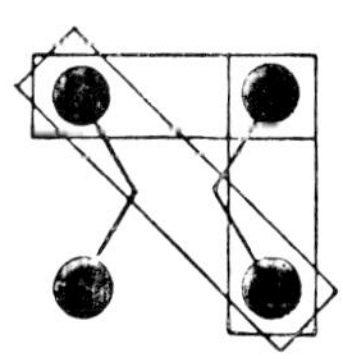

Inferior rectus
Superior obliquus

Superior rectus
Superior obliquus

Fig. 13. Correlation between the responses of the six semicircular canals to angular acceleration and the ensuing reflex contractions of the six eye muscles. Solid circles: excited; crossed circles: inhibited; open circles: unaffected; *a.v.* anterior vertical canals; *p.v.* posterior vertical canals; *l.h.* left horizontal canal; *r.h.* right horizontal canal (From LOWENSTEIN and SAND, 1940a)

on the canal crista is correct, the hair cells in the vertical canal ampullae should point towards the canal and away from the utriculus or vestibular cavity. This is in fact the case (LOWENSTEIN et al., 1964). GROEN (1960) has proposed a simple embryological explanation for this apparent oppositeness in hair-cell arrangement.

Figures 10 and 11 show that the hair cells in the horizontal and those in the anterior vertical canal point in the same direction, as if the two cristae developed from a common anlage. The fact that the two cristae come to lie at opposite sides of the utricular opening makes excitatory utriculo-petal cupula-endolymph action dependent on ampulla-leading movement in the case of the vertical canal and on ampulla-trailing movement in the case of the horizontal canal.

The statement that semicircular canals respond preponderantly to accelerations taking place in their own plane is approximately true for the horizontal canal only in the elasmobranch labyrinth (Lowenstein and Sand, 1940a). Its latitude ranges about 15–20° on either side of its plane. Beyond this the threshold of response rises steeply. The vertical canals have a considerably wider latitude in the dogfish, *Scylliorhinus canicula*. They respond with a raised threshold to rotation in a plane perpendicular to their own. Thus the anterior vertical canal of the dogfish responds well to angular acceleration in a horizontal plane when the head of the animal is in a normal position. The response is characterized by increased activity on contralateral acceleration and inhibition of activity on ipsilateral acceleration, which is the reverse of the response of the homolateral horizontal canal. In the same circumstances, the posterior vertical canal yields an increase in activity on ipsilateral and inhibition on contralateral acceleration, i.e. a discharge picture identical with that of the homolateral horizontal canal except for the raised threshold. It is interesting that these out-of-plane responses of the vertical canals are much less pronounced in *Raja clavata* (unpublished observation). It is therefore not permissible to generalize from the situation in the dogfish. However, Lowenstein and Sand (1940a) attempted to correlate the responses of all six semicircular canals on horizontal rotation and refer them to the known responses of the six eye muscles normally associated with the activity of these canals. They found that during horizontal acceleration the activity of the horizontal canals leads to antagonistic behaviour of the horizontal eye muscles, while the simultaneous responses of the vertical canals results in a simultaneous rise in tonus in both vertical and both oblique eye muscles (Fig. 13). One might be tempted to speculate that such synergic behaviour could provide a fixed pivot for the eyeball during its horizontal nystagmic activity. Lorente de Nó (1931) took kymographic recordings of the simultaneous activity of all six eye muscles of the rabbit during horizontal rotation and found exactly this type of synergic behaviour in the vertical and oblique muscles.

VIII. Labyrinths without Horizontal Canals

This is perhaps an appropriate point to introduce the question of the absent horizontal canal in the cyclostomes *Myxine* and *Lampetra* or *Petromyzon*.

As can be seen from Fig. 1, the cyclostome labyrinths contain two ampullae joined by a wide endolymph-filled space in *Myxine* and by two limbs of "semicircular canal" with a relatively large diameter in *Lampetra*. The two ampullae are considered to be homologues of the ampullae of the anterior and posterior vertical canals of gnathostome vertebrates (Lowenstein et al., 1968). There is no trace of the horizontal canal or its ampulla. Observation of the swimming behaviour of these animals reveals that their movements in the horizontal plane are well controlled in a manner normal for a fish of their body shape, even though optical orientation is either absent (*Myxine*) or indifferent (*Lampetra*). Passive angular acceleration in the horizontal or yawing plane elicits typical low-threshold impulse responses against the background of resting activity (LOWENSTEIN, 1970a). The responses are localized in the two "vertical" ampullae. The anterior ampulla reacts to contralateral acceleration with an increase in the discharge rate, and the posterior ampulla reacts in this way to ipsilateral acceleration; these are the "adventitious responses" observed in the vertical ampullae of the dogfish (LOWENSTEIN and SAND, 1940a). Besides responding in this manner to yawing movement, the two ampullae of the cyclostome labyrinth show the normal responses to head-up and head-down and lateral tilting movements, the anterior ampulla responding with an increased discharge rate to nose-down and side-down, the posterior to nose-up and side-down swings. LOWENSTEIN et al. (1968) found features accounting for all these responses in the ultrastructure, i.e. the shape and spatial disposition of the two trifid cristae and the topography of hair-cell orientation on them.

IX. Type of Unit Responses

We have so far based our argument on one type of canal response, i.e. the upward or downward modulation of the frequency of a resting discharge. This mode of behaviour is very commonly found in single-unit recording. But there are other types of unit behaviour in a population of hair cells. After isolation of a single spontaneously firing unit in the stationary preparation it is common to find that an excitatory swing not only increases the discharge frequency of this unit but also brings in responses from a number of additional units. These are spontaneously silent and are recruited into activity by angular acceleration. A third type of unit found quite frequently fires at a rather high rate (over 30 impulses per second) but in a way different from the high-frequency firing of an injured or dying nerve fibre. The activity of such units often either completely fails to respond to acceleration or responds exclusively to acceleration in the inhibitory direction by a lowering or abolition of impulse discharge.

It is questionable whether these response types arise from morphologically distinguishable types of sensory cell. We know there are two such cell types in the higher vertebrates, flask-shaped type I and cylindrical type II cells (WERSÄLL, C.I.). They do not only differ in shape but also in the mode of innervation. In the lower vertebrates, cells resembling type II only are found, but some dimorphism in the diameter of the stereocilia has been described in the elasmobranch labyrinth (LOWENSTEIN et al., 1964), and in the labyrinth of the lamprey two types of kinocilia are found in the hair cells in different parts of the labyrinth. Furthermore, the distribution of diameters of dendrites associated with hair cells has been found to be at least bimodal. HALLPIKE and HOOD (1953) drew attention to the existence of the so-called colossal fibres demonstrated by CAJAL (1909) and LORENTE DE NÓ (1926) side by side with fibres of smaller diameter in the cristae. The candelabra fibres described in the labyrinth of the lamprey (LOWENSTEIN et al., 1968) are colossal fibres innervating a number of hair cells and extending over a considerable area of the crista. Responses from this kind of fibre, which is a large composite functional unit, will obviously be different from those from fibres with a more restricted or even one-to-one type of rapport with the sensory cells.

The responses from a hair cell within any one crista are directionally uniform, and claims of units yielding excitatory responses to acceleration in two opposite directions and units yielding inhibitory responses to acceleration in both directions (GERNANDT, 1929) are not compatible with the uniform polarization of crista cells. The author has investigated many hundreds of single-unit preparations of the isolated elasmobranch labyrinth, and none has responded in a direction opposite to the bulk of the population of units (cf. ROSS, 1936). The findings of workers who have recorded from second- or third-order central nervous units and have observed two oppositely responding classes of response from units in the yawing plane (GERNANDT, 1949; ADRIAN, 1943; SCHOEN, 1957) can only be explained by central nervous convergence of responses from units situated either in the cristae of horizontal canals on opposite sides of the head or to units from the homolateral anterior vertical canals (see above). The information now available on the ultrastructure shows quite clearly that all hair cells on a crista point in the same direction. Sometimes the orientation of the hair cells becomes less strict right at the lower edge of the crista, but the number of cells involved is insignificant. The back-to-back or front-to-front arrangement of hair cells characteristic for the lateral line cristae or some of the otolith maculae is definitely absent in the cristae of the semicircular canals.

Let us now return to the above-mentioned three types of behaviour of canal units. The spontaneously silent type of unit which becomes recruited into activity during acceleration in the excitatory direction is often characterized by high-amplitude impulses and might therefore be imagined to stem from cells innervated by large-diameter nerve fibres. The possibility that some cells may be deployed in a specific area of the crista, e.g. along its central ridge can therefore not be excluded, but they would definitely conform with the general directionality of the crista in question.

There is a mechanism which could account for all three reaction types being exhibited by the same hair cell after a change in one or the other basic parameter of function. When a polarizing current is routed through the nerve twig of an isolated preparation of a horizontal semicircular canal of the elasmobranch labyrinth, the behaviour of a single unit can be modified by the direction and strength of the current (LOWENSTEIN, 1955). It is possible to select a unit with a moderately high resting discharge and to ascertain on turntable or torsion swing (GROEN et al., 1952) that its response to oppositely directed excitatory and inhibitory accelerations is symmetrical over a limited range of stimulus intensity. A unit of this kind can be thought of as lying on the straight part of an S-shaped characteristic (Fig. 14). If it were subjected to an ascending (excitatory) polarizing current the frequency of its impulse discharge would rise steeply, and after some adaptation settle down at a rate considerably higher than that of its original resting discharge. If this unit were then subjected to angular accelerations, the effects of galvanic polarization and acceleration would sum and, given a sufficient degree of polarization, the unit would behave like a unit with a high resting discharge which is little affected by excitatory acceleration but extremely sensitive to acceleration in the inhibitory direction. It might now be described as lying at the upper non-linear part of the characteristic curve. Conversely, if our unit were subjected to a descending (inhibitory) polarizing current its resting discharge would disappear, i.e. it would be silenced. If

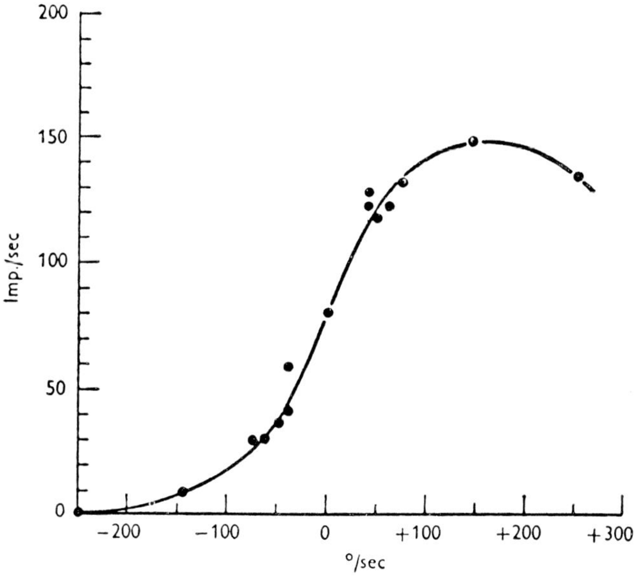

Fig. 14. Impulse responses from a three-unit preparation of the horizontal semicircular canal in the isolated surviving labyrinth of the ray (*Raja clavata*). "Characteristic" curve of response frequency plotted against "mechanical impulse" (Groen, Lowenstein and Vendrick, 1952)

tested on turntable or torsion swing its behaviour would now resemble that of a spontaneously silent unit with obvious responses only to excitatory acceleration.

It is therefore not unreasonable to suppose that the differences between the three types of unit found in a crista are different in "bias" and that such units are in fact intraconvertible. The factor controlling the bias may be the degree of basic membrane polarization in or near the synaptic sites of the hair cell, and may be imagined in the normal organ to be under the control of the efferent innervation. The interruption of the efferent supply in an isolated preparation could easily be responsible for the permanency of type characteristics in the behaviour of the units recorded from under these conditions. *In vivo* the whole population of hair cells might be under the influence of continuous efferent adjustment correlated with the requirements of the moment.

X. Mechanical Analysis

The mechanical analysis of the parameters involved in the mode of functioning of semicircular canals is dealt with elsewhere (Mayne, G.I.; Jones, C.II.). It might be useful to recall the contribution made in this field by experimenters on the peripheral organ itself. On the basis of direct observation of the behaviour of the cupula, Steinhausen (1931) described the cupula-endolymph system as an over-critically damped torsion pendulum. The cupula of the pike labyrinth takes at least 20 sec to return to its resting position after maximal deviation under the impact of a mechanical "impulse". Steinhausen's work led to the description of the behaviour of the cupula-endolymph system in terms of a differential equation, the constants of which have been the object of extensive experimentation in a number of laboratories (MAYNE, G.I.). GROEN et al. (1952) contributed to our knowledge on this subject by determining the constants in experiments on the isolated surviving labyrinth of the elasmobranch fish *Raja clavata*. This preparation is suitable for the determination of constants in an open-loop situation, i.e. uninfluenced by feedback regulation derived from the central nervous system. On the other hand it must be kept in mind that the preparation's suitability for quantitative evaluation is limited by at least two circumstances. Firstly, the interruption of the blood supply may in due course induce changes in the physical and chemical make-up of endolymph and cupula, affecting the viscosity and elastic properties of the system. Secondly, the fact that access to the ampullary nerves is gained through an opening in the perilymphatic space may lead to distortion of the response picture, especially in responses to relatively high-intensity mechanical impulses.

A torsion swing was used to determine the phase shift between the mechanogram of the swing and the plotted course of change in impulse frequency from single-unit preparations direct from the responses of single- or even multifibre preparations in suitable cases after integration by means of a counting-rate meter. A phase shift of 90° reveals the natural frequency of the system. With swing frequencies much higher or much lower than the natural frequency of the cupula-endolymph system, significant deviations from the 90° phase shift were measured, allowing assessment of the average value of the quotient of the cupula-restoring couple at unit angle over the moment of inertia of the endolymph ($\frac{\Delta}{\Theta}$).

When a number of correction factors were taken into account $\frac{\Delta}{\Theta} = 1.0\ \mathrm{sec}^{-2}$ appeared a justifiable value. The second constant is represented by the quotient of the moment of friction at unit angular velocity (π) over Θ the moment of inertia of the endolymph. The average value of $\frac{\pi}{\Theta}$ was found to be $36\ \mathrm{sec}^{-1}$.

In a second series of experiments, the preparation was mounted on a turntable and subjected to a range of intensities of "mechanical impulse" by sudden breaking of prolonged rotations covering a range of constant velocities both in the excitatory and in the inhibitory direction. In response to the mechanical impulse the discharge frequency of the preparation shown during constant velocity rotation (basic discharge frequency) was instantaneously increased or decreased and then returned gradually to the basic level. This gradual return yielded so-called decay curves in which the logarithm of the difference of the discharge frequency from the basic frequency was plotted against time. These curves were found to be straight over a considerable range and their slope was used in calculation of the quotient $\frac{\pi}{\Theta}$. The average of the values obtained in this way fell well within the corresponding average values for $\frac{\pi}{\Theta}$ obtained in the experiments on the torsion swing.

A theoretical calculation of $\frac{\pi}{\Theta}$ based on a measured value of 0.68 mm for the diameter of the horizontal semicircular canal and on an assumed value of 1.0 g cm^{-3} for the density of the endolymph and 0.010 c.g.s. units for its viscosity yielded a value of 35 sec^{-1}. This tallies well with the value of 36 sec^{-1} obtained in the torsion swing experiments and encouraged the authors to propose $\ddot{\zeta} + 35\dot{\zeta} + \zeta = 0$ as a differential equation describing the behaviour of an average cupula-endolymph system in the horizontal canal of the elasmobranch labyrinth in the experimental conditions outlined above. How this equation compares with similar equations proposed for the human labyrinth on the basis of nystagmographic measurements and subjective data is fully discussed in the article by MAYNE (G.I.). It may suffice here to say that v. EGMOND et al. (1949) computed values of 10 and 1 respectively for $\frac{\pi}{\Theta}$ and $\frac{\Delta}{\Theta}$ (L and P) in MAYNE's terminology, whereas NIVEN and HIXON (1961) arrived at an average value of 16 for $\frac{\pi}{\Theta}$. MAYNE points out that all these values for $\frac{\pi}{\Theta}$ are an order of magnitude lower than the value computed by SCHMALTZ (1931) but comes to the conclusion that "the basic concept of the STEINHAUSEN model as an integrating accelerometer, although probably oversimplified in its present form, will survive further investigation".

XI. Semicircular Canals and Linear Accelerations

The "classical" assumption that semicircular canals respond exclusively to angular accelerations has recently come under fire from various sources (LANSBERG et al., 1965; BENSON and BODIN, 1965; CRAMPTON, 1966; GUEDRY, 1966; BENSON, 1966; YOUNG, 1967; BENSON et al., 1967; STEER, JR., 1967; BODIN, 1968). Two main observations have led to this challenge. Firstly, during constant-velocity rotation of the human subject around a horizontal longitudinal axis the nystagmus of the horizontal eye muscles, assumed to originate in the horizontal canals which lie in the plane of rotation in this case, continues during the whole period of constant-velocity rotation instead of decaying as soon as constant velocity is attained. It was thought that this was a response to the vector of linear (gravitational) acceleration sweeping over the ampullae once per rotation. The second observation is that the expected decay time of nystagmus during constant-speed rotation around the vertical longitudinal axis varies with the subject's distance from the centre of rotation. In this case the stimulus responsible for the modification of the decay time was thought to be the centrifugal linear acceleration acting in a constant radial direction on the horizontal semicircular canals which in this case too lie in the plane of rotation.

As these observations involve the registration of reflex responses, the possibility cannot be excluded that they represent modifications of the nystagmic response of otolithic or kinesthetic origin. Whether or not semicircular canals respond to linear acceleration could be answered most directly by the study of the impulse response in the branches of the eighth nerve before they enter into synaptic connection with other pathways in the vestibular ganglia and nuclei.

Use of the isolated labyrinth preparation (LOWENSTEIN and SAND, 1940b) has been suggested. Its limitations have been set out above in a different context (see X). It would, therefore, be desirable to record from the unopened labyrinth with chronic electrodes implanted in the eighth nerve distal to the cell bodies of the primary sensory neurons. Whether this is technically possible under conditions of stimulation on accelerating devices is an open question. The experiments of GUALTIEROTTI (1965) come nearest to fulfilling these conditions, but he recorded almost exclusively from utricular endings. The experiments by MONEY (1966) on the albino cat with genetically undeveloped utriculi are the only hint that results similar to those reported by GUEDRY (1966) can be obtained in the absence of otolithic interference. Confirmation of the validity of the findings by post-mortem histology is eagerly awaited.

Meanwhile, a series of preliminary experiments has been carried out on the isolated elasmobranch labyrinth (LOWENSTEIN, unpublished except for a preliminary report to the Bárány Society at Uppsala (1968) (LOWENSTEIN, 1970b). After studying the effect of a rotating vector of linear acceleration on receptor units in the utriculus and in the lagena, which gave low-threshold responses to this type of stimulus (by means of a counterrotating accelerator), the author found that the horizontal and anterior vertical canals also respond, but with a much higher threshold. The response picture obtained would be compatible with the continuous elicitation of phasic responses in the eye muscles during constant-speed rotation. Usually responses appear at linear accelerations of over 0.5 g. It was realized that such preparations should respond to the gravitational stimulus of a tilt from normal, as in fact they do. This response of the semicircular canals to positional change had been reported by LEDOUX (1949) in the isolated labyrinth of the frog. I had also observed it on many occasions during experiments on the elasmobranch preparation, but had hitherto interpreted it as a sign of the onset of functional deterioration. Recently, however, I obtained static responses of this kind, especially from the vertical canal, in the nose-down position of the head as early as 15 min after interruption of the blood supply by decapitation. At present, it looks as if susceptibility of the semicircular canal to linear acceleration cannot be excluded when the stimulus intensity is approximately 1 g or over.

The susceptibility of semicircular canals to linear acceleration has been postulated on theoretical grounds (STEER, 1967). The rationale behind such arguments is the fact that in a torus of uneven diameter and with elastic walls, linear acceleration results in shifts in pressure distribution that could affect the position and shape of the cupula (roller-pump action). An account of the mathematical treatment is beyond the scope of this article, however.

XII. The Otolith Organs

The analysis of the function of the otolith-bearing end organs has been incomparably more difficult than the experimental work on the semicircular canals. Experiments with direct mechanical stimulation of otolith organs (KUBO, 1906; MAXWELL, 1924; ULRICH, 1935; TRINCKER, 1959) have yielded useful information on the mode of functioning of otolith organs, especially on the role of shearing displacement, despite the fact that the effect of such artificial mechanical stimulation can be restricted to a specific organ within the labyrinth only with great difficulty. Experiments based on separate elimination were more successful. DE KLEIJN and MAGNUS (1921), HASEGAWA (1931) and DE KLEIJN and VERSTEEGH (1932) used centrifugation to remove otoliths from their sensory epithelia in some cases without causing overt damage to the cristae of the semicircular canals, and observed the ensuing deficiency phenomena in the spontaneous and reflex behaviour of the animal (see also IGARASHI and NAGABA, 1967; PARKER et al., 1967). The many, often conflicting results included evidence for the subordinate importance of the sacculus macula (see LOWENSTEIN (1936) for review). In most vertebrates the utriculus, in the pars superior of the labyrinth, appears to be capable of controlling the whole of the labyrinthine gravity responses. In the pars inferior of the non-mammalian labyrinth the lagena rather than the sacculus is implicated in the elicitation of gravity responses (see XIII).This does not necessarily exclude, in some animals, the participation of the sacculus, the macula of which has a divided innervation derived from the ramus superior and inferior of the eighth nerve.

A. Elimination Experiments

Prior to the advent of the electrophysiological technique, TAIT and MCNALLY (1934) made a very detailed and reliable analysis of the function of the various parts of the labyrinth in the frog, based on operative interruption of the nerve supply to the individual end organs followed by exhaustive reflex tests and post-mortem histology. The results obtained with what the authors call bi-de-utriculate frogs, i.e. frogs in which the two utriculi *only* were put out of action are important and will be discussed here at some length. In this condition *all* static reactions are lost. This makes efficient participation of the semicircular canals in the control of static responses appear unlikely. On the other hand, the "dynamic responses" controlled by the canals, i.e. responses to angular acceleration, are intact. However, the absence of the utriculi causes overcompensation during rapid accelerated tilts, which is not observed in animals with intact utriculi. A tremor of the head during fast spontaneous movements is another consequence of the absence of "damping" by the utriculi. The absence of gravity sensors also results in a strong tendency to seek contact with the substrate or solid objects during locomotion in water. Finally, a tendency to "fall asleep" in deep water and a decrease in the frequency of respiratory movements is attributed by the authors to a "tonus" deficit caused by the loss of the utriculi.

Conversely, in so-called bi-soli-utricular animals, i.e. animals in which all end organs except the two utriculi were eliminated, all static reflexes are intact. Rapid tilting about horizontal axes leads to vehement head and body movements *in* and not against the direction of the imposed movement. Instead of compensating for the passive movement they totally upset the animal. In view of the fact that these violent and compensatory movements are absent in animals after total loss of all labyrinthine end organs the authors attribute them to the intact utriculi. The utriculi would in this case respond to fast angular acceleration in the opposite direction to the response of the semicircular canals. In the normal animal these reactions of the utriculi would have the damping effect postulated above on the basis of the findings with bi-de-utriculate frogs. Altogether MCNALLY and TAIT's experiments are a rich source of information on the mode of collaboration between semicircular canals and otolith organs.

The article byMAYNE (G.I.) deals with the systems analysis of this collaboration. Assuming certain physical properties of the semicircular canals and of otolith organs, such as critical or overcritical damping MAYNE introduces block diagrams in which the ultimate processing of the peripheral information from both types of end organ is allotted to various types of integrating systems and band-pass filters in the ascending pathway including the various vestibular centres, basing his argument on the classic assumption of the exclusive sensitivity of the semicircular canal to angular accelerations as opposed to a wide-range receptivity of the otolithic system including angular linear and "constant" gravitational stimuli.

B. Electrophysiological Approach

The argument rests in part on the electrophysiological data described by LOWENSTEIN and ROBERTS (1950) for the isolated surviving labyrinth of the ray (*Raja clavata*). The electrophysiological pioneer work of ROSS (1936) on the labyrinth of the frog must, however, be mentioned in this context. The experiments were carried out in ADRIAN's laboratory at Cambridge and were a follow-up of the work of TAIT and MCNALLY of which ROSS had first-hand experience. The paper describing his results is a classic example of his meticulously critical approach to the interpretation of technically excellent recordings. The interpretation of the responses from the semicircular canals suffers from the fact that he did not recognize the functional significance of the resting discharge (see VII). In the work on the otolith organs the origin of the responses from the utriculus and sacculus is correctly traced because ROSS, being aware of the work of ASHCROFT and HALLPIKE (1934a and b), assumed that the vibration-sensitive units were situated in the sacculus and attributed all units sensitive to slow tilting and linear acceleration to the utriculus. He points out correctly that the utricular sense endings respond with increased activity to tilts about more than one axis, but in one direction only. However, within a given utriculus some units respond to ipsilateral and others to contralateral tilt. ROSS found two types of gravity-sensitive receptors in the stump of the posterior ramus of the eighth nerve besides units responding to vibration and angular acceleration, but refrained from assigning these responses to any specific end organ within the complex of four end organs innervated by the posterior branch. We now know that the gravitational responses must have originated in the lagena. One technical aspect of ROSS's work is worthy of special mention. Although he experimented on the isolated head and consequently under conditions of interrupted blood supply, his recording electrode made contact with slivers of nerve proximal to their entry into the cranial cavity and it is therefore reasonable to assume that the perilymphatic space remained inviolate. The price paid for this was a lack of certainty in localization of the origin of recorded responses, especially so far as the pars inferior of the labyrinth was concerned.

Among the receptor units sensitive to position and linear acceleration, ROSS distinguished units responding to out-of-level tilting from others that responded when the preparation returned to normal (into-level response). The units responding exclusively to into-level tilts were found in the posterior ramus only. A search for units that responded differently to slow and rapid tilting, i.e. to units that might be responsible for the anti-compensatory responses seen by TAIT and MCNALLY in bi-soli-utricular frogs was unsuccessful. MAYNE (G.I.) has demonstrated that this reflex behaviour need not be referred to special peripheral mechanisms.

The isolated preparation of the elasmobranch labyrinth (LOWENSTEIN and ROBERTS, 1950) offers the advantage of direct access to the various vestibular nerve branches close to the sensory epithelium. The precise localization of the origin of the impulse response is therefore never in doubt. However, single-unit preparations from the utriculus, sacculus and lagena are naturally more difficult to obtain

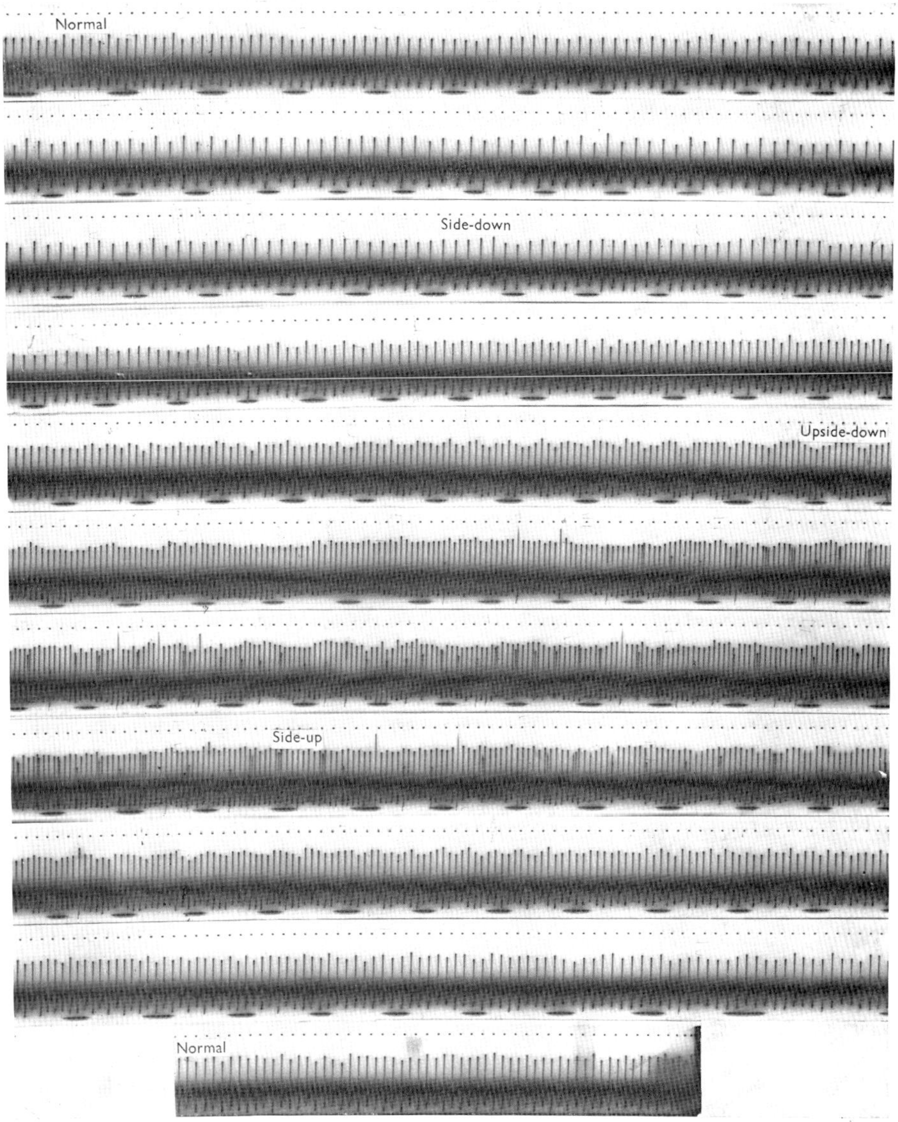

Fig. 15. Continuous record of the response from two end organs of the utriculus of the isolated surviving labyrinth of the ray (*Raja clavata*) to a full-circle lateral tilt. Time marker at top of record 24/sec. Rotation signal at the bottom: 1 gap/3°. Constant speed of tilting 10°/sec approximately. The maximum discharge frequency lies near the side-up and the minimum near the side-down position (From LOWENSTEIN and ROBERTS, 1950)

than similar preparations from semicircular canals. There is a much shorter length of nerve available for pick-up and the pick-up electrode comes to lie very close to the wall of the membraneous labyrinth. Preparations tend to be microphonic, and fluid short circuits are frequently established during tilting. In single-unit preparations the course of change in the discharge frequency can be assessed directly from the film record. In multifibre preparations the integrated total voltage is measured on a counting rate meter. In more recent work this meter is used in conjunction with a pen recorder giving a write-out in terms of change in total voltage output.

Before the behaviour of individual receptor units is discussed, let us recall the overall localization of gravity-sensitive endings. Such units were found in the otolith-covered main portion of the macula utriculi, in roughly the posterior third of the otolith-covered macula sacculi and in the whole of the otolith-covered macula lagenae. The unloaded lacinia utriculi, roughly the anterior two thirds of the otolith-covered macula sacculi and the unloaded macula neglecta were found to yield low-threshold vibration responses in the absence of responses to angular acceleration and tilting (LOWENSTEIN and ROBERTS, 1951). The "gravity" responses recorded from the posterior third of the macula sacculi were very similar to those recorded from the macula utriculi, whereas the macula lagenae contained units behaving antagonistically to those of the utriculus.

The majority of utricular units showed minimum discharge activity near the normal horizontal position in space, whereas lagena units were maximally active near this and also sometimes near the horizontal "upside-down" position of the skull.

Figure 15 shows the impulse activity of a single utricular unit during an uninterrupted constant-velocity (10°/sec) tilt about the horizontal longitudinal axis (lateral tilt) plotted as a graph in Fig. 16. The dotted curve in Fig. 16 corresponds to the course of events recorded in the continuous film strip (Fig. 15). It will be seen that the plot reaches a clear minimum approximately half-way between normal and 90° side-down and a maximum in a correspondingly intermediate position between upside-down and 90° side-up. After a full-circle tilt in one direction the preparation was made "to retrace its course" during a full-circle tilt in the opposite direction. The important feature of this second tilt is that it yielded a "phase shift" of approximately 90° in the sine-like frequency plot, so that in this case the maximum came to lie approximately half-way between normal and side-up and the minimum in a correspondingly intermediate position between upside down and side-down. The course of the two curves indicates clearly that we are dealing here with a receptor monitoring a constant-velocity tilt in a direction-dependent manner. Otolith organs can be described as differential-density accelerometers. A constant-velocity tilt subjects such an organ to two different changes, apart from the angular acceleration from rest to constant-velocity tilt. Firstly, it brings about a sinusoidal change in the magnitude of the component of the otolith "weight" acting tangentially to the surface of the macula according to the expression $(m_2-m_1)\ g \sin a$, where m_2-m_1 expresses the difference in density between otolith and endolymph, g gravitational acceleration and a the angle of tilt from the normal. The adequate stimulus is now generally considered to be the shearing of the bases of the hair processes of the sensory cell by forces

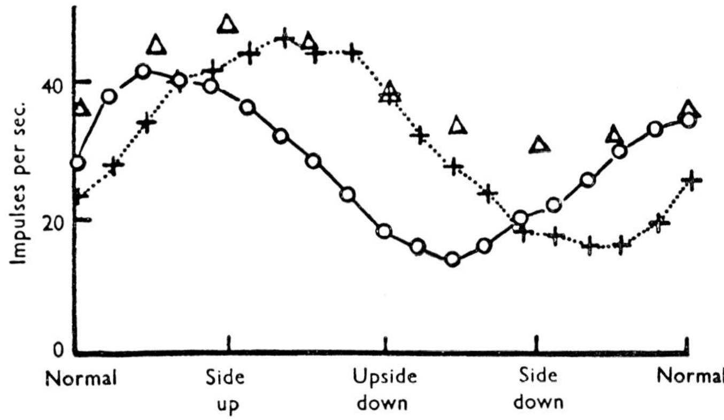

Fig. 16. Plot of response from the utriculus (see Fig. 15). The discharge frequencies of two full-circle lateral tilts in opposite directions. The continuous curve to be read from left to right. The superimposed frequency readings marked by triangles were taken during an interrupted full-circle tilt after 30 sec rest in each position. Interpretation in text (From LOWENSTEIN and ROBERTS, 1949)

acting tangentially to the apical cell surface. This was in fact the original interpretation by BREUER (1891). During the intervening history of vestibular research different hypotheses were proposed in which pressure on the hair cell, traction on the hair processes or changes in the hydrostatic pressure were proposed as the adequate stimulus (MAGNUS, 1924; QUIX, 1925; WITTMAAK, 1929). None of these hypotheses has stood the test of time, and the ultrastructural evidence coupled with experiments on the lateral line with imposed mechanical movement of the cupula of the hair cells combined with simultaneous recording of the impulse responses to such movements have made it abundantly clear that tangential shearing is, in fact, the adequate stimulus (GÖRNER, 1963; HARRIS and MILNE, 1966). The work of v. HOLST and his school provided elegant experimental evidence for this by plotting tilting and centrifugal stimulation against optostatic responses in fishes. It experimentally verified a stimulus-response relationship obeying the expression (m_2-m_1) g sin a for the integrated response derived from the utriculus (v. HOLST, 1950).

During our constant-velocity lateral tilt (Figs. 15 and 16) the utricular otolith organ was subjected to two mechanical changes:

1. A change in the tangential component of the weight of the otolith, i.e. the shearing force parallel to the apical surface of the hair cell from zero in the normal position to $m_2-m_1 \times 1$ g in the 90° side-down-position-to zero in upside down-to $m_2-m_1 \times 1$ g in the 90° side-up position-to zero in the normal position. This sinusoidal change of position should produce a sinusoidal change in the frequency of the impulse discharge with peak values (maximum and minimum) in the 90° side-up and 90° side-down position respectively.

In the preparation under review this did not happen during the uninterrupted constant-velocity tilt. Instead, the peak values occurred 45° out of phase in advance of the expected position. The appropriate position of the peaks (maxima and minima) did in fact appear in the experiment in which the tilting movement was interrupted and the impulse frequency recorded 30 sec after tilting was stopped. The triangles show the discharge frequencies which yield the sinusoidal relationship with maxima and minima in the 90° positions. This specific sensory cell thus showed a dual mode of response. It acted as a true static position monitor under the influence of constant gravitational acceleration. When there was a constant change in the effective tangential component of g during the uninterrupted constant-velocity tilting movement it responded to the dynamic situation with a phase advance in the sinusoidal response curve. MAYNE (G.I.) describes such a cell as a mixed-response Type 3 cell. In my experience this type of behaviour is very common among otolithic units. When recording simultaneously from a population of cells, the peaks of the dynamic response may be sharpened by recruitment of units of high threshold whose limited response range may lie relatively close to the normal and upside-down position, i.e. close to the positions of the steepest rate of change in the sine curve. There are, in fact, a relatively large number of units with narrow maxima and a more or less constant discharge activity for the rest of the full circle. They are unlikely to be discovered or chosen for recording when the experimenter selects single-unit preparations for the purpose of an analysis of quantitative stimulus-response relationships. Hence they do not figure in examples described by LOWENSTEIN and ROBERTS; units showing modulation of activity over the full circle were selected for the above reason. When recordings are taken from multi-unit preparations the "range fractionation" by narrow-range units becomes evident, especially when the discharge is monitored acoustically by loudspeakers.

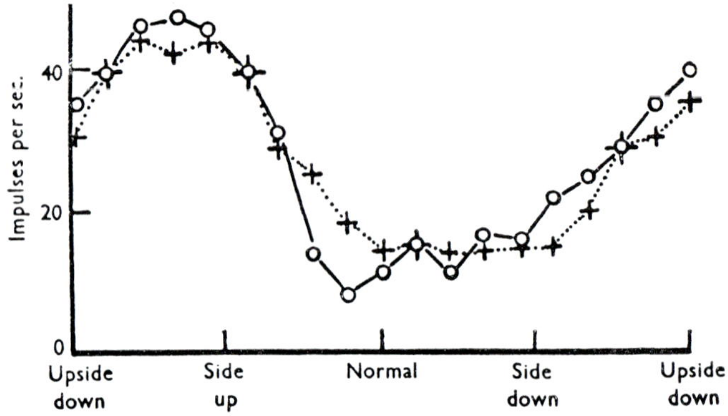

Fig. 17. Plot of response from the utriculus of the ray (*Raja clavata*) to two full-circle lateral tilts in opposite directions. The continuous curve to be read from left to right and the dotted curve from right to left. Interpretation in text (From LOWENSTEIN and ROBERTS, 1949)

Units are not infrequently found in which the discharge picture cannot be dissected into dynamic and static components (Fig. 17). Here the plot is derived from an uninterrupted constant-velocity tilt and from a point-by-point measurement of the "adapted response" to maintained positions around the full circle. One may say that one is dealing with a pure positional (static) receptor devoid of a phasic or dynamic element. This unit shows a fairly broad maximum in an intermediate position between the upside-down and side-up positions and shows complete coincidence of the plots for consecutive tilts in opposite directions. A step-by-step analysis of the adapted activities was not carried out in this case, but we can probably assume that a curve like this would not diverge significantly from the plots describing the response to constant-velocity rotation. MAYNE (loc. cit.) describes a unit like this as Type 1. It is interesting to note that this unit does not discriminate between the normal and the side-down position, which both lie within a very broad minimum. The deviation of the maximum from the 90° side-up position (greatest value of m_2–m_1 g sin a) must in this case be attributed to anatomical features, i.e. to the functional polarization of the hair cell within the macula, as it clearly does not represent a dynamic phase shift.

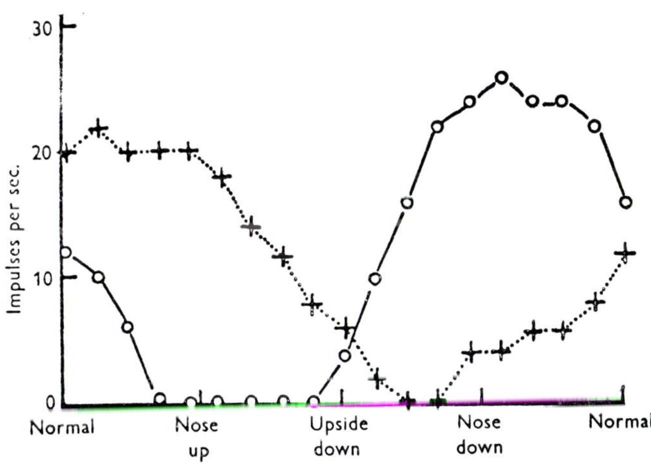

Fig. 18. Plot of response from the utriculus of the ray (*Raja clavata*) to two full-circle fore-and-aft tilts in opposite directions. The continuous curve to be read from left to right and the dotted curve from right to left. Interpretation in text (From LOWENSTEIN and ROBERTS, 1949)

Whether the macula contains units which are purely dynamic and unresponsive to position as such is an obvious question. Figure 18 illustrates the behaviour of a unit of this kind (Type 2 of MAYNE, loc. cit.). The plots for consecutive full-circle tilts in opposite directions show a phase shift of approximately 180°, i.e. whereas maximum activity in the fore-and-aft tilt is attained near the nose-down position, it occurs near the nose-up position during the oppositely directed tilt and vice versa for the minimum. The normal and upside-down positions are characterized by an intermediate level of activity. In this case the plot of a test for the static behaviour is available (Fig. 19). The adapted discharge levels of the unit in maintained positions lie near the basic level of activity in every case. A unit of this nature is obviously unable to monitor position as such. It would be interesting to know where such units are positioned in the macula in relation to the otolith. Unfortunately this information is not obtainable. Purely "dynamic" hair sensilla have been found by COHEN (1955) in the statocyst of the lobster. They were identified as thin thread hairs not loaded with otolith material and projecting freely into the statocyst from its median wall. The majority of otolith-loaded sensilla behaved like true position receptors with relatively narrow activity maxima.

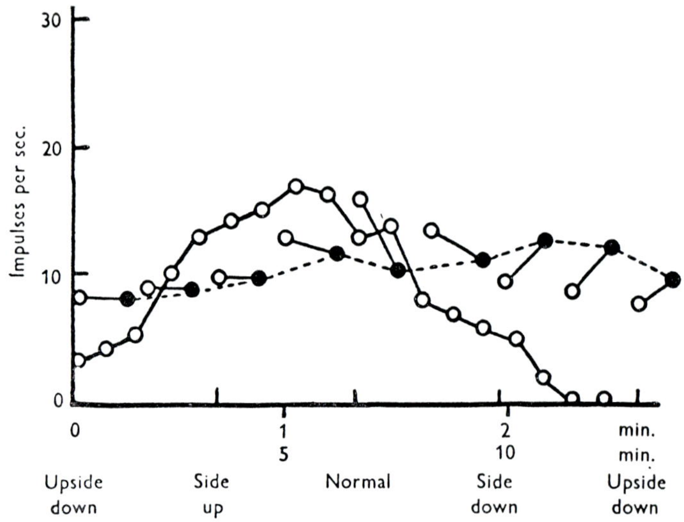

Fig. 19. Plot of response from the utriculus of the ray (*Raja clavata*) to a full-circle lateral tilt, to be read from left to right. Superimposed are the frequency readings during an interrupted tilt in the same direction. Open circles: frequency on reaching position; black circles: frequency after 1 min rest in position. The latter readings are connected by a dotted line to show basic discharge level. Interpretation in text (From LOWENSTEIN and ROBERTS, 1949)

It is abundantly clear that a given macula represents an ordered mosaic of sensory units whose orientation within the macula map is responsible for the mode of their response. More will be said below about such maps and their elucidation by ultrastructural research. Two factors are relevant to our present discussion. Firstly, the same hair cell or group of synergic hair cells can respond to tilt both about the longitudinal and about the transverse axis of a fish or about the frontal, occipital and the bitemporal axes of Man (lateral and fore-and-aft tilts respectively). Let us assume that the excitatory direction of deflexion of the hair bundle points diagonally forward. The consequences of this orientation would be an increase in discharge activity both on nose-down and on homolateral downwards tilt. The absence of data from preparations showing maxima in or near the side-down position given by LOWENSTEIN and ROBERTS (1950) is a technical matter connected with access to a very limited region of the utriculus macula. This is a marginal region of the macula in which a preponderance of hair cells with the excitatory deflexion of the hair bundle directed diagonally inwards might therefore be expected. ADRIAN (1943), recording from the vestibular nucleus of the cat, showed that neurons identified by their typical response to tilting as opposed to angular acceleration respond with an increase in discharge activity to side-down and others to side-up tilting. Similar results were obtained by SCHOEN (1957) in experiments on central vestibular neurons in fishes.

The range of responses obtained from the part of the sacculus macula that is preponderantly sensitive to tilting rather than vibration was similar to that described for the utriculus and no more need be said about the sacculus.

In contrast, the lagena yielded a different type of response. It is characterized by a narrow-peaked maximum near the normal position, with relatively low-level activity elsewhere round the full circle (Fig. 20). These units are so common that they could be used for the identification of the lagena as their origin, when recordings were taken from the posterior ramus centrally to the confluence of the lagena nerve with the saccular part of the nerve. This type of unit obeying the expression $(m_2-m_1)\ g \cos \alpha$ is therefore antagonistically poised against the overall utricular activity. In the ray the macula lagenae lies in a near-vertical plane, i.e. at right angles to the macula utriculi. In the normal position the orientation of the hair cells is such that a fair proportion of the hair bundles should be fully deflected in the excitatory direction. Narrow-peaked units with broader maxima are also found, and the subdivision into the three functional types proposed by MAYNE is also applicable to this end organ.

MACNAUGHTON and MACNALLY (1946) described experiments from which they concluded that, when all other labyrinthine end organs are functionally eliminated by nerve severance, the lagena can furnish a frog with the ability to right itself and they suggest that the lagena has a function antagonistic to that of the utriculus.

SCHOEN and v. HOLST (1950) investigated the function of the lagena and its relation to that of the utriculus in a bony fish (*Gynocorymbus ternetzii*) and found that its tonic response to gravity was maximal in the normal position. In a rather involved and not altogether convincing argument the authors postulate that apart from acting as a source of labyrinthine tonus, in the normal fish the lagena had very little if anything to do with equilibration. It is true, however, that in the minnow (*Phoxinus laevis* L.) the operative elimination of the pars inferior of the labyrinth, which includes a large lagena, has no noticeable influence on the observable postural reflexes of eyes and fins even in a fish blinded by transection of the optic nerve (LOWENSTEIN, 1936), whereas there is a certain possibility that it participates in the responses to auditory stimuli in this type of fish (v. FRISCH, 1936). Otolith organs, being sensors for linear acceleration, are naturally capable of reacting to sound and have been found to act as receptors for vibrational stimuli (see v. FRISCH, 1936; ASHCROFT and HALLPIKE, 1934a and b; ROSS, 1936; LOWENSTEIN and ROBERTS, 1951; ENGER, 1968).

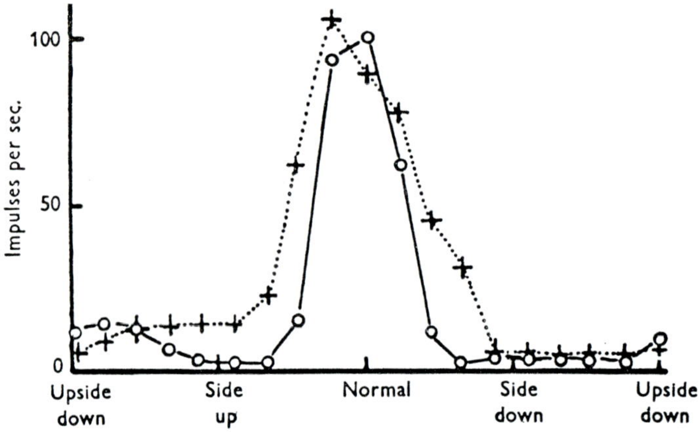

Fig. 20. Plot of response from the lagena of the ray (*Raja clavata*) to two full-circle lateral tilts. The continuous curve to be read from left to right, the dotted curve from right to left. Interpretation in text (From LOWENSTEIN and ROBERTS, 1949)

In general, otolith organs are dual-purpose mechanoreceptors and their specific function depends on anatomical circumstances such as specific exposure to pathways of sound conduction or protection from them. It is possible that a certain type of orientation of sensory cells in the macula epithelium is specifically associated with vibration reception. For instance, the macula is divided into two halves with the hair cells uniformly polarized in one half and oriented in the opposite direction in the other, the two halves being arranged back to back (Figs. 10, 11, and 12).

XIII. Hair-Cell Maps

At this point it may be useful to examine the hair-cell maps in the various otolith organs.

Figures 10, 11, and 12 show samples of hair-cell maps compiled from electron microscope surveys of otolith organs in the ray (LOWENSTEIN et al., 1964), the bony fish *Lota vulgaris* (FLOCK, 1964), and a cell-by-cell representation of the entire hair-cell population in the cyclostome *Lampetra fluviatilis*, the river lamprey (LOWENSTEIN et al., 1968). These maps have made it abundantly clear that a macula cannot convey a massive and uniformly directed unitary signal to the central nervous system as was envisaged by the early workers and fairly recently by v. HOLST and his school (v. HOLST, 1950). Instead, the afferent signals form a complex pattern of often oppositely directed groups of signals in accordance with the topographic arrangement of the polarized hair cells which at any given moment and in any given spatial orientation of the macula are undergoing deflexion of their hair processes in one direction or another under the influence of the tangential "flow" of the otolith mass. The picture is further complicated by the fact that maculae are not plane surfaces but are curved and thus extend into more than one spatial plane. In his theoretical exposition of labyrinth function, MYGIND (1948) compared a macula to the curved palm of a hand holding an irregularly shaped heavy object, and the influx of afferent information to the tactile sensation which results from turning the hand. We are aware of a changing pattern of contact with the complex contours of the object and localize these accurately as the object rolls in the palm of our hand. In this situation the tactile sense, depending chiefly on an apparently random network of free nerve endings, performs a feat of pattern recognition which the orderly arrangement of polarized sensors in a macula is bound to surpass. The difference is that we become aware of tactile sensation but remain ignorant of labyrinthine afference.

MAYNE (G.I.) draws a parallel between pattern resolution in otolith organs and place-representation of pitch discrimination in the cochlea, and postulates that each dynamic and static situation is associated with "a unique pattern" of information. These patterns are not necessarily rigidly determined. They are more probably in a continuous state of flux and depend on the successive stimulus configurations. This pattern of dependence is often referred to as hysteresis and is due to almost inextricably complex interaction between purely neurological functional parameters, such as adaptation and possibly marginal inhibition, and the very probable mechanical compliance of the macula otolith complex; the consequence of this interaction may well be "mechanical accommodation". There is no reason to assume that lower and higher vestibular centres cannot cope with such a situation. In comparison, continuous cross-reference between information from the semicircular canals and information from the otolith organs seems relatively simple. MAYNE (G.I.) deals with this aspect of information processing in detail. No more need be said about it here (see also JONKEES, 1967).

XIV. The Consequences of Weightlessness

However, a new question transcending the analysis of the "natural" range of functions of the labyrinthine end organs arises from the imposition of weightlessness upon a sense organ designed to deal with conditions of almost constant gravitational acceleration of 1 g. In fact, the otolith organs may be considered to furnish the central nervous system with reference levels against which the directional significance of signals from the semicircular canals is currently assessed. How are the otolith organs affected by weightlessness? GUALTIEROTTI and GERATHEWOHL (1965) have recorded the impulse activity in single units in the eighth nerve of the frog during parabolic flight. A balanced tungsten microelectrode (GUALTIEROTTI and BAILEY, 1968) was implanted in the eighth nerve of a curarized frog and the preparation was mounted with full live support (in oxygenated water). The resting discharge from single otolith-controlled units showed relatively large fluctuations in frequency. However, significant changes occurred in response to tilting before and after weightlessness in parabolic flight. The results can be summarized as follows: there is a sudden increase above the resting discharge frequency when weightlessness follows upon a high-g period (2–3 g). Furthermore, there is initially a larger response to acceleration and a sudden decrease in activity before its restoration on return to 1 g. Finally, there is a substantial increase in the overall activity in the fibre after a number of short-interval parabolae. Experiments under conditions of prolonged weightlessness would be necessary before it was possible to decide whether the changes in activity are in fact related to weightlessness or to the cessation of the antecedent hight-g stimulation (see XV.). There is in fact no *prima facie* reason to postulate a complete abolition of resting activity in weightlessness. There is some experimental evidence (HASEGAWA, 1931; PARKER et al., 1967) that a macula from which the otolith has been removed may still be able to act at least as a source of "tonus". The experiments of HASEGAWA were not sufficiently rigorous to prove the continued outflow of excitation from a macula deprived of its otolith. However, recent ultrastructural studies of the hair cell support this assumption. Recently DOHLMAN (personal communication) has removed the cupulae from canal cristae in the pigeon and found that the resting discharge was not abolished by this procedure, whereas the responses to angular acceleration disappeared. The resting activity is not the consequence of a continuous mechanical stimulus of the hair processes, but is due to a gradual release of transmitter substance at a "leaking" synapse between hair cell and primary sensory neuron. This mechanism is very probably independent of gravity. It is true that under these circumstances the influx of "resting" excitation will not be modulated gravitationally when the head turns relatively slowly in space, i.e. the information from the semicircular signalling angular accelerations is unsupported by otolithic reference to the spatial coordinates. Visual information, which always plays a significant part in this process, has to take over to a larger extent in these circumstances.

It must not be forgotten, however, that some dynamic components in otolith function are definitely unaffected by weightlessness. The otoliths retain their function as differential density sensors for non-gravitational angular and linear acceleration. Linear translations in planes in which they produce a tangential momentum of the otolith on the macula are still sensed in the absence of gravitational pull. The otolith is possibly less stable and therefore liable to overshoot in the absence of frictional resistance, and its mechanical sensitivity to linear translations may well be increased (GUALTIEROTTI and GERATHEWOHL, 1965). Furthermore, we have so far neglected to take into account the sinusoidal oscillatory linear acceleration of the otolith which takes place during rapid full circle tilts about the centre of the head, because the magnitude of this stimulus is insignificant compared with that due to the gravitational component to which it acts at right angles. This must be distinguished from the potentially much more pronounced effects of centrifugal forces to which the otolith is bound to continue to respond in weightlessness. Again, the change in frictional parameters due to weightlessness of the otolith has to be taken into account. In the author's experience with many hundreds of preparations, the course of the impulse responses from the utriculus is less predictable during tilts passing through the upside-down position than when the organism is in a near-upright position, where the otolith "rests" on the sensory epithelium. In fact the upside-down position appears to be unstable. This has also been observed in studies examining the counter-rolling of the eye during full-circle tilts (GRAYBIEL and KELLOG, 1966; see also JONKEES, 1967).

It is therefore inadmissible to assume that weightlessness produces the same effects as functional elimination of the otolith organs. The overall configuration of the flux of information from the labyrinth is bound to be very much changed, and this probably leads to a set of "illusions" with which the organism learns to cope. If it were definitely established that semicircular canals normally respond to linear accelerations, we should have to accept that the canal signals may also be significantly modified by the absence of gravitational acceleration, and signals which are normally filtered out or suppressed are no longer forthcoming in weightlessness. The situation is complex but need not be considered too complex for the central nervous system when other clues, especially visual ones, are available. The impairment of static compensatory adjustment of the position of the eyes in the orbit is, however, a factor that may interfere with the efficiency of visual orientation.

XV. Postscript

Since the completion of this article there has been a major breakthrough in the electrophysiological analysis of single-unit responses from vestibular semicircular canal- and otolith-controlled sense endings in mammals (GOLDBERG and FERNANDEZ, 1972; FERNANDEZ and GOLDBERG, 1971a, b; FERNANDEZ, GOLDBERG and ABEND, 1971; VIDAL, JEANNEROD, LIFSCHITZ, LEVITAN, ROSENBERG and SEGUNDO, 1971; LOE, TOMKO and WERNER, 1972). The animals in which such recordings have now been obtained are squirrel, monkey, and cat.

These experiments represent a considerable achievement as the technical difficulties inherent in direct recording from the first-order vestibular neurons in mammals had been considered almost insurmountable. Access to the nerve branches innervating semicircular canals and the otolith organs was gained only after ablation of parts of the cerebellum by suction in all cases. In all probability this involves a serious impairment of the efferent system and the functionally closed-loop status of the preparations.

In this short postscript it is only possible to summarize those of the results that have yielded substantially new information on some of the important functional parameters of vestibular end organs.

In general the extension of the analysis of the mode of functioning of the vestibular hair cell both in semicircular canals and in otolith organs to mammals has fully confirmed the validity of the findings and interpretations presented in the main body of this article.

Particular aspects of the new work can be summarized as follows:

A. Semicircular Canals

The remarkable feature of the semicircular canals of the squirrel monkey is the high frequency of their resting discharge with up to 200 impulses/sec and an average of some 90/sec. Among the units studied there are both regularly and irregularly firing types. Some units adapt little in response frequency during constant stimulation, while others adapt quite considerably. The authors express the degree of adaptive behaviour in a so-called adaptation index the highest value of which is equivalent to one fifth of the primary response. The time constants found for both the horizontal and the vertical semicircular canal units were short, in the region of 5 sec. A time constant suggested for the adaptive process ranges from 30 sec to above 80 sec. The sensitivity of units ranged from 0.5 to 4.0 impulses sec^{-1}/degrees sec^{-2}. Adapting units tended to be more sensitive than non-adapting ones. For short periods of stimulation the response was a linear function of the stimulus. In this context it may be of interest that in experiments on first-order neurons associated with the anterior semicircular canal of the pigeon CORREIA and LANDOLT (1973) found an average time constant of 3.33 ± 0.38 sec and on the whole a linear stimulus-response relationship. However, the authors believe that one unit obeyed a power-function law with an exponent $n = 0.19$.

B. Otolith Organs

As in the case of the semicircular canals, the average resting discharge frequencies in otolith-controlled units is high. The discharge pattern in the majority of units is regular. However, units characterized by an irregular discharge pattern are attributed both to the utriculus and to the sacculus, and there is a lower proportion of such irregular units in the otolith organs than in the semicircular canals. As in the semicircular canals, irregular discharge behaviour is thought to be the property of WERSÄLL's Type I cells, which are innervated by large-diameter axons. In the regularly discharging units the sensitivity appears to be positively correlated with the resting discharge frequency.

Despite the observed differences between units in various functional parameters, the authors found no evidence for strict bimodality or segregation into distinct populations of hair cells, and they are inclined to attribute such differences in behaviour to a possibly continuous spectrum in the mode of afferent innervation in terms of the diameters of the axons synapsing with hair cells situated in various regions of the sensory epithelia.

Finally, the authors come to the conclusion that in the squirrel monkey the response of the otolith-controlled units is approximately a linear function of the effective force.

The reports on the work on the otolith-controlled endings in the cat by VIDAL et al. and LOE et al. (loc. cit.) differ in certain important aspects of observation and of interpretation. The authors agree that there are both regularly and irregularly firing units, and they also agree on the relative statistical distribution of the two types among the units analyzed, i.e. a preponderance by approximately 80% of units with a low coefficient of variability, a percentage distribution tallying well with that described for the otolith organs of the squirrel monkey.

It is also agreed that the units can be divided into preponderantly static and preponderantly dynamic ones, with units characterized by an intermediate behaviour type in between. However, LOE et al. having deliberately selected units with a low coefficient of variation and with a preponderantly "static" response picture, make no contribution towards an analysis of "dynamic or intermediate" units.

The chief difference between the findings of the two research groups relates to what VIDAL et al. call "multivaluedness" in the output of units, related to specific spatial orientations reached on chronologically different occasions in the same serial lateral tilting test between normal and 10° side-down and normal and 10° side-up positions. The authors attribute this behaviour to the possible action of forces like "stiction", that may prevent complete relaxation of the otolith membrane under static as opposed to dynamic conditions.

LOE et al. tilted their selected units over a wider range of angles up to 360° and do not report "multivaluedness" but emphasize the relative fixity of maximum- and minimum-discharge positions in the case of their specially selected units with preponderant static behaviour and under the condition of very low-velocity tilting movements.

Finally, perhaps the most important discrepancy in the findings of the three research groups relates to the assessment of the nature of the stimulus-response relationship in otolith-controlled sense endings. FERNANDEZ et al. and VIDAL et al. describe this relationship as approximately linear, at least over a relatively restricted stimulus range, whereas LOE et al. claim that the relationship is best fitted by a power function, i.e. it can be expected to yield a straight-line graph when the logarithms of both the stimulus and the response are plotted. They therefore suggest the following power-function equation as a suitable model for the stimulus-response relationship for data corrected for phase shift: $f - f_0 = K(\sin(\theta - \theta_0) + 1.0)^n$, where K is a constant of proportionality and n reflects the curvature of the power function ranging from 0.9 to 1.6.

A postscript to this article would not be complete without a mention of the successful orbital flight of two bullfrogs achieved meanwhile by Gualtierotti and collaborators, in which the behaviour of four otolith-controlled units was telemetered for 6 days under conditions of "weightlessness" and in response to remote-controlled centrifugal linear accelerations. So far only preliminary results of this experiment, code name OFO A (Orbiting Frog Otolith A), are available, and the data analysis is not yet complete. It appears certain, however, that the otolith organ responds to "weightlessness" by regular periodic fluctuations between over- and under-activity on a time scale measured in tens of hours, and that this reflects the intervention of a central nervous regulating mechanism, which finally appears to contribute to the restitution of the normal basic activity level of the organ. There are also corresponding fluctuations in the sensitivity of the organ to acceleratory stimulation.

In conclusion, the time that has elapsed since the completion of this article has been characterized by lively work on models in the field of vestibular function carried out in a number of centres. This is dealt with and documented in the atricle by Mayne in this volume.

References

Adrian, E.D.: Discharges from vestibular receptors in the cat. J. Physiol. (Lond.) **101**, 389–407 (1943).

Adrian, E.D.: The physical background of perception. Oxford: Clarendon Press 1947.

Ashcroft, D.W., Hallpike, W.C.S.: On the function of the saccule. J. Laryng. **49**, 450–460 (1934a).

Ashcroft, D.W., Hallpike, W.C.S.: Action potentials in the sacculus nerve of the frog. J. Physiol. (Lond.) **81**, 23–34P (1934b).

de Beer, G.R.: How animals hold their heads. Proc. Linn. Soc. (Lond.) **159**, 125–139 (1947).

Benson, A.J.: Modification of per- and post-rotational responses by the concomitant linear acceleration. NASA SP **115**, 199–213 (1966).

Benson, A.J., Bodin, M.A.: Comparison of the effect of the direction of the gravitational acceleration on post-rotational responses in yaw, pitch and roll. RAF Inst. Aviat. Med. Rpt. 348, Farnborough/England 1965.

Benson, A.J., Guedry, F.E., Jones, G.M.: Evidence for artificial stimulation of the semicircular canal by rotation of a linear acceleration vector. Proc. 38th Annual Meeting Aerospace Med. Assoc. (1967).

Bodin, M.A.: The effect of gravity on human vestibular responses in pitch. J. Physiol. (Lond.) **196**, 74–75P (1968).

Breuer, J.: Neue Versuche an den Ohrbogengängen. Pflügers Arch. ges. Physiol. **44**, 134–152 (1889).

Breuer, J.: Über die Funktion der Otolithen-Apparate. Pflügers Arch. ges. Physiol. **48**, 195–306 (1891).

Carlström, D.: A crystallographic study of vertebrate otoliths. Biol. Bull. Woods Hole **125**, 441–463 (1963).

Christiansen, J.A.: On hyalouronate molecules in the labyrinth as mechano-electric transducers and as molecular motors acting as resonators. Acta oto-laryng. (Stockh.) **57**, 33–49 (1964).

Citron, L.D., Exley, D., Hallpike, C.S.: Formation, circulation and chemical properties of the labyrinthine fluids. Brit. med. Bull. **12**, 101–104 (1956).

Cohen, M.J.: The function of receptors in the statocyst of the lobster (Homarus americanus). J. Physiol. (Lond.) **130**, 9–34 (1955).

Correia, M.J., Landolt, J.P.: Spontaneous and driven responses from primary neurons of the anterior semicircular canal of the pigeon. Advanc. Oto-rhino-laryng. **19**, 134–148 (1973).

Crampton, G.H.: Does linear acceleration modify cupula deflection? NASA SP **115**, 169–184 (1966).

Crum-Brown, A.: On the sense of rotation and the anatomy and physiology of the semicircular canals of the internal ear. J. Anat. (Lond.) **8**, 327–331 (1873/4).

Dohlman, G.: Some practical and theoretical points in labyrinthology. Proc. roy. Soc. Med. **50**, 779–790 (1935).

Dohlman, G.: Some aspects of the mechanism of vestibular hair cell stimulation. Confin. neurol. (Basel) **20**, 169 (1960).

Dohlman, G., Boord, R.L.: The effect of cupula removal on the activity of ampullary structures in the pigeon. Acta oto-laryng. (Stockh.) **57**, 507–516 (1964).

van Egmond, A.A.J., Groen, J.J., Jonkees, L.B.W.: The mechanics of the semicircular canal. J. Physiol. (Lond.) **110**, 1–17 (1949).

Enger, P.S.: Hearing in fish, pp. 4–17. Ciba Found. Symp. on Hearing Mechanisms in Vertebrates. London: Churchill 1968.

Engström, H., Lindeman, H.M., Ades, M.W.: Anatomical features of the auricular sensory organs. NASA SP **115**, 33–46 (1966).

Ewald, J.R.: Physiologische Untersuchungen über das Endorgan des Nervus Octavus. Wiesbaden: Bergmann 1892.

Fernández, C., Goldberg, J.M.: Physiology of peripheral neurons innervating semicircular canals of the Squirrel Monkey. II. Response to sinusoidal stimulation and dynamics of peripheral vestibular system. J. Neurophysiol. **34**, 661–675 (1971).

FERNNÁDEZ, C., GOLDBERG, J.M., ABEND, W.K.: Response to static tilts of peripheral neurons innervating otolith organs of the Squirrel Monkey. J. Neurophysiol. **35**, 978–997 (1972).

FISCHER, M.H.: Die Funktion des Vestibularapparates (der Bogengänge und Otolithen) bei Fischen, Amphibien, Reptilien und Vögeln. In: Handb. Norm u. Pathol. Physiol. Vol. 11/1, pp. 797–867. Berlin: Springer 1926.

FLOCK, Å.: Structure of the macula utriculi with special reference to directional interplay of sensory responses as revealed by morphological polarization. J. Cell Biol. **22**, 413–431 (1964).

FLOCK, Å.: Ultrastructure and function in the lateral line organs. In: Lateral Line detectors. P. CAHN, Ed. pp. 163–197. Bloomington, London: Indiana University Press 1967.

FLOURENS, P.: Recherches expérimentales sur les propriétés et les fonctions du système nerveux, dans les animals vertébrés, 2ed. Paris 1824.

VON FRISCH, K.: Über den Gehörsinn der Fische. Biol. Rev. **11**, 210–246 (1936).

GERNANDT, B.: The effect of the centrifugal force upon the nerve discharge from the horizontal canal. Acta physiol. scand. **21**, 61–72 (1950).

GIBBONS, I.R.: The relationship between the fine structure and the direction of beat in gill cilia of the lamellibranch mollusc. J. biophys. biochem. Cytol. **11**, 179–205 (1961).

GIRARD, L.: L'attitude normale de la tête determinée par le labyrinth de l'oreille. Oto-rhino-laryng. int. **14**, 517–537 (1930).

GOLDBERG, J.M., FERNÁNDEZ, C.: Physiology of peripheral neurons innervating semicircular canals of the Squirrel Monkey. I. Resting discharge and response to constant angular accelerations. J. Neurophysiol. **34**, 635–660 (1971).

GOLDBERG, J.M., FERNÁNDEZ, C.: Physiology of peripheral neurons innervating semicircular canals of the Squirrel Monkey. III. Variations among units in their discharge properties. J. Neurophysiol. **34**, 676–684 (1971).

GOLTZ, F.: Über die physiologische Bedeutung der Bogengänge des Ohrlabyrinthes. Pflügers Arch. ges. Physiol. **3**, 172–192 (1870).

GÖRNER, P.: Untersuchungen zur Morphologie und Electrophysiologie des Seitenlinienorgans vom Krallenfrosch (Xenopus laevis Daudin). Z. vergl. Physiol. **47**, 316–338 (1963).

GRAHE, K.: Die Funktion der Bogengangsapparates und der Statolithen beim Menschen. In: Hand. norm. u. pathol. Physiol. Bd. 11, S. 909. Berlin: Springer 1926.

GRAY, E.G., PUMPHREY, R.J.: Ultrastructure of the insect ear. Nature (Lond.) **181**, 618 (1958).

GRAYBIEL, A., KELLOGG, R.S.: The inversion illusion in parabolic flight: it's probable dependence on otolith function. NASA SP **115**, 15–24 (1966).

GRIBENSKI, A.: Contribution à l'étude fonctionelle des canaux semi-circulaires chez la grenouille (Rana esculenta). J. Physiol. (Lond.) **55**, Suppl. 4, 1–95, (1963).

GROEN, J.J.: Problems of the semicircular canal from a mechanico-physiological point of view. Acta oto-laryng. (Stockh.) Suppl. **163**, 59–67 (1960).

GROEN, J.J., LOWENSTEIN, O., VENDRIK, A.J.H.: The Mechanical analysis of the responses from the end-organs of the horizontal semicircular canal in the isolated elasmobranch labyrinth. J. Physiol. (Lond.) **117**, 329–346 (1952).

GUALTIEROTTI, T., BAILEY, P.: A neutral buoyancy micro-electrode for prolonged recording from single nerve units. Electroenceph. clin. Neurophysiol. **25**, 77–81 (1968).

GUALTIEROTTI, T., GERATHEWOHL, S.J.: Spontaneous firing and responses to linear acceleration of single otolith units of the frog during short periods of weightlessness during parabolic flight. NASA SP **77**, 221–229 (1965).

GUEDRY, F.E., JR.: Influence of linear and angular accelerations on nystagmus. NASA SP **115**, 185–198 (1966).

HALLPIKE, C.S.: On the case for repeal of Ewald's second law. Acta oto-laryng. (Stockh.) Suppl. **159**, 7–14 (1961).

HALLPIKE, C.S., HOOD, J.D.: The speed of the slow component of ocular nystagmus induced by angular acceleration of the head: its experimental determination and application to the physical theory of the cupular mechanism. Proc. Roy. Soc. B **141**, 216–230 (1953).

HARRIS, G.G., MILNE, D.C.: Input-output characteristics of the lateral-line sense-organs of Xenopus laevis. J. acoust. Soc. Amer. **40**, 32–42 (1966).

HASEGAWA, T.: Die Veränderung der labyrinthären Reflexe bei zentrifugierten Meerschweinchen. Pflügers Arch. ges. Physiol. **229**, 205–225 (1931).

HOAGLAND, H.: Electrical responses from the lateral line nerves of catfish. J. gen. Physiol. **16**, 695–714 (1933a).

HOAGLAND, H.: Quantitative analysis of responses from lateral line nerves of fishes, II. J. gen. Physiol. **16**, 715–732 (1933b).

HOAGLAND, H.: Electrical responses from lateral line nerves of fishes, III. J. gen. Physiol. **17**, 77–82 (1933c).

HOAGLAND, H.: Electrical responses from the lateral line nerves of fishes, IV. The repetitive discharge. J. gen. Physiol. **17**, 195–209 (1933d).

VON HOLST, E.: Die Arbeitsweise des Statolithenapparates bei Fischen. Z. vergl. Physiol. **32**, 60–120 (1950).

IGARASHI, M., NAGABA, M.: Vestibular end-organ damage in squirrel monkeys after exposure to intensive linear accelerations. NASA SP **152**, 63–82 (1967).

IGARASHI, M.: Dimensional Study of the vestibular end organ apparatus. NASA SP **115**, 47–54 (1966).

JONKEES, L.B.W. On the otoliths: Their function and the way to test them. NASA SP **152**, 307–330 (1967).

DE KLEIJN, A., MAGNUS, R.: Labyrinthreflexe auf Progressivbewegungen. Pflügers Arch. ges. Physiol. **186**, 39–60 (1921).

DE KLEIJN, A., VERSTEEGH, C.: Labyrinthreflexe nach Abschleuderung der Otolithenmembranen bei Meerschweinchen. Pflügers Arch. ges. Physiol. **232**, 454–465 (1932).

KUBO, I.: Über die vom N. acusticus ausgelösten Augenbewegungen Pflügers Arch. ges. Physiol. **115**, 457–482 (1906).

LANSBERG, M.P., GUEDRY, F.E., JR., GRAYBIEL, A.: Effect of changing the resultant linear acceleration relative to the subject on nystagmus generated by angular acceleration. Aerospace Med. **36**, 456–460 (1965).

LEDOUX, A.: Activité électrique des nerfs des canaux semi-circulaires du saccule et de l'utricule chez la grenouille. Acta oto-rhino-laryng. belg. **3**, 335–349 (1949).

LOE, P.R., TOMKO, D.L., WERNER, G.: The neural signal of angular head position in primary afferent vestibular nerve axons. J. Physiol. (Lond.) **230**, 29–50 (1973).

LORENTE DE NÓ, R.: Die Grundlagen der Labyrinthphysiologie. Skand. Arch. Physiol. **49**, 251 (1926).

LORENTE DE NÓ, R.: Ausgewählte Kapitel aus der vergleichenden Physiologie des Labyrinthes. Die Augenmuskelreflexe beim Kaninchen und ihre Grundlagen. Ergebn. Physiol. **32**, 73 (1931).

LOWENSTEIN, O.: The equilibrium function of the vertebrate labyrinth. Biol. Rev. **11**, 113–145 (1936).

LOWENSTEIN, O.: The tonic function of the horizontal semicircular canals in fishes. J. exp. Biol. **14**, 473–482 (1937).

LOWENSTEIN, O.: Labyrinth and Equilibrium. Symp. Soc. exp. Biol. **4**, 60–82 (1950).

LOWENSTEIN, O.: The effect of galvanic polarization on the impulse discharge from sense endings in the isolated labyrinth of the thornback ray (Raja clavata). J. Physiol. (Lond.) **127**, 104–117 (1955).

LOWENSTEIN, O.: The electrophysiological study of the responses of the isolated labyrinth of the lamprey (Lampetra fluviatilis) to angular acceleration, tilting and mechanical vibration. Proc. Roy. Soc. B **174**, 419–434 (1970a).

LOWENSTEIN, O.: Electrophysiological experiments on the isolated surviving labyrinth of elasmobranch fish to analyse the responses to linear accelerations. Wenner-Gren Center International Symposium Series, **15**, 35–41. Oxford: Pergamon Press 1970b.

LOWENSTEIN, O., ROBERTS, T.D.M.: The equilibrium function of the otolith organs of the thornback ray (Raja clavata). J. Physiol. (Lond.) **110**, 392–415 (1949).

LOWENSTEIN, O., ROBERTS, T.D.M.: The localisation and analysis of the responses to vibration from the isolated elasmobranch labyrinth. A contribution to the problem of the evolution of hearing in the vertebrates. J. Physiol. (Lond.) **114**, 471–489 (1951).

LOWENSTEIN, O., SAND, A.: The activity of the horizontal semicircular canal of the dogfish, Scyllium canicula. J. exp. Biol. **13**, 416–428 (1936).

LOWENSTEIN, O., SAND, A.: The individual and integrated activity of the semicircular canals of the elasmobranch labyrinth. J. Physiol. (Lond.) **99**, 89–101 (1940).

LOWENSTEIN, O., OSBORNE, M.P., WERSÄLL, J.: Structure and innervation of the sensory epithelia of the labyrinth in the thornback ray (Raja clavata). Proc. Roy. Soc. B **160**, 1–12 (1964).

LOWENSTEIN, O., OSBORNE, M.P., THORNHILL, R.A.: The anatomy and ultrastructure of the labyrinth of the lamprey (Lampetra fluviatilis L.). Proc. Roy. Soc. B **170**, 113–134 (1968).

LOWENSTEIN, O., THORNHILL, R.A.: The labyrinth of Myxine: anatomy, ultrastructure and electrophysiology. Proc. Roy. Soc. B **176**, 21–42 (1970).

MACH, E.: Grundlinien der Lehre von den Bewegungsempfindungen. Leipzig: Engelmann 1875.

MACNAUGHTON, I.P.J., MCNALLY, W.J.: Some experiments which indicate that the frog's lagena has an equilibrium function. J. Laryng. **61**, 204–214 (1946).

MAGNUS, R.: Körperstellung. Berlin: Springer 1924.

MAGNUS, R., DE KLEIJN, A.: Funktion des Bogengangs- und Otolithenapparates bei Säugern. In: Handb. d. norm. u. pathol. Physiol. Bd. **11**, S. 868–908. Berlin: Springer 1926.

MAXWELL, S.S.: Labyrinth and equilibrium. Philadelphia and London: Saunders 1923.

MAXWELL, S.S.: On the localization of otolith function. Laryngoscope (St. Louis) **34**, 849–853 (1924).

MCNALLY, W.J., TAIT, J.: Ablation experiments on the labyrinth of the frog. Amer. J. Physiol. **75**, 155–179 (1925).

MCNALLY, W.J., TAIT, J.: Some results of section of particular nerve branches to the ampullae of the four vertical semicircular canals of the frog. Quart. J. exp. Physiol. **23**, 147–196 (1933).

MILLAR, R.H., CIONA, L.M.B.C.: Memoirs, Vol. 35. Liverpool 1953.

MURRAY, R.W., Potts, W.T.W.: The composition of the endolymph perilymph and other body fluids of elasmobranches. Comp. Biochem. Physiol. **2**, 65–75 (1961).

MYGIND, G.H.: Static function of the labyrinth. Attempt at a synthesis. Acta oto-laryng. (Stockh.) Suppl. **70**, 1–114 (1948).

PARKER, D.E., COVEL, W.P., v. GIERKE, H.E.: Behavioral loss and otoconia displacement in guinea pigs following linear acceleration. NASA SP **152**, 83–97 (1967).

PUMPHREY, R.J.: Hearing. Symp. Soc. exp. Biol. **4**, 3–18 (1950).

QUIX, F.M.: Die Otolithenfunktion in der Otologie. Z. Hals-, Nas.- u. Ohrenheilh. **8**, 516 (1924).

RAUCH, S., KÖSTLIN, A.: Aspects chimiques de l'endolymphe et de la perilymphe. Pract. oto-rhino-laryng. (Basel) **20**, 287–291 (1958).

RETZIUS, G.: Das Gehörorgan der Wirbeltiere. Stockholm: Samson and Wallin 1881.

ROSS, D.A.: Electrical studies on the frog's labyrinth. J. Physiol. (Lond.) **86**, 117–146 (1936).

SCHÖN, L.: Microableitungen einzelner zentraler Vestibularisneurone von Knochenfischen bei Statolithenreizen. Z. vergl. Physiol. **39**, 399–417 (1957).

SCHÖN, L., v. HOLST, E.: Das Zusammenspiel von Lagena und Utriculus bei der Lageorientierung der Knochenfische. Z. vergl. Physiol. **32**, 552–571 (1950).

SMITH, C.A., LOWRY, O.H., WU, M.-L.: The electrolytes of the labyrinthine fluids. Laryngoscope (St. Louis) **64**, 141–153 (1954).

SPOENDLIN, H.H.: Ultrastructural Studies of the labyrinth in Squirrel monkeys. NASA SP **77**, 7–22 (1965).

STEER, R.W., JR.: The influence of angular and linear acceleration on the human semicircular canal, Mass. Inst. Tech. Sc. D. Thesis, M.V.T.-67-3, 1967.

STEINHAUSEN, W.: Über den Nachweis der Bewegung der Cupula in der intakten Bogengangsampulle der Labyrinthes bei der natürlichen rotatorischen und calorischen Reizung. Pflügers Arch. ges. Physiol. **228**, 322–328 (1931).

STENSIÖ, E.: The Downtonian and Devonian vertebrates of Spitzbergen I. Oslo: Dybwad 1927.

TAIT, J., MCNALLY, W.J.: Some features of the action of the utricular maculae (and of the associated action of the semicircular canals) of the frog. Phil. Trans. B **224**, 241–286 (1935).

TRENDELENBURG, W., KÜHN, A.: Vergleichende Untersuchungen zur Physiologie der Ohrlabyrinthes der Reptilien. Arch. Anat. Physiol. Suppl. 1908, pp. 160–188.

TRINCKER, D.: Neuere Untersuchungen zur Electrophysiologie des Vestibularapparates. Nautrwissenschaften **46**, 344–350 (1959).

TRINCKER, D.: Physiologie des Gleichgewichtsorgans. In: Hals-Nasen-Ohrenheilkunde, Bd. 3/1, S. 311–361. Stuttgart: Thieme 1965.

ULRICH, H.: Die Funktion der Otolithen geprüft durch die mechanische Beeinflussung des Utriculusotolithen am lebenden Hecht. Pflügers Arch. ges. Physiol. **235**, 545–553 (1935).

VIDAL, J., JEANNEROD, M., LIFSCHITZ, W., LEVITAN, H., ROSENBERG, J., SEGUNDO, J.P.: Static and dynamic properties of gravity-sensitive receptors in the cat vestibular system. Kybernetic **9**, 205–215 (1971).

VINNIKOV, YA.A.: Evolution of the gravity receptor. Estratto da Minerva Otorinolaryngologica. **24**, 1–48 (1974).

WERSÄLL, J., GLEISNER, L., LUNDQUIST, P.-G.: Ultrastructure of the vestibular end organs. In: Myotatic, Kinesthetic and Vestibular Mechanisms, pp. 105–120. London: Churchill 1967.

WITTMAAK, K.: Über den Erregungsvorgang in der Cupula. Arch. Ohrenheilk. **139**, 1 (1930).

WOLSKY, A.: Stimulationsorgane: Biol. Rev. **8**, 370–417 (1933).

WOHLFAHRT, T.A.: Anatomische Untersuchungen über das Labyrinth der Elritze (Phoxinus laevis L.). Z. vergl. Physiol. **17**, 659–685 (1932).

C. Peripheral Mechanisms

Chapter I.

Morphology of the Vestibular Sense Organ*

By

J. Wersäll and D. Bagger Sjöbäck, Stockholm

With 60 Figures

Contents

---

* Supported by Swedish Medical Research Council grant nr B71–12 X–720–06–09. The technical assistance of Miss Birgitta Björkroth and Miss Lieselotte Jakobson is cordially acknowledged.

I. Introduction

The labyrinth in vertebrates is a bilateral system of membranous sacs and channels filled with fluid, the endolymph, and surrounded by fluid, the perilymph. A capsule of cartilage or bone encapsulates and resembles grossly the membranous labyrinth. The labyrinths can schematically be divided into two forms, the static form and the statoacoustic form (DE BURLET, 1934).

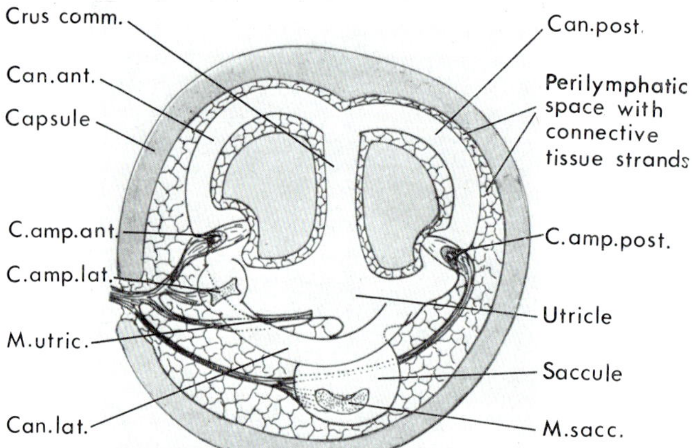

Fig. 1. Schematic drawing of a labyrinth of the static type, showing the relation between the labyrinthine membrane and the bony capsule (from DE BURLET, 1934)

The more primitive static labyrinth (Fig. 1) is provided with three semicircular canals. Each canal has a widened part, the ampule, containing a sensory area, the crista ampullaris. The canals communicate with an elongated sac, the utricle, which in turn opens into a second sac, the saccule. In both the utricle and the saccule, part of the floor is occupied by a sensory area, the macula utriculi and the macula sacculi. Each sensory area of the labyrinth is supplied by a branch of the eighth nerve. All branches unite to form the main branch of the eighth nerve, which leaves the capsule through a common opening. The membranous labyrinth is connected to the capsule by connective tissue strands which pass through the perilymphatic space and anchor the labyrinth to the walls of the capsule.

The statoacoustic labyrinth contains one or more sensory areas, each lying in an endolymphatic chamber connected to the saccule. Two more openings appear in the capsule of the labyrinth. One of these openings is covered by a mobile footplate of an accessory stapes or columella. This opening connects with the second opening, which is covered by a connective tissue membrane, via a perilymphatic channel devoid of connective tissue strands. Movements of the columellal footplate are transmitted to the new sensory area via the perilymphatic space and the thin-walled endolymphatic chamber facing the perilymphatic channel. The secondary membrane-covered opening levels out the pressure changes formed by the movements of the columella footplate.

The utricle and three semicircular canals with their ampules form the superior static part of the labyrinth. The saccule and the endolymphatic chambers connected with the saccule beside the utricle form the inferior part of the labyrinth, which is related to the acoustic function of the labyrinth.

The utricle and semicircular canals show little variation among the vertebrates apart from the cyclostomes, whereas the saccule and its outpocketing show considerable anatomical variations which correspond to functional variations.

II. Embryological Remarks

The labyrinth develops from a thickening in the ectoderm. The ectodermal thickening invaginates to form a vesicle, the otocyst. In some fishes the otocyst is permanently connected with the ectoderm surface via a duct, the endolymphatic duct. In other species this duct is closed and a separate closed duct forms the new endolymphatic duct and sac. In some fishes and amphibia the otocyst is formed from an epithelial protrusion which grows down into the epidermis and forms the otocyst.

The various parts of the labyrinth are formed by means of a complicated reorganization of the otocyst (STREETER, 1906) (Fig. 2). A fold growing into the

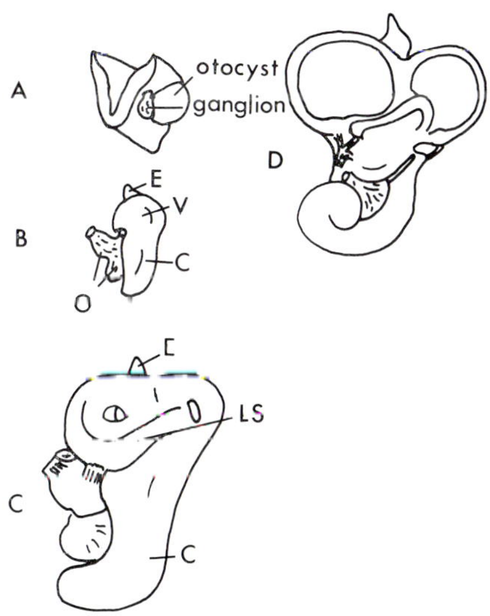

Fig. 2. Schematic drawing of development of the mammalian labyrinth (redrawn from Streeter). A: late somite embryo showing formation of the otocyst close to the neural fold. B: 9-mm stage with formation of the endolymphatic sac (E) and division of vestibular region (V) and cochlea region (C). C: 17 mm, demonstrating how at this stage the lateral semicircular canal (LS) starts to divide and the cochlear region begins to curve. D: 20-mm stage: the various parts of the labyrinth are clearly distinguished with free semicircular canals and endolymphatic duct and sac formed as well as a cochlea

otocyst divides it into a pars superior and a pars inferior. In the pars superior, opposite walls of the otocyst form deep inpocketings until the walls come into contact with each other and fuse. The remaining canals form the semicircular canals and the utricle. The two vertical canals are thought to be formed from a common anlage in which the pocket formation appears in two places, thus forming two channels with a common part. This common part forms the common crus, the crus commune, whereas at the other end the two canals widen to form ampules which end in the utricle.

The connection between the saccule and the utricle is thin in most animals, and in some cases closed by a valve. This thin duct, the utriculo-saccular duct, is also in communication with the endolymphatic duct (Engström, 1951).

Secondary outpocketings from the saccule form the lagena and the cochlea as well as their sensory areas the macula lagenae, the macula neglecta, the papilla basilaris and the organ of Corti (Retzius, 1881, 1884).

Some of the ganglion cells forming the nervus octavus come from the neuronal ganglion crest which separates early from the neuronal tube, and others from cells migrating from the ectoderm after the neural tube has closed.

The cartilaginous or osseus capsule of the labyrinth is formed secondarily to the membranous labyrinth by condensation of the mesenchyme surrounding the labyrinth. The perilymphatic space appears first as fluid spaces between the mesenchymal cells, which later form a communicating space with only thin strands of connective anchoring tissues passing through the spaces.

III. Gross Structure of the Membranous Labyrinth

A. The Cyclostome Labyrinth

The labyrinth of cyclostomes is considerably different from the labyrinth of higher vertebrates and a separate description of the cyclostome labyrinth as it appears in petromyzon and myxine thus seems justified.

The anatomy of these labyrinths was accurately described by Retzius (1881), and de Burlet and Versteeg (1930) gave a description of the petromyzon labyrinth. Recently Lowenstein and Thornhill (1970) have described the morphology and the fine structure and physiology of the myxine labyrinth, and Lowenstein, Osborne and Thornhill (1968) the anatomy and ultrastructure of the lamprey labyrinth.

1. Myxine

The labyrinth of the myxine is formed by an oblique, sagitally positioned ring. The medial part of the ring contains a macula communis. Anterior and posterior to this are the slightly widened ampules, each containing a crista ampullaris. The ampules open into the two canals, which fuse dorsally to complete the ring (Fig. 3).

The membranous labyrinth is enclosed by a kidney-shaped capsule consisting of cartilage except for its median aspect, which is formed by a membrane of connective tissue (Lowenstein and Thornhill, 1970). The capsule is penetrated by the branches of the eighth nerve supplying the sensory areas located on the macula communis and the two cristae ampullares (Fig. 4).

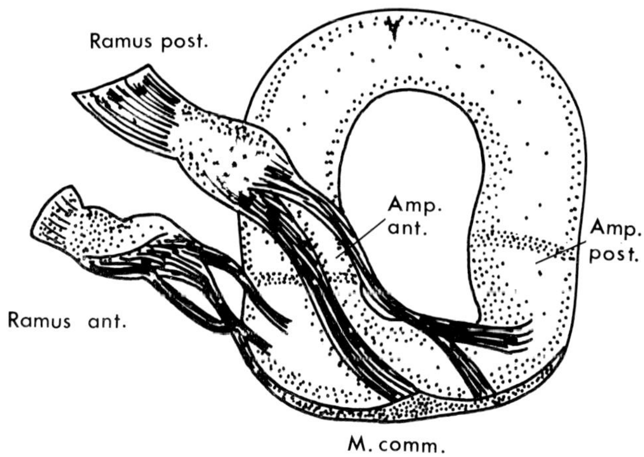

Fig. 3. Schematic drawing of the Myxine labyrinth, demonstrating the one semicircular canal and two ampules as well as the relation between the innervating nerve branches and the macula communis (Redrawn from RETZIUS)

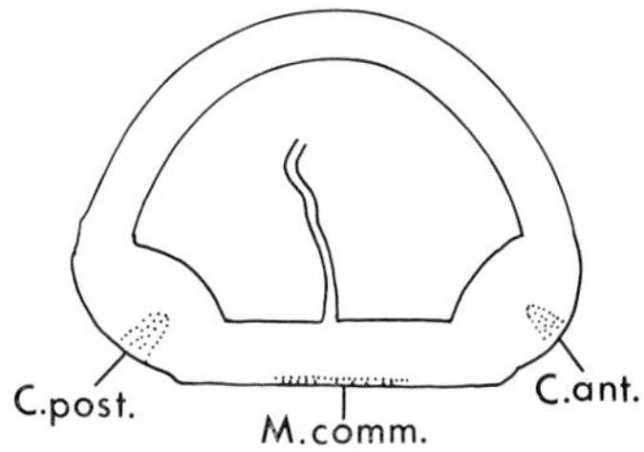

Fig. 4. Schematic drawing of the Myxine labyrinth, demonstrating the location of the crista anterior and posterior as well as of the macula communis (Redrawn from DE BURLET, 1934)

The labyrinth of the myxine differs from those of the gnathostomes in that only two ampullar cristae are present. Each crista forms an annular ridge around the inner wall of the ampule and is innervated by a branch of the eighth nerve. A cupula proper is apparently not present. The macula communis forms a continuous sheet covering the median part of the ventral wall of the labyrinthine ring. The entire macula is covered by a mass of statoconia embedded in a fibrous matrix.

The macula communis and the two cristae are covered by a sensory epithelium containing sensory cells and supporting cells. The structure and orientation of these cells will be described in conjunction with the sensory cells of other labyrinths.

2. The Petromyzon

The membranous labyrinth of the petromyzon is considerably more complicated than that of the myxine. Two semicircular canals are present, the anterior and posterior canals. Each canal widens at one end into an ampule, which in turn communicates with the elongated sac forming the median part of the labyrinth. It also communicates with one of the two ciliated chambers which are unique structures appearing only in the petromyzon labyrinth (Fig. 5).

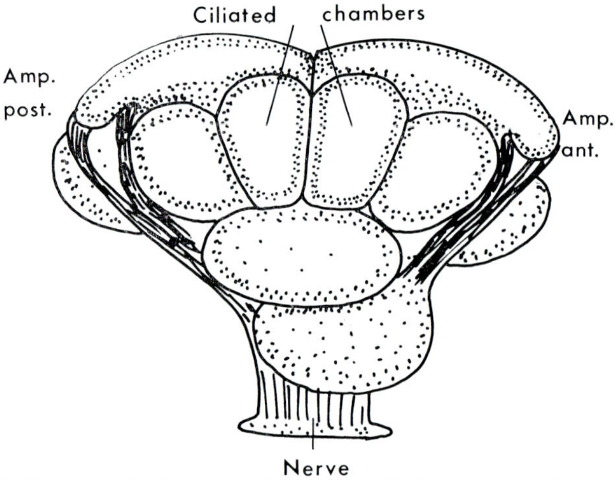

Fig. 5. Schematic drawing of petromyzon labyrinth with its two separate semicircular canals (from RETZIUS redrawn)

The ciliated chambers form two parts of the central cavity of the labyrinth which is partially divided by an incomplete ciliated chamber. As described by DE BURLET and VERSTEEG (1930), the ciliated chambers are lined with ciliated cells except for their central wall. The powerful cilia of these cells keep the endolymph in the chambers in constant movement. The ciliated chambers are divided into two compartments by an invagination of the wall of the chamber, and the two compartments have opposite rotations of the endolymphatic movements. However, the ciliated chambers, which DE BURLET considers are formations of the utricle and the common crus of the canals, have an extensive area of communication with the semicircular canals and the sac of the labyrinth. The endolymph in these compartments is undisturbed by the movements.

LOWENSTEIN and THORNHILL (1970) described three arms forming the cristae ampullares of the two ampullae, projecting from the ampullary wall into the lumen of the ampulla and covered with sensory epithelium: one basal arm along the bottom of the ampulla, one vertical and one horizontal arm. The three arms run in planes roughly perpendicular to each other. The vertical and horizontal arms correspond to the transverse crista of RETZIUS (1881) and the basal arm to the longitudinal crista.

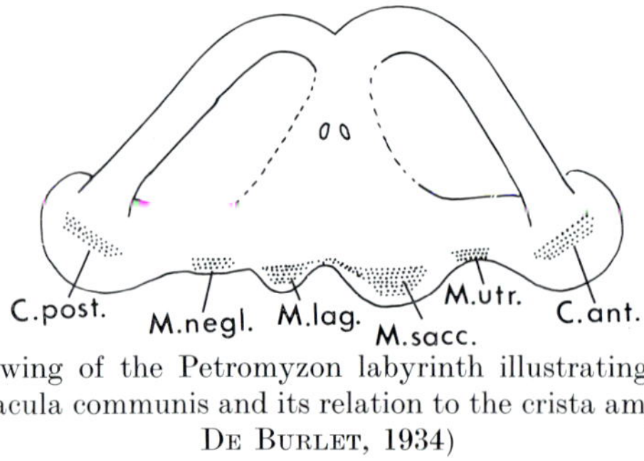

Fig. 6. Schematic drawing of the Petromyzon labyrinth illustrating the separation of the various parts of the macula communis and its relation to the crista ampullaris (Redrawn from DE BURLET, 1934)

Except for the macula neglecta, the maculae of the lamprey labyrinth form a macula communis occupying the base of the labyrinth (Fig. 6). Although this macula is covered by an uninterrupted layer of otoconia embedded in a fibrous matrix, it is possible to distinguish an anterior horizontal macula, the macula utriculi, a vertical macula, the macula sacculi, and a posterior horizontal macula, the macula lagenae. The macula dorsalis or macula neglecta lies in a separate recess on the dorsomedian face of the labyrinth.

B. Comparative Morphology of the Semicircular Canals

As already mentioned, the labyrinth of the myxine forms a circle where each of the two ampullae is in contact with one half of the united semicircular canal. In petromyzons two canals can be distinguished, which end with a common crus in the macula carrying the otosaccus (Fig. 6).

The elasmobranches are characterized by three semicircular canals which in some elasmobranches are widely separated. In the most primitive form the two vertical canals are connected to the macula bearing otosaccus only by a very thin canal. The horizontal canal ends with its two openings in the anterior vertical canal (Fig. 7). Thus there is no common crus. The study of various other elasmobranches and chondrostei reveals successive closing up of the free ends of the vertical semicircular canals till fusion takes place with formation of a common crus (Fig. 8). In cases where fusion has taken place, the posterior opening of the horizontal canal ends in the crus commune or the utricle. Even among the bony fishes some variation is seen, with separate endings of the three semicircular canals in the utricle or a high ending of the posterior crus of the horizontal canal in the common crus.

There are both inter- and intraspecies differences in the length and diameter of the semicircular canals, including differences in the ratio between the two dimensions. Very long canals are found in elasmobranches and many birds. On the other hand, frogs and some mammals, have thick, short canals. The

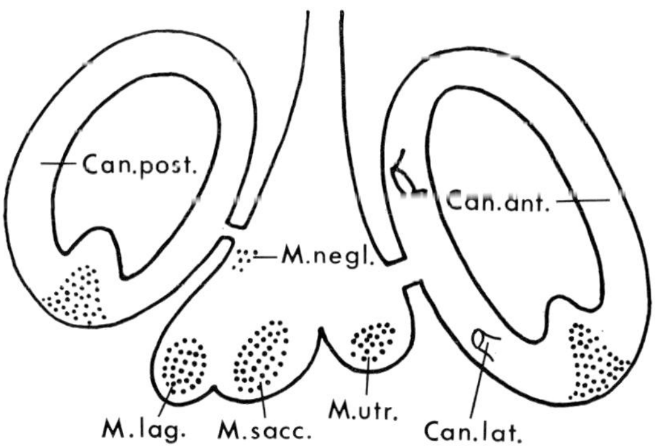

Fig. 7. Schematic drawing of the labyrinth of ray. The anterior and posterior semicircular canals are completely separate; only the openings of the lateral canal are illustrated. The macula lagenae, the macula sacculi and the macula utriculi are only partly separated (From DE BURLET, 1934)

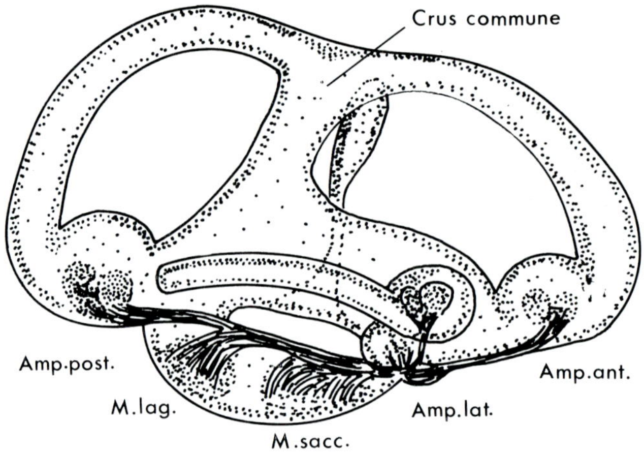

Fig. 8. Schematic drawing of a chondrostial labyrinth illustrating the development of the common crus

horizontal canal is generally thinner in fishes than the vertical canals. In pigeon, the anterior vertical canal is almost twice as long as the posterior vertical canal.

Whether these variations between species have any physiological significance is hard to say. It seems likely, however, that the isolated canals of the elasmobranches prevent foreign bodies from reaching the ampullae through the endolymphatic duct, which in these animals is in more or less open communication with the seawater (DE BURLET, 1934).

C. Comparative Morphology of the Utricle and Saccule

1. The Utricle

The utricle is a structure which varies very little throughout phylogenetic development. It is an elongated sac in most animals, which receives the opening of the anterior vertical canal at its anterior end, where a slightly widened part, the utricular recess, is found in its floor and contains the utricular macula. The posterior end of the utricle receives the opening of the posterior vertical ampulla. Its middle upper surface has an opening for the common crus of the vertical canals, and its lateral wall receives the crus simplex of the horizontal canal. This opening is located slightly posterior to the opening of the crus commune. A thin canal connects the middle part of the floor of the utricle with the saccular duct and the endolymphatic duct (Fig. 1).

This picture is somewhat different in elasmobranches, as mentioned above; the semicircular canals are more or less separate structures connected with the utricle only by thin ducts, and the utricle and saccule with their diverticula form a widely communicating sac, the otosaccus, which contains the various sensory areas of the macular type (Figs. 7, 9). In some fishes the connection between the utricle and saccule is said to be closed. In some mammals a valve partly occludes the saccule from the utricle (ENGSTRÖM, 1951).

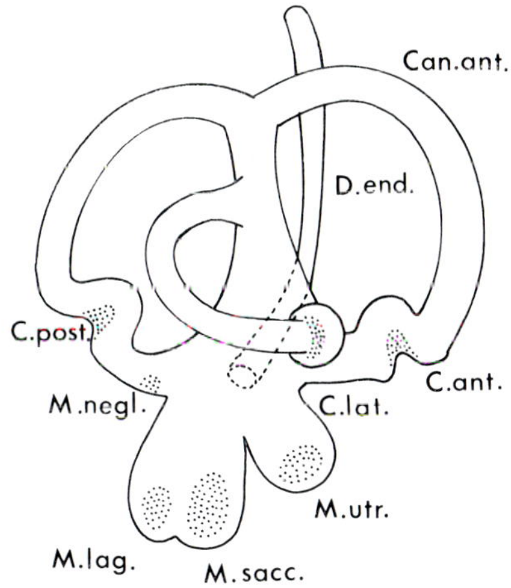

Fig. 9. An elasmobranch fish with a common crus and the ending of the lateral canal in the common crus. The macula utriculi is moved towards the anterior ampulla (Redrawn from DE BURLET, 1934)

2. The Saccule

The saccule varies widely in size and configuration. The macula sacculi proper and the outpocketings of the saccule vary in size, forming a number of sensory areas, some of which have unknown functions.

The saccule has not been observed in the myxine. In petromyzons the vertical macula protrudes into an outpocketing of the otosaccus which can be considered a homolog to the saccule. A separate macula lagena can also be observed in these animals (Fig. 6).

The saccule is only partly separated from the utricle in elasmobranches, and together with the utricle it forms the otosaccus, which is separate from the semicircular canals and connected with them only by thin canals. An outpocketing forming a lagena is only partly demarcated from the wall of the saccule (Figs. 7, 9).

The size of the saccule relative to the semicircular canals and to the lagena varies widely in ganoids and teleosts (Fig. 10). In some cases the saccule protrudes upward and fills the space inside the horizontal canal, as in the *Gobius niger* where the lagena is a small sac located ventrally and far to the rear. In the *Amia calva* the opposite is the case. Here the lagena is considerably larger than the saccule. In the *Amia calva* the saccule and the lagena are very small compared to the superior part of the labyrinth.

Amphibia are provided with a sacculus projection from the medial wall of the saccule close to the connection between the utricle and the saccule. This recess is called recessus amphibiorum, and the sensory area of the recess the papilla amphibiorum (Fig. 10). This sensory area is directed ventrally. In most amphibia another recess, the recessus papillae basilaris, is found posterior to the macula lagenae; in certain reptiles, in birds, and in mammals this recess forms the cochlear duct.

The recessus amphibiorum and the recessus papillae basilaris lie close to the perilymphatic duct system, which is widely developed in the amphibia. Some

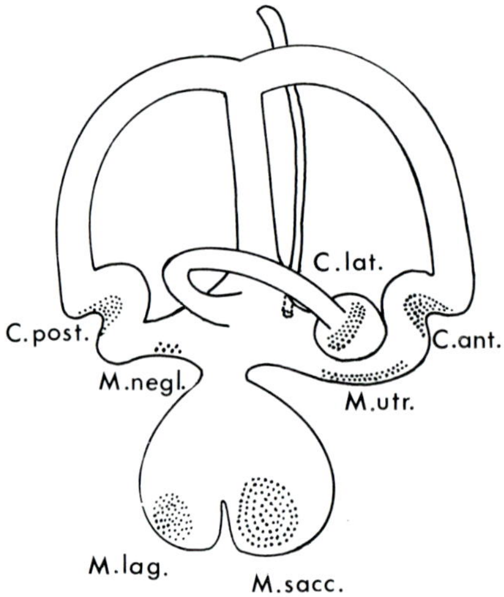

Fig. 10. Schematic drawing of a bony fish; the lateral canal ends in the utricle and the macula utriculi is located in a utricle recess in the anterior part of the utricle

amphibiae, like the salamander, have the papilla amphibiorum but not the papilla basilaris. In reptiles, an important difference is seen in the wall of the recessus papillae basilaris in that the membrane facing the perilymphatic space is thinned out, forming a membrana basilaris.

The papilla basilaris is small compared with the lagena in amphibia (Fig. 11). In reptiles a gradual change is found, so that in crocodiles the papilla basilaris is large compared with the lagena. In this case the recess of the papilla basilaris forms a long tube, the cochlear duct, which thus appears for the first time in the crocodiles. The papilla basilaris is also larger than the lagena in turtles and snakes, in which the lagena and the papilla basilaris lie in a common cavity, with the lagena located peripherally and the papilla basilaris closer to the saccule.

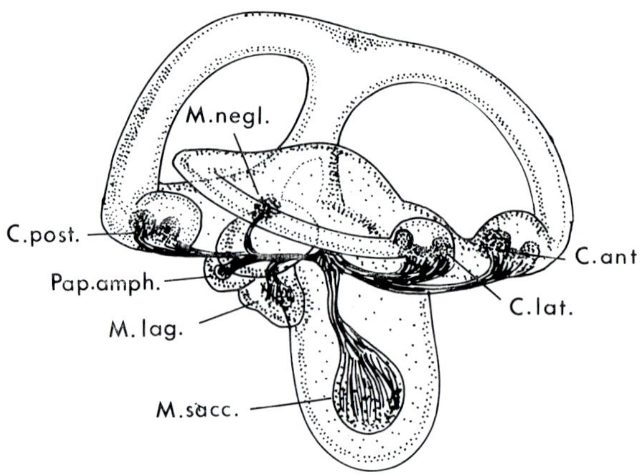

Fig. 11. Schematic drawing of a frog labyrinth, illustrating the large sacculi and the separation of the lagena and papilla amphibiorum from the sacculus (Redrawn from Retzius)

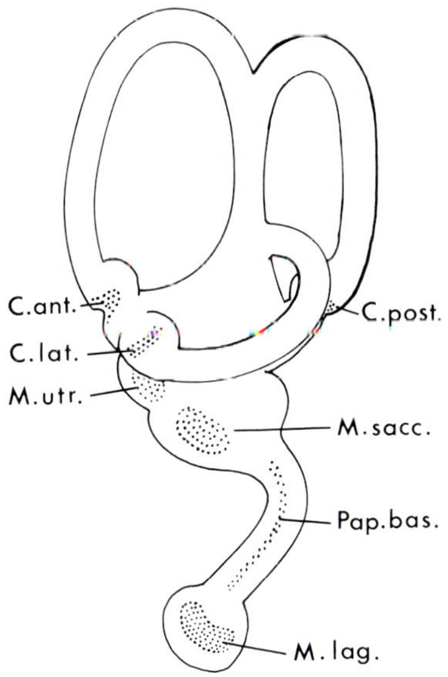

Fig. 12. Schematic drawing of a bird labyrinth, illustrating the displacement of the macula lagenae away from the saccule with formation of a papilla basilaris

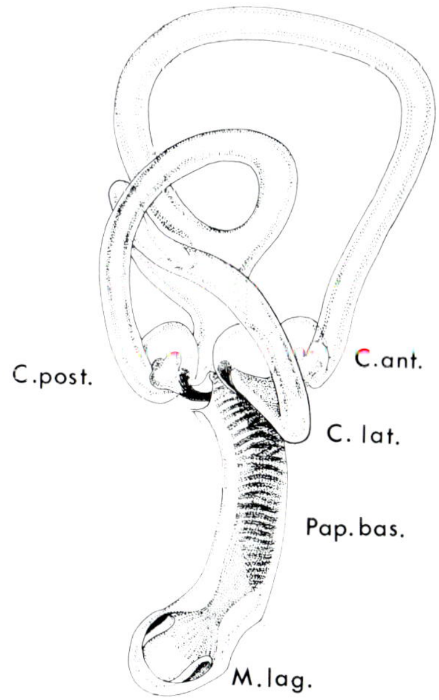

Fig. 13. Schematic drawing of a bird labyrinth, illustrating the often complicated relation between the three semicircular canals in some birds (Redrawn from RETZIUS)

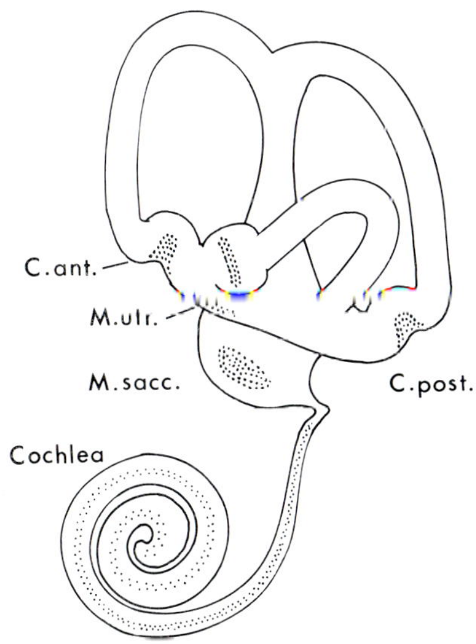

Fig. 14. Schematic drawing of the mammalian labyrinth with a fully developed cochlea

The lagena in crocodiles and birds is displaced into a somewhat widened blind sac forming the end of the cochlear duct (Figs. 12, 13). The curvature of the cochlear duct is slight in birds, and is much more pronounced in mammals, where a varying number of coils form a complete cochlea. The lagena, which is still present in the monotremata, is not found in higher mammals. The basilar membrane which appears at the reptilian stage of evolution is still more pronounced in birds and mammals, where the sensory epithelium is in the form of the papilla basilaris in birds and the organ of Corti in mammals (Fig. 14). The membrane opposite to the basilaris membrane is rich in vessels, forming a membrana vasculosa. The scanning light microscope reveals the existence of dark cells in this membrane; these resemble other dark-staining cells in the labyrinth, which have been described by many authors as secretory cells and were early studied and mapped by IWATA (1924).

The two labyrinths are connected by the canalis communicans transversus in many bony fishes. This canal, which connects the sacculi of the two labyrinths, is a part of Weber's apparatus, which conducts vibrations from the swimbladder to the inner ear.

IV. Structure of the Labyrinthine Wall

If we disregard the sensory epithelia, which will be considered in greater detail later, the wall of the labyrinth is composed of an epithelial layer and a connective tissue layer.

The epithelium is a one-layered epithelium. In some areas of the labyrinth, including the semicircular canals proper, certain areas of the utricle, the roof

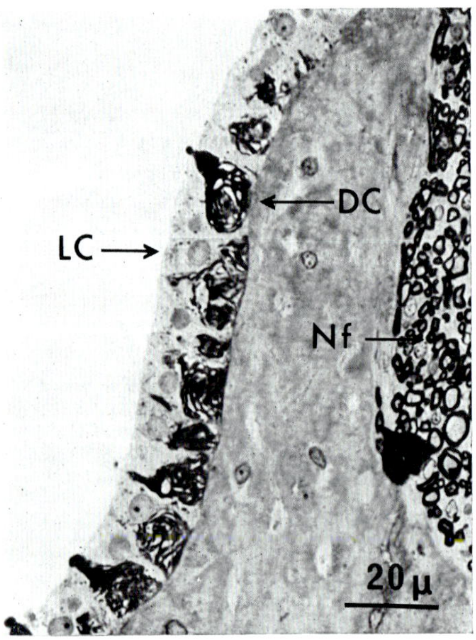

Fig. 15. Light micrograph showing a section of the crista ampullaris from a lizard, illustrating the light cells (LC) and dark cells (DC) along the utricular side of the crista. Nf: nerve fibers in the crista

of the ampullae, and the saccule, the epithelium is undifferentiated and squamous. In other areas the epithelium is differentiated into a secretory epithelium with certain types of cells.

A. The Dark Cells

The epithelial cell type which has been most studied is the so-called dark cell type. These cells were described as early as 1876 by Mayer and Kuhn in teleost fishes and in the frog. Iwata (1924) described secretory areas in the bat. Ultrastructural analysis of these cells in the utricle by Smith (1956, 1967, 1970) revealed that they are provided with extensive basal infoldings of the plasma membrane resting on the basement membrane of the epithelium. The nucleus is displaced towards the surface, and the surface facing the endolymphatic space is provided with microvilli of varying lengths (Figs. 15–17). Multiple pinocytotic vesicles close to the surface are suggestive of fluid passage through the cells, and large numbers of mitochondria in the basal protrusion of the cell suggest a high metabolic activity around the basal protrusions and infoldings. The fine structure of these cells in the neighboring crista ampullaris has been analyzed by Kimura, Lundquist and Wersäll (1963). Kimura (1969) demonstrated the widespread

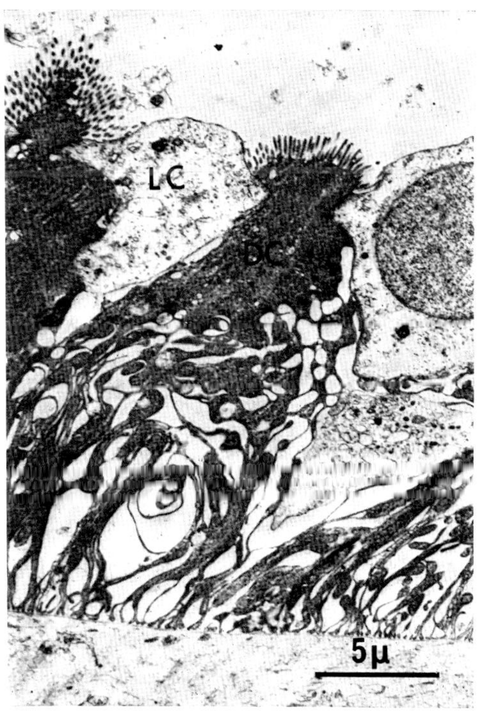

Fig. 16. Electron micrograph illustrating light cells (LC) and dark cells (DC) in the lateral wall of the crista ampullaris from a lizard. Observe the fine microvilli on the surface of the dark cell and the many cellular protrusions resting as feet on the basement membrane

localization of the dark cells in the guinea-pig labyrinth, and also found these cells in similar localizations in bat, oppossum, cat, Rhesus monkey, and man. Although a certain variation in the pattern of distribution was found, the dark cells were found in the walls of all ampullae.

Between the dark cells and the sensory epithelium is a layer of tall cylindrical cells containing secretory granules; Kimura et al. (1963) called these the transitional cells. On the utricular side of the crista ampullaris lateralis the dark cells form a continuous layer around the opening to the utricle from the roof of the ampulla to its bottom. The entire posterior endolymphatic wall of the utricle is lined with dark cells. On the anterior wall of the utricle the dark cells are not found within the immediate periphery of the macula. Instead, this area is lined with a well-defined layer of cuboidal cells. A dark-cell epithelial lining is found

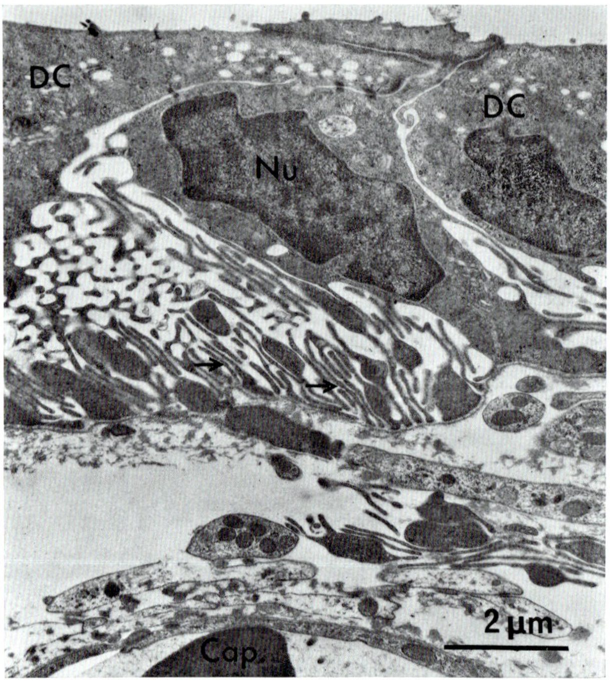

Fig. 17. Dark cells from the utricular side of the crista ampullaris lateralis from a guinea-pig. Nu: nuclei in a dark cell. A number of pinocytotic vesicles are found close to the surface. A large number of basilar protrusions from the cells containing mitochondria (arrows) are resting on the basement membrane. A capillary is seen immediately below the basement membrane

on the lateral wall of the common crus. Dark cells are not, however, found in the wall of the saccule. In lizards the dark cells alternate with light cells. The surface of the dark cells protrudes over the surface covered with abundant microvilli (Figs. 15, 16).

As the dark cells are structurally similar to the ion-transporting epithelia of the renal tubules, ciliary plexus, choroid plexus, and salt-secreting glands, they have been thought to be involved in the endolymphatic circulation. NAKAI and HILDING (1968) reported evidence of ATPase activity on the surface of the folded membranes and suggested that endolymph is formed by a passage of ions and water between the cells. DOHLMAN (1965) considered that dark cells had a secretory function in the labyrinth of pigeon.

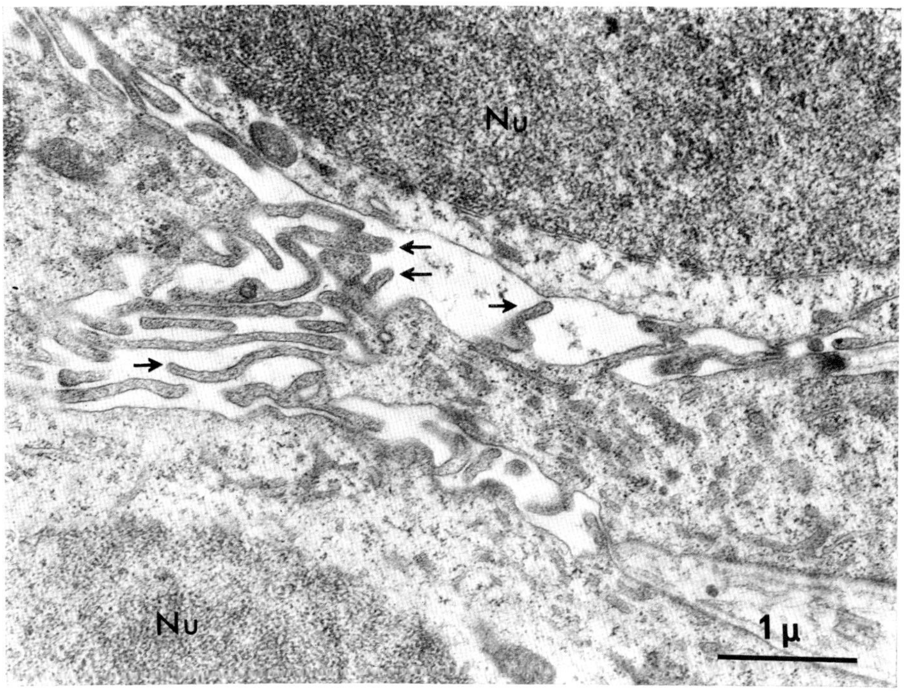

Fig. 18. A large number of microvilli protrusions are found between the intermediate cells on the sides of the crista ampullaris as well as between the planum semilunatum cells. Nu: nucleus. Arrows indicate intercellular protrusions of the cells. Electronmicrograph

SMITH (1970) stresses the appearance of lateral infoldings between some of the cells in the labyrinth, including the transitional cells in the periphery of the crista epithelium (Fig. 18). She suggests that the dark cells with basal infoldings represent a tissue fluid to endolymph transport, whereas the transport in or between the cells with lateral infoldings should be from the endolymph to the tissue fluid. Alternatively, she suggests that the basal infolded cells may transfer sodium from endolymph, in which case the directional flow would be in the opposite direction.

The planum semilunatum, which is the area forming a semilunar surface of rather tall columnar cells containing granules in the ampullar wall at the ends of the cristae, has also been discussed as a possible source of products secreted into the endolymph. In the horizontal ampulla there is usually only one planum in one end of the ampulla (Wersäll, 1956; Bairati and Iurato, 1960).

Hilding and Wersäll (1962) showed higher concentrations of nonspecific cholinesterase in the area of the planum semilunatum. Although much work has been done on the morphology of the variety of cells found in the labyrinthine wall, the unavailability of sufficiently good methods for the study of the activity of the cells has made it difficult to clarify their function.

It seems likely, however, that it is not only the striae vasculares in the cochlea, where present, or the tegmentum vasculosum that are responsible for the production of the endolymph, but that endolymph production is a complicated process which certainly involves most of the cell types in the labyrinth.

V. The Topographic Organization of the Sensory Areas

The sensory areas are best grouped according to the covering structure in which the sensory hairs are more or less embedded. Thus they can be divided into cupula-covered structures: cristae ampullares and macula neglecta; otolith-covered structures: macula utriculi, macula sacculi, macula lagenae; tectorial membrane-covered structures: the papilla basilaris and the organ of Corti. The present paper does not go into the fine structure of the organ of Corti and the papilla basilaris, which will be dealt with in a later volume.

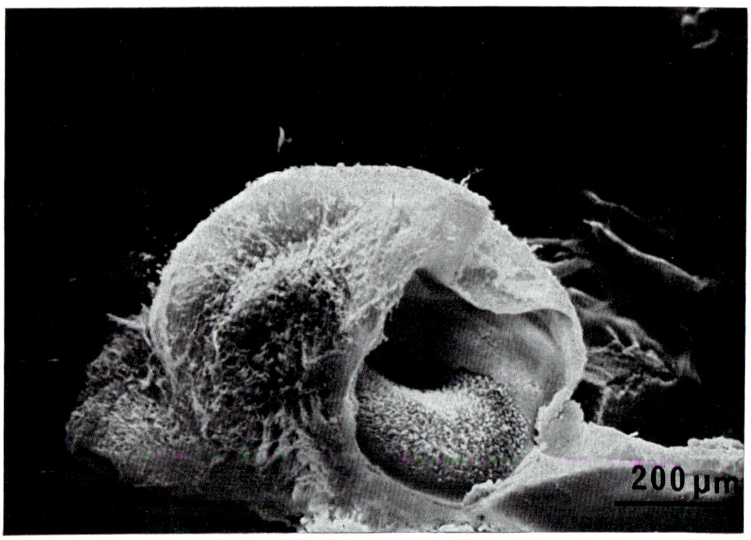

Fig. 19. The crista ampullaris forms a septum transversing the base of the ampulla. An opening in the ampullar wall demonstrates the localization of the crista ampullaris in a guinea-pig ampulla. Scanning electron micrograph

A. The Crista Ampullaris

The crista ampullaris is a transverse septum running across the ampulla more or less perpendicular to the plane of the canal (Fig. 19). The top of this septum is covered by a sensory epithelium, on which a gelatinous structure rests, the so-called cupula filling out the space between the summit of the crista and the ampullar roof (Fig. 20). The height of the crista varies, as does the area of the crista covered with sensory epithelium. Frogs and fishes have a comparatively small sensory epithelium compared to the large ampule and the high crista, while mammals have large parts of the crista covered with sensory epithelium (Figs. 21–24) (WERSÄLL et al., 1965).

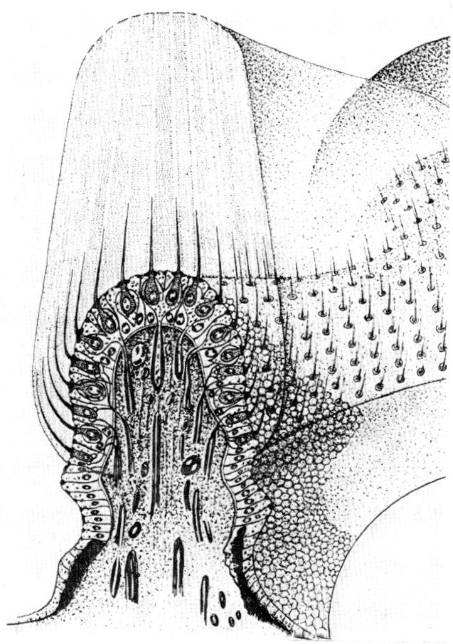

Fig. 20. Schematic drawing of the crista ampullaris in the guinea-pig labyrinth illustrating the sensory cells and their relation to the innervating nerve fibres. The sensory hair bundles from the hair cells protrude into channels of the cupula resting on top of the crista surface

Although the crista in fishes is often supplied by two separate nerve branches, each supplying half of the crista, it is in reptiles that a division of the cristae of the vertical canals into two parts is observed. In some reptiles this division is marked only by a lack of sensory epithelium in one part in the middle of the crista. In other reptiles, as in birds, protrusion is found on the utricular as well as the canal side of the crista covered by cylindrical nonsensory epithelium, the septum cruciatum.

This division of the crista into two halves is exceptional in mammals. It is, however, found in cat and in bat. The floor of the ampule forms a shallow groove at the base of each side of the crista. In cristae where a septum cruciatum divides

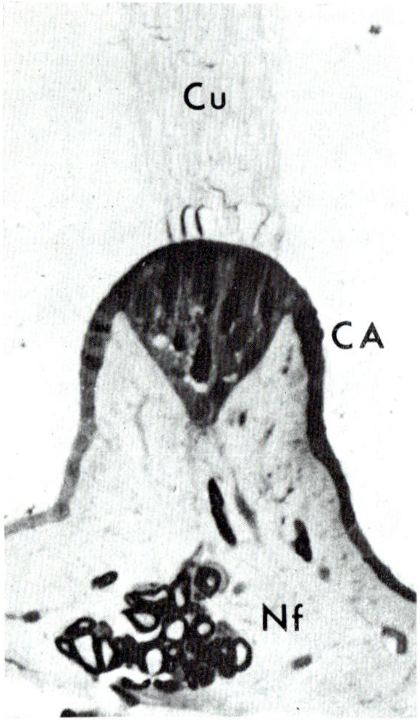

Fig. 21. Crista ampullaris from a frog ampulla with a cupula resting on top of the sensory epithelium from which sensory hairs seem to protrude

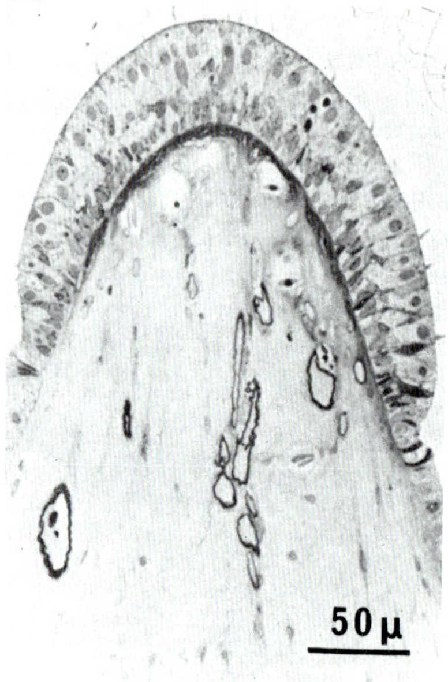

Fig. 22. Crista ampullaris from a ray labyrinth with a large number of sensory cells

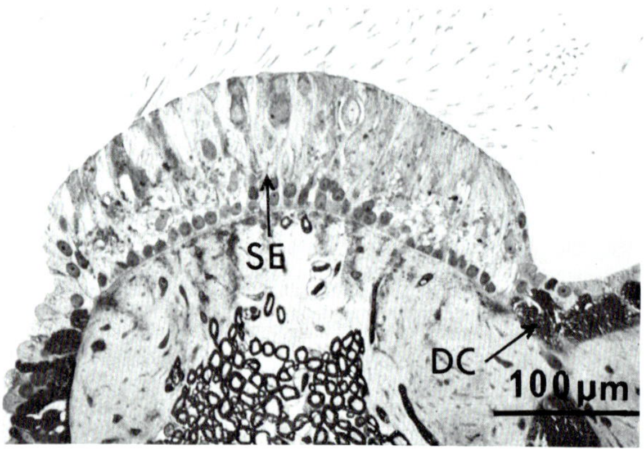

Fig. 23. Crista ampullaris from a lizard ampulla. *SE*: sensory epithelium, *DC*: dark cells on the utricular side of the epithelium

the crista into two halves, even the grove is divided. In these cases fluid displacement in the canals follows two completely separate paths on the two sides of the crista.

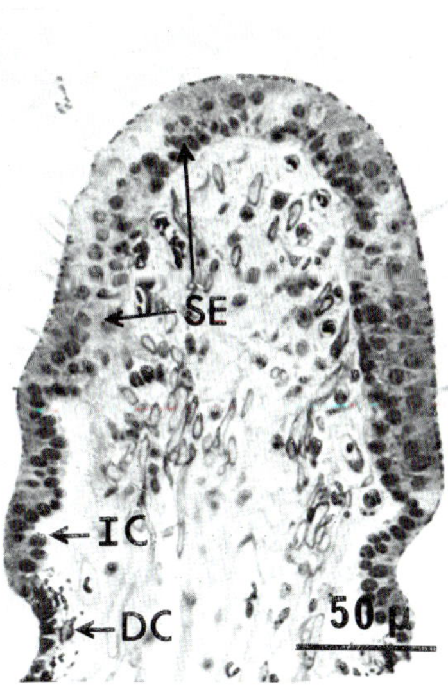

Fig. 24. Crista ampullaris from a guinea-pig ampulla with sensory epithelium (SE), intermediate cells (IC), and dark cells (DC). Compare with the schematic drawing (Fig. 20)

B. The Macula Neclecta

The macula neglecta (Figs. 7, 9–11), which resembles the crista ampullaris in many ways, was first found in the utricle of birds by RETZIUS (1884). This end organ is always found in fishes, sometimes in duplicate. Its localization varies from the area immediately behind the junction of the utricle and the saccule to a situation located lower down under the opening of the common crus. A special situation is found in sharks, where the macula densa is located in the tube connecting the posterior vertical canal with the rest of the labyrinth. The sensory epithelium of the macula neglecta is covered by a cupula which completely fills out the tube around the macula in the shark and has the appearance of a dome over the macula in other animals. The structure has also been called the crista quarta, which stresses its relation to the cristae ampullares rather than to the otolith-carrying maculae (LOWENSTEIN et al., 1964). The macula neglecta is not found in amphibia and is only found in some mammals (GATSEK, 1966). It is fairly regularly found in cats. Amphibia have a different type of sensory area, which is called the papilla amphibiorum and is located in the upper part of the recessus sacculi. Like the macula neglecta it is covered by a cupula-like structure. It is thought to function mainly as an acoustic receptor.

C. The Macula Utriculi, the Macula Sacculi and the Macula Lagenae

Although variations are seen in the size and general shape of the macula utriculi and sacculi as well as in the size of the covering layer, the plane of orientation of the main surface of the macula is fairly constant (WERNER, 1933, 1940, 1960; LINDEMAN, 1962, 1970).

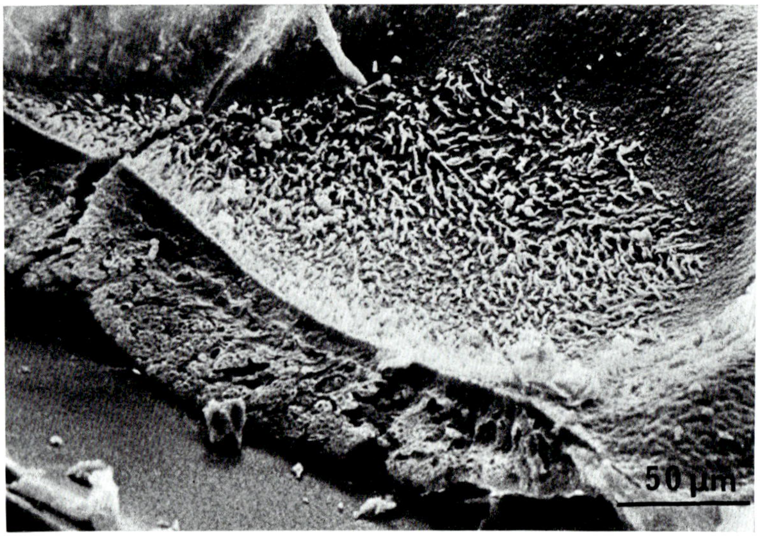

Fig. 25. In most labyrinths the macula utriculi is spoon-shaped. This macula was fractured during preparation. The hair bundles on the surface are seen as thin tufts protruding from the macular surface. The otoconium membrane was removed. Scanning electron micrograph

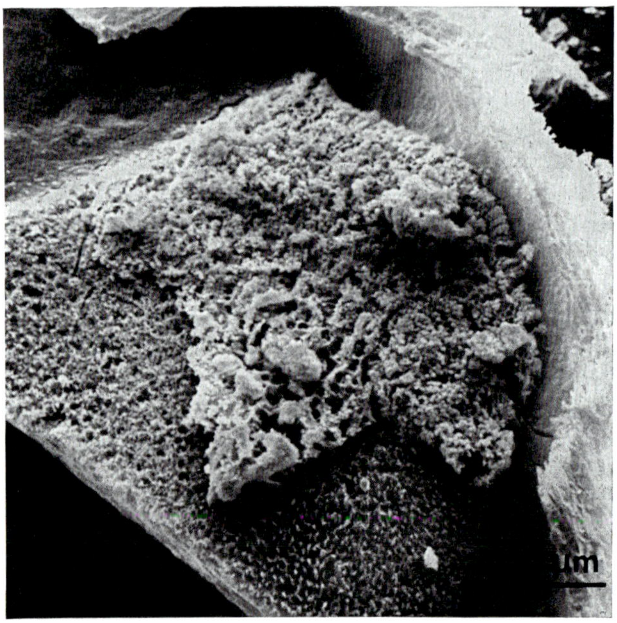

Fig. 26. A part of the otoconium membrane was left intact on the surface of this macula utriculi from a monkey. Scanning electron micrograph

1. The Macula Utriculi

The macula utriculi, which originally forms part of the otosaccus (Figs. 7–9), is found on the floor of the anterior part of the utricle in bony fishes and higher vertebrates (Figs. 10, 11). The main orientation of the macula is in the plane of the horizontal canal. Some of the anterior part of the utricle is often separated from the rest of the utricle as the recessus utriculi. The macula is roughly heart-shaped, with a slightly spoon-shaped depression on its surface (Fig. 25). In mammals, the anterior end is elevated at a wide angle to the main surface (WERNER, 1933, 1940, 1960).

2. The Macula Sacculi and the Macula Lagenae

The *macula sacculi* is found on the medial wall of the saccule. Its plane is roughly vertical. The *macula lagenae* forms a continuation of the macula sacculi in fishes and amphibia. The surface is, however, bent in such a way that its spatial orientation is difficult to define (Fig. 60). With the development of the *papilla basilaris* the macula neglecta is pushed in a peripheral direction, a development which is found in crocodiles but is more pronounced in birds, where the cochlea separates the lagena from the saccular macula. The lagena is not found in mammals (RETZIUS, 1881, 1884; JOERGENSEN, 1970).

The cover of the maculae is composed of a combination of hard substance and a gelatinous covering layer. The hard substance is composed of calcium carbonate crystals and foreign material in sharks, where there is an open communication between the labyrinth and the seawater. In ganoids and teleost fishes the hard substance forms a compact stone, the statolith. The statolith is often larger than the sensory epithelium. It is fixed to the epithelium surrounding the macula by a gelatinous embedding substance (WERNER, 1960).

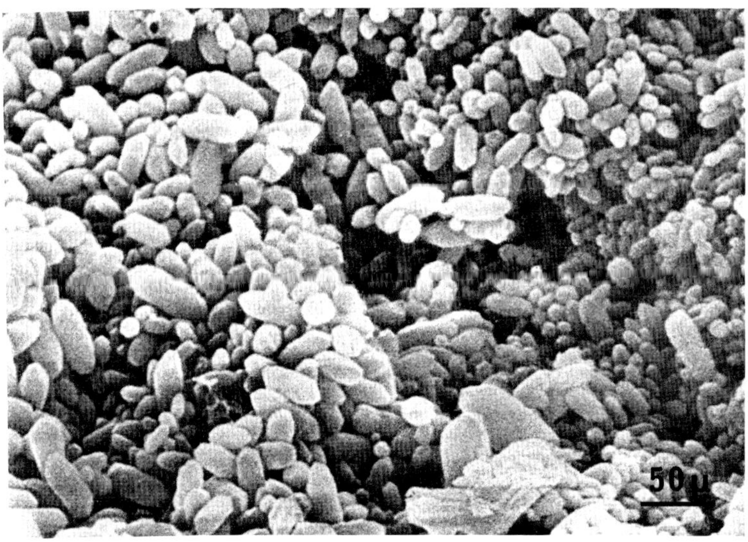

Fig. 27. The hexagonal configuration of the otoconia in the otoconium membrane from a guinea-pig macula utriculi is clearly seen on this scanning electron micrograph

The otoconium membrane of amphibia, birds, and mammals is composed of otoconia i. e. crystals formed by calcite of aragonite in a gelatinous embedding substance (Figs. 26–27). The lagena is like the macula sacculi and utriculi covered by a statolith or an otolothic membrane respectively (CARLSTRÖM, 1963; CARLSTRÖM and ENGSTRÖM, 1955; CARLSTRÖM et al., 1953).

VI. The Minute Structure of the Sensory Epithelia

A. General Structure

The sensory areas are covered by a sensory epithelium. The basic structure of this epithelium is the same throughout the phylogenetic development from the myxine to the mammalian labyrinth. The sensory cells are secondary receptor cells, i.e. they receive a stimulus from the surrounding medium and transform the effect of the stimulus via synapses to nerve endings of the innervating nerve fibers inside the epithelium (WERSÄLL and FLOCK, 1965; FLOCK, 1971). The

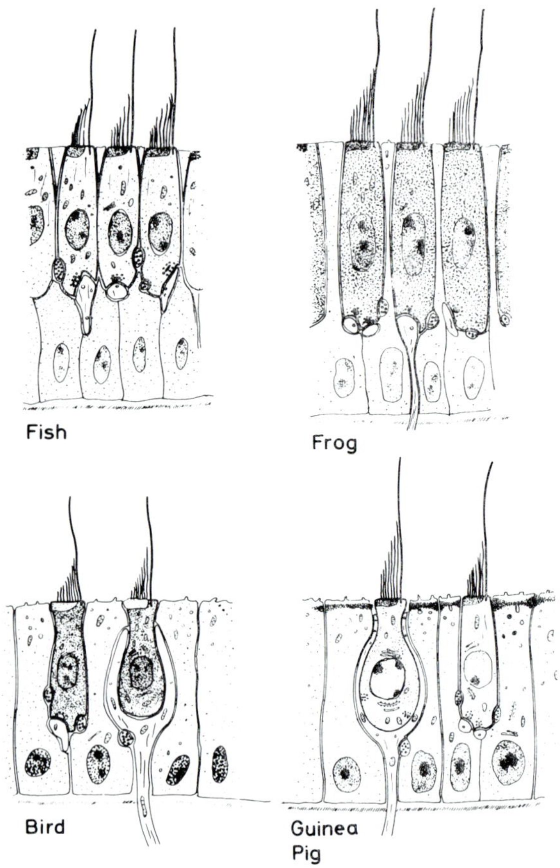

Fig. 28. Schematic drawing illustrating the various types of sensory epithelia in fish, frog, bird, and guinea pig. Fish and frogs have only one type of cylindrical haircells and supporting cells, whereas birds and mammals and lizards have two types of sensory cells

sensory cells are cylindrical, globular, or flask-shaped. They reach from the surface through part of the epithelium but never to the basement membrane of the epithelium. The distal part of each sensory cell is surrounded by the distal part of a number of *supporting cells*. These cells reach from the surface down to the basement membrane, where neighboring supporting cells are in close contact with each other and only separated by nerve fibers penetrating the basement membrane on their way to the sensory cells. The basal part of the supporting cells is generally broad and contains the nucleus. The middle part, which protrudes between the sensory cells, is often flattened out to a thin prismatic portion extending to the epithelial surface. A specially developed sensory epithelium is found in birds, lizards, and mammals, where two types of sensory cells are found, haircells of type I and of type II (WERSÄLL, 1956; WERSÄLL et al., 1967; VINNIKOV 1965).

B. Fine Structure of the Sensory Cells

Sensory cells in all sensory areas of the labyrinth are provided with a hair bundle protruding from the flat cell surface and their structure is basically the same in all animals (Figs. 28–30).

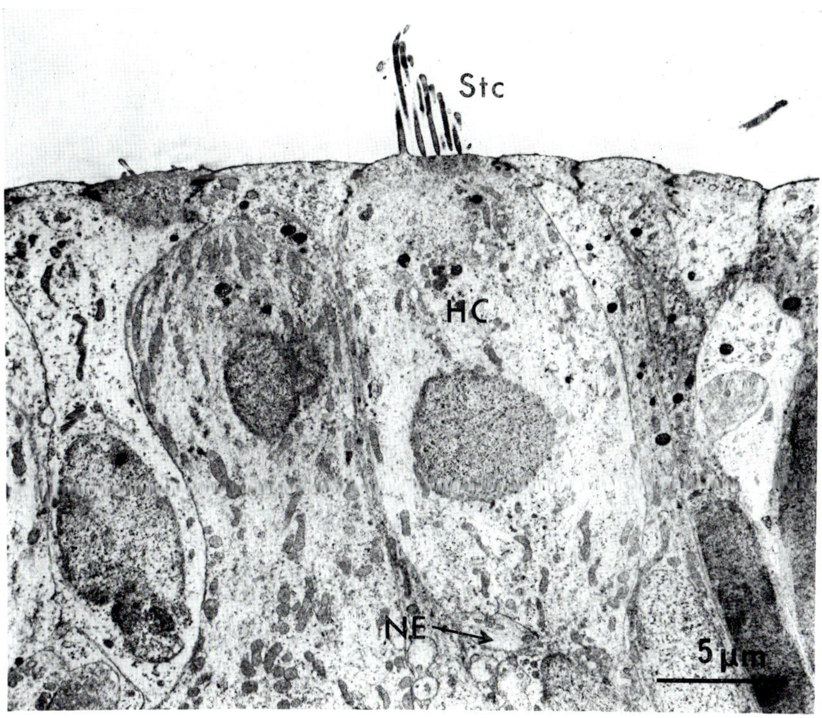

Fig. 29. The cylindrical hair cells in the ray labyrinth are provided with a hair bundle on the cell surface. In this picture only the stereocilia are seen. Afferent and efferent nerve endings (NE) attached to the bottom of the cell

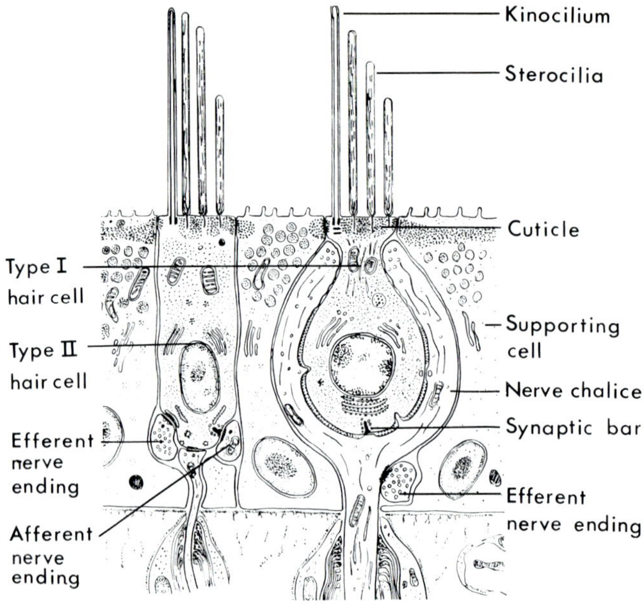

Fig. 30. Schematic drawing of the two types of sensory cells in the mammalian labyrinth showing the fine structure organisation of the type I and the type II sensory cells and their innervation

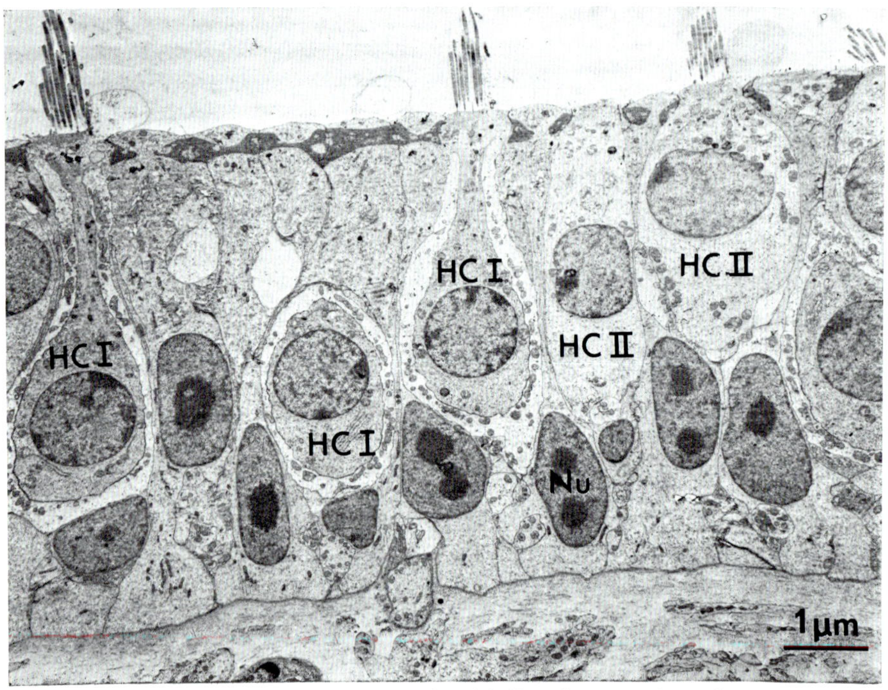

Fig. 31. Survey picture of the macula utriculi epithelium from a guinea-pig macula utriculi illustrating type I and type II haircells. Haircells of type I (HCI) are surrounded by a large nerve chalice, whereas the type II haircells (HCII) are innervated by small nerve terminals attached to the bottom of the haircell. Sensory hair bundles are seen to protrude from the cell surface of each cell. Transmission electron micrograph

Immediately below the plasma membrane a cuticle is located, which is composed of densely packed granules forming an opaque plate extending somewhat varying depths into the cell. The cuticle is best developed in birds and mammals and forms a rather thin and somewhat irregular plate in cyclostomes and fishes. The cuticle covers most of the distal part of the cell, but leaves a small area on one side open; at this point the cytoplasm of the cell is in direct contact with the plasma membrane of the cell surface. This open part contains the basal body of a kinocilium which protrudes at various distances over the cell surface (Figs. 30, 31). A globular protrusion of cell cytoplasm, possibly a fixation artifact, is often seen in the same area.

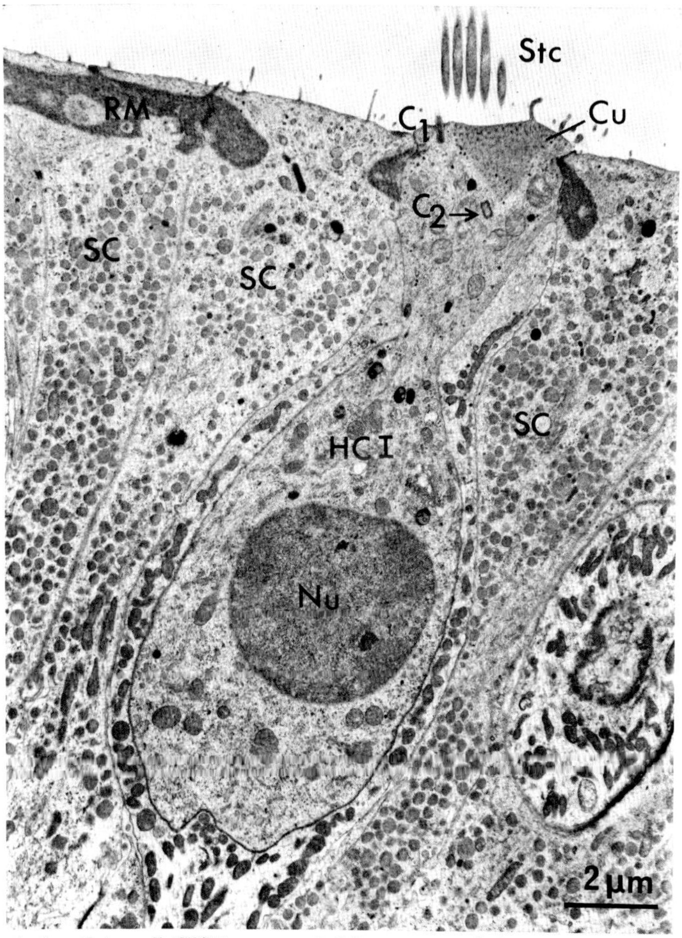

Fig. 32. The hair cell type I (HCI) surrounded by a nerve chalice enclosing the major part of the cell surface. Spherical nucleus (Nu) is found in the lower part of the cell. Stereocilia (Stc) protrude from the cuticle (Cu). A kinocilium protrudes from a basal body or a centriole C_1, whereas the second centriole of the cell is found below the cuticle C_2. A reticulum membrane (RM) is formed in the top of the supporting cells (SC). Each supporting cell contains a very large number of granules

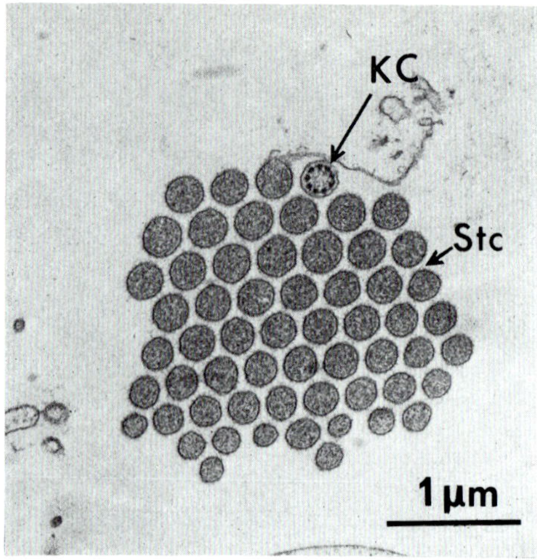

Fig. 33. Cross-section from a hair bundle close to the cell surface illustrating the regularity in the arrangement of the stereocilia (Stc) and the kinocilium (KC) located in the periphery of the hair bundle. The sensory hairs are arranged in hexagonal figures in the bundle, which also has a similar hexagonal shape transmission electron micrograph (TEMG)

The structure of the *kinocilium* and its basal body varies in various species. In cyclostomes, frogs, and fishes the kinocilium is composed of nine peripheral double-tubular fibrils surrounding two single-tubular fibrils (Figs. 33, 34) (WERSÄLL et al., 1965; FLOCK, 1965; LOWENSTEIN et al., 1970). The fibril bundle is surrounded by a triple-layered plasma membrane. The structure of the distal shaft of the cilium is thus identical with that of the vibratile cilia in various ciliated cells. The diameter of the cilium varies from 0.2–0.3 μm. The basal part of the cilium forms a neck with a slightly larger diameter than the shaft proper (Fig. 35). The two central filaments end in the neck. The peripheral double filaments continue into the cell, where a third, short, tubular filament is added to the other two in such a way that a triple-tubuled cylinder is formed, with a structure closely resembling that of a centriole (Figs. 35, 36). A dense spoke protrudes from each triple tubule and extends obliquely outward towards the plasma membrane, giving the appearance of a paddle wheel when a section is made through this area parallel to the plasma membrane and the surface. A basal foot protrudes from the basal body on the side facing away from the central part of the cuticle. A second body built like a centriole is often found below the basal body. This centriole often lies with its axis in right angles to the surface of the cells (Fig. 36).

The central two tubular filaments of the kinocilium and the basal foot are not present in myxine (LOWENSTEIN et al., 1970). In the kinocilium of mammals the peripheral nine fibrils are regularly found. The tubular nature of the filaments is often difficult to identify in the central two filaments. These filaments often appear as compact filaments, and although two filaments are usually found, sometimes they are reduced to one filament, or the central filaments are missing

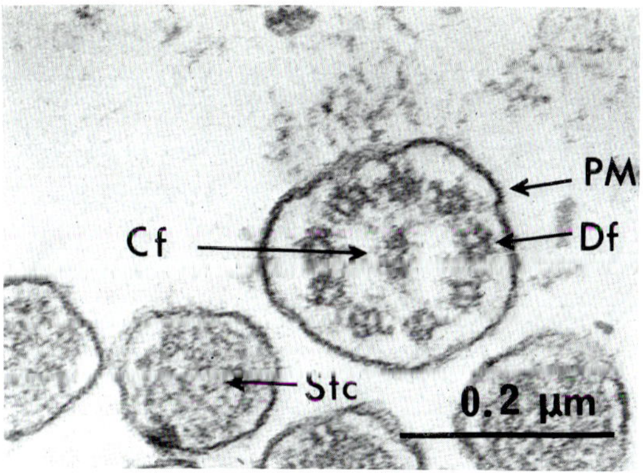

Fig. 34. Part of a cross-sectioned hair bundle from a guinea-pig crista ampullaris illustrates the fine structure of the kinocilium and a few stereocilia. The kinocilium is composed of a filament bundle with nine double tubular filaments (Df) surrounding two central filaments (Cf). The filaments are surrounded by a plasma membrane (PM). The central filaments are often irregular in mammalian labyrinths. Stc: stereocilium (TEMG)

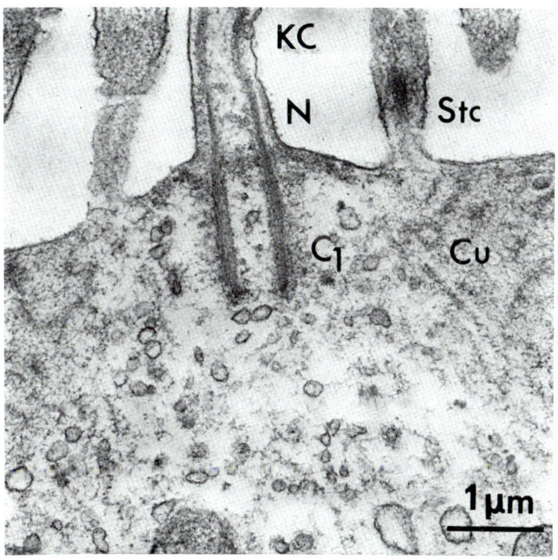

Fig. 35. A section through part of the apical portion of a sensory cell of a guinea-pig labyrinth illustrates the basal body or centriole of the kinocilium (C_1) and protruding kinocilium proper with its neck portion. The centriole is located in the opening in the cuticle (Cu). Stc: stereocilium (TEMG)

(HAMILTON, 1970). The basal body in mammals usually lacks the basal foot, but the spokes protruding from the triple tubular of the centriole are present.

The length of the kinocilium varies from a few microns in the macula sacculi to 30–40 µm in the cristae ampullares of frog. The kinocilium of the papilla basilaris and of the macula sacculi in frog are provided with a peripheral swelling

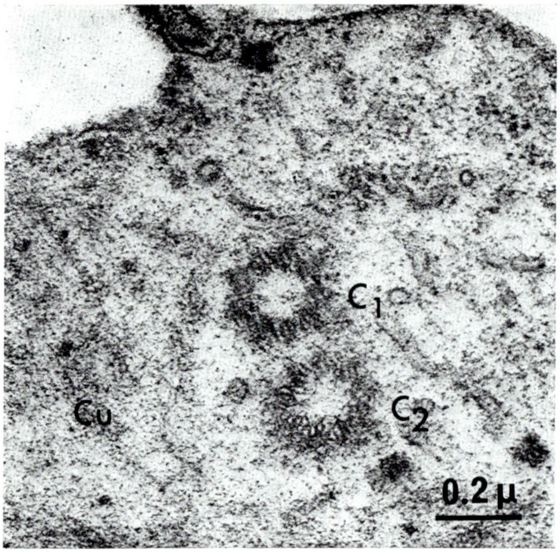

Fig. 36. Sometimes the two centrioles are located very close together, as in this picture which shows the cross-section of the two centrioles located in the periphery of the cuticle of the sensory cell from the guinea-pig labyrinth

closely attached to the covering substance (Flock, 1971; Hillman, 1971). Otherwise the kinocilia are often found lying in bends outside the periphery of the stereocilial bundle and without apparent attachment to this bundle.

A spiral structure on the surface of the kinocilium is observed with the scanning electron microscope. The structural counterpart of this spiral structure has, however, not yet been identified under the transmission electron microscope.

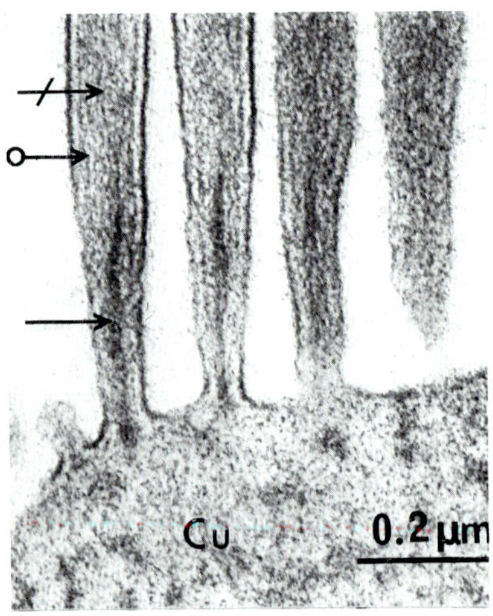

Fig. 37. Part of base of four stereocilia from a guinea-pig sensory cell illustrating the central fibrillar core of a stereocilium,–/→ which is separated from the plasma membrane by a thin osmiophilic layer (O→). The basilar filaments fuse to form a rootlet which protrudes into the cuticle. (→) Cu: cuticle (TEMG)

The *stereocilia* are composed of a central core of fibrils 40–60 Å in diameter surrounded by a triple-layered plasma membrane (Fig. 37). The filaments fuse close to the plasma membrane of the sensory cell and form a basal rootlet which protrudes into and sometimes passes through the cuticle and into the cytoplasm below the cuticle (Fig. 38). A zone around the rootlet in the cuticle is less dense than the rest of the cuticle. The diameter of the stereocilia in most species is 0.2 μm. Stereocilial bundles with stereocilia of different thicknesses have, however, been reported in the ray (LOWENSTEIN et al., 1964) and in the macula lagenae of birds (JOERGENSEN, 1970). In these animals there are thus a few sensory cells with bundles containing stereocilia only 0.1 μm thick. The diameter of the stereocilia reduces at the plasma membrane to a diameter less than one third of its maximum diameter in the cell.

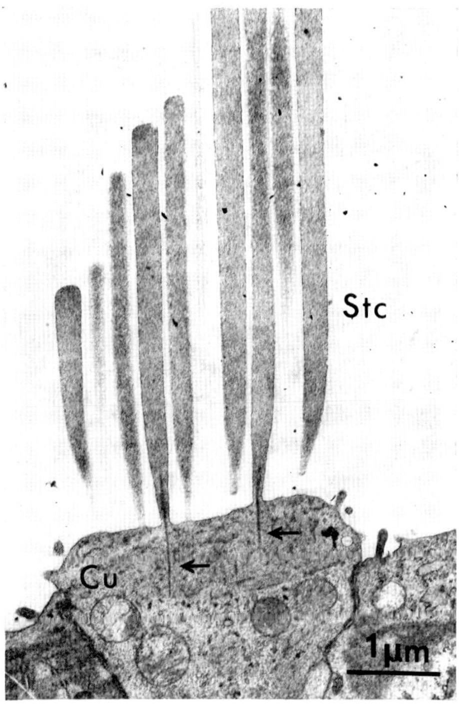

Fig. 38. Hair bundle from type I haircell from a guinea-pig labyrinth, illustrating the rootlets (arrows) protruding from the stereocilia (Stc) down into the cuticle (Cu) (TEMG)

The length of the stereocilia decreases gradually as the distance from the kinocilium increases (ENGSTRÖM, 1958). The arrangement in the stereocilial bundle is extremely regular, as observed by scanning electron microscopy (Fig. 39) or in transverse sections through the bundle close to the cell surface studied with the transmission electron microscope. A cross-section through a hair bundle close to the cell surface reveals that the sensory hairs are closely packed and separated

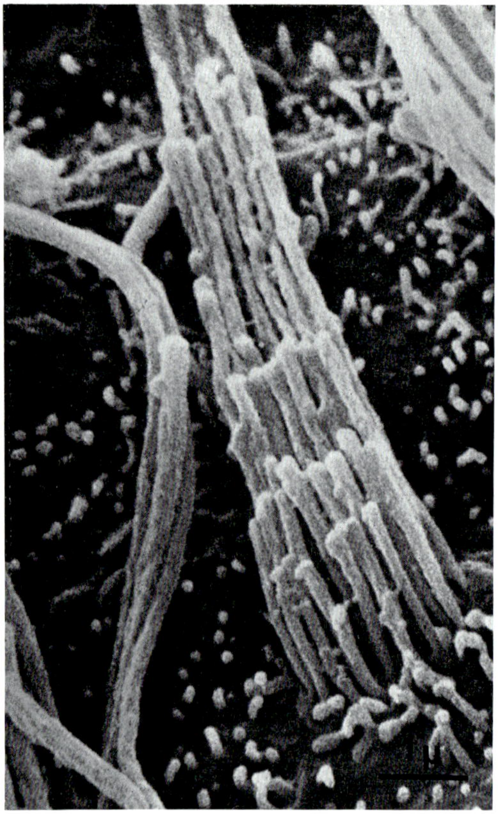

Fig. 39. Hair bundles from the crista ampullaris in guinea-pig ampulla, illustrating the gradual shortening of the sensory hairs with increasing distance from the kinocilium. Each row of sensory hairs is of approximately the same length. Microvilli on top of supporting cells surround the sensory hair bundle (SCEG)

by a space which might be as small as 200 Å or even less (Fig. 40). The stereocilia are arranged in straight rows in such a way that regular hexagonal figures are formed with the circle of six cross-sectioned stereocilia surrounding a central one. The whole bundle is often hexagonal. However, some bundles are rectangular. On one side a number of stereocilia are missing from the hexagonal figure of the bundle, forming a W-shaped opening in which the kinocilium is located. Scanning electron microscope pictures reveal that the decrease in lenght from the kinocilium proceeds row by row, in such a way that all stereocilia in one row across the bundle are of approximately the same length (Fig. 41). There are several arrangements in the orientation of the bundle. The most common bundle is one in which the kinocilium is in line with the central cilium in the hexagonals described above. There are bundles, however, in which the kinocilium is oriented by a line perpendicular to one side of the hexagon. Occasionally two kinocilia are seen on the same bundle, either on the same side or on opposite sides (Flock, 1964).

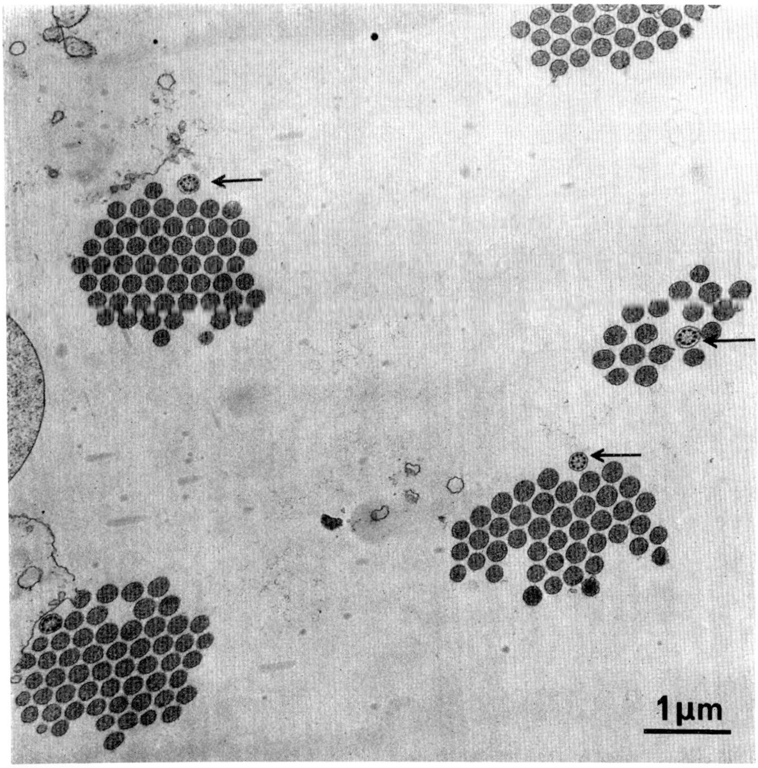

Fig. 40. Cross-section through hair bundles of the guinea-pig macula utriculi showing that the hair-bundle arrangement is fairly regular. The kinocilium is located on one side of the bundle. One arrow, however, indicates one kinocilium located in the middle of the bundle (TEMG)

The relationship of the kinocilium to the stereocilia varies considerably from one sensory area to another. In the cyclostome lamprey (Lowenstein et al., 1968) they are clearly differentiated. In one type of bundle the kinocilium is 3–5 µm long and only a little longer than the adjacent stereocilia. In the second type of hair bundle the kinocilium is approximately 10 µm long and is straight and stiff; the number of stereocilia is significantly smaller than in the first type. We observed the same type of differences between hair bundles in the macula neglecta of the shark, where most bundles are of the first type but a considerable number in the periphery of the macula neglecta are of the second type (Fig. 12).

The sensory cells in the vestibular sensory epithelia have a nucleus, the localization of which varies in different epithelia (Figs. 21–24). The mitochondria are rod-shaped or ovoid, and appear in fairly large numbers. In most cells there is a concentration of the mitochondria below the cuticle and around the nerve-ending region. The mitochondria of the sensory cells are significantly larger than those in the supporting cells.

The *Golgi apparatus* in the shape of cisternae of smooth endoplasmic reticulum and granules varies in its development and is best developed in mammalian hair-cells (Fig. 43). Ribosomes are found in clusters in all vestibular sensory cells. In birds and mammals the distribution of the ribosomes varies in different sensory

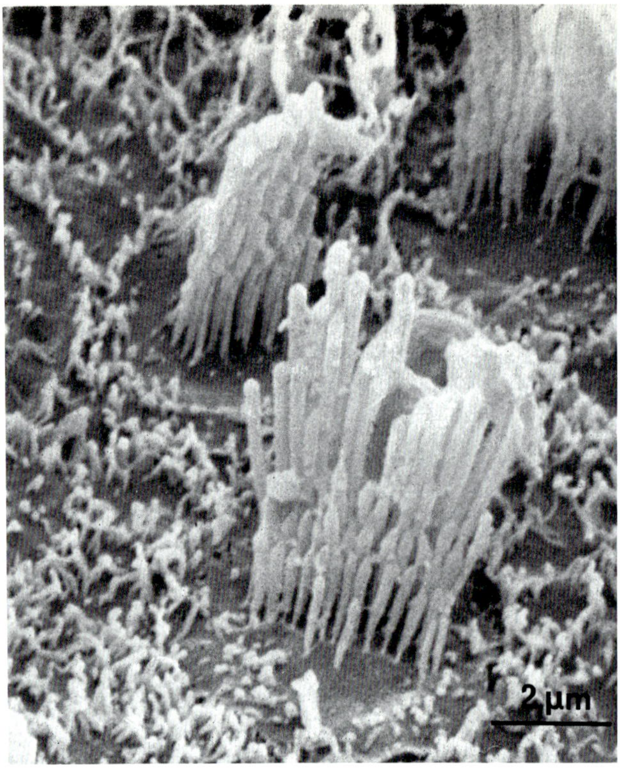

Fig. 41. Scanning electron micrograph illustrating a number of sensory hair-bundles from the macula utriculi of a shark. Closest to the observer is a bundle of rectangular type. Gradual shortening of hair towards the observer and the regular arrangement in the bundle are clearly observed

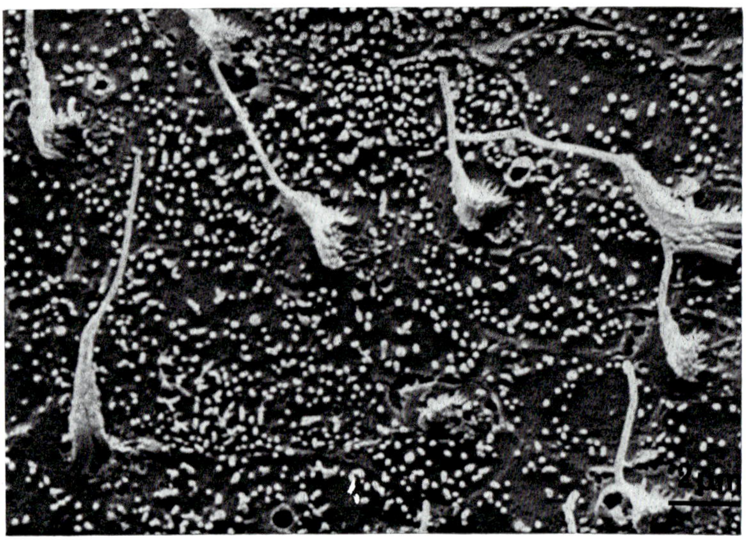

Fig. 42. Some hair bundles are composed of a long kinocilium and comparative short stereocilia, as in this picture taken from the surface of macula neglecta in a shark (SEMG)

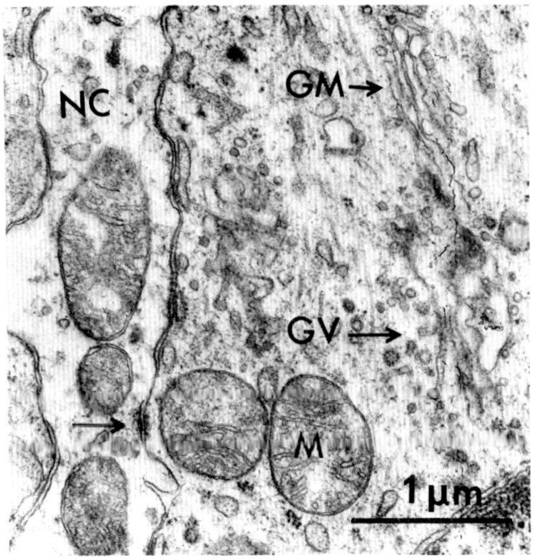

Fig. 43. Golgi membranes and Golgi vesicles (GV) are regularly observed in most sensory cells in the supranuclear region of the sensory cell. This picture is taken from a portion of haircell type I from a guinea-pig. NC: nerve chalice. M: mitochondria. Arrow indicates a thickening of the membranes in contact between the nerve chalice and the sensory cell

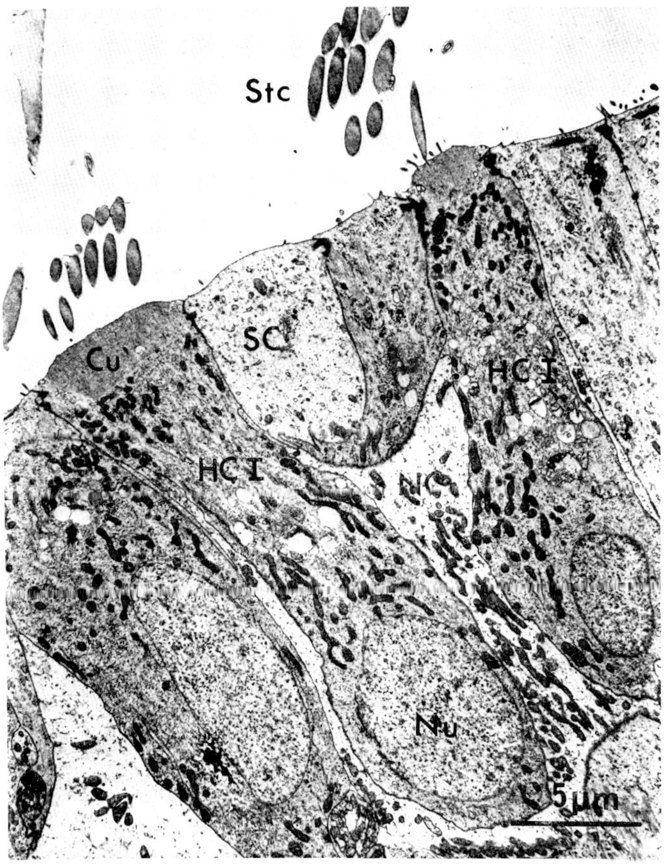

Fig. 44. Hair cells of type I and supporting cells in the crista ampullaris epithelium from a lizard. The stereocilia (Stc) protrude from the surface. The kinocilium of the bundles is not seen in the picture. *Cu*: Cuticle. *NC*: Nerve chalice. *SC*: Supporting cell distal part (TEMG)

cell types. In sensory cell type I (WERSÄLL, 1956) there is often a system of flat, communicating cisternae in the subnuclear part of the cell where the outsides of the cisternae are covered with ribosomes. The structure of this area of ribosome-covered endoplasmic reticulum is similar to the Nissle substance in ganglion cells. In the cylindrical type II sensory cell the ribosomes are found in clusters or along membranes or tubules, distributed irregularly throughout the cells.

The type I sensory cells in birds and mammals are different in shape from all other sensory cells (Figs. 44–46). They are flask-shaped, with a wide distal part in which the cuticle is located, a thin neck and a wider basal part containing the nucleus. The neck of a type I sensory cell contains a large number of microtubules connecting the subcupular area with the supranuclear part of the cell (Fig. 47). Various types of dense bodies are found in sensory cells in various animals. In mammals there are a number of dark membrane-covered bodies with a diameter of about 0.3 μm in the subcupular space, which are probably lysosomes. In the frog there are larger irregular bodies in varying numbers, presum-

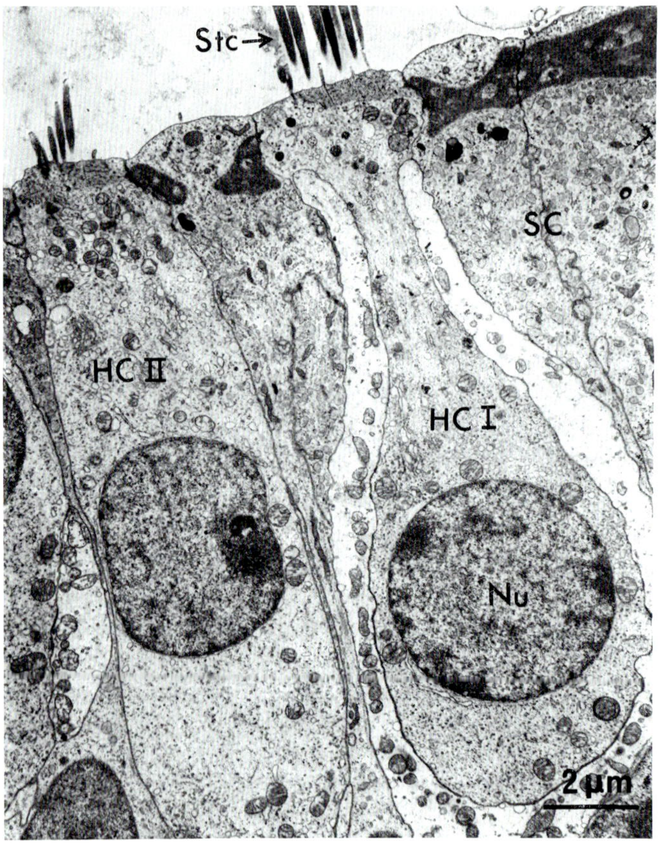

Fig. 45. The two types hair cells of the guinea-pig macula utriculi. HC I and HC II. *SC*: Supporting cells. *Stc*: Stereocilia. *Nu*: Nucleus in the type I haircell. The layering in the maculae differs from that in the crista. Thus in the maculae the nuclei of the type II haircells are often located more peripherally in the epithelium than those of the type I haircells (TEMG)

ably pigment granules. Multivesiculated bodies are found in varying numbers in the subcupular space (WERSÄLL et al., 1965).

The sensory cells of the lamprey are unique in their structural organization. They have a striated body running from the cuticular plate to the base of the cell, which is composed of fibrils with a periodicity of 1100–1300 Å. The filaments are about 50 Å in diameter (LOWENSTEIN and OSBORNE, 1964; LOWENSTEIN, OSBORNE and THORNHILL, 1968).

The sensory cells contain synaptic structures in the synaptic area in contact with the innervating nerve fibres. These structures, which should be looked upon as part of the synaptic complex, are closely related to the type of nerve ending attached to a certain area of the cell and will be discussed again later with reference to the innervation of the sensory cells.

C. Supporting Cells

The structure of the supporting cells between the sensory cells varies from species to species. A few microvilli are found on the cell surface in all species.

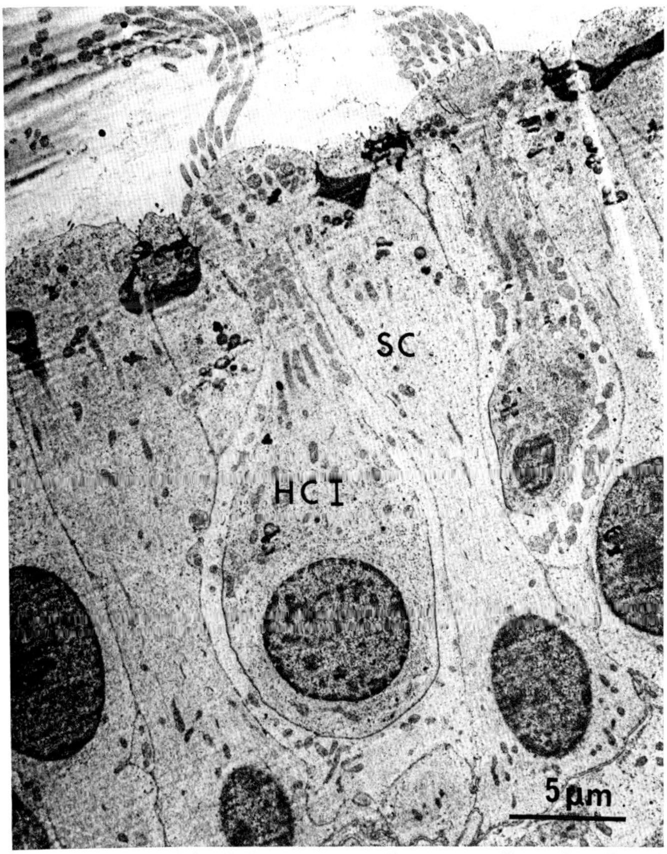

Fig. 46. Even in the human labyrinth two types of sensory cell are found in the vestibular epithelia. The structure of the type I sensory cell illustrated in the picture is similar to that in the guinea-pig. The granula content of the human supporting cells is sparse (TEMG)

In cyclostomes, elasmobranches, fishes, and frogs a ciliary rod appears as a short kinocilium projecting from the center of the supporting cell surface. It has a basal body and a basal foot, and has the normal kinocilial 2–9 arrangement. In birds and mammals so short a cilium is much more unusual but a centriole is normally found close to the surface in the supporting cell.

The mitochondria of the supporting cells are long, thin, and dense, with their orientation normally perpendicular to the epithelial surface of the cell. The Golgi membranes, the flat, thin cisternae of smooth endoplasmic reticulum, normally occupy the central, thin part of the cell. Very dense osmiophilic droplets, presumably lipids, have been found in the supporting cells of the lamprey labyrinth. Fibrils of tonofibrillar type have sometimes been found, usually accumulated in the basal part of the cells.

Irregular strands of ribosome-covered endoplasmic reticulum are found in varying amounts in the supporting cells. Mammalian labyrinths have supporting cells containing large amounts of single membrane-covered granules about 0.2 μm wide (Fig. 32). Granules of this type are not found in the supporting cells located between the haircells in the labyrinths of other species. Specific granula-containing cells presumably of secretory type, however, are found in parts of the labyrinth in lower species. There is a ring of tall granula-containing cells round the cristae ampullares in the ray (LOWENSTEIN et al., 1964), and tall columnar cells with secretory granules and vacuoles are found in the area around the sensory epithelium of the saccule in the same animal.

In birds and higher animals, a well-developed supporting structure is found in the sensory epithelium, the so-called membrana reticularis. This is a system of rings of dense substance located in the distal part of the supporting cells close to the endolymphatic surface of the cells. It is about 0.25 μm deep (WERSÄLL, 1956). The supporting cells are joined to each other and to the sensory cells at the surface in a manner found both in the organ of Corti and in the vestibular system (Fig. 47). In mammals there is a rather variable distance between the dense layers of the two opposing cell membrances. The distance between two supporting cells is fairly constant (SMITH, 1967), whereas the distances between supporting cells and haircells vary widely between about 80 Å to 175 Å. At the base of the supporting cells there is a close approximation to the basement membrane on which the cells are resting but a very varying distance with formations of rather wide spaces in some species (frogs) further away from the basement membrane.

VII. Innervation

A. The Eighth Nerve and its Ganglion Cells

The vestibular ganglion cells supplying the vestibular sensory epithelia with *afferent fibres* are bipolar cells located in the vestibular ganglion in the cartilage or bone capsule surrounding the labyrinth. The nerve fibers in the eighth nerve of the myxine are exceptional in that the nerve fibers going to the sensory epithelia are nonmyelinated. The Schwann cells, which in the myxine nerve envelop one or more nerve fibers, contain larger collagenous fibers and thinner tonofilaments.

1. Ganglion Cells and Afferent Fibers

There are two types of vestibular ganglion cells in the lamprey (LOWENSTEIN et al., 1968). Large neurons are located along the branch of the eighth nerve or in the labyrinthine capsule. The largest of these cells reach a diameter of 200 μm. Their neurons are not myelinated but wrapped in a sheath of Schwann cells. The small bipolar cells range in diameter from 20–25 μm. They are always located within the labyrinthine capsule. Several neurons from small ganglion cells are wrapped in the same Schwann-cell sheath in a manner reminiscent of the wrapping of unmyelinated nerve fibers generally found in vertebrates. The ganglion cells and nerve fibers of elasmobranches and bony fishes, frogs, lizards, birds and mammals are myelinated (WERSÄLL, 1960; BALLANTYNE and ENGSTRÖM, 1969).

2. Efferent Fibers

Efferent fibers run from nerve cells in the medulla to the vestibular sensory epithelium in fish, birds and mammals (GAISEC. 1960, 1966; ROSSI, 1965). In frog some of the fibers have been found to originate from cells in the cerebellar cortex (HILLMAN, 1969). Unmyelinated fibers, at least some of which are sympathetic, have been found in all vestibular nerves examined. Preliminary observations on the ganglion and nerves of cats have revealed the appearance of sympathetic fibers with the fluorescence method (DENSERT, 1971).

3. Nerve Branches of the Eighth Nerve

The separation of the eighth nerve into separate branches is intimately related to the development of the different sensory areas as well as the localization of these sensory areas in the labyrinth. The separation of the macula communis into an anterior part and a posterior part also means a division of the eighth nerve into an anterior and a posterior branch, the ramus anterior and the ramus posterior. The ramus anterior innervates the anterior and horizontal crista and the macula utriculi, while the varying number of sensory areas formed by the posterior part is innervated by the ramus posterior of the macula communis.

The macula sacculi has different locations in the vestibule in different species, and the branch or branches innervating the macula sacculi are thus the ones which vary most widely in the whole labyrinth. DE BURLET's drawings (1934) illustrate this variation very well and there seems to be no reason whatsoever to draw any physiological conclusion about the architecture of the saccular branches and their relation to the anterior and posterior ramus.

Thus, in the lizard *Iguana* the saccule is supplied from the ramus posterior only (Fig. 47), in crocodile (Fig. 48) from both the anterior and posterior branches, in the *Cheldyra* turtle by one branch from each ramus plus an intermediate branch (Fig. 49), in chameleon from one intermediate branch only (Fig. 50), in mammals from both branches and in frog from the anterior branch.

The peripheral branches of the vestibular nerve and its connections with the cochlear and facial nerve have been studied by RETZIUS (1884), HARDY (1934), DE BURLET (1924, 1934), OORT (1918), RASMUSSEN (1963) and GAISEC (1966). The superior branch of the vestibular nerve supplies the anterior vertical and horizontal ampulla and the utricle, as well as the anterior superior part of the saccular macula.

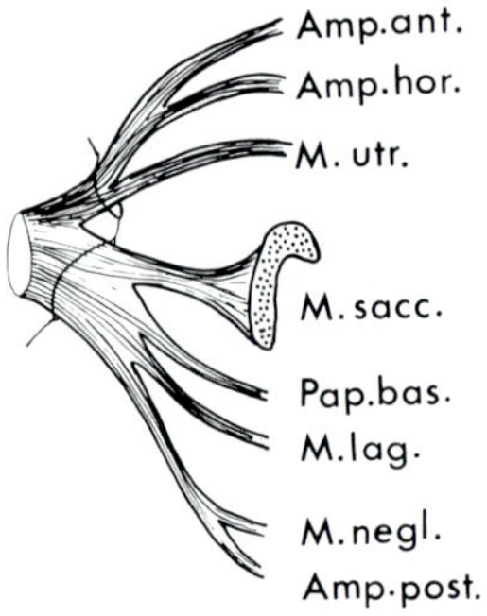

Fig. 47

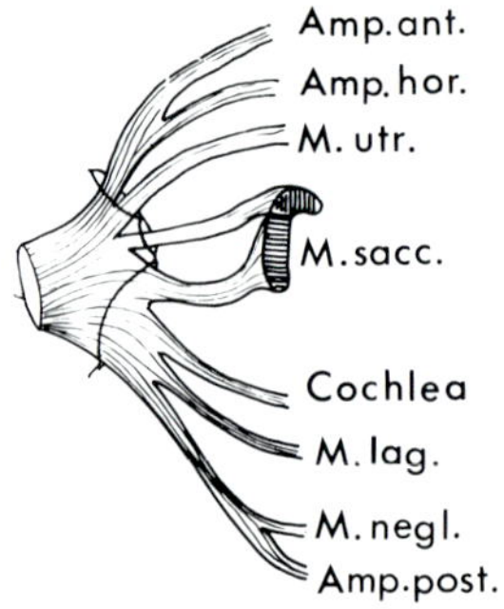

Fig. 48

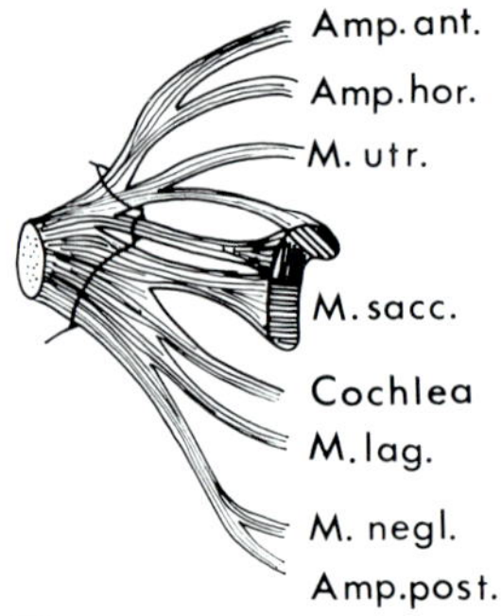

Fig. 49

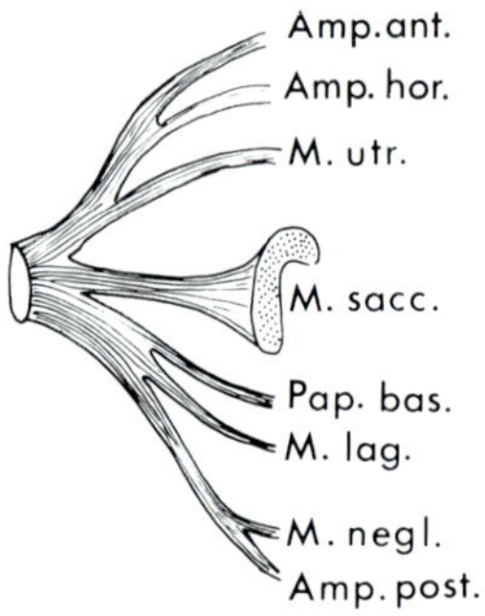

Fig. 50

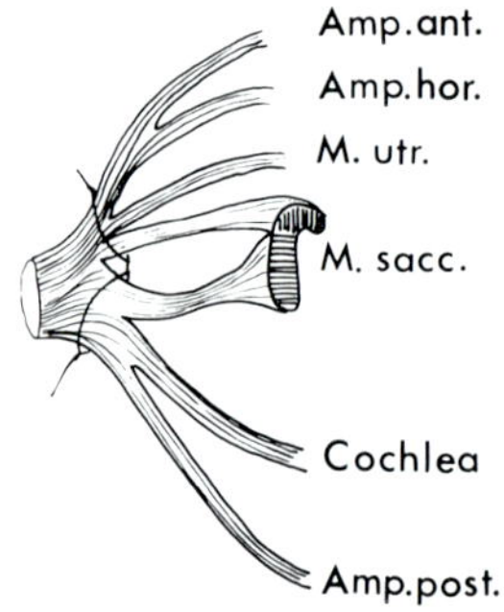

Fig. 51

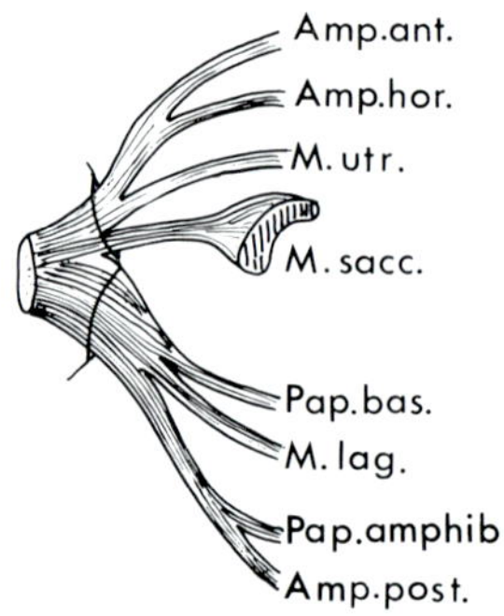

Fig. 52

Figs. 47–52. The branching of the vestibular nerve is mainly dependent on the location of the sensory areas and their spatial relations within the labyrinth. This is especially clear when the nerve supply to the saccular macula is studied, as in this series of pictures from De Burlet (1934) (Redrawn). In the lizard *Iguana* these saccular nerve comes from the posterior ramus of the vestibular nerve (47). In the crocodile two branches innervate the macula, one from the posterior ramus of the nerve and one small separate bundle (48). The turtle has three branches (49). The chameleon has a special branch for the macula sacculi (50), the mammals one branch from each ramus (51) and the frog one branch only from the anterior ramus of the nerve (52)

The inferior branch of the vestibular nerve supplies the main part of the saccular macula and the posterior ampulla. The efferent nerve fibers cross over to the cochlear nerve via the vestibulocochlear anastomosis of Corti (Rasmussen, 1963). Communicating branches are also found between the facial nerve and the cochlear and vestibular nerve respectively.

The vestibular nerve contains a slightly varying number of fibers. Gacec and Rasmussen (1961) found 7093–10027 fibers in guinea pig and 14200–24000 in man (Rasmussen, 1940). Engström and Rexed (1940) found that 88.5% of the fibers in the vestibular nerve were 2–9 μm thick, 71.2% 8–13 μm, and 4.2% less than 2 μm thick. Gacec and Rasmussen (1961) found that 51% of fibers in guinea pig were less than 2.5 μm in diameter, 42% were 2.5–5 μm and 7% 5–8 μm thick. The distribution of fibers of varying caliber in the distal part of the whole nerve is consistent with the figures given for the posterior vertical canal by Wersäll (1956).

4. Structure and Distribution of Nerve Endings

The innervation of the sensory cells of the cristae and the various parts of the macula communis in the myxine seem to have the same morphologic pattern (LOWENSTEIN and THORNHILL, 1970). Only one type of nerve ending is found. The nerve fibers enter at the base of the epithelium and run between sensory and supporting cells to end in a small swelling in close proximity to the sensory cell. The nerve endings contain mitochondria and numerous dense granules. Some vesicles have been observed in and outside the endings. The dense bodies observed in some sensory cells close to the nerve endings were similar in structure to synaptic bodies found in other species.

The innervation of the cyclostome *Lampreta fluviatilis* has a considerably more complicated pattern (LOWENSTEIN, OSBORNE and THORNHILL, 1968). Three main types of nerve endings were distinguished in the epithelia. Their frequency of occurrence and distribution varied from area to area. Thus, sensory afferent endings of type I, inhibitory efferents of type II, and a third type of unknown function, possibly afferent, were described. The afferent nerve endings, which were associated with a typical synaptic bar with associated structures in the sensory cell, were crowded with mitochondria or contain numerous vesicles and a few mitochondria. The efferent endings contained a profusion of synaptic vesicles but very few mitochondria. In the area of contact between the efferent endings and the sensory cells, accessory membranes had developed within the sensory cell. A third type of ending was described as "numerous small diameter nerve fibers at the base of the sensory cells in the region of the crista." It does not, however, seem unlikely that these fibers were not endings, but thin interconnecting fibers in the widespread arborization of the peripheral nerve branches which had dilated to form the true nerve endings or swellings.

Except for the third type of so-called endings, the description of the nerve endings in the lamprey is strikingly reminiscent of the system of terminal nerve fibers and nerve endings found throughout the phylogenetic series apart from birds and mammals. Each nerve fiber reaching the sensory epithelium divides into a number of terminal branches which supply a number of sensory cells with nerve terminals, and each sensory cell can be innervated by several nerve fibers. The afferent nerve endings contain a large number of mitochondria, sparse vesicles and some fine neurofilaments, whereas the efferent nerve terminals are filled with synaptic vesicles.

The synaptic structure in the cells is also uniform in cyclostomes, fishes, and amphibia (WERSÄLL, 1956; ENGSTRÖM and WERSÄLL, 1958a, b, IURATO, 1962; SMITH, 1956, 1967; WERSÄLL et al., 1965). Each sensory cell contains a number of synaptic bodies, which are spherical or pear-shaped and usually have a number of dense feet which rest on the plasma membrane of the sensory cell at the area of contact with a nerve ending. Each synaptic body is surrounded by a large number of vesicles (Figs. 53, 54, 55, 56).

A number of coated vesicles are usually found in the neighborhood of the synapse with the afferent fiber. In frog, these coated vesicles seem to be part of a system of coated vesicles and tubules located in the cytoplasm of the sensory cell around the synaptic area of afferent synapse and closely related to pinocytotic grooves and vesicles on the plasma membrane surface of the sensory cell

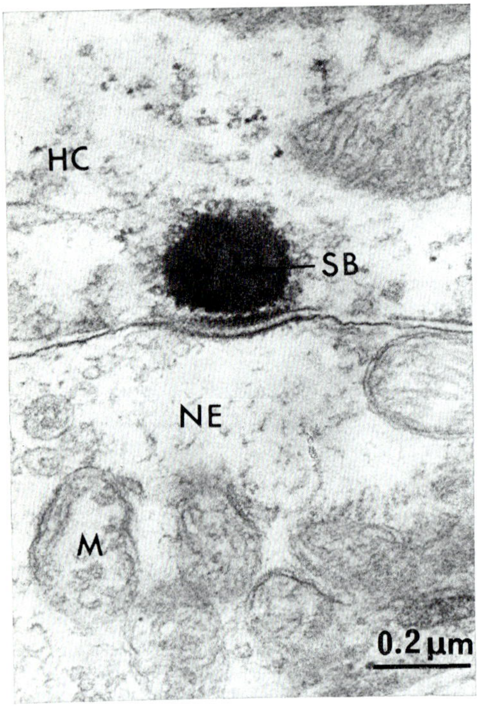

Fig. 53

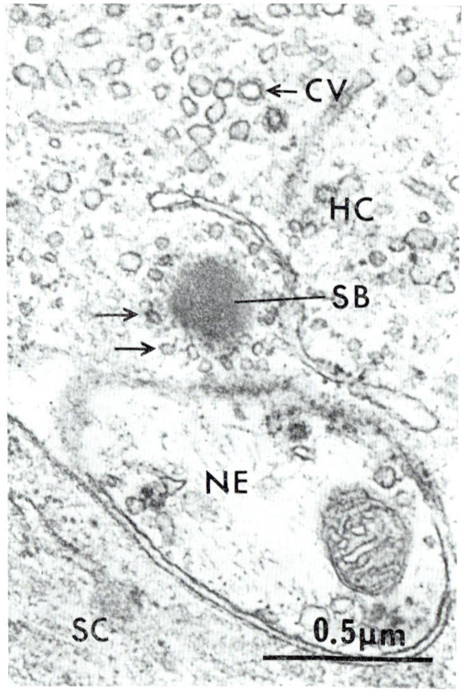

Fig. 54

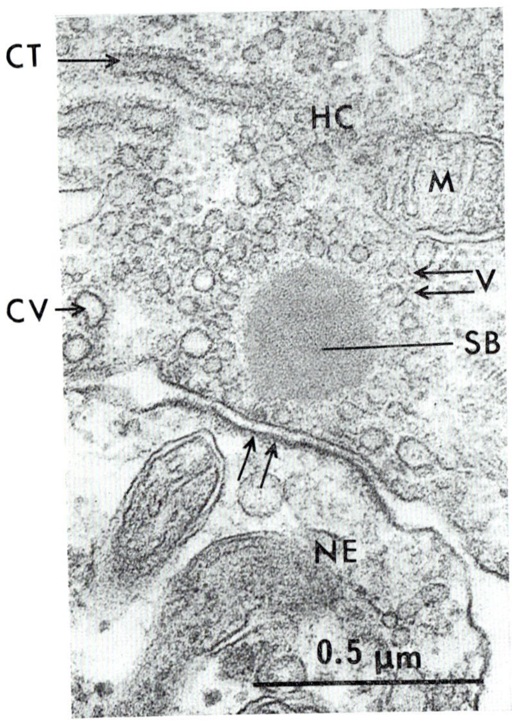

Fig. 55

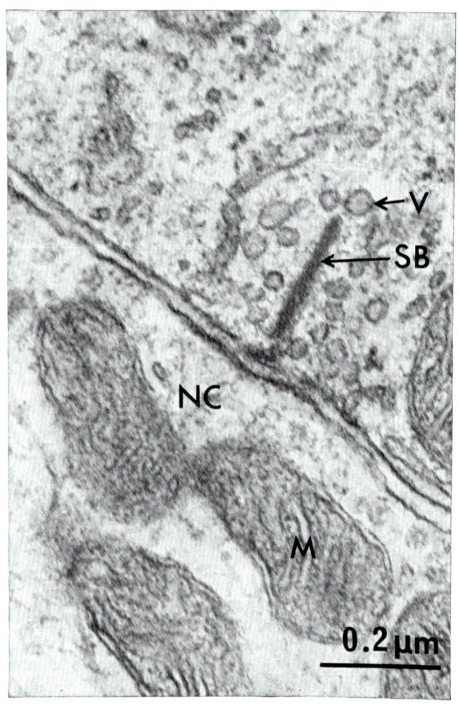

Fig. 56

surrounding the synaptic space between the nerve ending and the sensory cell (Fig. 55).

The accessory membranes found in the synapse between the efferent nerve endings and the sensory cell are shaped like flat cisternae surrounded by a thin smooth membrane closely approaching the plasma membrane of the sensory cell at the synaptic junction (Fig. 57) (LOWENSTEIN et al., 1969; WERSÄLL, 1956; WERSÄLL et al., 1965). The efferent nerve endings are sometimes found to contain accumulations of synaptic vesicles close to the synaptic space, and vesicles sometimes open into the space. Dark substance can also be found in the nerve endings attached to the plasma membrane on the surface facing the sensory cell.

There is some variation in the size of nerve endings. Some of the endings, in fact, are attached to a large surface of one or more sensory cells, resembling an early stage in the development of the nerve chalices in higher animals.

In birds and mammals a distinct difference is found between nerve endings supplying type I sensory cells, which are a special type of sensory cell found only in birds and mammals, and the type II sensory cells which are cylindrical cells

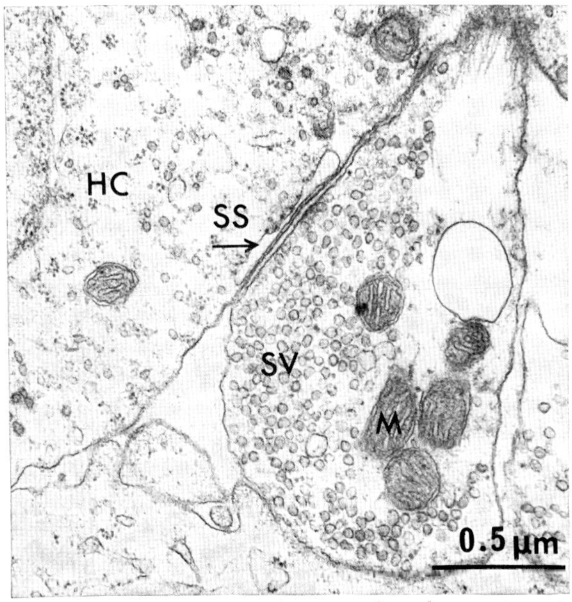

Fig. 57. The efferent nerve endings contain a large number of synaptic vesicles (SV) accumulated towards the haircell and mitochondria located away from the hair cell. A synaptic sac is found on the hair cell side of the synaptic membrane (SS) (TEMG)

Figs. 53–56. The hair cell contains one or more synaptic bodies located very close to the plasma membrane in the synapse between the haircell and each afferent nerve ending. In elasmobranchs, bony fishes, lizards, and birds this body is dense, more or less spherical, and surrounded by vesicles. This body is seen in the ray (53), lizard (54), frog (55). In the mammals (56) this synaptic body is shaped like a bar or a sheath, as in the guinea pig where a bar is resting with a foot on the plasma membrane. One or more dense bars run on the inside of the plasma membrane parallel with the membrane and in close contact with the membrane between the body and the membrane. *HC*: Haircell. *SB*: Synaptic body. *NE*: Nerve ending. *M*: Mitochondrion. *CV*: Coated vesicle. *CT*: Coated tubules. *V*: Vesicles. *NC*: Nerve chalice (TEMG) resembling those found in lower animals (Figs. 30–32, 44–47) (WERSÄLL, 1956; WERSÄLL et al., 1965; VINNIKOV, 1965, 1971; ROSENHALL, 1970).

The type I sensory cells are enclosed by a nerve chalice enclosing the major part of the cell. The chalice contains fine neurofilaments, mitochondria and some vesicles, apart from the most apical end which is usually filled with a large number of vesicles. The synaptic space between the sensory cell type I and the nerve chalice varies in width and structure. Most of the space located basally in the midplane of the nucleus of the cell is thus about 250 Å wide. The triple-layered membrane of the sensory cell is easily distinguished from that of the nerve chalices, and a granular substance is attached to the outermost layer of both the nerve chalice and the sensory cell membrane (Fig. 58) (WERSÄLL, 1956). At some points in this area, however, the sensory cell is invaginated to shallow grooves in which the granular substance in the synaptic space disappears and the synaptic space is reduced so that in some specimens points of fusion are observed between apposing layers of the plasma membrane of the sensory cell, and that of the nerve chalice (Fig. 59) (SPOENDLIN, 1965). In other areas no grooves are found, but a close apposition is found between the membranes where single vesicles with similar diameters are found on one or both sides of the contact within both the nerve chalice and the sensory cell (Fig. 58). In some places synaptic rods are observed (WERSÄLL and FLOCK, 1965). Above the level of the equator of the nucleus the synaptic space is highly irregular. The granular substance in the synaptic space has disappeared and the synaptic space has an irregular appearance with wide variations in the distance between the apposing plasma membranes. The functional importance of these varying contact points and synaptic structures has been discussed, and the possibility of electrical synaptic points has been discussed (SPOENDLIN, 1966).

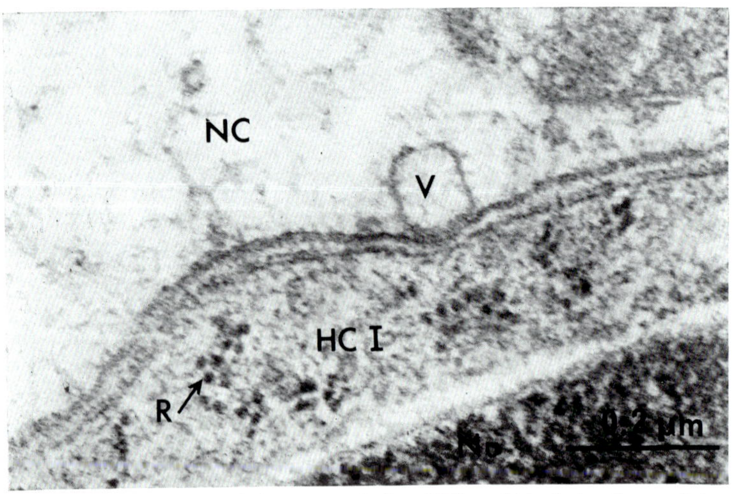

Fig. 58. The plasma membrane of the nerve chalice (NC) and the haircell type I is separated by a wide space in large areas of the synaptic contact between the nerve chalice and the hair cell. A granular substance coats the side of the plasma membrane facing this space. In some areas the plasma membranes come in closer apposition within limited areas; characteristic vesicles (V) are sometimes found on the nerve chalice side of the membrane, and sometimes in both the nerve chalice and the haircell (TEMG)

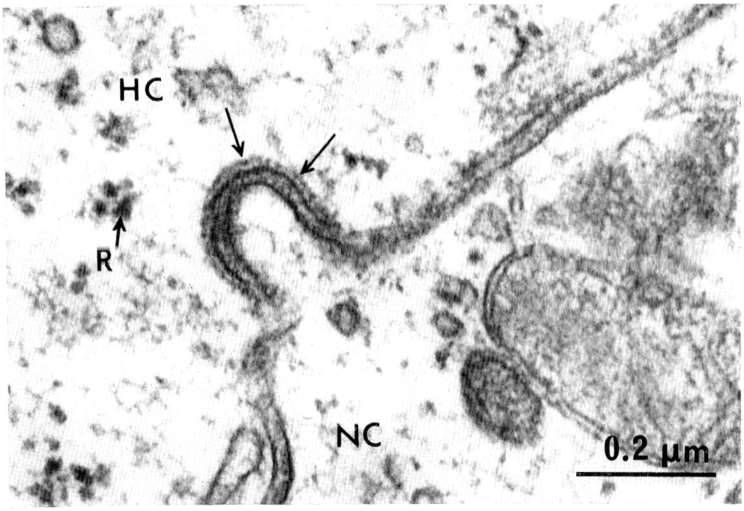

Fig. 59. In some areas of contact between nerve chalice (NC) and hair cell, (HC) a dense line between the plasma membrane layers indicates a partial fusion of the membranes (TEMG)

The type II sensory cells are innervated by nerve terminals from small fibers of medium size, with several afferent and efferent nerve terminals on the bottom of each cell. The afferent terminals are like those of lower animals, containing sparse vesicles and fine neurofilaments and a large number of mitochondria. The sensory cells of type II are supplied with synaptic rods of varying length, resting on the plasma membrane at the synapse. The synaptic rods are surrounded by synaptic vesicles. Several synaptic rods are sometimes found within the synapse of one nerve ending. The efferent nerve endings are filled with synaptic vesicles, and in the synaptic area the sensory cells contain accessory membranes of the synaptic sac type (WERSÄLL, 1956; ENGSTRÖM, 1958; ENGSTRÖM and WERSÄLL, 1958a, b).

VIII. Morphological Polarization of the Vestibular Sensory Areas

The directional sensitivity of the vestibular receptors was originally described in the semicircular canals by EWALD (1892), and was functionally analyzed by recording from single nerve fibers by LOWENSTEIN and SAND (1940) and GROEN, LOWENSTEIN and VENDRIK (1952) in the ray, and in the frog by LEDOUX (1951, 1956). The possibility of a morphological correlate to these physiologic findings has been discussed by VILSTRUP (1950) and by WERSÄLL (1956). LOWENSTEIN and WERSÄLL (1959) found a correlation between the orientation of the sensory hair bundle of the ampullar sensory receptors in the ray and the function of the receptors with the kinocilium of the bundle located on the side of the hair bundle facing in the direction of displacement when the cupula undergoes excitatory deflection. FLOCK and WERSÄLL (1962) found that the lateral canal sense organ containing cells with the sensory hair bundles was oriented in opposite directions with regard to the orientation of the kinocilium. On the basis of these findings and of earlier physiological findings on the microphonic potentials and single-fiber recordings from sensory cells (Sand, 1937; Kuijpers, 1956) the following hypothesis was proposed with regard to the function of the hair cells: "The response of the haircell is determined by the direction from which the stimulus approaches the hair bundle. The morphological polarization of the sensory hair bundle and of the top of the cell is an indicator of this discrimination system." This hypothesis was extended to cover all sensory cells of the acoustic lateralis system by Flock et al. (1962) and Duvall et al. (1966) when they demonstrated that although the sensory cells of the organ of Corti have no kinocilium proper in the fully developed stage, they have a centriole located on one side of the sensory hair bundle. Thus it was suggested that the directional sensitivity of the organ of hearing and equilibrium is correlated with the orientation of the polarized sensory cells.

Flock (1965) further analyzed the importance of the sensory-cell orientation in the lateral canal end organ with regard to the microphonic potential output from the cells when stimulated by displacement of the sensory hair bundle in various directions.

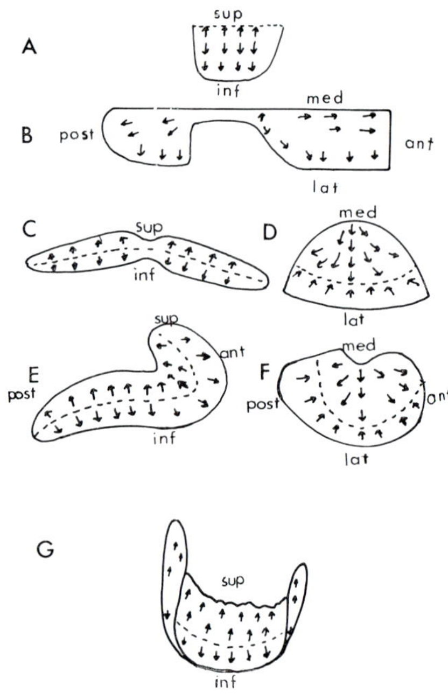

Fig. 60. The orientation of the sensory epithelia in the vestibular end organs have a characteristic pattern determined by the location of the kinocilium of the hair bundle, indicated by arrows in the schematic drawings. A–B: Macula communis from lamprey, redrawn after Lowenstein et al. (1968). A: The macula sacculi part of the macula communis. B: The horizontal main part of the macula. The posterior part corresponds to the macula lagenae, the anterior part to the macula utriculi. C: Macula sacculi from bony fish. D: Macula utriculi from bony fish. C and D redrawn from Wersäll et al. (1965). E: Macula sacculi in mammals. F: Macula utriculi in mammals. G: Lagena in bird (Redrawn from Joergensen, 1970)

These early findings have demonstrated the possibility of analyzing the directional sensitivity of the sensory epithelium of the acoustico-lateralis system by means of studies of the orientation of the hair bundle (Fig. 60). FLOCK (1964) described a significant pattern in the orientation of the sensory hair bundles in the macula utriculi of the bony fish, *Lota vulgaris*. The main orientation was from medial to lateral, but there was a fan-shaped divergence from this main line towards the anterior and posterior direction respectively. A dividing line was found along the lateral and posterior border, along which the cells were found to change their orientation by 180°, so that cells on opposite sides of this line were oriented in opposite directions. LOWENSTEIN, OSBORNE and WERSÄLL (1964) found that the sensory cells in the macula sacculi of the ray changed orientation along a line going along the whole macula sacculi but with the kinocilia of the sensory cells facing away from that line. SPOENDLIN (1964, 1965) described the orientation of the sensory cells in the vestibular sensory epithelia of the squirrel monkey. He found that the dividing line of the macula utriculi and the macula sacculi along which the sensory cells changed their orientation 180° corresponding to the striola described by WERNER (1933, 1960). SPOENDLIN (1965) and LINDEMANN (1969a, b) studied the otoconium membrane on the surface of the macula utriculi and found that the otoconium layer, in accordance with WERNER'S findings, was thinnest over the striola region and that the largest otoconia were found in the lateral part of the macula utriculi outside the striola. LINDEMANN (1969a, b) described a thicker layer of small otoconia in the striola region in the macula sacculi and a concentration of sensory cells of type I in the striola region confirming ENGSTRÖM'S and WERSÄLL'S (1958a) and SPOENDLIN'S (1965) findings.

The macula lagenae in birds was studied by JOERGENSEN (1970). He found that the sensory cells on the upper side of the striola were oriented with the kinocilia on the dorsal side of the bundle. In the striola, some of the haircells were polarized at right angles to the rest of the cells. In the ventral part of the lagena the kinocilium was located on the ventral side of the bundle, except for some cells on the lower edge of the epithelium which were reversely polarized (Fig. 60).

JOERGENSEN (1970) suggests four types of polarization on the vestibular epithelia: 1) The utriculus type, with the polarization fan-shaped with or without a border of conversely polarized cells; 2) The sacculus type with the sensory cells in one half of the macula polarized in the opposite direction to those in the other half; 3) The neglecta type with the kinocilium oriented facing in all directions; 4) The crista type with the sensory cells polarized in one direction, also found in the organ of Corti. There is also the lateral line organ type, with each sensory cell polarized in the opposite direction to its neighboring sensory cells.

Although our knowledge of the comparative anatomical aspects of the orientation pattern of the vestibular sensory epithelia is by no means complete, it seems that the suggested scheme of groups of polarization will be helpful in discussion of the polarization and its functional significance in various sensory areas in different species. There is no doubt that the possibility of analyzing the morphological polarization and correlating it with the directional sensitivity, as demonstrated by physiological methods, will be of the utmost importance for the single cell recording studies on the vestibular sensory cells now under way in various laboratories.

References

Bairati, A., Iurato, S.: The ultrastructural organization of "plana semilunata". Exp. Cell Res. **20**, 77–83 (1960).

Ballantyne, J., Engström, H.: Morphology of the vestibular ganglion cells. J. Laryng. **83**, 19–42 (1969).

Burlet, H.M., de: Zur Innervation der Macula Sacculi bei Säugetieren. Anat. Anz. **58**, 26–32 (1924).

Burlet, H.M., de: Vergleichende Anatomie des Stato-akustischen Organs. In: Handbuch der vergleichenden Anatomie der Wirbeltiere. Berlin: Urban & Schwarzenberg 1934.

Burlet, H.M., de, Versteegh, C.: Über Bau und Funktion des Petromyzonlabyrinthes. Acta oto-laryng. (Stockh.) Suppl. **13**, (1930).

Carlström, D.: Crystalographic study of the vertebrate otoliths. Biol. Bull. **125**, 441–463 (1963).

Carlström, D., Engström, H., Hjort, S.: Electron microscopic and X-ray defraction studies of statoconia. Laryngoscope (St. Louis) **63**, 1052–1057 (1953).

Carlström, D., Engström, H.: The ultrastructure of statoconia. Acta oto-laryng. (Stockh.) **45**, 14–18 (1955).

Densert, O.: Unpublished observations.

Dohlman, G.F.: The mechanism of secretion and absorption of endolymph in the vestibular apparatus. Acta oto-laryng. (Stockh.) **59**, 275–288 (1965).

Duvall, A.J., Flock, Å., Wersäll, J.: The ultrastructure of the sensory hairs and associated organelles of the cochlear inner hair cells, with references to directional sensitivity. J. Cell Biol. **29**, 497–505 (1966).

Engström, H.: Microscopic anatomy of the inner ear. Acta oto-laryng. (Stockh.) **40**, 5–22 (1951).

Engström, H.: On the double innervation of the sensory epithelia of the inner ear. Acta oto-laryng. (Stockh.) **49**, 109–118 (1958).

Engström, H.: The innervation of the vestibular sensory cells. Acta oto-laryng. (Stockh.) Suppl. **163**, 30–40 (1961).

Engström, H., Wersäll, J.: The ultrastructural organization of the organ of Corti and of the vestibular sensory epithelia. Exp. Cell Res. **5**, 460–492 (1958).

Engström, H., Wersäll, J.: Structure and innervation of the inner ear sensory epithelia. Int. Rev. Cytol. **7**, 535–585 (1958).

Engström, H., Rexed, B.: Über die Kaliberverhältnisse der Nervenfasern im N. stato-acusticus des Menschen. Z. mikr.-anat. Forsch. **47**, 448 (1940).

Ewald, J.R.: Physiologische Untersuchungen über das Endorgan des Nervus octavus. Wiesbaden: Bergmann 1892.

Flock, Å.: Structure of the macula utriculi with special reference to directional interplay of sensory responses as revealed by morphological polarization. J. Cell. Biol. **22**, 413–431 (1964).

Flock, Å.: Sensory transduction in hair cells. In: Handbook of Sensory Physiology, vol. I. Principles of Receptor Physiology. Berlin–Heidelberg–New York: Springer 1971.

Flock, Å., Kimura, R., Lundquist, P.-G., Wersäll, J.: Morphological basis of directional sensitivity of the outer hair cells in the organ of Corti. J. acoust. Soc. Amer. **34**, 1351–1355 (1962).

Flock, Å., Wersäll, J.: A study of the orientation of the sensory hairs of the receptor cells in the lateral line organ of fish, with special reference to the function of the receptors. J. Cell Biol. **15**, 19–27 (1962).

Gaisec, R.R.: Efferent component of the vestibular nerve. In: Neural mechanisms of the auditory and vestibular systems. pp. 176–284, G. L. Rasmussen and W. F. Windle, Eds. Springfield: Thomas 1960.

Gaisec, R.R.: The macula neglecta in the feline species. J. comp. Neurol. **116**, 317–323 (1961).

Gaisec, R.R.: The vestibular efferent pathway. In: The Vestibular System and its Diseases. Philadelphia: Univ. Pennsylvania Press 1966.

Gaisec, R.R., Rasmussen, G.L.: Fiber analyzis of the stato-acoustic nerve of guinea pig, cat and monkey. Anat. Rev. **139**, 455–463 (1961).

GROEN, J.J., LOWENSTEIN, O., VENDRIK, A.J.H.: The mechanical analysis of the responses from the end organs of the horizontal semicircular canal in the isolated elasmobranch labyrinth. J. Physiol. (Lond.) **117**, 329–346 (1952).

HAMILTON, D.W.: The cilium on mammalian vestibular hair cells. Anat. Rec. **164**, 253–258 (1970).

HARDY, M.: Observations on the innervation of the macula sacculi in man. Anat. Rec. **59**, 403–418 (1934).

HILDING, D.A., WERSÄLL, J.: Cholinesterase and its relation to the nerve endings in the inner ear. Acta oto-laryng. (Stockh.) **55**, 205–217 (1962).

HILLMAN, D.E.: Light and electron microscopic study of the relationships between the cerebellum and the vestibular organ of the frog. Exp. Brain Res. **9**, 1–15 (1969).

HILLMAN, D.E.: Morphological basis for a mechanical linkage in otolithic receptor transduction in the frog. Science **174**, 416–419 (1971).

IURATO, S.: The sensory cells of the membraneous labyrinth. Arch. Otolaryng. **75**, 312–328 (1962).

IIELOF, R., SPOOR, D., DE VRIES, H.: The microphonic activity of the lateral line. J. Physiol. (Lond.) **116**, 137–157 (1952).

IWATA, N.: Über das Labyrinth der Fledermaus mit besonderer Berücksichtigung des statischen Apparatus. Aichi J. Exp. Med. **1**, 42–173 (1924).

JOERGENSEN, J.M.: On the structure of the macula lagenae in birds with some notes on the avian maculae utriculi and sacculi. Vidensk. Medd. dansk naturh. Fören. **133**, 121–147 (1970).

KIMURA, R.S.: Distribution, structure and function of dark cells in the vestibular labyrinth. Ann. Otol. (St. Louis) **78**, 542–561 (1969).

KIMURA, R., LUNDQUIST, P.-G., WERSÄLL, J.: Secretory epithelial linings in the ampullae of the guinea pig labyrinth. Acta oto-laryng. (Stockh.) **57**, 517–530 (1963).

KUIJPERS, J.W.: The microphonic effect of the lateral line organ. Publ. Biophys. Groop. Groningen 1956.

LEDOUX, A.: Novelle technique pour l'étude de l'activité etectarique des nerfs labyrinthiques. Rev. Laryng. (Bordeaux) Suppl. **265** (1951).

LEDOUX, A.: Réponses électriques de l'ampoule du canal semicirculaire à la stimulation calorique. Acta oto-laryng. (Stockh.) **46**, 290 (1956).

LINDEMANN, H.H.: Studies on the morphology of the sensory regions of the vestibular apparatus. Ergeb. Anat. Entwickl.-Gesch. **42**, 1–113 (1969).

LOWENSTEIN, O., OSBORNE, M.P.: Ultrastructure of the sensory hair cells in the labyrinth of the ammoccete larva of the lamprey, *Lampreta fluviatilis*. Nature (Lond.) **204**, 197–198 (1964).

LOWENSTEIN, O., OSBORNE, M.P., THORNHILL, R.A.: The anatomy of and ultrastructure of the labyrinth of the lamprey. (*Lampreta fluviatilis L.*). Proc. roy. Soc. B **170**, 113–134 (1968).

LOWENSTEIN, O., OSBORNE, M.P., WERSÄLL, J.: Structure and innervation of the sensory epithelia of the labyrinth in the Thornback Ray (*Raja clavata*). Proc. roy. Soc. B **160**, 1–12 (1964).

LOWENSTEIN, O., SAND, A.: The individual and integrated activity of the semicircular canals of the elasmobranch labyrinth. J. Physiol. (Lond.) **99**, 89–101 (1940).

LOWENSTEIN, O., THORNHILL, R.A.: The labyrinth of Myxine: anatomy, ultrastructure and electrophysiology. Proc. roy. Soc. B **174**, 419–434 (1970).

LOWENSTEIN, O., WERSÄLL, J.: A functional interpretation of the electron microscopic structure of the sensory hairs in the cristae of the elasmobranch *Raja clavata* in terms of directional sensitivity. Nature (Lond.) **184**, 1807–1810 (1954).

LUNDQUIST, P.-G.: The endolymphatic duct and sac in the guinea pig. Acta oto-laryng. (Stockh.) Suppl. **201**, 1–108 (1965).

NAKAI, J., HILDING, D.A.: Vestibular endolymph-producing epithelium. Acta oto-laryng. (Stockh.) **66**, 120–128 (1968).

OOORT, H.: Über die Verästelung der Nervus octavus bei Säugetieren. Anat. Anz. **51**, 272–280 (1918/19).

Rasmussen, A.T.: Studies of the eighth cranial nerve in man. Laryngoscope (St. Louis) **50**, 67–83 (1940).

Rasmussen, G.L., Gaisec, R.: Concerning the question of an efferent fiber component of the vestibular nerve of the cat. Anat. Res. **130**, 361–362 (1958).

Rasmussen, G.L.: Further observations of the efferent cochlear bundle. J. comp. Neurol. **99**, 61–74 (1963).

Retzius, G.: Das Gehörorgan der Wirbeltiere. I. Das Gehörorgan der Fische und Amphibien. Stockholm: Centraldruckerei 1881.

Retzius, G.: Das Gehörorgan der Wirbeltiere. II. Das Gehörorgan der Reptilien, der Vögel und der Säugetiere. Stockholm: Centraldruckerei 1884.

Rosenhall, U.: Some morphological principles in the vestibular maculae in birds. Arch. klin. exp. Ohr.-, Nas.- u. Kehlk.-Heilk. **197**, 154–182 (1970).

Rossi, G.: The efferent innervation of the inner ear. Historical bibliographical survey. Laryngoscope (St. Louis) **75**, 212–235 (1965).

Sand, A.: The mechanism of lateral sense organs of fishes. Proc. roy. Soc. Biol. **123**, 472–495 (1937).

Saxtén, A.: Histological studies on the endolymph secretion and resorption in the inner ear. Acta oto-laryng. (Stockh.) **40**, 23–31 (1951).

Smith, C.A.: Microscopic structure of the utricle. Ann. Otol. (St. Louis) **65**, 450–469 (1956).

Smith, C.A.: Utricle and saccule. In: Submicroscopic structure of the inner ear. S. Iurato, Ed. Oxford and London: Pergamon Press 1967.

Smith, C.A.: The extra-sensory cells of the vestibule. In: Biochemical Mechanisms in Hearing and Deafness. Springfield: Charles C. Thomas 1970.

Spoendlin, H.: Organization of the sensory hairs in the gravity receptors in utricle and saccule of the squirrel monkey. Z. Zellforsch. **62**, 701–716 (1964).

Spoendlin, H.: Ultrastructural studies of the labyrinth in squirrel monkeys. In: First Symposiom on the role of the vestibular organs in the exploration of space. NASA report SP-77. Washington: U.S.G.G.O. 1965.

Spoendlin, H.: Some morphofunctional and pathological aspects on the vestibular sensory epithelia. In: Second Symposium on the role of the vestibular organs in the exploration of space. NASA report SP-115. Washington: U.S.G.G.O. 1966.

Streeter, G.L.: On the development of the membraneous labyrinth and the acoustic and facial nerves in the human embryo. Amer. J. Anat. **6**, 139–165 (1906).

Werner, Cl. F.: Die Differenzierung der Maculae im Labyrinth, insbesondere bei Säugetieren. Z. Anat. Entwickl.-Gesch. **99**, 696–709 (1933).

Werner, Cl. F.: Das Labyrinth. Leipzig: Georg Thieme 1940.

Werner, Cl. F.: Das Gehörorgan der Wirbeltiere und des Menschen. Leipzig: VEB Georg Thieme 1960.

Wersäll, J.: Studies on the structures and innervation of the sensory epithelium of the cristae ampullares in the guinea pig. Acta oto-laryng. (Stockh.) Suppl. **126**, 1–85 (1956).

Wersäll, J.: Electron micrographic studies of vestibular hair cell innervation. In: Neural Mechanisms of the Auditory and Vestibular Systems. Springfield: Charles C. Thomas 1960.

Wersäll, J., Flock, Å.: Functional anatomy of the vestibular and lateral line organs. In: Contributions to sensory Physiology, Vol. I. New York: Academic Press Inc. 1965.

Wersäll, J., Flock, Å., Lundquist, P.-G.: Structural basis for directional sensitivity in cochlear and vestibular sensory receptors. Cold Spr. Harb. Symp. quant. Biol. **30**, 115–145 (1965).

Wersäll, J., Lundquist, P.-G.: Morphological polarization of the mechanoreceptors on the vestibular and acoustic systems. In: Second Symp. on the role of the vestibular organs in the explorations of space. NASA report SP-115. Washington: U.S.G.G.O. 1966.

Vilstrup, T.: Studies on the structure and function of the semicircular canals. Copenhagen: Munksgaard 1950.

Vinnikov, J.A., Govardovski, V.I., Osipuva, I.V.: Substructural organization of the organ of gravitation utricle of the pigeon. Biophysics **10**, 705–716 (1965).

Vinnikov, J.A.: The Gravity Receptor. Cosmik Biology 1971.

Chapter II.

The Functional Significance of Semicircular Canal Size

By

G. Melvill Jones, Montreal

With 4 Figures

Contents

I. Introduction

A striking feature of the semicircular canal is its small size. In man the radius of curvature of the endolymphatic canal is about 3.3 mm and the internal radius of the lumen 0.15 mm. Furthermore, as will emerge below, it is of more than passing interest that on the whole these dimensions show relatively little change with the size of the animal. Thus, it can be calculated from the data of Jones and Spells (1963) that on average for all animals examined, a 1000-fold increase in body weight (and hence presumably about a 10-fold increase in linear dimensions of the body) is associated with increases of canal radius of curvature and internal radius by factors of only 1.7 and 1.4 respectively. It seems that natural selection in evolution has met with some constraint tending to keep the physical dimensions of these small end-organs within rather closely prescribed size limits, and it is therefore pertinent to enquire into the kind of physiological consequence which might derive from such constraint.

Bearing in mind the usually accepted principle that inertial forces due to angular acceleration generate Newtonian fluid flow in the endolymphatic canal, in a tube as small as that of the canal the ratio of viscous forces to those due to inertia becomes very high. Consequently, patterns of flow generated by normal head movement become dominated by viscous damping, associated with fluid flow with a Reynolds number of less than one. Indeed, as indicated by VAN EGMOND et al. (1949), the damping is more than 10 times the critical value in the combined cupula-endolymph mechanical system. Two important functional features emerge from this fact.

A. Limitation of Cupular Angle

First, due to very heavy viscous drag, the actual volume flow of fluid round the canal circuit associated with normal head movements must always be very small; sufficiently small, that is, to permit accurate transduction of the volume displacement of fluid by means of a water-tight "swing-door" cupula having limited angular excursion in the ampulla. Anticipating the analytical treatment of later sections, a rough approximation of the actual cupular angle per unit head angular velocity can be assessed from the numerical data of JONES and SPELLS and equations (2) and (3) below. The mean of internal radii (r) from the five human specimens quoted is 0.0145 cm. This value agrees well with that of 0.0144 cm calculated from the regression line of Fig. 4 for a man weighing say 80 kg. If we assume 20% shrinkage due to formalin fixation in the prepared specimens, this gives a probable living value for r of 0.0174 cm. Then, as pointed out below, the gain of the angular velocity transducing system is given by the ratio $\frac{I}{C}$, which from equations (2) and (3) becomes:

$$\frac{I}{C} = \frac{2}{8} \cdot \frac{\rho}{\eta} \cdot r^2$$

where
I = moment of inertia of the endolymph
C = moment of friction per unit angular velocity of relative endolymph flow
ρ = fluid density
η = fluid viscosity

According to MAYNE (1965) and NEWMAN (1967) this value is too large by a factor of 2 since moment of inertia cannot be taken all round the circuit as was assumed by VAN EGMOND et al. (1949) in their derivation of equation (3). If this is true then numerically it is more correct to write

$$\frac{I}{C} = \frac{1}{8} \cdot \frac{\rho}{\eta} \cdot r^2$$

for the gain of the system in terms of the angle of fluid displacement round the canal circuit per unit angular velocity of the skull.

Physiologically, of course, it is the angle of cupular deflection per unit angular velocity which signifies, and the probable ratio of this to $\frac{I}{C}$ can also be assessed from the data of JONES and SPELLS. They point out that the approximate volume swept per unit angular deflection of the cupula in the ampulla is given by $\frac{V}{\pi}$ where V is the ampulla volume, and that the volume of endolymph flowing per unit angular displacement of endolymph round the canal circuit is given by $\pi r^2 R$ where R is the radius of curvature of the canal.

Equating these two values gives

$$\frac{V}{\pi} = \pi r^2 R,$$

and the ratio of angle of fluid circulation in the endolymphatic tube (θ_e) to cupular angle (θ_c) is given by

$$\frac{\theta_e}{\theta_c} = \frac{\pi^2 r^2 R}{V}.$$

The value of $\frac{r^2 R}{V}$ was calculated from measurements on 44 different species and found to be 0.0509 (S.D. 0.0264). Substitution of this value gives

$$\frac{\theta_e}{\theta_c} = 0.0509\ \pi^2 \simeq 0.5.$$

Thus the expression for cupular angle (θ_c) per unit input of head angular velocity ($\dot{\theta}_i$) is now given by

$$\frac{\theta_c}{\dot{\theta}_i} = 0.5 \times \frac{I}{C} = \frac{0.5}{8} \cdot \frac{\rho}{\eta} \cdot r^2.$$

Then for $\rho = 1.0$; $\eta = 0.006$ (c.g.s.); r = 0.0174 cm we have an overall gain of,

$$\frac{\theta_c}{\dot{\theta}_i} = \frac{0.5}{8} \times \frac{1}{0.006} \times (0.0174)^2$$

$\simeq 0.0032$ degrees of cupular deflection per degree per sec of head angular velocity.

This value is very much smaller than that of about 0.1 arrived at by VAN EGMOND et al. (1949), although somewhat larger than corresponding values of about 5×10^{-4} estimated by OMAN and YOUNG (1972) for MAN and 6×10^{-4} estimated by MELVILL JONES and MILSUM (1971) for the cat from measurements of cat canal dimensions made by FERNÁNDEZ and VALENTINUZZI (1968).

These small values illustrate the point at issue, namely that owing primarily to the small size of the canal, actual cupular displacements must be very small in natural life. For example during a maximum head angular velocity of $\pm 800°$/sec (HALLPIKE and HOOD, 1953) cupular angles would only be on the order of one degree.

B. The Significance of Laminar Flow

The second and perhaps most important single feature emerging from the small size of the canal arises from the low Reynold's number of the system which, as already mentioned, is probably less than one. This ensures that such flow as does occur must behave in accordance with the Hagen-Poiseuille law of laminar flow in small circular pipes. As a result, the *velocity* of *relative* flow becomes strictly proportional to the inertial force driving it and hence also to the angular acceleration of the head, at least insofar as parabolic flow obtains for the greater part of any movement. Thus

$$\text{Velocity of relative fluid flow} \propto \text{Head angular acceleration},$$

and hence if linearity obtains,

$$\text{Displacement of endolymph} \propto \text{Head angular velocity}.$$

With the small volume flows realized in practice, this implies a close relation between cupular angle in the ampulla and instantaneous head angular velocity in the relevant plane. As will emerge below, and as concluded from the detailed analytical treatments of VAN EGMOND et al. (1949), JONES and SPELLS (1963), MAYNE (1965), this simple conclusion, heavily dependent as it is upon the particular size of the endolymphatic canal, apparently embodies a fundamental principle in the physiological operation of the canal system.

However, the simple issue tends to be complicated by two additional factors, namely the time required to reach steady flow conditions during angular acceleration and the effects of cupular elasticity which always generates an additional restoring force when the cupula is deflected from its datum position.

The various interacting factors at this point become too involved to allow further appraisal of the matter without recourse to formal mathematical treatment. The methods employed below follow closely those of JONES and SPELLS (1963), whose anatomical measurements of actual canal dimensions over a wide range of species are also employed in order to compare theoretical predictions with observed findings. It should be mentioned that the observational findings quoted here were derived mainly from prepared specimens and elegant stereoscopic and scaled photographs of prepared specimens collected by A. A. GRAY (1907) and O. GRAY (prepared specimens preserved at the Museum of the Royal College of Surgeons, London). Of course, as already mentioned, the process of fixing in formalin probably caused some shrinkage in these specimens, but this is immaterial to the main theme of the following arguments, since the latter are based largely upon comparative rather than actual dimensions.

II. Criteria for Dynamical Similarity

In order to examine the functional significance of canal dimensions quantitatively, it is convenient to obtain criteria for dynamical similarity which are dependent only upon dimensionless ratios and therefore independent of actual size. For this purpose equation (8) in Mayne's chapter on Physics of Canal may be restated here in the more general form derived by dimensional analysis. It will be recalled that this equation relates the relative angle of fluid flow round the canal circuit (and its first and second derivatives with respect to time) to angular acceleration of the whole canal in its own plane. Six quantities are taken into account, namely the relative angle of fluid displacement round the circuit of the endolymphatic canal (θ_e), time (t), the input angular acceleration of the whole system ($\ddot{\theta}_i$), the relevant moment of inertia of the endolymph (I), the moment of friction per unit angular velocity of relative endolymph flow (C), and the moment of cupular restoring force per unit relative angular displacement of the fluid round the canal circuit (K). These quantities can be expressed dimensionally in terms of mass (M), length (L) and time (T) as follows:

$$\theta_e = \text{(dimensionless)}$$
$$t = (T)$$
$$\ddot{\theta}_i = \frac{1}{T^2}$$

$$I = (ML^2)$$

$$C = \frac{ML^2}{T}, \text{ derived from } \left[\frac{\left(\text{force} = \frac{ML}{T^2}\right) \times \left(\text{moment arm} = L\right)}{\text{Angular Velocity} = \left[\frac{1}{T}\right]}\right]$$

$$K = \frac{ML^2}{T^2}, \text{ derived from } \left[\frac{\left(\text{force} = \frac{ML}{T^2}\right) \times \left(\text{moment arm} = [L]\right)}{\text{Angular displacement} = \text{dimensionless}}\right]$$

From these relations only two fundamental dimensional units emerge, namely $[ML^2]$ and $[T]$. As a result, four independent dimensionless groups are required for the general relationship between the relevant quantities to be adequately expressed (see π theorem, BRIDGMEN, 1931). These may be chosen as

$$\frac{I}{Ct};\ \frac{I\ddot{\theta}_i}{K};\ \ddot{\theta}_i t^2;\ \theta_e$$

and hence:

$$F\left(\frac{I}{Ct}, \frac{I\ddot{\theta}_i}{K}, \ddot{\theta}_i t^2, \theta e\right) = 0$$

or

$$\theta_e = F\left(\frac{I}{Ct}, \frac{I\ddot{\theta}_i}{K}, \ddot{\theta}_i t^2,\right) \tag{1}$$

is the equation for θ_e given by dimensional analysis.

From this it is evident that if equal angular deviations of contained fluid, θ_e, are to occur at identical times t in response to a given time history of θ_i, then $\frac{I}{C}$ and $\frac{I}{K}$ must remain constant; hence this is the condition required for dynamical similarity as regards the angular displacement of endolymph round the canal circuit.

In order to examine the influence of canal physical dimensions upon these fundamental terms it is necessary first to evaluate the inertial (I), viscous (C) and elastic restoring (K) coefficients in terms of basic physical parameters. VAN EGMOND et al. (1949) give

$$C = 8\pi^2 \eta R^3 \tag{2}$$

and

$$I = 2\pi^2 \rho r^2 R^3 \tag{3}$$

whilst JONES and SPELLS (1963) give

$$K = \pi r^2 \mu R \tag{4}$$

where

R = radius of curvature of endolymphatic canal
r = internal radius of the lumen of the endolymphatic tube
ρ = fluid density
η = fluid viscosity
and μ = the pressure exerted by the cupula per unit angular deflection of fluid round the circuit.

There are reservations attached to these relations. First it is assumed that steady-state conditions obtain and hence transient effects are not taken into account. However, these are probably very rapid (time constant around 5 msec in man) (see previous chapter) and are unlikely to exert any significant influence during natural head movements. Second, as already mentioned, there is some conflict of opinion regarding the effective "control volume" to be taken into account in a fluid circuit in which the tube is thin in some parts and thick in others, as in the canal-utricle combination (VAN EGMOND et al., 1949; MAYNE, 1965; NEWMAN, 1968). But in the current context the differences of opininion are not particularly relevant, in view of the comparative nature of the present arguments. Thirdly, it is tacitly assumed that the thin canal always occupies about the same proportion of the circuit, which in reality is manifestly not the case in all animal species. No doubt the variability of this factor between species will account in part for the observed variability to be found in the plotted points of

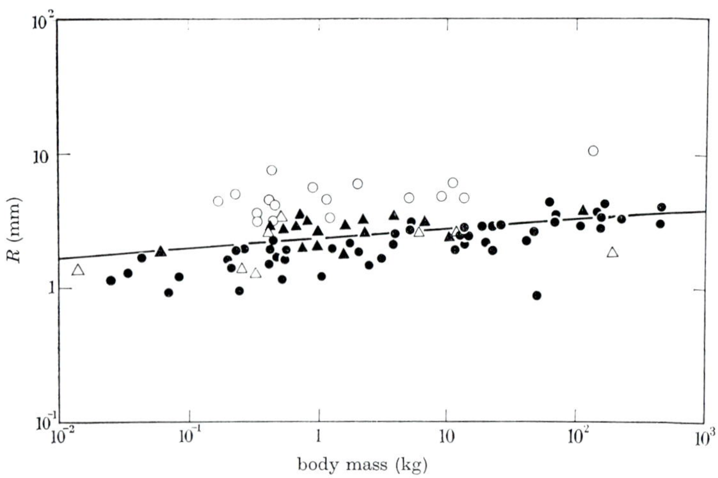

Fig. 1. Change in canal radius of curvature (R) with animal body mass measured in 93 specimens obtained from 87 species. ● Mammals; ○ Fishes; ▲ Birds; △ Reptiles (Figs. 1 to 4 reproduced from JONES and SPELLS, 1963)

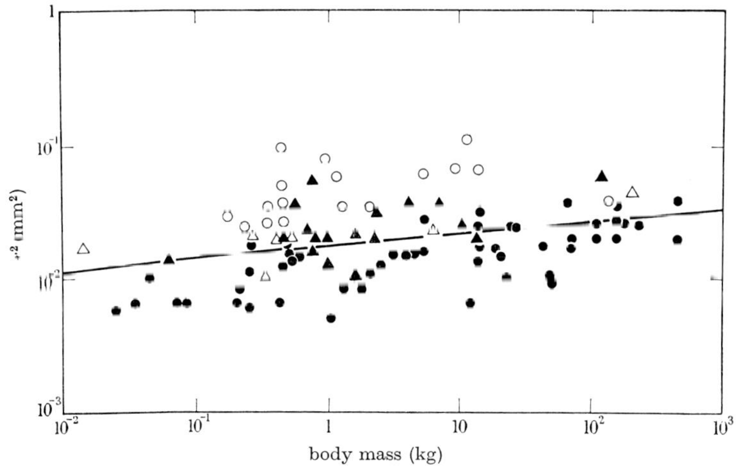

Fig. 2. Change in the square of internal radius of endolymphatic canal $(r)^2$ with body mass. Same specimens as in Fig. 1. Key as in Fig. 1

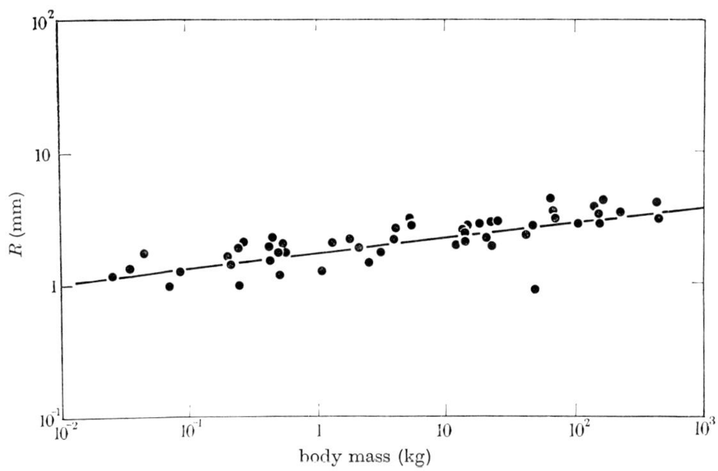

Fig. 3. Change in canal radius of curvature (R) with body mass measured in 51 specimens obtained from 87 species of mammals alone

Figs. 1 to 4. But such an effect will presumably have its influence largely averaged out in collective data from many species, as appears to have been the case in Figs. 1 to 4 from the statistical validity attributable to the relevant calculated regression lines (see Table 1 and associated text).

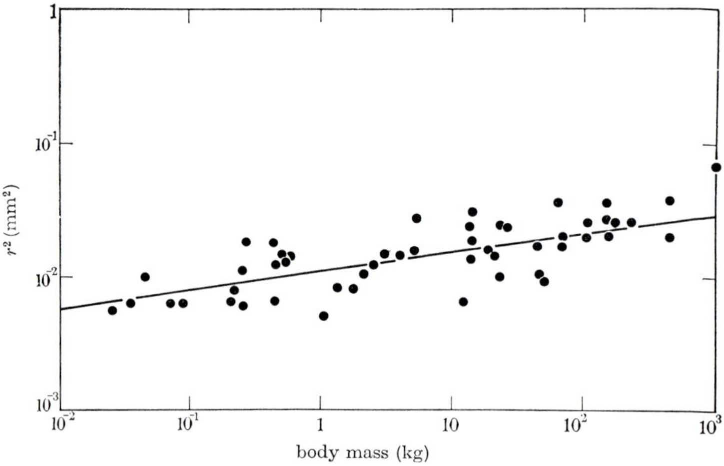

Fig. 4. Change in the square of internal radius of endolymphatic canal $(r)^2$ with body mass for mammals alone. Same specimens as in Fig. 3

With these reservations, and substituting for I, C and K from equations 2, 3 and 4,

$$\frac{I}{C} \propto \frac{\rho}{\eta} \cdot (r^2) \tag{5}$$

$$\frac{I}{K} \propto \frac{\rho}{\mu} \cdot (R^2). \tag{6}$$

Thus, since it has already been shown that for similarity $\frac{I}{C}$ and $\frac{I}{K}$ must remain invariant, it follows that both the radius of curvature (R) and the internal tube radius (r) should remain independent of animal size for equal response to rotational movement. This conclusion somewhat naively assumes that there is no interspecific variation in ρ, η and μ. This may be broadly true for ρ and η but μ is likely to vary with detailed anatomical structure. Indeed MAYNE (1965) has suggested that systematic changes in μ might be expected on theoretical grounds. However, the general assumption can be allowed to stand here since the present object is to examine the effects of size alone.

This general conclusion therefore gives some insight into the relatively very small variation in canal size seen in all mammalian species (see Figs. 3 and 4), or for that matter throughout the animal kingdom (Figs. 1 and 2). It is true that fishes have noticeably larger canals for a given body weight than other animals, but this matter will be discussed below in more detail.

The figures clearly indicate that although on the whole canal dimensions are indeed constrained to change very little with animal size, there certainly are finite changes having high statistical significance. The regression lines calculated for (R) and $(r)^2$ for all animals represented in Figs. 1 and 2 (93 specimens from 87 species) and for mammals alone (41 specimens from 46 species) as in Figs.3

and 4 have slopes which are positive at the 0.1% level of significance. Indeed it can be seen at a glance from the figures that the incremental changes in canal dimensions with body size are real and highly systematic.

III. Matching the Canal Response to Patterns of Head Movement

Evidently the simplest case in which (R) and (r) do not change at all is not realized in practice. But, again from dimensional considerations, it might be expected that the larger the animal the more sluggish would be its natural movement. In this case similar cupular motions will only occur in different time scales related by

$$\frac{t_2}{t_1} = \lambda,$$

where λ is a nondimensional quantity depending in some way on the ratio of two body masses m_1 and m_2, and t_1 and t_2 are the respective times for equal cupular deflection.

It follows also that since $\ddot{\theta}i$ is dimensionally $(\frac{1}{T^2})$,

$$\frac{\ddot{\theta}_{i_1}}{\ddot{\theta}_{i_2}} = \lambda^2.$$

Returning now to equation (1), the new conditions for similarity in this more complex case are that $\frac{I}{\lambda C}$ and $\frac{I}{\lambda^2 K}$ should remain constant. But in this case, since λ, although nondimensional, can be regarded as having a magnitude dependent on some function of animal body mass, these relations are no longer independent of animal size. Thus, referring to equations 5 and 6,

$$\frac{I}{C} \propto \lambda \propto r^2 \tag{7}$$

and $$\frac{I}{K} \propto \lambda^2 \propto R^2$$

or $$\sqrt{\frac{I}{K}} \propto \lambda \propto R, \tag{8}$$

and therefore $$\lambda \propto r^2 \propto R.$$

These conclusions imply that for similarity in the different time scales associated with the head movements of animals of different size, R and r^2 should vary in proportion to the same function, λ, of body mass, and hence should always remain proportional to one another. It is on the basis of this prediction that the data for R and r are plotted on ordinates as R and r^2 in Figs. 1 to 4. It is striking how closely this prediction is adhered to. The slopes of curves for R and r^2 against body mass are hardly distinguishable from one another. Statistically they do not differ from one another at the 5.0% level of significance.

A. Relation beetween λ and Body Mass

It has been postulated above that λ varies as some function of body mass. The form of this function might be examined initially by assuming complete geometrical similarity between animals of all sizes. In all cases, head angular acceleration will be determined by the ratio of the moment due to neck muscle action divided by the moment of inertia of the head. Dimensionally, head moment of inertia $\propto L^5$ (i.e. mass $\propto L^3 \times \text{radius}^2 \propto L^2$), whilst the moment due to neck muscle action might be considered $\propto L^3$ to a first approximation (area of muscle cross-section $\propto L^2 \times$ radius arm $\propto$ L). Then for the simple case of complete geometrical similarity between all animals,

$$\ddot{\theta}_i \propto \frac{L^3}{L^5} = L^{-2}.$$

Since for a given angular excursion $\dot{\theta}_i \propto \sqrt{\ddot{\theta}_i}$, we can write

$$\dot{\theta}_i \propto L^{-1} \propto M^{-\frac{1}{3}},$$

where M is the dimension of mass ($M \propto L^3$ for the case of geometrical similarity).

Thus in this case, head angular velocity would vary in proportion to $M^{-\frac{1}{3}}$.

In view of the above assertion that in natural head movement angular deviation of endolymph, θ_e, is at all times directly related to head angular velocity, and in view of the limited excursion available to the cupula, it seems appropriate that the sensitivity, or gain (G) of the system should increase inversely as the average head angular velocity. The slower the average head movement, the greater should be the cupular response per unit angular velocity of stimulus in order to utilize the available angular excursion in the ampulla to best advantage. With this assumption therefore,

$$\frac{1}{\dot{\theta}_i} \propto G \propto M^{\frac{1}{3}}$$

or, since the gain of the system is given by the ratio $\frac{I}{C}$ (JONES and SPELLS, 1963) and since $\frac{I}{C} \propto \lambda$, we have from equations (7) and (8)

$$\lambda \propto M^{\frac{1}{3}} \propto r^2 \propto R.$$

Hence for the case of simple geometric similarity both R and r^2 should vary as $M^{\frac{1}{3}}$, and the slope of the log, log regression lines in Figs. 1 to 4 should be +0.33. The results quoted in Table 1 show that this is not the case.

B. Likely Changes in Patterns of Head Movement with Animal Size

A clue to this discrepancy may be found in the observation of D'ARCY THOMPSON (1942) that with increasing size, the neck of animals tends to become more than proportionately thick. This eventuality would not only tend to reduce the otherwise inevitable slowing of angular head movement with increase of animal size, but would also cater for the maintenance of a constant mechanical stress in the neck due to head weight. In view of this latter observation perhaps a more realistic assumption than strict geometric similarity would be that the stress (force per unit area) in the neck due to head weight is independent of animal size.

Then as before, head moment of inertia $\propto L^5$. But this time (neck radius)^2 $\propto$ head mass $\propto L^3$. Hence the turning moment is now $\propto$ (neck radius)$^2 \times$ (neck radius) $= L^3 \times L^{\frac{3}{2}}$. Thus in this case

$$\ddot{\theta}_i \propto L^3 \cdot L^{\frac{3}{2}} \cdot L^{-5} = L^{-\frac{1}{2}} \propto M^{-\frac{1}{6}},$$

and again as before, bearing in mind that $\dot{\theta}_i \propto \sqrt{\ddot{\theta}_i}$,

$$\frac{1}{\dot{\theta}_i} \propto G \propto M^{\frac{1}{12}}$$

or since the gain (G) $= \frac{I}{C} \propto \lambda$

$$\lambda \propto M^{\frac{1}{12}} \propto r^2 \propto R. \tag{9}$$

Hence in this more realistic case both r^2 and R would be expected to vary as functions of $M^{\frac{1}{12}}$, and the slopes of the log, log regression lines in Figs. 1 to 4 to be around 0.083.

Table 1. *Calculated slopes of regression lines in Figs. 1 to 4* (From Jones and Spells, 1963)

	No. of Specimens	Slopes of log, log regression lines R	r^2
All Species (Figs. 1 and 2)	93	0.076 ($\pm$0.040)	0.095 ($\pm$0.055)
Mammals (Figs. 3 and 4)	51	0.116 ($\pm$0.030)	0.143 ($\pm$0.042)

The actual slopes of calculated regression lines in the figures are given, with their 95% confidence limits in brackets, in Table 1, in which it is seen that although the value derived theoretically above closely approximates those found for all species examined by Jones and Spells (1963), the corresponding values for mammals were somewhat higher. Mayne (1965) has suggested the higher value might be expected on the grounds that head movements might be constrained by the rule that maximum inertial stresses caused by head oscillation should be constant for all animals, to avoid brain damage, for example. On the basis of this thoroughly reasonable assumption he derives a value of 0.167, and it is of interest that the actual values for mammals in Table 1 lie roughly midway between the two theoretical ones derived by Jones and Spells and Mayne.

IV. Functional Interpretations

A. The Influence of Internal Radius (r)

The close conformity which emerges above between actual and theoretical changes in r and R with animal size suggests rather strongly that generally speaking, the angular velocity transducing property of canal hydrodynamics has been matched to the likely changes in head angular velocity with animal size by small but altogether appropriate changes in critical canal dimensions. As head movements become slower with increasing animal size, the required increase in gain ($G = \frac{I}{C} \propto r^2$) of velocity transduction is largely accounted for by small changes in the internal diameter of the endolymphatic canal. But the theory predicts that for similarity the canal radius of curvature (R) must also change, but always in proportion to the square of internal tube radius $(r)^2$, and this too is apparently closely adhered to in fact. What then is the functional significance of change in R?

B. The Influence of Canal Radius of Curvature (R)

To answer this we must return to equations (5) and (6), from which it can be seen that

$$\frac{C}{K} \propto \frac{\eta}{\mu} \cdot \left(\frac{R^2}{r^2}\right),$$

or assuming η and μ constant,

$$\frac{C}{K} \propto \frac{R^2}{r^2}.$$

But if $r^2 \propto R \propto \lambda$

$$\text{then also} \quad \lambda \propto \frac{R^2}{r^2} \propto \frac{C}{K}. \tag{10}$$

Thus from equations (7), (9) and (10), theory requires that in general

$$\lambda \propto \frac{I}{C} \propto \frac{C}{K} \propto M^n \tag{11}$$

where n is some value between about 0.08 and 0.16 according to the particular assumptions on which the theory is based.

As already seen $\frac{I}{C}$ gives the gain of the velocity-transducing system. But from Chapter (MAYNE, Physics of Canal) it is also seen that in practice $\frac{I}{C}$ closely approximates the "inertia-viscosity" time constant of the canal, which in turn is the reciprocal of the upper cut-off frequency of its angular velocity-transducing characteristic. Also, $\frac{C}{K}$ closely approximates the cupular restoring time constant which in turn is the reciprocal of the lower cut-off frequency of the velocity transducing characteristic of the canal. The essential point is that during movements containing frequencies within these two cut-off values the canal functions essentially as an angular velocity transducer; whilst for oscillatory movements above or below these frequencies this is no longer the case.

On the basis of the above argument it can now be seen from equation (11) that similarity requires both upper and lower cut-off frequencies to vary inversely as λ and hence also inversely as M^n. Thus, as animal size increases, not only does the gain increase as M^n, but also both upper and lower cut-off frequencies associated with velocity transduction must decrease proportionately with the increase of gain; or symbolically,

$$\lambda \propto G \propto \frac{1}{\omega_1} \propto \frac{1}{\omega_2} \propto M^n,$$

where ω_1 = upper cut-off frequency $\simeq \frac{C}{I}$ radians/sec

and ω_2 = lower cut-off frequency $\sim \frac{K}{C}$ radians/sec.

This means that for similarity, the band-width of frequencies of head movements within which the canal operates as a reliable angular velocity-measuring device is apparently shifted up and down inversely as (body mass)^n by the ingenious device of changing r^2 and R (and hence also $\frac{R^2}{r^2}$) always approximately in proportion to one another and to (body mass)^n. This implies that the very small changes observed in r and R are alone largely sufficient to maintain the canal system within its velocity-transducing frequency range despite changes in animal size.

It seems that strong evolutionary pressure has been brought to bear in such a way as to maintain dynamical similarity through altogether appropriate changes in r and R, even though the actual magnitude of change in dimensions is far smaller than those of the whole body. For example, according to the assumptions of Jones and Spells (1963) the appropriate change in gain is apparently brought about according to the relation $r^2 \propto M^{\frac{1}{12}}$ and therefore $r \propto M^{\frac{1}{24}} \propto L^{\frac{1}{8}}$, where L is some representative linear body dimension, such as length. That is to say, theory predicts that the diameter of the endolymphatic tube should vary as the $\frac{1\text{th}}{8}$ root of animal length and the observational data cited in Figs. 1 and 2 indicate that this is indeed generally approximately true throughout the range of species examined.

A subsidiary point of interest is raised by the relatively large values of r and R observed for a given body mass in fishes (see Figs. 1 and 2). From the data of Jones and Spells (1963) typical values for a mammal and a fish each of 10 kg mass would be r = 0.12 and 0.23, and R = 2.3 and 6.0 respectively. Perhaps these increased dimensions cater for the reduced angular velocity and lower frequencies of angular head movement to be expected at a given body mass owing to the head being relatively fixed with respect to the body. Other contributory factors might be the special mode of propulsion and the physical characteristics of the fluid in which the fishes move (Ten Kate, Van Barneveld and Kupier, 1970; Howland and Masci, 1973). Whatever the cause, it is interesting to find that the changes in magnitude of r and R with body mass tend to obey the same general law as that deduced above, namely that $r^2 \propto R \propto M^n$. Calculated regression lines from the few data available for the fishes (17 specimens) give $n = 0.10$ for R and 0.12 for r^2, although the statistical significance attached to these values is below the 5% level as may be judged visually from Figs. 1 and 2.

In conclusion it may be stated that a general law appears to have emerged from the above data, i.e. that in the canal there is a strong tendency for the internal radius of the endolymphatic canal (r) and the radius of curvature of its thin section (R) to approximate the relation:

$$r^2 \text{ (or R)} = Am^n$$

where A is a constant, m the body mass and n a small value lying somewhere between about 0.08 and 0.16. By means of this relationship suitable adjustments are brought about in both gain and frequency response to maintain accurate angular velocity transduction despite changes in the likely range of head movements brought about by size, habitat and mode of movement.

References

BRIDGMAN, P.W.: Dimensional analysis (2nd ed.), Chapter 4. London: Oxford University Press 1931.

EGMOND, A.A.J., VAN GROEN, J.J., JONGKEES, L.B.W.: The mechanics of the semicircular canal. J. Physiol. (Lond.) **110**, 1–17 (1949).

FERNÁNDEZ, C., VALENTINUZZI, M.: A study on the biophysical characteristics of the cat labyrinth. Acta oto-laryng. (Stockh.) **65**, 293–310 (1968).

GRAY, A.A.: The Labyrinth of animals (vols. I and II). London: J. and A. Churchill 1907.

GRAY, O.: Prepared specimens preserved at the Museum of the Royal College of Surgeons, London, England.

HALLPIKE, C.S., HOOD, J.D.: The speed of the slow component of ocular nystagmus induced by angular acceleration of the head: its experimental determination and application to the physical theory of the cupular mechanism. Proc. roy. Soc. B **141**, 216–230 (1953).

HOWLAND, H.C., MASCI, J.: The functional allometry of semicircular canals, fins, and body dimensions in the juvenile centrarchid fish, *Lepomis gibbosus* (L.). J. Embryol. exp. Morph. **29**, 721–743 (1973).

JONES, G. M., SPELLS, K. E.: A theoretical and comparative study of the functional dependence of the semicircular canal upon its physical dimensions. Proc. roy. Soc. B **157**, 403–419 (1963).

MAYNE, R.: The functional parameters of the semicircular canals. Tech. Report GERA–1056, Goodyear Aerospace Corpn. Arizona. Also in report under NASA contract No. NAS9-4460 1965.

MELVILL JONES, G., MILSUM, J.H.: Frequency-response analysis of central vestibular unit activity resulting from rotational stimulation of the semicircular canals. J. Physiol. (Lond.) **219**, 191–215 (1971).

NEWMAN, B.G.: Theoretical study of semicircular canal hydrodynamics. Division of Aeronautics, Dept. of Engineering, McGill University, Montreal 1967.

OMAN, C.M., YOUNG, L.R.: Physiological range of pressure difference and cupular deflections in the human semicircular canal: Theoretical considerations. In "Basic aspects of central vestibular mechanisms", Ed. BRODAL, A., POMPEIANO, O. 529–536. Amsterdam: Elsevier Publishing Co. 1972.

TEN KATE, VAN BARNEVELD, H.H., KUPIER, S.W.: The dimensions and sensitivities of semicircular canals. J. exp. Biol. **53**, 501–514 (1970).

THOMPSON, W. D'ARCY: On growth and form (2nd ed.), Cambridge: University Press 1942.

Chapter III.

Histochemistry and Metabolism of the Inner Ear

By

G. F. DOHLMAN, Toronto (Canada)

Contents

I. Introduction

The goal of all histochemical and cytochemical work is "the quantitative chemical analysis of the cell, its parts and extracellular products, *in situ* and in the living state" (GLICK, 1954) and the establishment of the mechanism for breaking down food supplies into simple compounds and ultimately into carbon dioxide and water. These are some of the energy-supplying functions that the cell performs as a part of the whole organism.

One characteristic common to every living system is the capacity to act and also the possibility of controlling its actions. In view of the diversity of the processes to be excited, controlled, and regulated by the living cell, one would expect it to be extremely complex. As is well known, nearby this whole complexity is coded as genetic information along the deoxyribonucleic acid (DNA) molecules of the cell nucleus, and this information determines the structure of the complementary lengths of ribonucleic acids (RNA). Among these, "messenger RNA" determines the structure of proteins, primarily enzymes, which catalyze all reactions in living organisms, and ribosomal or "transfer RNA" is engaged in the synthesis of protein for use within the individual cell. The synthesis of proteins from amino acids requires "work", a process represented by an ordered input of energy; this energy is supplied by the stepwise breakdown of large specific molecules into carbon dioxide and water.

The food available to the organism is originally ingested in the form of proteins, fats and polysaccharides; these are large molecules, most of which cannot penetrate through cell membranes; they are therefore split into fragments by the addition of water, i.e. by hydrolysis. The most important of such products finally brought to the cells by way of the circulating blood are the monosaccharides, primarily glucose, which thus provides the bulk of the material for metabolism and energy production of the cell. The amino acids derived from the breakdown of food proteins are the building blocks for the proteins that the cell requires to replace its own enzymes and organelles, also for special functions of secretion and absorption, and for reproduction. The main function of lipids and some carbohydrates, such as glycogen, is to provide reserves for special requirements. These functions are made possible by the oxidation — reduction reactions that occur during the decomposition of the glucose molecule. In this process glucose is phosphorylated and, after rearrangement in the molecule, splits into two triose phosphates. In the presence of dehydrogenases and other enzymes, each triose phosphate is oxidized to pyruvic acid. This phase of the reaction can occur in the absence of oxygen. In the second phase of glucose decomposition, which occurs only in the presence of oxygen, the pyruvic acid is first decarboxylated as CO_2 is given off, then again oxidized and decarboxylated with different enzymes, further carbon dioxide and water being given off in the process.

The first reaction, the phosphorylation of glucose to glucose-6-phosphate, is catalyzed by hexokinases. The enzyme phosphogluco-isomerase then brings about isomerization to fructose-6-phosphate. These products are next phosphorylated to fructose-1,6-diphosphate by phosphofructokinase at the expense of adenosine triphosphate (ATP). A second series of reactions splits these breakdown products into phosphodihydroxyacetone and 3-phosphoglyceraldehyde, catalyzed by aldolase and triosephosphate isomerase. In the next step of anaerobic glycolysis, 3-phosphoglyceraldehyde is oxidized to 3-phosphoglyceric acid, with nicotine-adenine-dinucleotide (NADH) and ATP as end products. At the same time, inorganic phosphate becomes the terminal phosphoryl of ATP. In this reaction 3-phosphoglyceric acid can be isomerized to 2-phosphoglyceric acid by the enzyme phosphoglyceromutase and further dehydrated by enolase, thereby producing a high-energy compound, phosphoenolpyruvate, which leads through phosphorylation to the product pyruvic acid with lactate as an end-product in the oxidation of NADH. It is significant that the activity ratios of five of the enzymes engaged in these reactions are virtually constant in a wide range of species and tissues. There is some reason to believe that this pathway of anaerobic glycolysis is the oldest and most primitive of all energy-trapping systems.

The further transformation of pyruvate can follow one of several pathways, depending on the presence or absence of oxygen and specific enzymes. In these transformations pyruvic acid can condense with dicarboxylic oxaloacetic acid to form tricarboxylic citric acid, which suggests that citric acid might regenerate oxaloacetic acid by decarboxylation to CO_2, so establishing a cycle in which pyruvate would be used up and CO_2 given off. In this process, succinic, fumaric and malic acids would constitute intermediate products (KREBS and JOHNSON, 1937). This is now variously known as the KREBS, citric-acid, or tricarboxylic-acid cycle.

The entire pathway, from glucose to pyruvic acid and through the citric-acid cycle, can be bypassed by means of the aerobic pentose shunt reactions, leading to decarboxylation of glucose-6-phosphate to form ribulose phosphate and the reorganization of ribulose through phosphoglyceraldehyde to form hexose. In this way it is possible for six molecules of glucose-6-phosphate to be reorganized into five molecules of glucose-6-phosphate and six of carbon dioxide. No matter which pathway is used to metabolize these biological substances the reaction nearly always passes pyridine nucleotides as hydrogen acceptors. Two of these compounds are known to be of major importance: nicotine adenine-dinucleotide (NAD) and nicotinamide-adenine-dinucleotide phosphate (NADP) (previously called diphosphopyridine nucleotide or DPN and triphosphopyridine nucleotide or TPN). These pyridine nucleotides are then reduced to NADH and NADPH and are again oxidized to NAD and NADP and water with concurrent release of energy. These redox reactions involve the transfer of electrons: an atom that receives electrons is said to be reduced and the donor oxidized. The oxidation of the reduced pyridine nucleotides occurs in several steps, and only in the last step of this "electron transport chain" is there reaction with atmospheric oxygen, mediated by Warburg's "Atmungsferment," cytochrome oxidase. This complex enzymatic process leads to the production of compounds containing phosphate bonds, mostly in the form of adenosine triphosphate (ATP) and adenosine diphosphate (ADP), from which other compounds are synthesized either with the simultaneous engagement of potassium and sodium ions in the cell membrane or with the presence of calcium or magnesium ions in the mitochondria.

Since ATP plays a role in virtually all major biological phenomena, an estimate of the amount of energy provided by a single ATP molecule would be useful. However, free energy is not the property of an individual molecule but of a given mixture of substrate-enzyme product in any given reaction. Therefore, there is no single value for a so-called "high-energy substance" such as ATP (DuPraw, 1970). The actual energy relationship can best be visualized if ATP is regarded, not as an energy source, but as an energy *carrier* in the steady-state system of a living cell, the hydrolysis of ATP in a solution containing a mixture of ATP, ADP, and phosphate being the energy source. Some of this energy is used to reverse ATP hydrolysis and other *energy-consuming* reactions, and this creates a situation in which the system never really approaches equilibrium but simultaneously harbors several reactions, both energy-releasing and energy-consuming. In such a system the ratios of ATP, ADP, and phosphate may remain constant, but energy is continuously flowing through the ATP-ADP system from one part of the environment to another part. Thus it is obvious that the total energy flux is more or less independent of the number of ATP molecules that act as energy *carriers* in this energy flow.

This perspective makes it obvious that what we can see, and what histochemistry can give, is just a flashlight view of some of the elements which themselves flow or carry building blocks in the mainstream of cellular metabolic processes. If all the cells in an organ like the inner ear only needed one metabolism for their basic survival, all cells might show the same histochemical distribution and staining density of their constituents and enzymes (Vosteen, 1960). As soon as the cells have any other function to fulfill, secretion, ion or water transport, reproduction, etc., the energy supplies of the cell must be increased, and this will become apparent in enhanced metabolism and increased staining of most of the oxidation — reduction enzymes of the cell, reflecting an increase in the respiration rate, the cytochemically measured rate of catalysis by the enzymes, etc. In the early days of histochemical research it was hoped that, if enough differences in distribution and quantity of enzymes were recorded, a pattern of data would emerge that was characteristic for specific functions of the cells e.g. the haircells (LOWRY, 1953). These expectations have in general not been fulfilled. Instead, the knowledge accumulated, supported by cytochemistry, has indicated that the first part of the decomposition of glucose in the cell takes place in the cytoplasm, and the second part is effected by enzymes in the mitochondria of the cell. This means that a cell rich in mitochondria has correspondingly greater possibilities for a channeled breakdown of pyruvic acid into CO_2 and water than a cell with only a few mitochondria. The staining of the enzymes engaged in this process will thus also depend on the morphological distribution of these cell organelles. In addition, cells that contain mitochondria with extensive cristae also show a higher oxygen consumption than cells with few cristae in their mitochondria. Thus the higher metabolic rate of the cell is apparent in the denser histochemical staining of the enzymes that break down the intermediate products in the citric acid cycle: succinic, fumaric, and malic acid. These histochemical findings are accompanied by a higher oxygen consumption. Both these results correspond directly to the morphologically higher density of mitochondria and the extent of the development of mitochondrial cristae. It is estimated that each living cell contains about 3,000 different enzymes, each with a distinct function of enhancing a specific chemical reaction (DUPRAW, [126]). However, of these 3,000 enzymes, only a few hundred are visible under the light microscope, and only ten or twenty in the electron microscope. Thus, histochemistry can provide only a limited, static picture of a few pieces in the jigsaw puzzle of continuously progressing cell reactions.

The function of the mitochondria is so important for the whole metabolic mechanism of the cell that it seems appropriate to mention some facts about these organelles. The mitochondria consist of about 75% protein and 25% lipids. Morphologically, they are wrapped in an outer membrane and have an inner membrane so wrinkled that it appears as "cristae" in section. These cristae have a rim of "elementary particles" on their inner surface. It has been shown that the functional molecules involved in electron transport and oxidative phosphorylation are arranged in replicate, highly ordered assemblies, constituting the internal membranes of the mitochondria. The mitochondria must have a large supply of enzymes at their disposal to perform these important functions.

The important specific enzymes found in mitochondria are pyruvate oxidase, all the enzymes of the citric cycle, the enzymes catalyzing beta-oxidation of fatty acids, all the components of the electron-transport chain and the enzymes of coupled phosphorylation. In addition, there are subsidiary enzymes such as adenyl kinase, betahydroxybutyrate dehydrogenase, α-glycerophosphate dehydrogenase, and other enzymes that catalyze transamination of amino acids and synthesis of protein, phosphatides and, in some mitochondria, also fatty acids. Altogether over 70 enzymes and 14 co-enzymes have been recorded (LEHNINGER, [88a]). However, mitochondria do not contain enzymes of anaerobic glycolysis;

these occur only in solution in the extramitochondrial cytoplasm. The availability of substrates, the disposition of products, and the orderly occurrence of enzymes are all subject to precise control, and thus a controlled influx of matter and energy is balanced against a controlled outflow.

Many factors are involved in controlling the system of enzyme-catalyzed reactions in the cells. Some known controlling elements are the concentration of substrate and product and changes in pH. Many enzyme-catalyzed chemical modifications have also been shown to provide a mechanism for the amplification of regulatory signals. Such activations by very low concentrations of the modifying enzyme can induce profound changes in the metabolic pattern of a cell. The specific effector may be a hormone, e.g. epinephrine, which activates the degration of glycogen.

Furthermore, it has been shown that mitochondria act as "perfect osmometers" by allowing the passage of water through the membranes while remaining impermeable to many ions and macromolecules. Since the essential function of the mitochondrion is to take up various substrates together with oxygen and to release carbon dioxide, water and phosphoryl energy, the permeability of their membranes is of particular interest. The observed generally low permeability of mitochondria membranes has been interpreted as being important to prevent indiscriminate oxidation of essential cell components (LEHNINGER, 1964). Their impermeability to substrates like NADH, citric-acid-cycle intermediates and ATP implies an efficient mechanism for transportation of phosphoryl energy thanks to their passive permeability to the *products* of phosphorylation without the transfer of ADP and ATP themselves. It has been suggested that phosphoryl transfer could be accomplished by an enzyme, adenylate kinase, which occurs in the mitochondrial membrane and which might catalyze the transfer of phosphoryl from intramitochondrial ATP to extramitochondrial adenosine monophosphate (AMP). As already mentioned, mitochondria are osmotically sensitive structures which swell in hypotonic media. However, there is another type of swelling of mitochondria, which occurs in isotonic media but depends on oxidative phosphorylation (RAAFLAUB, 1954). This metabolism-dependent swelling can increase the volume of mitochondria by 4–5 times, which results in an influx of water, uncoupling of phosphorylation, and an increase in membrane permeability, and hence the temporary release of mitochondrial contents such as ATP. Besides these processes, there is still another phenomenon that is important for the function of the mitochondria. It has been shown (LEHNINGER, 1964) that an active mitochondrial contraction can be produced even in the absence of metabolic activity, e.g. by the addition of ATP, fatty acids or α-glycerophosphate (NEUBERT, 1962). This is a very sensitive reaction, and it has been calculated that as many as 2,400 molecules of water may be extruded by each molecule of ATP hydrolyzed. This is not an osmotic mechanism but an active mechanical event, like muscle contraction. Such movements of the mitochondria have also been seen in the intact living cell observed by phase-contrast microscopy. All these reactions are reversible, which again indicates their importance in the regulation of the metabolic processes of the cell.

It may be easier to appreciate the functional importance of the work done by the mitochondria and the significance of their strategic location in specialized cells, particularly the dark cells in the inner ear, against the background of these processes. A report with special reference to the histochemistry of the ear, see SCHÄTZLE [143].

After these general remarks, it seems pertinent to give an account of the contribution histochemistry can make to this subject, particularly as it affects the inner ear.

II. Enzyme Histochemistry of the Ear

The localization of enzymes in the different tissues and cells of the inner ear started with VOSTEEN's investigation (1956) of succinic dehydrogenase distribution in the cochlea, and has been continued mainly by German investigators (VOSTEEN, v. WESTERNHAGEN, MÜSEBECK, SCHÄTZLE, and others) with the aid of a soluble tetrazolium salt reduced by the enzyme to insoluble formazan deposits. The cells of the spiral ganglion showed many formazan precipitations, as did the epithelium of the limbus cells, the vascular stria, the hair cells, and the region under the external spiral sulcus, indicating high functional activity in these regions.

VOSTEEN [188] applied protracted acoustic stimulation and showed that the succinic dehydrogenase activity decreased. When the duration of sound stimulation was extended, the damage to the structures of the stimulated part of the cochlear elements increased, with damaged enzyme activity starting in the nerve ending under the hair cells. When intermittent tone stimuli were used, there was only insignificant damage to the organ of Corti. VOSTEEN interpreted these findings as indicating exhaustion of the enzymatic respiratory process and not primarily mechanical destruction of the hair-cell structure.

Succinic dehydrogenase activity has since been investigated by several other scientists, who have confirmed VOSTEEN's findings (BECK and MICHLER, 1960; VINNIKOW and TITOVA, 1963; IMOKAWA, 1959; GERHARDT, 1961). SCHÄTZLE and MÜSEBECK (1962) and IMOKAWA and KOIDE (1959) used different inhibitors which caused a weaker reaction due to the inactivation of sulfydryl groups of the enzymes. The succinic dehydrogenase activity was shown to be strong in the basal turn of the cochlea, increasing towards the apex (KOIDE et al., 1962; KAWAMATO and KAKIZAKI, 1962; KOIDE, 1958, 1958; KOIDE et al., 1964).

NOMURA and BALOGH (1964) incubated sections for succinic dehydrogenase after EDTA decalcification of the bone. They found a relatively low activity in cristae and maculae. In the planum semilunatum and the dark-cell regions the reaction was more intense. MIRA and DAL NEGRO (1969) and v. WESTERNHAGEN (1968) came to the conclusion that decalcification had removed some of the enzyme activity in such experiments.

NAKAI (1965) and NAKAI and HILDING (1968, 1968) investigated the vascular stria and the organ of Corti by electron microscopy after incubation with tetranitrophenyltetrazol blue, which showed the succinic dehydrogenase activity localized to the mitochondria, especially the mitochondrial cristae. Accordingly, the cells with the highest density of mitochondria, such as the marginal cells of the vascular stria, also showed the strongest reaction. In none of these experiments was any stain found in the cupulae or tectorial membrane.

Vosteen (1957, 1960, 1964, 1970) also investigated several other respiratory enzymes, e.g. the DPN (diphosphopyridine nucleotide) and TPN (triphosphopyridine nucleotide) diaphorases [renamed nicotinamide-adenine-dinucleotide = NAD and nicotinamide-adenine-dinucleotide-phosphate = NADP]. These diaphorases showed a high activity in the hair cells, with a weaker activity in the vascular stria. The nerve endings showed a negative reaction to NAD and low activity of NADP. Most of these findings were later confirmed by Gerhard [17] and Nomura and Balogh [113]. Nakai and Hilding [111c] and Koide et al. [82] used neotetrazol for their investigations on guinea pigs. The reaction indicated a marked NAD-diaphorase activity in the vascular stria and spiral ligament. The intensity of the reaction was strongest in the basal turn, decreasing towards the apex. The intensity was the same in all hair cells, however, throughout the cochlea. Nomura and Balogh (1964), Nomura et al. (1970), and Mira (1966) found a strong reaction of both diaphorases in the vestibular apparatus in the hair cells and the epithelium of the transitional cells.

By electron-microscope studies Nakai and Hilding (1968) investigated the NADH-diphorase activity in the guinea-pig cochlea. The diaphorase activity was found in the cristae mitochondriales and accordingly in the hair cells, where mitochondria are situated, and in the Deiters' cells and specifically in the vascular stria. Lim [90] made similar investigations with the same finding in the hair cells, some stria cells, Reissner's membrane, and the connective tissue cells in the spiral ligament and limbus spiralis. In limbus spiralis some cells showed especially high activity which others (Voldrich [185], Lim [91]) have also assumed to be due to an active phase of cyclic activity in their supposed secretory function. The afferent nerve endings were diffusely stained, whereas at the efferent endings the formazan was conspicuously precipitated along the synaptic cleft.

Furthermore, lactate dehydrogenase was found by Vosteen (1957, 1960) to be present in hair cells and to a lesser degree also in the vascular stria, and concluded that this might indicate that the hair cells had a capacity for anaerobic glycolysis which Vosteen assumed to be absent in other cells in the ear, which might explain the greater resistance to hypoxia in the hair cells than in other cells, such as the cells of the stria, which might be damaged by a low oxygen supply. Vosteen also found glutamate-dehydrogenase and α-glycerophosphate dehydrogenase in the same locations as lactate dehydrogenase.

In a study of lactate dehydrogenase isoenzymes (by means of agar electrophoresis) in man, guinea pigs, rabbit, cat, and rat, Lotz and Kuhl [93] were able to isolate 5 isoenzymes. These enzymes have specific relations to the aerobic or anaerobic metabolism of the cell. The authors found a predominance of the aerobic enzyme fraction in guinea pigs, rabbits and cats in the stria and the organ of Corti.

Like the dehydrogenases of the citric-acid cycle, cytochrome oxidase is localized in the mitochondria [22, 23]. The dehydrogenases are probably located in the matrix of the mitochondria in the space between the cristae, whereas the cytochrome chain and the enzymes of coupled phosphorylation are bound to the cristae (Barrnett and Palade [6]). Vosteen [187, 190, 191, 192] demonstrated the presence of cytochromeoxidase in the cochlea, mainly in the same locations as the succinic dehydrogenase. Thus the activity was especially high in the mitochondria dense cells of the vascular stria and the cells of the spiral sulcus with their continuations into the spiral ligament.

The hair cells were intensely stained. These findings have since been confirmed by IMIKOWA (1959), GERHARDT (1962), KOIDE et al. (1962), CONTI and BORGO (1964) and NOMURA and BALOGH (1964). CONTI and BORGO [23] investigated the influence of acoustic trauma on the intensity of the reaction to this respiratory enzyme. Their results seemed to indicate that a general decrease in cytochrome oxidase activity was produced in the hair cells as well as in the vascular stria cells. In the vestibular labyrinth NOMURA and BALOGH (1964) demonstrated an intense reaction in the hair cells of the cristae and macula sacculi, and somewhat weaker staining of the planum semilunatum.

Among other enzymes investigated in the inner ear, the phosphorylases, which regulate the breakdown process of glycogen, have been the subject of a biochemical study by THALMANN et al. (1968), who found phosphorylase activity in the hair cells, vascular stria and Reissner's membrane. These enzymes had also been investigated histochemically by VINNIKOV and TITOVA (1963), who found such activity in the hair cells and Deiters' cells.

Other enzymes have been investigated by SCHÄTZLE and v. WESTERNHAGEN [140, 141, 142, 147, 148, 149, 150], namely glucosaminidase, galactosidase, glucoronidase, monoamine oxidase, tyrosinase, peroxidase, and nonspecific esterases and lipases. Monoamine oxidase was found in high concentrations in the spiral ganglion cells, and in lower concentrations in the vascular stria. An intense reaction was shown in the hair cells. This enzyme is known to break down toxic products of protein metabolism which could therefore be of importance for the function of the inner ear, but investigations on this point have not been sufficiently extensive to indicate any influence on the metabolism of the inner ear structures.

Tyrosinase is of importance in pigment formation and must therefore be taken into account in consideration of the pigment metabolism in the ear. The enzyme was found mainly in the vascular stria, which normally contains pigment in many animal species. In the hair cells there was only a slight reaction, as also in Reissner's membrane. The limbus spiralis and the tectorial membrane were negative.

SCHÄTZLE and v. WESTERNHAGEN (1966) found nonspecific esterases and lipases in several structures of the cochlea. The hair cells showed only a slight reaction, whereas the epithelium of the spiral sulcus and the vascular stria showed a considerably higher activity, as did the cells of the limbus spiralis. In the vestibular apparatus the hair cells of the cristae and maculae showed an intense reaction to nonspecific esterase. The lipase reaction was positive in the transitional zone of the cristae, the dark-cell region and the planum semilunatum. This was confirmed in principle by the investigations by MIRA (1966) and MIRA and DAL NEGRO (1969).

In an attempt at quantitative estimation of the enzyme reactions, MATSCHINSKY and THALMANN (1967), and THALMANN et al. (1970) investigated many of the respiratory enzymes. The glycolytic enzymes hexokinase and fructokinase were found to be present in equal quantities in the organ of Corti and the vascular stria, but only 10–30% of these quantities were found in Reissner's membrane, whereas the enzymes of the citric-acid cycle, such as malic dehydrogenase, appeared in the vascular stria in concentrations 2–3 times higher than in the hair cells, and 5–10 times higher than in Reissner's membrane. As discussed earlier, this confirms the dependence of these enzymes on their location in the mitochondria.

The enzymes of the pentose shunt, glucose-6-phosphodehydrogenase and lactic dehydrogenase, seemed to be present in the organ of Corti in the same concentration as in the vascular stria.

Investigations on isolated semicircular canals with retained vascular supply (DOHLMAN and RADOMSKI, 1968) showed that the indifferent epithelium of the canal wall also had the capacity for active transport of ions. The investigations by KUIJPERS [85, 86], THALMANN (1970, 1971a, b, 1972, 1968; THALMANN 1970, et al. 1970) and MATSCHINSKY and THALMANN (1967, 1969, 1970) seem to have indicated that the membrane of the dark cells form the main ion pump for maintaining high potassium and low sodium concentrations in the endolymph. Accordingly, the vascular stria and in birds the tegmentum vasculosum had the highest K-NA-activated ATPase activity. This enzyme was ouabain-sensitive and was inhibited by this drug, resulting in a decrease both in microphonics and in endolymph potential. In addition, v. ILBERG and IMAMURA (1966) claimed that the isolated Reissner's membrane was also capable of active transport.

This ion-exchanging function of the dark cells is thus apparently sufficiently active to explain the concept of "radial flow" coined by LAWRENCE (1966), which implies that a leak in the membranous walls of the labyrinth can be compensated by the action of local dark cells protecting the hair cells.

It must be assumed that in the living animal ions are continuously diffusing through the membranous walls of the ear, potassium from the endolymph to the perilymph and sodium in the opposite direction, due to existing ionic concentration differences (CHOO and TABOWITZ, 1965, 1965; CITRON et al., 1957). The ability to balance this leakage of ions by an active ion transport in the opposite direction is apparently a function of all the living cells in the membranous wall as long as the cells are metabolically sustained by the bloodstream. If the blood supply is blocked, the differences in ion concentrations in the two fluid compartments, endolymph and perilymph, are rapidly equalled out. However, the main safeguard for maintaining the unique ionic pattern of the endolymph is the collar of dark cells (DOHLMAN, 1967, 1969), that is always located around or very close to all the sensory areas of the ear [27, 29, 94a, 94b].

In animal experiments with ototoxic drugs interest has centered mainly on the morphologic changes (GODZDZIK-ZOLNIERKIEWITZ, 1969; COX et al., 1964). However, using dihydrostreptomycin (200 mg/kg for 14 days) MÜSEBECK and SCHÄTZLE (1962, 1964) and MÜSEBECK (1963) were able to record a considerable decrease in succinic dehydrogenase activity in the vascular stria, whereas the enzyme activity and the morphologic appearance seemed to be unchanged in other structures, including the hair cells. KAKIZAKE (1968), FLAKS et al. (1962), and ISHII et al. (1968) attained a decrease of this same enzyme in the hair cells with kanamycin. GOZDZIK-ZOLNIERKIEWICZ (1969) showed that streptomycin 200 mg/kg for 10 days produced a decrease in succinic dehydrogenase only in the basal turn of the cochlea. No morphological changes were found in the cochlear structures with this dosage. If streptomycin was applied in the middle-ear cavity (v. WESTERNHAGEN and SCHÄTZLE, 1969), a considerable decrease was recorded in succinic dehydrogenase in the hair cells of the cristae and the maculae, whereas the reaction of the dark cells on the slopes of the cristae seemed to be unchanged.

The influence on the ATPase activity in the vascular stria and spiral ligament following the administration of kanamycin and streptomycin was studied by Jinuma et al. (1967). They found a decrease in activity of the membrane-bound K^+- and Na^+-dependent ATPase that serves the fluid transport through the membrane. The mitochondrial Mg-dependent ATPase was not reduced and could even be increased. This enzyme has been shown to take part in metabolic oxidative phosphorylation.

These results seem to be highly significant in the interpretation of the metabolic processes of the ear, again emphasizing the decisive importance of the dark cells in the function of the inner ear.

III. The Pigments

Pigment cells are normally found in the membranous wall of many mammals, including man. In the human ear, pigment cells are found in the vascular stria, Reissner's membrane, the modiolus and the region surrounding the cristae and maculae. Wolff (1931) showed that the pigment in the human labyrinth was melanin. Electron-microscope investigations by Rauch and Ruska (1965) indicated that only the light cells of the vascular stria contained this pigment, and not the dark, marginal cells. Beck (1961) demonstrated that acoustic stimulation did not change the density of pigment in the vascular stria. Haubrich and Schätzle (1970) found that cortisone injections to guinea pigs produced an increase of the pigment in the vascular stria, while Duvall (1968) produced severe damage to the vascular stria when the Reissner's membrane was partly destroyed, resulting in perilymph sodium diffusing into the scala media. This led to short-term cell destruction with the extrusion into the endolymph of cell debris containing melanin. A few weeks later new melanin-containing cells were found in the atrophic tissue of the spiral ligament. However, the function of the pigment cells in the ear remained unknown. In ophthalmology it is now generally accepted that drugs like chloroquine and the phenothiazines are the most important factors in the etiology of toxic retinopathy. In a study of the uptake of these drugs in melanin-containing tissues Ullberg et al. (1970) found that these tissues had a remarkable capacity for the accumulation and retention of drugs of these classes. Lindquist (1973) emphasized that chloroquine- and quinine-induced retinopathy and several other ocular pigment disturbances are known to be associated with deafness. In their work with ototoxic antibiotics Johnson and Hawkins (1972) came to the conclusion that the hair cell degeneration in these experiments might be due to an alteration in the endolymph secondary to atrophy of the vascular stria.

Lindquist (1973) made *in-vitro* measurements of the absorption of ototoxic drugs on melanin. A very high uptake was recorded for kanamycin, hydroxychloroquine, chloroquine and chlorpromazine. Quinine, dihydrostreptomycin, streptomycin and viomycin also had a high affinity for the pigment, while salicylic acid, PAS and isoniazid had none at all. Müsebeck and Schätzle (1962) and Ostyn and Tyberghein (1968) found that the vascular stria was always impaired when the sensory cells were affected. This seems to indicate that the accumulation of ototoxic drugs on the melanin in the inner ear might be an important factor in the development of ototoxic lesions (Lindquist, 1973).

IV. Lipofuscin

Another group of pigments, the lipofuscins, are regarded as the "wear-and-tear" pigments of the cells. In an electron-microscope study of the lipofuscin in the human inner ear, ISHII et al. (1967) studied the distribution and content of some of these enzymes. The lipofuscin was found in membrane-limited inclusions in all cells in the cochlea and the vestibular apparatus. The sensory and supporting cells contained numerous lipofuscin granules in the apical cytoplasm. The lipofuscin was demonstrated by means of Schmorl's test (ADAMS, 1958). Lipofuscin was found enclosed in lysosomes. The lysosomes contain many enzymes, more than 20 of which are known. The lysosomes are assumed to participate in a number of cell functions, e.g. the intracellular digestion of endogenous and foreign material, which explains the large variety of their enzymes. In the lysosomes the presence of acid phosphatase (BARKA and ANDERSON, 1962), β-glucoronidase and N-acetyl-β-glucosaminidase was shown (BLOOM et al., 1954) but not that of alkaline phosphatase (SCHÄTZLE et al., 1969). Lipofuscin granules were also shown to be strongly fluorescent in the cochlear cells as well as the vestibular cells. The fluorescent material was not found in newborns or young children but increased with age [67].

V. Visualization of Adrenergic Nerve Fibers in the Ear

A method was developed by FALCK (1962) to visualize the presence of noradrenaline. Freeze-dried tissue was fixed in formalin vapor, which produces an insoluble strongly fluorescent compound with noradrenaline. TERAYAMA et al. (1965, 1966) fixed adrenergic-nerve structures of the cochlea by this method and studied them by fluorescence microscopy. They found fluorescent nerve fibers on the outside of the muscle layer of the large blood vessels in the modiolus and in the branches of the acoustic nerve thin fibers, which seemed to accompany the blood vessels of the nerve. No adrenergic fibers were found in the organ of Corti, vascular stria or spiral ligament. SPOENDLIN and LICHTENSTEIGER (1965, 1966, 1967) also demonstrated two different systems of adrenergic fibers in the inner ear. Besides the perivascular plexus described by Terayama they detected a second system within the acoustic nerve; this system was independent of the blood vessels and was found in the bony spiral lamina where it was seen as a dense terminal plexus close to the habenula perforata. In the vestibular part the fluorescent fibers were shown to be attached to the nerve fibers and their course to be independent of the capillaries. Injections of nialamid, which inhibits the activity of monoamine oxidase, produced a marked increase of catecholamines in the adrenergic fibers, whereas the result of section of the VIII nerve seemed to indicate that the second adrenergic system comes from the central nervous system and is continuous to the receptors. The system independent of the blood vessels was traced to the superior cervical ganglion, whereas the fibers to the capillaries seemed to come from the inferior cervical ganglion. The authors point out that the adrenergic terminal plexus is localized close to the area where the myelin sheaths of the afferent cochlear nerve fibers begin and the first Ranvier node is located, i.e. where the action potentials of the fiber are assumed to be elicited. The release of noradrenaline was therefore believed to influence the threshold of these afferent nerve fibers from the sensory areas of the ear.

The adrenergic fibers attached to the vessels and capillaries did not seem to have any direct synaptic contact with the muscles of the vascular walls, however. As mentioned by SCHÄTZLE (1971), the capillary walls have been found to be surrounded and embraced by pericytes covering 40–50% of their outer surface (RAUCH and REALE, 1968). This suggests that the pericytes, which show filaments believed to be contractile elements, could have a function which regulates the capillary lumen and blood flow. The "varicosities" on the adrenergic fibers seen by SPOENDLIN (1965, 1967) by means of fluoroscopy, contained vesicles like those in the presynaptic space of nerve endings. TERAYAMA et al. (1965) investigated the diameter of these vesicles in the efferent nerve endings and in the adrenergic ones. The diameter of those in the efferent nerve endings was 930 Å, whereas those in the adrenergic nerve endings were 750 Å in diameter, indicating a morphologic difference probably corresponding to a difference in vesicle content and physiological function. (For adrenergic fibers to the inner ear see DENSERT [24]).

VI. Acetylcholin

The method of KOELLE and FRIEDENWALD (1949) for the demonstration of the presence of acetylcholinesterase (AChE) in nerve fibers and nerve endings was first used in the inner ear by CHURCHILL et al. (1956). They were able to show the distribution to the base of the outer and inner hair cells. By means of inhibition with DFP and incubation in butyrylthiocholine they showed that unspecific cholinesterase accounted for only an insignificant fraction of the total enzymes and that AChE made up the main bulk. The authors concluded therefore that the stained nerve and nerve endings must belong to the efferent system represented by Rasmussen's olivocochlear bundle. The density of reaction appeared higher at the inner hair cells, which was probably due to the higher density of nerve fibers in the inner than in the outer spiral bundle. The density of staining decreased from the base of the cochlea towards the apex. In other experiments, the cochlear nerve was cut with retention of the vascular supply to the cochlea. This resulted in degeneration of the efferent fibers with a convincing decrease of AChE but with normal hair cells in the organ of Corti. WERSÄLL et al. (1961) were able to localize the AChE activity in the organ of Corti to the region at the base of the hair cells, in an arrangement which seemed to indicate localization in the efferent endings (KANEKO and DALY, 1968) and also on the endolymphatic surface of the hair cells (1969). In the vestibular labyrinth, AChE was demonstrated at the level of the efferent nerve endings by means of the Holmstedt modification of Koelle-Friedenwalds method (DOHLMAN et al., 1958). In electron-microscope studies HILDING and WERSÄLL (1962) showed the localization of the stain in the efferent nerve endings of the type-II hair cells. This has been confirmed by other investigators (IRELAND and FARKASHIDY, 1961; ROSSI and CORTESINA, 1966; GACEK et al., 1965; ISHII et al., 1967; SPOENDLIN and GACEK, 1963).

VII. Protein Metabolism

Staining of the protein by the tetrazolium reaction is a crude method based mainly on the reaction with the sulfydryl and sulfide groups of the proteins (BARR-

NETT and SELIGMAN, 1954). A more refined method based on photometric quantitation enabled KRAUS and DOENNIG (1969) to detect that the protein content of the cells in the inner ear varied in concentration in the different cell groups. If the cell in the spiral ganglion was assumed to contain 100%, the cells of the vascular stria contained 79% and the hair cells 30%. This gives information only on the cell content of total protein. More meaningful information, however, is given by the injection of tritium-labeled amino acids which are then traced by autoradiography after incorporation into the proteins of the different tissues and cells. The number of radioactively exposed and developed silver grains that can be counted over the cells reflects the uptake of the injected labeled substance and the turnover of the proteins of the cell.

The synthesis of proteins in the cytoplasm occurs with the aid of ribonucleic acids (RNA) localized to the "rough endoplasmic reticulum" and the free ribosome particles or the aggregates of such as "polysomes." When electron microscopy reveals a well-developed endoplastic reticulum or many ribosomes in the cytoplasm of the cells, it can be concluded that these cells have a high RNA content and therefore also the potential capacity for high protein synthesis and rapid protein turnover. This led KRAUS and DOENNIG (1969) to create an index for the relation between protein content and RNA content as well as the relation between protein turnover and the RNA concentrations in the cell. They regarded this as an indicator of the specific rate of protein synthesis of the cell. However, investigations of the intensity of protein synthesis of cells in the inner ear seemed to indicate an unexpectedly high intensity of protein synthesis in some, the Boettcher, Deiters' and hair cells, whereas in other cells that are known from investigations with other methods to have a high rate of metabolism, e.g. the vascular stria cell, low values were found. This aroused the suspicion that the fixation and decalcification methods used might have removed some of the soluble protein or parts of the RNA thus making this method of estimation of the rate of synthesis unreliable (SCHÄTZLE, 1966).

The counting of silver grains in autoradiography has been much used to compare the protein metabolism of different cell groups (LEBLOND, 1965, 1969; MEYER ZUM GOTTESBERGE, 1960, 1961; PLESTER [123]; MAURER and KOBURG [99]; KOBURG and PLESTER [77]; MEYER ZUM GOTTESBERGE et al. [102].

All these studies indicated that activity in the hair cells was about half that in the spiral ganglion cells and that the value in the vascular stria was about 75% that of the ganglion cells.

This amino-acid uptake in different cochlear turns was investigated by KOBURG and MEYER ZUM GOTTESBERGE [79] with the aid of tritium-labeled phenylalanin. This showed a rate decrease of about 30% from the basal turn to the apex. According to the study by MEYER ZUM GOTTESBERGE et al. [102], the permeability of Reissner's membrane to ^{42}K increased from the basis towards the apex.

KOBURG and PLESTER [78] examined the tectorial membrane after the injection of tritium-labeled leucin. Unexpectedly, they found its activity was about 11% of that in the spiral ganglion, while that in the vascular stria was 62% and that in the organ of Corti 36%. BELANGER [9] had used ^{35}S-methionine in his protein investigations and was able to show that no silver grains were exposed over the tectorial membrane or the cupulae, indicating that no protein turnover could be recorded in these membranes. When ^{35}S was used as sulfate, the labeled sulfur was attached to the acid mucopolysaccharides, which BELANGER therefore believed to be constituents of the cupula and other gelatinous membranes.

IURATO [69] referred to the absence of hexuronic acid in this membrane and NAFTALIN [109] indicated the presence of mere traces of hexosamine, indicating that the content of mucopolysaccharides must at least be very low. SAITO and DALY [138] found 0.1% mucopolysaccharides per dry weight of the tectorial membrane in guinea pigs, besides which DOHLMAN [26, 27, 33, 34] has shown the presence of considerable amounts of and rapid turnover of sulfated mucopolysaccharides in the labyrinth in pigeon, but not in mammals. These substances were also traced to the secretory cells in the planum semilunatum by electron-microscope histochemical methods in pigeon (DOHLMAN [30, 31)]. TACHIBANA et al. [166] and SAITO [137, 138] have recently studied the disputed presence of acid mucopolysaccharides in the tectorial membrane. They demonstrated these substances in guinea pigs in electron-microscope histochemistry with ruthenium red stain. They used microspectrophotometry to measure the absorption of Alcian Blue by the acid mucopolysaccharides. It was also shown that some of these might be digested by hyaluranidase. They also performed electron-probe microanalysis of sulfur elements in the tectorial membrane and this analysis yielded positive results which, combined with those of digestion experiments, seemed to indicate that sulfur was present in the tectorial membrane in association with acid mucopolysaccharides.

The interdental cells of the limbus spiralis have attracted interest in recent years (ISHIYAMA et al. [68]; VOLDRICH [185]; LIM [89a, 91]; ARNOLD and VOSTEEN [4]).

These investigations have pointed out that the interdental cells are functionally quite active elements. MIRA [103] studied the distribution of some oxidative and hydrolytic enzymes to attain a better understanding of the functional characteristics of these cells. Hydrolytic enzymes like acid phosphatase were decidedly positive, oxidative enzymes such as succinic isocitric dehydrogenase showed strong activity, and lactic dehydrogenases NADH and NADPH showed moderate reactions. Alkaline phosphatase was always negative. It was characteristic for all enzymes studied that differences in intensity of reaction among the interdental cells were evident. Some cells showed a strong reaction while others were only lightly stained, which was interpreted as indicating a functional cycle of reactional activity, as suggested by VOLDRICH [185] and strongly supported by the finding of large secretory vacuoles by LIM [91]. These findings have been further supported by GERHARDT [47] and NOMURA and BALOGH [113] in their studies of succinic dehydrogenase and NADH and NADPH diaphorases. ISHII and BALOGH [66, 67c] found acid phosphatase [194] only in the supranuclear region of the cytoplasm of these cells. In an electron-microscope study, LIM [90] found NADH-diaphorase activity in some interdental cells. In another electron-microscope and histochemical study of the cells, ARNOLD and VOSTEEN [4] showed that the endoplasmic reticulum produced an amorphic substance that was packed by the Golgi complex into vesicles delivered into the endolymphatic space among the fibers of the tectorial membrane. This secretion was found to contain mainly neutral glycoproteids.

The protein content of the endolymph and perilymph has been the subject of several investigations. VILSTRUP and JENSEN [180, 181, 182] reported a high protein content in the endolymph of some fishes. VILSTRUP and KORNERUP [181] found that the protein content was considerably lower in mammals. The protein content of the perilymph, however, was 3–4 times higher than that of the endolymph. CHEVANCE et al. [14, 15] made electrophoretic studies of the perilymph proteins and found a high content of β-globulin but low γ-globulin values (FRITSCH [43]; PALVA [117, 118, 119]). Their chromatographic analysis of the perilymphatic amino acids in calf, guinea pig and man showed the presence of several amino acids. The absence of tryptophan seemed to be especially noteworthy, as it could not be found even after three days when a high dose of this amino acid had been injected intraperitoneally to guinea pigs. This was interpreted as indicating the presence of a barrier.

SILVERSTEIN [155, 156, 67a] investigated the labyrinthine fluids for their content of many enzymes, and found it to be relatively low in the peripheral labyrinth but very high in the endolymphatic sac, a result that is in keeping with the concept of the sac as a receptaculum of endolymph from the ear for absorption and digestion of debris [53, 38, 94b, 94c].

The study of protein by staining methods or autoradiography involves the assessment of one or other of the amino-acid building blocks of the protein. It could therefore be expected that a difference in pattern of absence or presence of a specific amino acid would give some information that could indicate a specific function or characteristic of a cell population. This, however, has been shown not to be the case; they are all incorporated, into the protein molecule in amounts which vary quite insignificantly [79, 154, 89].

The connective tissue of the inner ear has been studied by ALBERNAZ [2] and IURATO [69], who found that the membranous labyrinth contained less hydroxyproline than the connective tissue in many other parts of the body. MÜSEBECK and SCHÄTZLE [107] also demonstrated some differences in the histochemical staining of the spiral ligament by using the disulfide reaction of BARRNETT and SELIGMAN [6a].

The protein in the cells and tissues of the cochlea was studied by means of the tetrazolium reaction (DANIELLI [24]) by ZORZOLI [206, 207], who found a strong reaction in the tectorial membrane. SCHÄTZLE and WESTERNHAGEN [148] repeated these studies but found only a relatively low response in this membrane. When radiolabeled amino acids were used in the study of protein synthesis in guinea pigs, MEYER ZUM GOTTESBERGE [100], PLESTER [123], PLESTER et al. [124], and BELANGER [9] detected no silver grains over the tectorial membrane, which indicates at least a very slow turnover of proteins in this structure. PLESTER et al. [124] came to the same conclusion when using pigeons. In investigations on rabbits and guinea pigs SCHREINER [153] found a relatively high silver-grain density over the tectorial membrane.

The uptake of tritium-labeled uridine from the endolymph (WATANUKI [197]) and/or after intraperitoneal administration (WATANUKI et al. [196]) was recorded autoradiographically in guinea pigs. This amino acid is incorporated into the RNA molecule and was localized in the nuclei after 30 to 60 min in the cells of Reissner's membrane, the marginal cells of the vascular stria and especially in the epithelium of the spiral prominence. In Reissner's membrane a higher uptake was shown over the cells close to the modiolus than over the peripheral cells. This was interpreted as a sign of a higher RNA synthesis in what were assumed to be the newly formed cells in this central area of Reissners membrane, and led to the assumption that the cells from this position move toward the periphery as they age.

The DNA of the nucleus (DANIELLI [24] can be labeled by uptake of ^{3}H-thymidine, but only during the period when a cell is preparing for cell division by redoubling its amount of DNA. RUBEN [134] exploited this to investigate both the DNA metabolism during the development of the ear in mice and uptake of ^{3}H-uridine as a precursor to RNA by autoradiography. He found DNA incorporation in the organ of Corti, but only up to the 15th day of pregnancy, and in the crista until one day post partum. The injection of precursors to RNA ^{3}H-uridine was followed by an uptake in the same areas during the first postnatal week, while later hardly any uptake was recorded.

Using Gomori's chromealum-hematoxylin and the aldehyde fuchsin methods, WISLOCKI and LADMAN [204] showed that the cupulae, tectorial membrane and otolith membranes were stained, which was assumed to be due to a reaction with the sulfydryl groups of protein in these membranes. These results seem to be compatible with those obtained by IURATO [69], NAFTALIN [109], and DOHLMAN [28, 33] with these membranes. They came to the conclusion that most of these substances must be proteins of the keratin group.

VIII. Lipids

Lipids were demonstrated in the cells of the inner ear as early as 1863 by HENSEN [55]. In 1962 these observations were reconfirmed by TONNDORF [178] who used Nile blue. GERHARDT and PIEPLOW [48] studied the lipids by means of Sudan-III and Sudan-black-B staining in the guinea-pig ear. They found lipids in the cells of Hensen, in the vascular stria, in the Claudius cells and in the limbus. The tectorial membrane was negative. The authors came to the conclusion that the density of lipids present seemed to be parallel to the location of respiratory enzymes and thus dependent on the density of mitochondria. SCHÄTZLE and v. WESTERNHAGEN [148] reported a widespread distribution in nearly all cells in the inner ear as well as in the nerve sheaths in their study with Sudan black B. SCHIFF and CHRISTIENSEN-LOU [151] showed that the lipid globules in Hensen's cells contained cephalin and sphingomyelin but no lecithin, indicating that the phosphatides found are not derived from nerve tissue.

Electron-microscope studies have been performed by KIMURA et al. [73], SPOENDLIN [163], C.A. SMITH [159], WERSÄLL [199], DUVALL [37], and ISHIYAMA et al. [68] on droplets or membrane-enclosed corpuscles, which must be lipid or lipid-containing lysosomes. They were shown in practically all cells in the inner ear. This finding has also been confirmed by the present author in staining tests with Sudan black B.

IX. Carbohydrates

According to the foregoing discussion, carbohydrates are of prime interest for the metabolism of living tissues. The monosaccharides and the low-molecular-weight polysaccharides are water-soluble and are therefore removed during histological processing. Hence, only polysaccharides with more than two monosaccharides which are polymerized or polysaccharide — protein complexes can be visualized by histochemical methods. The neutral glucoproteids are accordingly characterized by a positive PAS reaction, whereas the acid glycoproteids show metachromasia and basophilia as well as a positive PAS reaction. The acid mucopolysaccharides give only metachromasia and basophilia.

The glycogen content of the cochlea of the guinea pig was examined in electron microscope studies by VOSTEEN [192] and by BALOGH [5]. Vosteen used the carmine staining method according to THEMANN [177]. The staining of the cytoplasm of the outer hair cells was especially prominent. In the nerve endings, as in cells of the spiral prominence and the spiral sulcus, the glycogen content was very low. Some glycogen granules were found in the cells of the vascular stria but hardly any in the spiral ligament. From these findings Vosteen drew the conclusion that glycogen was found mainly where the vascularization was slight and the oxygen supply consequently low. In these areas Vosteen observed that anaerobic metabolism predominated. Glycogen did in fact seem to be absent where the vascularization was assumed to be good and the oxygen supply high.

FALBE-HANSEN [41] made a comprehensive study of the glycogen content of the cells in the cochlea of rats. During fetal life, glycogen was found in the membrane of Reissner and in the vascular stria. Before 10 days post partem no glycogen could be found in the hair cells. A decrease in the glycogen content in Reissner's membrane and in the stria with increasing age was recorded, accompanied by an increase in Hensen cells, Deiters' cells and pillar cells. FALBE-HANSEN and THOMSEN [40] studied the glycogen in the inner ear of guinea pigs. They were able to show that the outer hair cells in the apical turns contained a high concentration of glycogen, whereas the concentration steadily decreased towards the basal turn, where very little or nothing could be found of this polysaccharide.

TAKAHASHI [167] and BALOGH [5] reported on the variations in glycogen content in different animal species. In guinea pigs they found glycogen only in the outer hair cells, decreasing from the apex to the basal turn as described by FALBE-HANSEN [41]. In mice it was found in higher concentrations in the cells of Deiters than in the outer hair cells. In cats no glycogen was found. From this it might be concluded that glycogen is a valuable nutritional reserve that shifts with the development of the animal or in accordance with the needs of different animal species.

In the tectorial membrane, metachromatic staining with toluidine blue was demonstrated by BELANGER [9, 10]. This indicated the presence of sulfo-mucopolysaccharides and was interpreted by BELANGER to mean that these membranes consisted of carbohydrates. His results were disputed by ZORZOLI [207] on the grounds that the membranes showed a negative Hale reaction with colloidal iron, which should have revealed the presence of acid mucopolysaccharides. JENSEN and VILSTRUP [70], KURATA [84], and IGARASHI and ALFORD [57], however, demonstrated that the cupula showed positive metachromasia, and DOHLMAN [27] found positive metachromasia and a positive reaction to colloidal iron and alcian blue. VILSTRUP et al. [181] gave a chemical proof of the presence of acid mucopolysaccharides in the fish endolymph. The observation of metachromasia, alcian blue and Hale-positive reactions by Schätzle and Müsebeck [145] confirmed this finding for the tectorial membrane. It was not possible to influence these reactions by pretreatment with ribonuclease or hyaluranidase, indicating what Igarashi and Kanda [57a] referred to as acid and neutral mucopolysaccharides. Schätzle and Müsebeck [145] also demonstrated by variations in pH the presence of one strongly acid and one less acid mucopolysaccharide. In the tectorial and other membranes they found a small fraction of strongly acid mucopolysaccharide, which was removed by hyaluronidase. These authors therefore regarded this polysaccharide as derived from the connective tissue and the rest as secreted from the epithelial cells in the walls of the membranous inner ear.

The glycomucoproteids were investigated by Zorzoli and Zorzoli [206], who found a positive PAS reaction in the tectorial membrane. This was confirmed by Plotz and Perlman [125] and Wislocki and Ladman [204] in rats and mice, and Schätzle and Westernhagen [148] in guinea pigs. Belanger [10] showed metachromasia with toluidine blue in rats, and also an autoradiographic uptake of sulfur [9], interpreted as reflecting the presence of sulfomucopolysaccharides. Igarashi and Alford [57] also produced metachromasia and a positive PAS reaction in the cupulae and tectorial membranes, and concluded that acid and neutral polysaccharides constituted these gelatinous membranes (Rambourg and Leblond [128, 129].)

Thus it was expected that some specific cells in these walls must reflect the process of polymerization to polysaccharides in a secretion. The organ of Corti and the vascular stria showed no metachromasia or staining with alcian blue. This indicated the absence of acid mucopolysaccharides in these cells (Chou [18]; Schätzle and Müsebeck (145]).

However, in 1953 and 1956, Belanger [9, 10] had claimed that radiolabeled sulfur (^{35}S as sulfate) was incorporated into the tectorial membrane as well as into the otolith membranes and the cupulae after 2–8 days. Belanger interpreted this uptake of sulfur in sulfate form to mean that it labeled carbohydrates whereas, when sulfur was injected as ^{35}S-methionine, no autoradiographic sign of uptake of this amino acid was recorded, indicating the absence of protein synthesis in the tectorial membrane and cupulae.

For similar autoradiographic investigations, Dohlman [26, 27] used different animals and injected ^{35}S as sulfate intravenously or intraperitoneally. The generally slow uptake of sulfur in the cupulae and otolithic and tectorial membranes, as found by Belanger [9], was confirmed when guinea pigs, cats, and mice were used for the experiments [29, 32]. When pigeons were used, however, the picture was quite different. As soon as 30 min after injection of ^{35}S-sulfate a considerable uptake of sulfur was observed in well-defined areas. The silver grains lay over the cells of the planum semilunatum and some were found in the endolymph. Fixation with formalin had precipitated the organic compounds of the endolymph and these precipitates in the endolymphatic space were labeled. The cupula was also diffusely covered with silver grains. Four hours after the injection the uptake had reached its peak, with very intense blackening of the planum semilunatum and the cupula, even when the autoradiographic sections were exposed only for a day or two. These observations were later confirmed by Be-

LANGER [9] in chickens. In the cochlea the uptake was considerably less, and was slower than in the planum semilunatum of the ampullae. The uptake in this part of the inner ear seemed to occur mainly in the light cells of the tegmentum vasculosum, the equivalent of the vascular stria and Reissner's membrane in mammals. The secretion from these cells into the endolymph did not precipitate as did that in the labyrinth, and therefore appeared as an evenly distributed labeled uptake. This suggests that the endolymph is different in the two parts of the inner ear: the labeled ^{35}S is taken up rapidly and intensely as a substance which precipitates to cloudy patches in the labyrinth, and evenly but slowly in the cochlear endolymph. The secretion of the light cells in the tegmentum was similar to the secretion produced by the light cells on the slope of the cristae in the ampullae. In the endolymphatic sac, however, the activity became intense after 2–4 days. This indicates a relatively slow flow of endolymph to the endolymphatic sac. This investigation suggests a species-specific difference in the constitution of the mucopolysaccharides and the bonding of sulfur in birds as opposed to the mammals investigated. In order to study the secretion from the planum semilunatum, which is assumed to contain mucopolysaccharides, these cells were studied by histochemical methods [164, 13, 45]. Inner ears from pigeons were subjected to staining with colloidal iron using the Hale method [13, 45], with ruthenium red and alcian blue. The sections were investigated by light and electron microscopy. The colloidal-iron method seemed to produce the best detailed pictures on examination by electron microscopy, and showed that the planum semilunatum cells were the main suppliers of stained acid mucopolysaccharides, to some extent aided by the light cells on the slope of the cristae (DOHLMAN [26]). These cells did not show any staining in the subnuclear part of the cells, indicating that any uptake of simple soluble saccharides must have been washed away during the processing. The inner concave cisternae of the supranuclear Golgi apparatus were stained with colloidal iron. From these cisternae small vesicles stained to varying degrees were detached on their way to the surface of the cell, where they could be found in direct communication with the stained endolymph content. The acid mucopolysaccharide secretion in the fluid was precipitated by the fixatives as stringlike and cloudlike masses, which were sometimes found in direct contact with the cupulae. In the cupula and the tectorial and otolith membranes it became evident that these "gelatinous membranes" consisted of a fibrillar ground substance that could not be stained with colloidal iron. Iron-stained substances had been precipitated onto the walls of the cupular meshwork of the ground substance and were also found in the cloudy material within the "canals" of these membranous structures. From this it is clear that the ground substance is not a mucopolysaccharide but is probably a protein of the keratingroup, as presumed from the chemical analysis (cf. NAKAI and HILDING [111 b]).

In these investigations it has been possible to establish the presence or absence of the proteins, and specifically of their sulfydryl groups by histochemical methods [6 a]. In addition, lipids or carbohydrates such as glycogen and other polysaccharides have been demonstrated in the cells or extracellular fluids by specific staining methods [12, 13]. This gives a picture indicating the presence and to some degree also the amount of these substances as integral parts of the cells. Further, electron microscopy has made it possible to localize the stained substances to specific organelles or parts of organelles. However, only with the support of autoradiography is it possible to observe and record the pathways and speed of the processes of protein production, the creation of nucleic acids or the secretion of polysaccharides.

It is obvious from the results of histochemical investigations on the metabolic enzyme activity in the inner ear that the enzyme distribution of the cells in the membranous walls is not basically different from that of most other cells. There are, however, differences in the density of the respiratory enzymes, generally in accordance with the morphological density of special organelles, especially the mitochondria, where most of these enzymes are located. The hair cells have been shown to have access to enzymes belonging to the anaerobic pentose shunt, which makes them more independent of possible variations in oxygen supply. The dark cells that perform the heavy work of removing sodium from the endolymph and supplying a high concentration of potassium against a high electrical and concentration gradient have, as expected, a high density of mitochondria for this energy-consuming work. As a consequence, the highest activity of the respiratory enzymes is generally found where the dark cells are prevalent. In accordance with the function of these cells, their cell membranes show an intense sodium-potassium-activated ATPase activity [111a, 111b]. Because of this functional pattern, the dark cells are the most important cells in the endolymphatic system, maintaining the electrolyte pattern essential to the normal functioning of the hair cells. The indication that the hair cells generator potential arises from an increase in conductance to an ion with an equilibrium potential between 30 and 35 mV (ALKON and BAK [3]) suggests a mechanism by which the hair cell would be dependent on the ionic environment and at the same time places the sensory function of the cells in its proper context within the whole sequence of production of the endolymph potential and the unique electrolytic pattern of the endolymph.

References

1. ADAMS, C.W.M.: Histochemical mechanisms of the Marchi reaction for degenerating myelin. J. Neurochem. **2**, 178 (1958).
2. ALBERNAZ, P.L.: Histochemistry of the connective tissue of the cochlea. Laryngoscope (St. Louis) **71**, 1–18 (1961).
3. ALKAN, D.L., BAK, A.: Hair cell generator potential. J. gen. Physiol. **61**, 619–637 (1973).
4. ARNOLD, W., VOSTEEN, K.H.: Zur sekretorischen Aktivität der Interdentalzellen des Limbus spiralis. Acta oto-laryng. (Stockh.) **75**, 192–202 (1973).
5. BALOGH, K.: Electron microscopic localization of glycogen in the organ of Corti. 3. Intern. Congr. of Histochem. Cytochem. New York: Springer 1968.
6a. BARRNETT, R.J., SELIGMAN, A.M.: Histochemical demonstration of sulfhydryl and disulfide groups of proteins. J. nat. Cancer Inst. **14**, 769 (1954).
7. BECK, C.: Das Pigment der Stria vascularis. Arch. Ohr.-, Nas.-, u. Kehlk.-Heilk. **179**, 51–58 (1961).
8. BECK, C., MICHLER, H.: Feinstrukturelle und histochemische Veränderungen an den Strukturen der Cochlea beim Meerschweinchen nach dosierter Reinton-Beschallung. Arch. Ohr.-, Nas.-, u. Kehlk.-Heilk. **174**, 496 (1960).
9. BELANGER, L.F.: Autoradiographic detection of S^{35} in the membranes of the inner ear of the rat. Science **118**, 520 (1953).
10. BELANGER, L.F.: On the intimate composition of membranes of the inner ear. Science **123**, 1074 (1956).
13. BURSTONE, M.S.: Enzyme Histochemistry. New York-London: Academic Press 1962.

14. Chevance, L.G., Galli, A., Jeanmaire, Y.: Contribution a l'étude biochimique de la périlymphe chez l'homme et certains mammifères. Ann. Oto-laryng. (Paris) **72**, 950 (1955).
15. Chevance, L.G., Gally, A., Jeanmaire, J.: Immuno-electro-phoretic study of the human perilymph. Acta Oto-laryng. (Paris) **52**, 41 (1960).
16. Choo, Y.B., Tabowitz, D.: The formation and flow of the cochlea fluids. I. Studies with radioactive sodium (Na^{22}). Ann. Oto-laryng. (Paris) **73**, 92–100 (1965).
17. Choo, Y.B., Tabowitz, D.: The formation and flow of the cochlea fluids. II. Studies with radioactive potassium (K^{42}). Ann. Oto-laryng. (Paris) **74**, 140–145 (1965).
18. Chou, Y.T.Y.: A cytological and histochemical study of the stria vascularis of the guinea pig's ear. Quart. J. micr. Sci. **102**, 75–82 (1961).
19. Cox, E.C., White, J.R., Flaks, J.G.: Streptomycin action and the ribosoma. Proc. nat. Acad. Sci. (Wash.) **51**, 703 (1964).
20. Churchill, J.A., Schuknecht, H.F., Doran, R.: Acetylcholinesterase activity in the cochlea. Laryngoscope (St. Louis) **66** (1956).
21. Citron, L., Exley, D., Hallpike, L.: Formation, circulation and chemical properties of the labyrinthine fluids. Proc. roy. Soc. Med. **50**, 697 (1957).
22. Conti, A., Borgo, M.: Studio istochimico sul comportamento dell attivita citocromoossidasica nei tessuti ed organi di pertinenza otorinolaringoiatrica III. Minerva otorinolaring. **14**, 26–30 (1964).
23. Conti, A., Borgo, M.: Behavior of cytochrome oxydase activity in the cochlea of the guinea pig following acoustic stimulation. Acta oto-laryng. (Stockh.) **58**, 321–329 (1964).
24. Densert, O.: The effect of 6-hydroxydopamine on the rabbit cochlea. Acta Oto-laryng. (Stockh.) (in press).
25. Dohlman, G.F., Farkashidy, J., Salomm, F.: Centrifugal nerve fibres to the sensory epithelium of the vestibular labyrinth. J. Laryng. **78**, 784 (1958).
26. Dohlman, G.F., Ormerod, F.C., McLay, D.: The secretory epithelium of the internal ear. Acta oto-laryng. (Stockh.) **50**, 243 (1959).
27. Dohlman, G.F.: Secretion and absorption of endolymph. Ann. Otol. (St. Louis) **73**, 708 (1964).
28. Dohlman, G.F., Boord, R.: The effects of cupula removal in the activities of ampullary structures in the pigeon. Acta oto-laryng. (Stockh.) **57**, 507 (1964).
29. Dohlman, G.F.: Secretion and absorption of the endolymph. Third Symposium on the Role of the Vestibular Organs in Space Exploration, p. 101–124, 1967.
30. Dohlman, G.F.: Excretion and absorption of endolymph in the vestibular apparatus, Ciba Foundation Symposium on Myotatic, Kinestetic and Vestibular Mechanisms, 1967.
31. Dohlman, G.F.: Mechanismus des Ionenaustausches, der Sekretion und der Exkretion der Endolymphe bei der Taube. Arch. klin. exp. Ohr.-, Nas.-, u. Kehlk.-Heilk. **194**, 400 (1969).
32. Dohlman, G.F.: Investigations on the Presence of Acid Mucopolysaccharides in the Endolymph of Pigeons. Proceedings of the Barany Society, 1970.
33. Dohlman, G.F.: The attachment of the cupulae, otolith and tectorial membranes to the sensory cell areas. Acta oto-laryng. (Stockh.) **71**, 89–105 (1971).
34. Dohlman, G.F.: The mechanism of secretion and absorption of endolymph in the vestibular apparatus. Acta oto-laryng. (Stockh.) **59**, 275–287 (1965).
35. Dohlman, G.F., Radomski, M.V.: The ion selective function of the epithelium of the membranous canal walls. Acta oto-laryng. (Stockh.) **66**, 409–416 (1968).
36. Godzdzik-Zolnierkiewicz, T.: Outer and inner hair cells in streptomycin poisoning. Laryngoscope (St. Louis) **79**, 125–133 (1969).
37. Duvall, A.Y.: Ultrastructure of the lateral cochlear wall following intermixing of fluids. Ann. Oto-laryng. (Paris) **77**, 317–331 (1968).
38. Duvall, A.Y., Quick, C.A.: Tracers and endogenous debris in delineating cochlear barriers and pathways. Ann. Oto-laryng. (Paris) **78**, 1042–1057 (1969).
40. Falbe-Hansen, J., Thomson, E.: Histochemical studies on glycogen in the cochlea of the normal guinea pig. Acta oto-laryng. (Stockh.) **56**, 429–436 (1963).
41. Falbe-Hansen, J.: On glycogen in the cochlear duct of foetuses and young of albino rats. Acta oto-laryng. (Stockh.) **63**, 340–346 (1967).
42. Flaks, J.G., Cox, E.C., White, J.R.: Inhibition of polypeptide synthesis by streptomycin. Biochem. biophys. Res. Commun. **7**, 385 (1962).

43. FRITSCH, Y.H., JOLLIFF, C.R., SCHLLESSER, H.F.: Problems of human perilymph. Ann. Oto-laryng. (Paris) **78**, 888–891 (1969).
44. GACEK, R.R., NOMURA, Y., BALOGH, K.: Acetylcholinesterase activity in the efferent fibres of the stato-acoustic nerve. Acta oto-laryng. (Stockh.) **59**, 541–559 (1965).
46. GERHARDT, J.Y.: Zur Methodik der Succinodehydrogenasedarstellung in der Meerschweinchenschnecke. Arch. Ohr.-, Nas.-, u. Kehlk.-Heilk. **178**, 158–162 (1961).
47. GERHARDT, H.J.: Zur Verteilung der DPN- und TPN-Diaphorase in der Meerschweinchenschnecke. Arch. Ohr.-, Nas.-, u. Kehlk.-Heilk. **181**, 16 (1962).
48. GERHARDT, H., PIPLOW, G.: Zur Lipidverteilung in der Meerschweinchenschnecke. Arch. klin. exp. Ohr.-, Nas.-, u. Kehlk.-Heilk. **189**, 21–32 (1967).
49. GLICK, D.: Methods of biochemical analysis. Vol. 18, 20. Interscience New York, London, Sydney, Toronto: Publ. J. Wiley & Sons, Bull., 1954.
51. GRAF, K., PORETTI, G.: Die Entstehung der Perilymphe. Pract. oto-rhino-laryng. (Basel) **12**, 351 (1950).
52. GOZDZIK-ZOLNIERKIEWICZ, T.: Outer and inner hair cells in streptomycin poisoning. Laryngoscope (St. Louis) **79**, 125 (1969).
53. HAUBRICH, Y.: On the metabolism of the saccus endolymphaticus. Arch. klin. exp. Ohr.-, Nas.-, u. Kehlk.-Heilk. **187**, 622 (1966).
54. HAUBRICH, Y., SCHÄTZLE, W.: Zur Frage histochemischer Veränderungen der Meerschweinchenschnecke unter dem Einfluß von Diuretica. Arch. klin. exp. Ohr.-, Nas.-, u. Kehlk.-Heilk. **196**, 319–323 (1970).
55. HENSEN, V.: Zur Morphologie der Schnecke des Menschen und der Säugetiere. Z. wiss. Zool. **13**, 481–518 (1863).
56. HILDING, D.A., WERSÄLL, Y.: Cholinesterase and its relation to the nerve endings in the inner ear. Acta oto-laryng. (Stockh.) **55**, 205–217 (1962).
57. IGARASHI, M., ALFORD, B.R.: Cupula, cupular zone of the otolithic membrane, and tectorial membrane in the squirrel monkey. Acta oto-laryng. (Stockh.) **68**, 420–426 (1969).
57a. IGARASHI, M., KANDA, I.: Fine structure of the otolithic membrane in the squirrel monkey. Acta oto-laryng. (Stockh.) **68**, 43 (1969).
58. IINUMA, T., MIZUKOSHI, O., DALY, J.F.: Possible effects of various ototoxic drugs upon the ATP hydrolyzing system in the stria vascularis and spiral ligament of guinea pigs. Laryngoscope (St. Louis) **77**, 159–170 (1967).
59. ILBERG, C.: Elektronenmikroskopische Überprüfung der Zugangswege zum Cortischen Organ. Arch. klin. exp. Ohr.-, Nas.-, u. Kehlk.-Heilk. **191**, 540–541 (1968).
60. ILBERG, C.: Elektronenmikroskopische Untersuchungen über Diffusion und Resorption von Thoriumdioxyd an der Meerschweinchenschnecke. Arch. klin. exp. Ohr.-, Nas.-, u. Kehlk.-Heilk. I: **190**, 415–425 (1968); II: **190**, 426–436 (1968); III: **192**, 163–175 (1968); IV: **192**, 384–400 (1968).
61. ILBERG, C., IMAMURA, C.: Ein methodischer Beitrag zu Permeabilitätsmessungen an der Reissnermembran. Arch. klin. exp. Ohr.-, Nas.-, u. Kehlk.-Heilk. **187**, 800–806 (1966).
62. ILBERG, C., SPOENDLIN, H.H., VOSTEEN, K.H.: Die Ultrastruktur und Funktion des Sulcus spiralis externus und der Prominentia spiralis der Meerschweinchenschnecke. Darstellung mittels Thorotrast. Arch. klin. exp. Ohr.-, Nas.-, u. Kehlk.-Heilk. **192**, 124–136 (1968).
63. IMOKAWA, M.: Histochemische Untersuchungen des Stoffwechsels des Innenohres. I. Beobachtungen über Dehydrogenase und Cytochrom c-Oxydase des Innenohres. Jibi Inkoka Rinsho **52**, 348–362 (1959).
64. IMOKAWA, M., KOIDE, Y.: Histochemical studies on the labyrinthine metabolism. II. The effects of metabolic inhibitors on the labyrinthine reaction and on the succinic dehydrogenase activity in the labyrinthine tissues. Jibi Inkoka Rinsho **52**, 356–362 (1959).
65. IRELAND, P., FARKASHIDY, J.: Studies on the efferent innervation of the vestibular end organs. Ann. Oto-laryng. (Paris) **70**, 490-503 (1961).
66. ISHII, T., BALOGH, K.: Acid phosphatase activity in the inner ear. Acta oto-laryng. (Stockh.) **62**, 185 (1966).

67. Ishii, T., Murakami, Y., Kimura, R.S., Balogh, K.: Electron microscopic and histochemical identification of lipofuscin in the human inner ear. Acta oto-laryng. (Stockh.) **64**, 17–29 (1967).

67a. Ishii, T., Silverstein, H., Balogh, K.: Metabolic activities of the endolymphatic sac. Acta oto-laryng. (Stockh.) **62**, 61–73 (1966).

67b. Ishii, T., Murakami, Y., Balogh, K.: Acetylcholinesterase activity in efferent nerve fibres of the human inner ear. Ann. Oto-rhino-laryng. **76**, 69–82 (1967).

67c. Ishii, T., Ishii, D., Balogh, K.: Lysosomal enzymes in the inner ears of kanamycin-treated guinea pigs. Acta oto laryng. (Stockh.) **65**, 449–458 (1968).

68. Ishyama, E., Weibel, I., Keels, E.B., Richardson, T.L.: Ultrastructure of the interdental cells in mammals. Acta oto-rhino-laryng. belg. **32**, 312 (1970).

69. Iurato, S.: Submicroscopic structure of the membranous labyrinth. I. The tectorial membrane. Z. Zellforsch. **52**, 105–128 (1960).

70. Jensen, C.E., Vilstrup, T.: On the Chemistry of human cupulae. Acta oto-laryng. (Stockh.) **52**, 383 (1960).

71. Johnson, L.G., Hawkins, Y.E.: Symposium on Basic Ear Research. II. Strial atrophy in clinical and experimental deafness. Laryngoscope (St. Louis) **82**, 1105 (1972).

72. Kakizaki, I.: Experimental studies on the toxic effects of kanamycin on the cochlea. J. Oto-laryng. Soc. Jap. **71**, 68–83 (1968).

73. Kimmra, R., Lundquist, P.G., Wersäll, J.: Secretory epithelial linings in the ampullae of the guinea pig labyrinth. Acta oto-laryng. (Stockh.) **57**, 517–530 (1964).

74. Kaneko, Y., Daly, Y.F.: Activity of acetylcholinesterase on the endolymphatic surface of outer hair cells. Acta oto-laryng. (Stockh.) **67**, 602–610 (1969).

75. Kaneko, Y., Daly, Y.F.: Actylcholinesterase on the nerve endings of outer hair cells and the tunnel radial fibres. Laryngoscope (St. Louis) **78**, 1566–1581 (1968).

76. Kawamato, K., Kakizaki, J.: A study on respiratory enzymes in the stria vascularis of the cochlea. J. Otorhinolaryng. Soc. Jap. **65**, 179–183 (1962).

77. Koburg, E., Plester, D.: Zur Größe des Eiweiß-Stoffwechsels der Gewebe der Cochlea. Autoradiographische Untersuchungen an Meerschweinchen mit H_3-Leucin und H_3-Lysin. Acta oto-laryng. (Stockh.) **54**, 319–335 (1962).

78. Koburg, E., Plester, D.: Zur Größe des Eiweiß-Stoffwechsels der Gewebe der Cochlea bei normalen Ratten mit chronischer Otitis media. Arch. Ohr.-, Nas.-, u. Kehlk.-Heilk. **179**, 332–387 (1962).

79. Koburg, E., Meyer zum Gottesberge, A.: Der Eiweiß-Stoffwechsel des Ganglion spirale des Meerschweinchens. Arch. Ohr.-, Nas.-, u. Kehlk.-Heilk. **183**, 280–284 (1964).

81. Koide, Y.: Introductory studies on the chemical physiology of the labyrinth. Acta med. biol. (Niigata) **6**, 1 (1958).

81a. Koide, Y., Imokova, M.: Histochemical studies on the labyrinthine metabolism. Zibi Rinsho (Jap.), 1958.

81b. Koide, Y., Yashikawa, Y., Morimoto, M.: Some oxidizing enzymes in the cochlea. Ann. oto-rhino-laryng. **71**, 96–104 (1962).

82. Koide, Y., Hondo, R., Yoshikawa, Y.: Distribution of some oxidizing enzymes in the cochlea. Acta oto-laryng. (Stockh.) **58**, 344–354 (1964).

84. Kurata, A.: The morphological and histochemical studies on otolith membranc of the guinea pig macula utriculi. J. Oto-rhino-laryng. Soc. Jap. **66**, 153–162 (1963).

85. Kuijpers, W.: Cation transport and cochlear function. Acta oto-laryng. (Stockh.) **67**, 200–205 (1969).

86. Kuijpers, W.V.D., Blenten, A.C., Bonting, S.L.: Cochlea function and sodium and potassium activated adenosine triphosphatase. Science **1957**, 943 (1967).

87. Kraus, J., Doennig, G.: Cytophotometrische RNA- und Eiweiß-Bestimmung am häutigen Innenohr des Meerschweinchens als Grundlagen zur Beurteilung des Eiweiß-Stoffwechsels und der Streptomycin-Ototoxizität. Arch. klin. exp. Ohr.-, Nas.-, u. Kehlk.-Heilk. **194**, 551–557 (1969).

88. Lawrence, M.: Histological evidence for localized radial flow of endolymph. Arch. Otolaryng. **83**, 406–412 (1966).

88a. Lehninger, A.L.: The Mitochondrion. New York: Benjamin 1964.

89. LEBLOND, C.P.: What radioautography has added to protein lore. Symp. Int. Soc. Cell Biol. **4**, 321–339 (1965).
89a. LIM, D.J.: Three-dimensional observation of the inner ear with the scanning electron microscope. Acta oto-laryng. (Stockh.) Suppl. **225**, 1–38 (1969).
90. LIM, D.J.: Ultrastructural localization of DPNH-diaphorase in the cochlea. Acta oto-laryng. (Stockh.) **69**, 32–45 (1970).
91. LIM, D.Y.: Morphology and function of the interdental cells. An ultrastructural observation. J. Laryng. **84**, 1241 (1970).
92. LINDQUIST, N.G.: Accumulation of drugs on melanin. Acta radiol. (Stockh.) Suppl. **325** (1973).
93. LOTZ, P., KUHL, K.D.: Die Lactatdehydrogenase des Innenohres. Arch. klin. exp. Ohr.-, Nas.-, u. Kehlk.-Heilk. **192**, 237–248 (1968).
94. LOWRY, O.H.: The quantitative Histochemistry of the Brain. J. Histochem. Cytochem. **1**, 420 (1953).
94a. LUNDQUIST, P.G., KIMURA, R., WERSÄLL, J.: Experiments in endolymph circulation. Acta oto-laryng. (Stockh.) Suppl. **188**, 198–201 (1963).
94b. LUNDQUIST, P.G., KIMURA, R., WERSÄLL, Y.: Ultrastructual organization of the epithelial lining in the endolymphatic duct and sac in the guinea pig. Acta oto-laryng. (Stockh.) **57**, 65–80 (1964).
94c. LUNDQUIST, P.G.: The endolymphatic duct and sac in the guinea pig. Acta oto-laryng. (Stockh.) Suppl. **201** (1965).
95. MATSCHINSKY, F.M., THALMANN, R.: Quantitative histochemistry of the organ of Corti, stria vascularis and macula sacculi of the guinea pig. I. Sampling procedures and analysis of pyridine nucleotides. Laryngoscope (St. Louis) **77**, 292–305 (1967).
96. Matschinsky, F.M., THALMANN, R.: Quantitative histochemistry of microscopic structures of the cochlea. Ann. Oto-laryng. (Paris) **76**, 638–646 (1967).
97. MATSCHINSKY, F.M., THALMANN, R.: Recent advances in the biochemistry of prominent cochlear structures. Excerpta Med. Int. Congr. Series **206**, 367 (1969).
98. MATSCHINSKY, F.M., THALMANN, R.: Energy metabolism of the cochlear duct. In: Biochemical Mechanisms in Hearing and Deafness. PAPARELLA, Ed. Springfield, Ill.: C.C. Thomas 1970.
99. MAURER, W., KOBURG, E.: Autoradiographie. In: S. RAUCH: Biochemie des Hörorgans. Stuttgart: Thieme 1964.
100. MEYER ZUM GOTTESBERGE, A.: Autoradiographische Untersuchungen über den Eiweiß-Stoffwechsel in der Schnecke und dem Nucleus N. cochlearis. Acta oto-laryng. (Stockh.) Suppl. **163**, 46–54 (1960).
101. MEYER ZUM GOTTESBERGE, A., PLESTER, D.: Autoradiographische Untersuchungen zum Stofftransport in der Cochlea des Meerschweinchens. Arch. Ohr.-, Nas.-, u. Kehlk.-Heilk. **178**, 145–150 (1961).
102. MEYER ZUM GOTTESBERGE, A., RAUCH, S. KOBURG, E.: Unterschiede im Metabolismus der einzelnen Schneckenwindungen. Acta oto-laryng. (Stockh.) **59**, 116–123 (1965).
103. MIRA, E.: Caratteristiche metaboliche degli epiteli differentiati delle region ampollari e maculari del labirinto posteriore di Cavia. Boll. Mal. Orecch. **84**, 25–44 (1966).
104. MIRA, E., DAL NEGRO, F.: Die histochemischen und histoenzymologischen Eigenschaften des Epithels der Übergangszone der Crista ampullaris. Arch. klin. exp. Ohr.-, Nas.-, u. Kehlk.-Heilk. **193**, 322–328 (1969).
105. MÜSEBECK, K., SCHÄTZLE, W.: Experimentelle Studien zur Ototoxicität des Dihydrostreptomycins. Arch. Ohr.-, Nas.-, u. Kehlk.-Heilk. **181**, 41–48 (1962).
106. MÜSEBECK, K.: Zum Wirkungsmechanismus der Streptomycin-Vergiftung des Ohres. Arch. Ohr.-, Nas.-, u. Kehlk.-Heilk. **182**, 583–587 (1963).
107. MÜSEBECK, K., SCHÄTZLE, W.: Die Verteilung der Sulfhydryle und der Disulfide in der Meerschweinchenschnecke. Arch. Ohr.-, Nas.-, u. Kehlk.-Heilk. **181**, 75–81 (1963).
108. MÜSEBECK, K., SCHÄTZLE, W.: Das Verhalten der sauren Mucopolysaccharide der Meerschweinchenschnecke nach Vergiftung mit Dihydrostreptomycin und mit einem Tetracyclin-Derivat. Arch. Ohr.-, Nas.-, u. Kehlk.-Heilk. **181**, 530–536 (1964).
109. NAFTALIN, L.: Some new proposals regarding acoustic transmission and transduction. Cold Spr. Harb. Symp. quant. Biol. **30**, 169–180 (1965).

110. Nakai, Y.: Histochemical study of the stria vascularis in the inner ear by electron microscopy. Ann. Oto-laryng. **74**, 326–337 (1965).

111. Nakai, Y., Hilding, D.: Electron microscopic studies of adenosine triphosphatase activity in the stria vascularis and spiral ligament. Acta oto-laryng. (Stockh.) **62**, 411–428 (1966).

111a. Nakai, Y., Hilding, D.: Adenosine triphosphatase distribution in the organ of Corti. Acta oto-laryng. (Stockh.) **64**, 477–491 (1967).

111b. Nakai, Y., Hilding, D.: Vestibular endolymph – producing epithelium. Acta oto-laryng. (Stockh.) **66**, 120–128 (1968).

111c. Nakai, Y., Hilding, D. A.: Oxidative enzymes in the cochlea. An electron microscopic and histochemical study of succinic dehydrogenases and dihydronicotinamid adenine dinucleotide diaphorase. Acta oto-laryng. (Stockh.) **65**, 459–467 (1968).

112. Neubert, K.: Die Basilarmembran des Menschen und ihr Verankerungssystem. Z. Anat. Entwickl.-Gesch. **114**, 539 (1962).

113. Nomura, Y., Balogh, K.: Localization of DPNH- and TPNH-diaphorase activity in the cochlea by various histochemical techniques. Laryngoscope (St. Louis) **74**, 1351 (1964).

114. Nomura, Y., Balogh, K.: Metabolic pathways in the vestibular labyrinth as revealed by histochemical techniques. Acta oto-laryng. (Stockh.) **57**, 484 (1964).

114a. Nomura, Y., Gacek, R. R., Balogh, K., Jr.: Efferent innervation of vestibular labyrinth; histochemical demonstration of acetylcholinesterase activity in the guinea pigs' inner ear. Arch. Otolaryng. **81**, 335–339 (1965).

115. Nomura, Y., Ishii, T., Ishii, D.: The histochemistry of the spiral prominence. Arch. klin. exp. Ohr.-, Nas.-, u. Kehlk.-Heilk. **195**, 266 (1970).

116. Ostyn, F., Tyberghein, J.: Influence of some streptomyces antibotics on the inner ear of guinea pigs. Acta oto-laryng. (Stockh.) Suppl. **234**, 1–91 (1968).

117. Palva, T., Raunio, V.: Disc-electrophoretic studies of human perilymph and endolymph. Acta oto-laryng. (Stockh.) **63**, 128 (1967).

118. Palva, T., Raunio, V.: Disc-electrophoretical studies of human perilymph. Ann. Oto-laryng. (Paris) **76**, 23 (1967).

119. Palva, T., Raunio, V.: The origin of perilymph albumin. Acta oto-laryng. (Stockh.) **66**, 136 (1968).

123. Plester, D.: Autoradiographische Untersuchungen des Eiweiß-Stoffwechsels in der Schnecke. Arch. Ohr.-, Nas.-, u. Kehlk.-Heilk. **176**, 668–672 (1960).

124. Plester, D., Koburg, E., Hempel, K.: Autoradiographische Untersuchungen der verschiedenen Gewebe des Innenohres. Ann. Histochim. **7**, Suppl. 2, 91–95 (1962).

125. Plotz, E., Perlman, H. B.: A histochemical study of the cochlea. Laryngoscope. (St. Louis) **65**, 291–312 (1955).

126. DuPraw, E. J.: Cell and Molecular Biology. New York-London: Academic Press 1970.

127. Raaflaub, J.: Komplexbindung durch Adenosintriphosphate. Helv. physiol. pharmacol. Acta **12**, C88–89 (1954).

128. Rambourg, A., Hernandez, W., Leblond, C. F.: Detection of complex carbohydrates in the Golgi apparatus of rat cells. J. Cell Biol. **40**, 395 (1969).

129. Rambourg, A., Leblond, C. P.: Staining of basement membranes and associated structures by the periodic acid Schiff and periodic acid – silver methenamine techniques. J. Ultrastruct. Res. **20**, 706–509 (1967).

130. Rauch, S.: Biochemie des Hörorgans. Stuttgart: Thieme 1964.

131. Rauch, S., Reale, E.: Die Pericyten (Rouget-Zellen) der Stria vascularis-Gefäße. Arch. klin. exp. Ohr.-, Nas.-, u. Kehlk.-Heilk. **192**, 82–90 (1968).

132. Rauch, S., Ruska, H.: Zur elektronenoptischen Struktur und Funktion der Stria vascularis. Arch. Ohr.-, Nas.-, u. Kehlk.-Heilk. **185**, 577–586 (1965).

133. Rossi, G., Cortesina, G.: Acetylcholinesterase activity in the efferent cochlear fibres after destruction of the organ of Corti and afferent fibres. Acta oto-laryng. (Stockh.) **61**, 488–494 (1966).

134. Ruben, R. J.: The synthesis of DNA and RNA in the developing inner ear. Laryngoscope (St. Louis) **79**, 1546–1556 (1969).

137. SAITO, H.: Biochemical and histochemical studies on acid mucopolysaccharides in the cochlea of guinea pigs. Jap. J. Otolaryng. **70**, 662 (1967).
138. SAITO, H., DALY, Y. F.: Quantitative analysis of acid mucopolysaccharides in the normal guinea pig cochlea. Acta oto-laryng. (Stockh.) **69**, 333 (1970).
139. SADE, J., ELIEZER, N.: Secretory otitis media and the nature of the mucociliary system. Acta oto-laryng. (Stockh.) **70**, 351–357 (1970).
140. SCHÄTZLE, W., v. WESTERNHAGEN, B.: Nachweis von Glucosaminidase in der Meerschweinchenschnecke. Arch. klin. exp. Ohr.-, Nas.-, u. Kehlk.-Heilk. **186**, 223–228 (1966).
141. SCHÄTZLE, W., v. WESTERNHAGEN, B.: Nachweis von Galactosidase in der Meerschweinchenschnecke. Arch. klin. exp. Ohr.,- Nas.-, u. Kehlk.-Heilk. **186**, 223–228 (1966).
142. SCHÄTZLE, W.: Histochemical demonstration of glucoronidase in the cochlea of the guinea pig. Arch. klin. exp. Ohr.-, Nas.-, u. Kehlk.-Heilk. **186**, 184–189 (1966).
143. SCHÄTZLE, W.: Histochemie des Innenohres. Munich-Berlin-Vienna: Urban & Schwarzenberg 1971.
144. SCHÄTZLE, W., MÜSEBECK, K.: Histochemische Untersuchungen zur Blockierung der Succinodehydrogenase in der Meerschweinchenschnecke. Arch. Ohr.-, Nas.-, u. Kehlk.-Heilk. **181**, 49–57 (1962).
145. SCHÄTZLE, W., MÜSEBECK, K.: Histochemische Untersuchungen zum Mucopolysaccharide- und Glucoprotein-Gehalt der Meerschweinchen Cochlea. Arch. Ohr.-, Nas.-, u. Kehlk.-Heilk. **181**, 297 (1963).
146. SCHÄTZLE, W., v. WESTERNHAGEN, B.: Vergleichende Untersuchungen zum histochemischen Nachweis alkalischer Phosphatase in der Meerschweinchenschnecke mit verschiedener Methodik. Arch. klin. exp. Ohr.-, Nas.-, u. Kehlk.-Heilk. **189**, 210–218 (1969).
147. SCHÄTZLE, W., v. WESTERNHAGEN, B.: Zur Fermentausstattung des peripheren Vestibularapparates. Arch. klin. exp. Ohr.-, Nas.-, u. Kehlk.-Heilk. **186**, 290–297 (1966).
148. SCHÄTZLE, W., v. WESTERNHAGEN, B.: Histochemischer Nachweis von Proteinbausteinen in den Strukturen des Innenohres. Arch. klin. exp. Ohr.-, Nas.-, u. Kehlk.-Heilk. **187**, 822–835 (1966).
149. SCHÄTZLE, W., v. WESTERNHAGEN, B.: Histochemische Untersuchungen zum Nachweis von Monoaminooxydase in der Meerschweinchenschnecke. Arch. klin. exp. Ohr.-, Nas.-, u. Kehlk.-Heilk. **189**, 51–58 (1967).
150. SCHÄTZLE, W., v. WESTERNHAGEN, B.: Über den Einfluß lokaler Pantocain-Applikation auf Fermente der Cochlea und des periferen Vestibularapparates. Arch. klin. exp. Ohr.-, Nas.-, u. Kehlk.-Heilk. **194**, 583–588 (1969).
151. SCHIFF, M., CHRISTIENSEN-LOU, H.: The nature of liquid globules in Hensen's cells. Ann. Oto-laryng. (Paris) **76**, 624–637 (1967).
151a. SCHINDLER, K., SCHNIEDER, E.A., WULLSTEIN, H.L.: Vergleichende Bestimmungen einiger Elektrolyte und Organischer Substanzen in der Perilymphe otosclerotischer Patienten. Acta oto-laryng. (Stockh.) **59**, 308–319 (1965).
152. SCHREINER, L.: Autoradiographische Untersuchungen zur Größe des Eiweiß-Stoffwechsels des peripheren Gleichgewichtsapparates beim Meerschweinchen. Klin. Wschr. **40**, 1016 (1962).
153. SCHREINER, L.: Experimentelle Untersuchungen über die Bildungsstätten und den Stoffaustausch der Perilymphe. Acta oto-laryng. (Stockh.) Suppl. 212 (1966).
154. SCHULTZE, B., CITOLER, P., HEMPEL, K., CITOLER, K., MAURER, W.: Cytoplasmic protein synthesis in cells of various types and its relation to nuclear protein synthesis. Symp. Int. Soc. Cell Biol. **4**, 107–142 (1965).
155. SILVERSTEIN, H.: Biochemical Studies of the inner ear fluids in the cat. Ann. Otolaryng. (Paris) **75**, 48–63 (1966).
156. SILVERSTEIN, H.: Biochemical and physiological studies of the endolymphatic sac in the cat. Laryngoscope (St. Louis) **76**, 498–572 (1966).
159. SMITH, C. A.: Utricle and Saccule. In: S. IURATO: Submicroscopic Structure of the Inner Ear. Oxford: Pergamon Press 1967.
160. SPOENDLIN, H., GACEK, R.: Electron microscopic study of the efferent and afferent innervation of the organ of Corti in the cat. Ann. Oto-laryng. (Paris) **72**, 660–686 (1963).

161. SPOENDLIN, H., LICHTENSTEIGER, W.: Die adrenergische Innervation des Labyrinthes, Pract. oto-rhino-laryng. (Basel) **27**, 371–372 (1965).

162. SPOENDLIN, H., LICHTENSTEIGER, W.: The adrenergic innervation of the labyrinth. Acta oto-laryng. (Stockh.) **61**, 423–434 (1966).

163. SPOENDLIN, H., LICHTENSTEIGER, W.: The sympathetic nerve supply to the inner ear. Arch. klin. exp. Ohr.-, Nas.-, u. Kehlk.-Heilk. **189**, 346–359 (1967).

164. SPOENDLIN, H.: Vascular stria and spiral prominence. In: S. IURATO: Submicroscopic Structures of the Inner Ear. Oxford: Pergamon Press 1967.

165. STOWARD, P.J.: A note on the use of p-fluorophenylhydrazin for the cytochemical demonstration of periodate-reactive muscosaccharides and polysaccharides in the electron microscope. Histochemie **15**, 93–94 (1968).

166. TACHIBANA, M., SAITO, H., MACHIMO, M.: Sulphated acid mucopolysaccharides in the tectorial membrane. Acta oto-laryng. (Stockh.) **76**, 37–46 (1973).

167. TAKAHASHI, K.: Study on the distribution of several chemical substances in membranous labyrinth of normal guinea pig. J. Oto-rhino-laryng. Soc. Japan **64**, 266–277 (1961).

168. TERAYAMA, Y., HOLZ, E., BECK, C.: Adrenergic innervation of the cochlea. Ann. Oto-laryng. (Paris) **75**, 69–86 (1966).

169. TERAYAMA, Y., HOLZ, E., BECK, C.: Fluorescenzmikroskopischer Nachweis adrenergischer Fasern in der Meerschweinchenschnecke. Mschr. Ohrenheilk. **99**, 513–518 (1965).

170. THALMANN, R.: Quantitative Microchemical Studies of Vestibular Sensory Struktures. Proc. Barany Society. (Amsterdam) (1970).

171. THALMANN, R.: Quantitative histo- and cytochemistry of the ear. In: Handbook of Auditory and Vestibular Research Methods. C.A. SMITH and Y. VERNON, Eds. Springfield, Ill.: C.C. Thomas 1971a.

172. THALMANN, R.: Metabolic features of auditory and vestibular systems. Laryngoscope (St. Louis) **81**, 1245 (1971b).

173. THALMANN, R.: Recent refinements of quantitative microchemical analysis of tissues and cells of the inner ear. Acta oto-laryng. (Stockh.) **73**, 161–174 (1972).

174. THALMANN, R., GLISMANN, L., MATSCHINSKY, F.M.: Activation of glycogen phosphorylase by ischemia in cochlear structures. 3rd Internat. Congr. Histochem. Cytochem. Berlin-Heidelberg-New York: Springer 1968.

175. THALMANN, Y., MATSCHINSKY, F.M., THALMANN, R.: Quantitative study of selected enzymes involved in energy metabolism of the cochlear duct. Ann. Oto-laryng. (Paris) **79**, 12 (1970).

176. THALMANN, R., THALMANN, Y., COMEGYS, T.H.: Dissection and chemical analysis of substructures of the organ of Corti. Laryngoscope (St. Louis) **80**, 1619 (1970).

177. THEMANN, H.: Elektronenoptische Untersuchungen über das Glykogen im Zellstoffwechsel. Stuttgart: Fischer 1963.

178. TONNDORF, J.: Intracochleäre Vitalfärbung. In: Rauch. Biochemie des Hörorganes. Stuttgart: Thieme 1964.

178a. TONNDORF, J., DUVALL, A.J., III, RENEAU, Y.P.: Permeability of intracochlear membranes to various vital stains. Ann. Oto-laryng. (Paris) **71**, 801–841 (1962).

179. ULLBERG, S., LINDQUIST, N.G., SJOESTRAND, S.E.: Accumulation of chorio-retinotoxic drugs in the foetal eye. Nature (Lond.) **227**, 1257 (1970).

180. VILSTRUP, T., JENSEN, C.E., KOEFOED, J.: Reports on the chemical composition of the fluids of the labyrinth. Ann. Oto-laryng. (Paris) **63**, 151 (1954).

181. VILSTRUP, T., VILSTRUP, G., JENSEN, C.E., KORNERUP, V.: Three reports on the chemical composition of the fluids of the labyrinth. Ann. Oto-laryng. (Paris) **63**, 151–163 (1954).

182. VILSTRUP, T., JENSEN, C.E., KOEFOED, Y.: Reports on the chemical composition of the fluids of the labyrinth. Ann. Oto-laryng. (Paris) **64**, 406 (1955).

183. VINNIKOV, J.A., TITOVA, L.K.: The presence and distribution of acid phosphatase in the organ of Corti in animals in a state of relative rest and upon auditory stimulation. Bull. exp. Biol. Med. **44**, 1212 (1958).

184. VINNIKOV, J.A., TITOVA, L.K.: Cytophysiology and cytochemistry of the organ of Corti: a cytochemical theory of hearing. Int. Rev. Cytol. **14**, 157–191 (1963).

185. Voldrich, L.: Morphology and function of the epithelium of the limbus spiralis cochleae. Acta oto-laryng. (Stockh.) **63**, 503 (1967).

186. Vosteen, K.H.: Die Darstellung der Bernsteinsäure-dehydrogenase in der Schnecke des Meerschweinchens. Arch. Ohrenheilk. **168**, 295–305 (1956).

186a. Vosteen, K.H.: Die Verteilung der Cytochrom-Oxidase in der Meerschweinchenschnekke. Zbl. all. Path. **97**, 66–69 (1957).

187. Vosteen, K.H.: Die Lokalisation verschiedener Atmungsfermente in der Schnecke. Arch. Ohr.-, Nas.-, u. Kehlk.-Heilk. und Z. Hals-, Nas.-, u. Ohrenheilk. **171**, 368–370 (1957).

188. Vosteen, K.H.: Die Erschöpfung der Phonoreceptoren nach funktioneller Belastung. Experimentelle histochemische Untersuchung zur Frage der Schalltransformation im Innenohr. Arch. Ohr.-, Nas.-, u. Kehlk.-Heilk. **172**, 489–512 (1958).

189. Vosteen, K.H.: Die Energieproduktion im Cortischen Organ. Acta oto-laryng. (Stockh.) Suppl. **163**, 54–55 (1960).

190. Vosteen, K.H.: The histochemistry of the enzymes of oxygen metabolism in the inner ear. Laryngoscope (St. Louis) **70**, 351 (1960).

191. Vosteen, K.H.: Neue Aspekte zur Biologie und Pathologie des Innenohres. Arch. Ohr.-, Nas.-, u. Kehlk.-Heilk. und Z. Hals-, Nas.-, u. Ohrenheilk. **178**, 1–104 (1961).

192. Vosteen, K.H.: Elektronenmikroskopische Untersuchungen über die Verteilung von Glykogen im Ductus cochlearis beim Meerschweinchen. Pract. oto-rhino-laryng. (Basel) **26**, 400–408 (1964).

193. Vosteen, K.H.: Passive and active transport in the inner ear. Arch. klin. exp. Ohr.-, Nas.-, u. Kehlk.-Heilk. **195**, 226–245 (1970).

194. Wachstein, M., Meisel, E., Ortiz, J.: Intracellular localization of acid phosphatase as studied in mammalian kidneys. Lab. Invest. **11**, 1243 (1962).

196. Watanuki, K., Hori, K., Kashiwazaki, H., Kaneko, Y., Kawamoto, S.: Some autoradiographic observations of the nucleic acid metabolism in the cells of Reissner's membrane. Arch. klin. exp. Ohr.-, Nas.-, u. Kehlk.-Heilk. **192**, 91–99 (1968).

197. Watanuki, K.: Some morphological observations of Reissner's membrane. Acta otolaryng. (Stockh.) **66**, 40–48 (1968).

198. Wersäll, J., Hilding, D., Lundquist, P.G.: Ultrastruktur und Innervation der cochlearen Haarzellen. Arch. Ohr.-, Nas.-, u. Kehlk.-Heilk. **178**, 106–126 (1961).

199. Wersäll, J.: Cristae Ampullares. In: S. Iurato: Submicroscopic Structures of the Inner Ear. Oxford: Pergamon Press 1967.

200. v. Westernhagen, B.W.: Histochemische Untersuchungen zur Wirkung der Salicylsäure auf das Innenohr. Arch. klin. exp. Ohr.-, Nas.-, u. Kehlk.-Heilk. **190**, 88–94 (1968).

201. v. Westernhagen, B.W., Schätzle, W.: Fermenthistochemische Untersuchungen an Meerschweinchen zum Einfluß des Otozin auf die ototoxische Wirkung des Streptomycins. Arch. klin. Ohr.-, Nas.-, u. exp. Kehlk.-Heilk. **194**, 558 (1969).

202. v. Westernhagen, B.W.: Innenohrveränderungen am Meerschweinchen nach chronischer Quecksilbervergiftung. Eine histochemische Studie. Arch. klin. exp. Ohr.-, Nas.-, u. Kehlk.-Heilk. **193**, 70–77 (1969).

203. Wise, G.E., Goldstein, L.: Electron microscope localization of nuclear RNA's that shuttle between cytoplasm and nucleus and nuclear RNA's that do not. J. Cell Biol. **56**, 129–138 (1973).

204. Wislocki, G.B., Ladman, A.J.: Selective and histochemical staining of otolithic membranes, cupulae and tectorial membrane of the inner ear. J. Anat. (Lond.) **89**, 3–12 (1955).

205. Wolff, D.: Melanin in the inner ear. Arch. Otolaryng. **14**, 195–211 (1931).

206. Zorzoli, G.C.E., Zorzoli, E.: Ricerche istochimiche sulla membrana tectoria del organo del Corti dell orecchio. Biol. lat. (Milano) **7**, 478–493 (1954).

207. Zorzoli, G.C.: Recherches histochimiques sur l'oreille interne du cobaye. C.R. Ass. Anat. **41**, 785–793 (1954).

Chapter IV

Morphological Aspects of the Efferent Vestibular System

By

R. R. Gacek, Boston, Mass. (USA)

With 5 Figures

Contents

I. Efferent Vestibular System (Anatomy)

Since Rasmussen in 1946 first clearly demonstrated anatomically the efferent neuron to the auditory labyrinth (Rasmussen, 1946, 1953), a tremendous interest has arisen in the physiology and function of such dual innervation of not only the labyrinth but other sense organs as well. Such efferent systems parallel the classical afferent sensory neural links from cortex to endorgan as indicated by the complete chain of descending (efferent) neurons which Rasmussen has presented for the auditory system (Rasmussen, 1964).

The peripheral efferent neuron to the vestibular portion of the labyrinth has been precisely described anatomically (Gacek, 1960, 1966, 1967); higher descending neurons have not yet been demonstrated. Therefore, the present discussion will concern the anatomy of only this peripheral efferent neuron to the vestibular sense organs.

Figure 1 summarizes the peripheral course and distribution of efferent vestibular fibers. The fibers enter the vestibular root in the brainstem. At that point they converge with the efferent cochlear fibers. In the vestibular nerve all the efferents are compactly arranged in bundles located in the central portion; the vestibular efferents occupy a dorsal position in these bundles. As the bundles course toward Scarpa's ganglion the efferent vestibular fibers split off and travel in the branches to each vestibular endorgan. In the peripheral segments of these branches they are scattered among the afferent fibers to the sensory epithelium. The efferent cochlear fibers leave the vestibular nerve at the saccular portion of Scarpa's ganglion via the vestibulo-cochlear anastomosis and enter the cochlea.

The most convenient site for evaluating the number and size of efferent nerve fibers to both halves of the labyrinth is within the vestibular nerve after it emerges

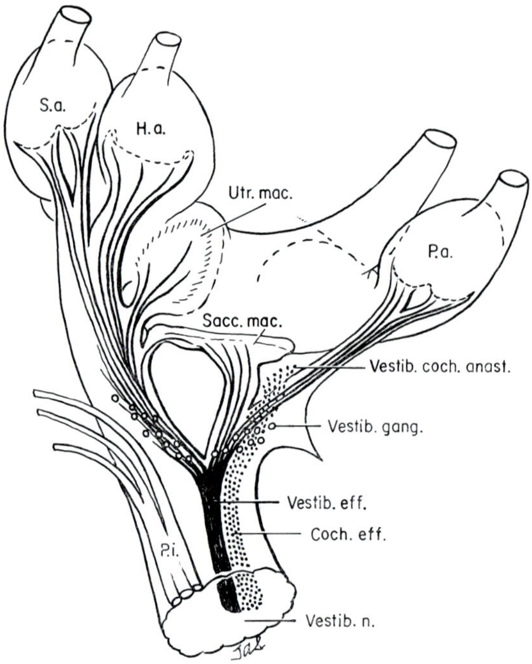

Fig 1. Drawing illustrating the peripheral course and distribution of efferent nerve fibers. Efferent vestibular fibers are represented by solid black lines while the efferent cochlear fibers are represented by dotted lines. *S.a.* = superior canal ampulla; *H.a.* = horizontal canal ampulla; *P.a.* = posterior canal ampulla; *P.i.* = pars intermedia (of facial n.)

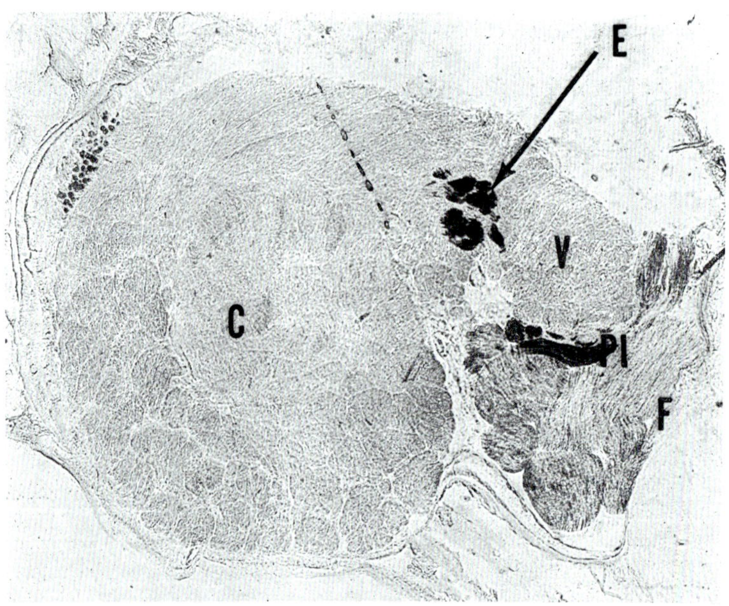

Fig. 2. Cross section through the nerves in the internal auditory canal of the cat. Acetylcholinesterase activity method localizes the efferent fiber bundles (E) in the center of the vestibular nerve (V). *C* = cochlear nerve, *PI* = pars intermedia, *P* = facial nerve

from the brainstem; this is the point at which all efferent fibers are compactly arranged. A cross section through the vestibular nerve illustrates this arrangement (Fig. 2). Normal nerve fiber staining methods allows an estimation of fiber diameters.

Axons of efferent neurons (vestibular and cochlear) at this level are of small diameter; their myelin sheath diameters measure from 2 μ to 3 μ. Central to this point the axons are slightly larger in diameter and as they are followed out peripherally to the sense organ the diameter is smaller. The size of these efferent axons indicates that their cells of origin are also relatively small. Rasmussen has identified the cell bodies of the crossed efferent cochlear fibers and described them as small multipolar cells dorso-medial to the accessory superior olivary nucleus (Rasmussen, 1946).

These anatomical facts are most important in the evaluation of methods utilized to demonstrate the existence and distribution of the efferent vestibular pathway in the laboratory animal. For example, it is a well-known pitfall that very small caliber nerve fibers (1 μ or less) are not consistently impregnated by protargol silver methods that are used after lengthy decalcification techniques such as would be necessary for the cat petrous bone. However, myelin techniques such as Sudan Black B can be used after decalcification to reliably demonstrate such small axons, and the question of unmyelinated axons in the vestibular nerve must be answered by electronmicroscopical methods. Furthermore, use of the retrograde degeneration technique to study the small neurons of the efferent system is severely limited by the difficulty in assessing equivocal changes in such small cells. Methods designed to label these small neurons *in vivo* have been developed to overcome this obstacle in localizing the cells of origin of the efferent system.

Direct unequivocal demonstration of efferent vestibular fibers to the labyrinth was first presented in 1958 (Rasmussen and Gacek, 1958) and 1959 (Gacek, 1960). The method utilized the phenomenon of peripheral axonal degeneration following injury to the efferent cell body or central (CNS) axonal segment. Following various lesions in the brainstem and allowing a short survival time (5–7 days because small nerve fibers degenerate more rapidly than large ones), the vestibular nerve and its branches were stained with Sudan Black and examined for axonal debris of degenerating efferent fibers. Since the lesions were located within the brainstem, injury to the labyrinthine blood supply was avoided.

Transection of the vestibular root lateral to the descending trigeminal root will produce degeneration of all efferent vestibular fibers to each endorgan. Retrograde degeneration of the afferent bipolar vestibular neurons does not occur following transection of its axons and therefore does not create a serious problem in identifying the degenerating fibers as efferent following vestibular root transection.

Methods utilizing the phenomenon of retrograde cell changes following labyrinthectomy or section of the vestibular nerve in young kittens have not been successful in localizing the cells of origin because unequivocal changes in small cells with little cytoplasm and Nissl substance are very difficult to assess. No changes have been found in larger cell bodies of the vestibular nuclei as a result of such lesions.

Brainstem material treated with the acetylcholinesterase localization technique consistently reveal a small area located in the caudal end of ventral Deiter's nucleus which shows very high activity and from which high Ache activity fibers can be followed into the vestibular root. Cytology of normal brainstems show that small neurons populate this area. ROSSI (ROSSI and CORTISINA, 1962) has suggested a similar area in the guinea pig brainstem (interposed nucleus) which may give rise to his "uncrossed efferent vestibular tract."

A method for labeling motor neurons in retrograde fashion with horseradish peroxidase has recently been described by KRISTENSSON and co-workers (1971). This technique has been adapted for use in demonstrating the small efferent vestibular neurons in newborn kittens (GACEK and LYON, 1974). When the peroxidase was placed into the vestibule of the labyrinth and 24 hours allowed for retrograde transport, the peroxidase was demonstrated colorimetrically only in small neurons located caudally in the vestibular nuclear area just lateral to the abducens nucleus. This was consistently found bilaterally indicating an equal ipsilateral and contralateral origin of the efferent vestibular component. The drawing in Fig. 3 illustrates the origin, course and termination of the vestibular efferent pathway.

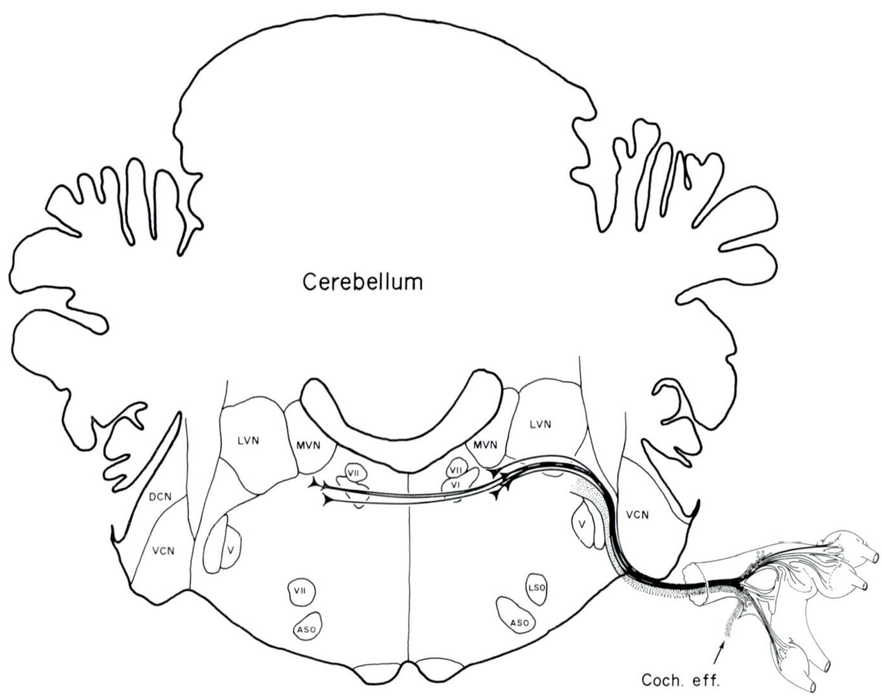

Fig. 3. Drawing of the central and peripheral course of the efferent vestibular pathway

The histochemical method localizing acetylcholinesterase activity has been very useful in demonstrating efferents and their endings because of the very high content of this enzyme in the efferent fibers while afferent fibers have a negligible amount. Various modifications of this method have been used to demonstrate such Ache localization in the vestibular sensory epithelium (DOHLMAN et al., 1958; HILDING and WERSÄLL, 1962; IRELAND and FARKASHIDY, 1961) and in the efferent nerve fibers themselves (GACEK et al., 1965; GACEK, 1967, NOMURA et al., 1965; ROSSI and CORTISINA, 1962). In fact, now the most accurate and complete way to illustrate the entire peripheral course of the efferent pathway utilizes such a histochemical method. By selectively staining these fine intact fibers out to the sense organ, segments of the axons are demonstrated which would be extremely difficult to see with degeneration methods (Fig. 4). Furthermore, it has revealed that branching of these individual fibers occurs before the sense organ is reached. Estimates of the number of efferent vestibular neurons must be made at a point more proximal than Scarpa's ganglion; that is, within the vestibular nerve trunk. These vestibular efferents number approximately three hundred (300).

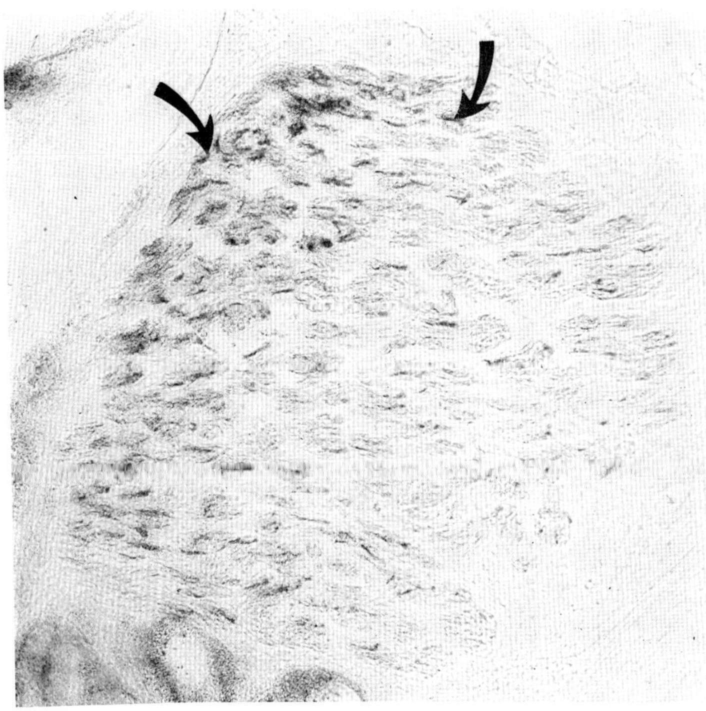

Fig. 4. Cross section through the peripheral part of superior division vestibular nerve shows scattered efferent fibers (arrows) demonstrated by Ache localization

It is well established experimentally in both the auditory (IURATO, 1962; KIMURA and WERSÄLL, 1962; SMITH and RASMUSSEN, 1963; SPOENDLIN and GACEK, 1963) and vestibular (SMITH and RASMUSSEN, 1967) endorgans that the two types of nerve endings described by ENGSTRÖM (ENGSTRÖM, 1958, 1961) and WERSÄLL (WERSÄLL, 1956) represent the two types of innervation to these sense organs. The vesiculated endings represent the terminals of the efferent nerve fibers while the non-vesiculated terminals are those of the afferent neurons.

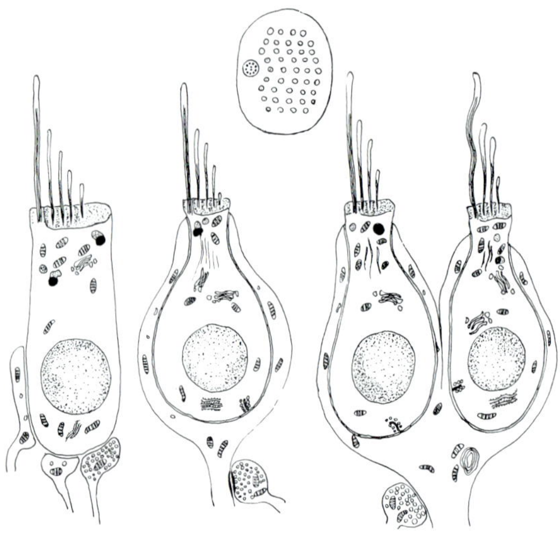

VESTIBULAR SENSORY CELLS

Fig. 5. Drawing summarizing the two types of vestibular hair cells. Type II hair cell is at the left and Type I represented by the remaining cells. The vesiculated nerve endings indicate efferent nerve terminals and non-vesiculated structures the afferent nerve endings (Courtesy of R. KIMURA)

Differences in function are implied not only by the two types of neuron systems but also by the fact that afferent terminals always make a direct contact with the peripheral hair cells (Type I and II), while efferent terminals make contact only with the Type II which is the phylogenitically older type of hair cell. Under Type I hair cells the efferent terminals contact the afferent nerve fibers or afferent terminals (Fig. 5).

Physiological investigations concerning the electrical activity and possible function of this system are discussed in the latter part of this chapter. From the anatomical viewpoint, however, it appears that such studies are very difficult to conduct and interpret because the efferent vestibular neuron is intimately associated with the afferent vestibular neurons throughout its entire course.

References

DOHLMAN, G.F., FARKASHIDY, J., SALONNA, F.: Centrifugal nerve nerve fibers to the sensory epithelium of the vestibular labyrinth. J. Laryng. **72**, 984 (1958).

ENGSTRÖM, H.: On the double innervation of the inner ear. Acta oto-laryng. (Stockh.) **49**, 109 (1958).

ENGSTRÖM, H.: The innervation of the vestibular sensory cells. Acta oto-laryng. (Stockh.) **163**, 30–41 (1961).

GACEK, R.R.: Efferent component of the vestibular nerve. In: Neural mechanisms of the auditory and vestibular systems. G. L. RASMUSSEN and W. F. WINDLE, Eds. Springfield, Ill.: Charles C. Thomas 1960.

GACEK, R.R., NOMURA, Y., BALOGH, K.: Acetylcholinesterase activity in the efferent fibers of the stato-acoustic nerve. Acta oto-laryng. (Stockh.) **59**, 541 (1965).

GACEK, R.R.: The vestibular efferent pathway. In: The vestibular system and its diseases. R. J. WOLFSON, Ed. Philadelphia: University of Penn. Press 1966.

GACEK, R.R.: Anatomical evidence for an efferent vestibular pathway. Third symposium on "The Role of the Vestibular Organs in Space Exploration". Naval Aerospace Medical Institute. Pensacola, Florida, Jan. 1967.

GACEK, R.R., LYON, M.: The localization of vestibular efferent neurons in the kitten with horseradish peroxidase. Acta Otol. **77**, 92–101 (1974).

HILDING, D., WERSÄLL, J.: Cholinesterase and its relation to the nerve endings in the inner ear. Acta oto-laryng. (Stockh.) **55**, 205–217 (1962).

IRELAND, P.E., FARKASHIDY, J.: Studies on the efferent innervation of the vestibular end-organs. Trans. Amer. otol. Soc. **49**, 20–30 (1961).

IURATO, S.: Efferent fibers to the sensory cells of Corti's organ. Exp. Cell Res. **27**, 162 (1962).

KIMURA, R., WERSÄLL, J.: Termination of the olivo-cochlear bundle in relation to the outer hair cells of the organ of Corti in the guinea pig. Acta oto-laryng. (Stockh.) **55**, 11 (1962).

KRISTENSSON, K., OLSSON, Y., SJÖSTRAND, J.: Axonal uptake and retrograde transport of exogenous proteins in the hypoglossal nerve. Brain Res. **32**, 399–406 (1971).

NOMURA, Y., GACEK, R.R., BALOGH, K.: Efferent innervation of vestibular labyrinth. Arch. Otolaryng. **81**, 335 (1965).

PETROFF, A.E.: An experimental investigation of the origin of efferent fiber projections to the vestibular neuroepithelium (Abstract). Anat. Rec. **121**, 352 (1955).

RASMUSSEN, G.L.: The olivary peduncle and other fiber projections of the superior olivary complex. J. comp. Neurol. **84**, 141 (1946).

RASMUSSEN, G.L.: Further observations of the efferent cochlear bundle. J. comp. Neurol. **99**, 61 (1953).

RASMUSSEN, G.L., GACEK, R.R.: Concerning the question of an efferent fiber component of the vestibular nerve of the cat (Abstract). Anat. Rec. **130**, 361 (1958).

RASMUSSEN, G.L.: Anatomic relationships of the ascending and descending auditory systems. In: Neurological aspects of auditory and vestibular disorders. W. S. FIELDS and B. R. ALFORD, Eds. Springfield, Ill.: Charles C. Thomas 1964.

ROSSI, G., CORTISINA, G.: Il "sistema efferente colinergicovestibolare". Sintesi storico-bibliografica e ricerche personali. Minerva otorinolaring. **12**, 1–63 (1962).

SMITH, C.A., RASMUSSEN, G.L.: Recent observations on the olivocochlear bundle. Ann. Otol. (St. Louis) **72**, 489 (1963).

Smith, C. A., Rasmussen, G. L.: Efferent nerve fibers to the vestibule of the chinchilla. Third Symposium on "The Role of the Vestibular Organs in Space Exploration." Naval Aerospace Medical Institute, Pensacola, Florida, Jan. 1967.

Spoendlin, H. H., Gacek, R. R.: Electron microscopic study of the efferent and afferent innervation of the organ of Corti in the cat. Ann. Otol. (St. Louis) **62**, 660 (1963).

Wersäll, J.: Studies on the structure and innervation of the sensory epithelium of the cristae ampullares in the guinea pig. Acta oto-laryng. (Stockh.) Suppl. **126**, (1956).

Chapter V.

Physiological Aspects of the Efferent Vestibular System*

By

W. Precht, Frankfurt a. M.

With 5 Figures

Contents

I. Introduction

The last article gives a full account of the anatomy of the efferent fibers supplying the peripheral vestibular apparatus. It is the aim of this paper to summarize the data relating to the *functional* properties of this system. Before going into details of the vestibular efferent system it is worthwhile mentioning a few studies on efferent systems to sensory organs other than the vestibular receptors, since the efferent control of vestibular receptors represents only a special case of centrifugal control of a sensory input. The control of sensory impulses can take place at different levels of a particular sensory pathway. For example, "higher" centers may act on *second order sensory* neurons *directly* or at a *presynaptic* level on the *afferent fibers* to modulate the incoming information in accordance with different functional requirements (for details and references see: Hernández-Peon, 1955; Granit, 1955; Rossi and Zanchetti, 1957; Hagbarth, 1960). The present Chapter, however, deals with another interesting aspect of centrifugal control of afferent sensory activity, i.e. the action of fibers of central origin on the *peripheral receptors* themselves. The presence of such fibers has been demonstrated anatomically as well as physiologically in various sensory systems. In the *retina* Granit (1955) first demonstrated reduction of the peripheral electrical activity as a consequence of electrical stimulation of certain central structures that are thought to give origin to efferent fibers. Similar effects were reported for the *olfactory* (Kerr and Hagbarth, 1955), *auditory* (Galambos, 1956; Fex, 1959, 1962; Desmedt and Monaco 1960, 1961) and lateral-line systems (Russel, 1968) when efferent fibers were stimulated.

* Manuscript completed Nov. 1971.

Neurons giving origin to efferent axons are, of course, also subjected to convergence of impulses arising in various related central structures, thus representing the final common path from the central nervous system to the receptor organs.

II. Physiological Evidence for Efferent Fibers to the Vestibular Receptors

SCHMIDT (1963) was the first to demonstrate directly the presence of *efferent* fibers in the vestibular nerve of the *frog* by detaching the distal end of the nerve from the labyrinthine receptors and recording single-unit activity from the proximal end of the nerve in response to adequate stimulation of the contralateral intact labyrinth and various extralabyrinthine sources. The efferent nerve fibers usually showed little or no spontaneous activity; furthermore, evoked activity in these fibers was demonstrated to be readily blocked by anesthesia, which usually had no appreciable effect on the afferent fiber activity (SCHMIDT, 1963; GLEISNER and HENRIKSSON, 1963). These findings have been confirmed in frog by LLINÁS et al. (1968) and LLINÁS and PRECHT (1969), by TRINCKER (1968) in guinea pig and by SCHMIDT et al. (1972) in goldfish. It was also shown that section of the vestibular nerve at its entrance into the brain stem abolishes, as expected, all activity in the efferent fibers recorded distal to the transection in the VIII nerve.

Stimulation of any of the three semicircular canals on the intact side evoked efferent spike activities in the contralateral nerve, whereas no effects have been seen after stimulation of the otolith organs (SCHMIDT, 1963). On the other hand, BERTRAND and VEENHOF (1964) found efferent activity generated by stimulation of the contralateral otolith system in rabbit; a finding that has been confirmed by KLINKE and SCHMIDT (1968) in goldfish. It also appears that adequate stimulation of the intact contralateral horizontal semicircular canals (utriculopetal deviation of the cupula) initiates a much larger number of efferent spikes than stimulation of any of the vertical canals (utriculofugal deviation of the cupula). The above findings imply that whenever a nerve fiber of the horizontal canal is found to be activated by utriculofugal stimulation of the ipsilateral horizontal canal (type-II response), this increase in frequency is caused by utriculopetal cupula deviation occurring at the same time in the *contralateral* horizontal canal. It seems, therefore, that the rule that in the horizontal canals only utriculopetal deviation causes frequency increase in nerve fibers is still valid (LOWENSTEIN and SAND, 1940). The evidence for an efferent feedback to an ampulla from itself is slight, although SCHMIDT (1963) has some evidence which implies the existence of such a projection in the posterior semicircular canal of frog. This finding has been confirmed by GLEISNER and HENRIKSSON (1963). Efferent impulses were also found to be elicited by stimulation of *extralabyrinthine* sources, e.g. by active or passive movements of the limbs or by gentle pressure on the eye in the region of the Gasserian ganglion (SCHMIDT, 1963).

In an attempt to measure the thresholds of efferent fiber activity to angular acceleration, GLEISNER and HENRIKSSON (1963) found that the firing frequency of efferent fibers rarely increased at accelerations of about $6°/sec^2$. In general, these findings were confirmed by PRECHT et al. (1971) although occasionally the

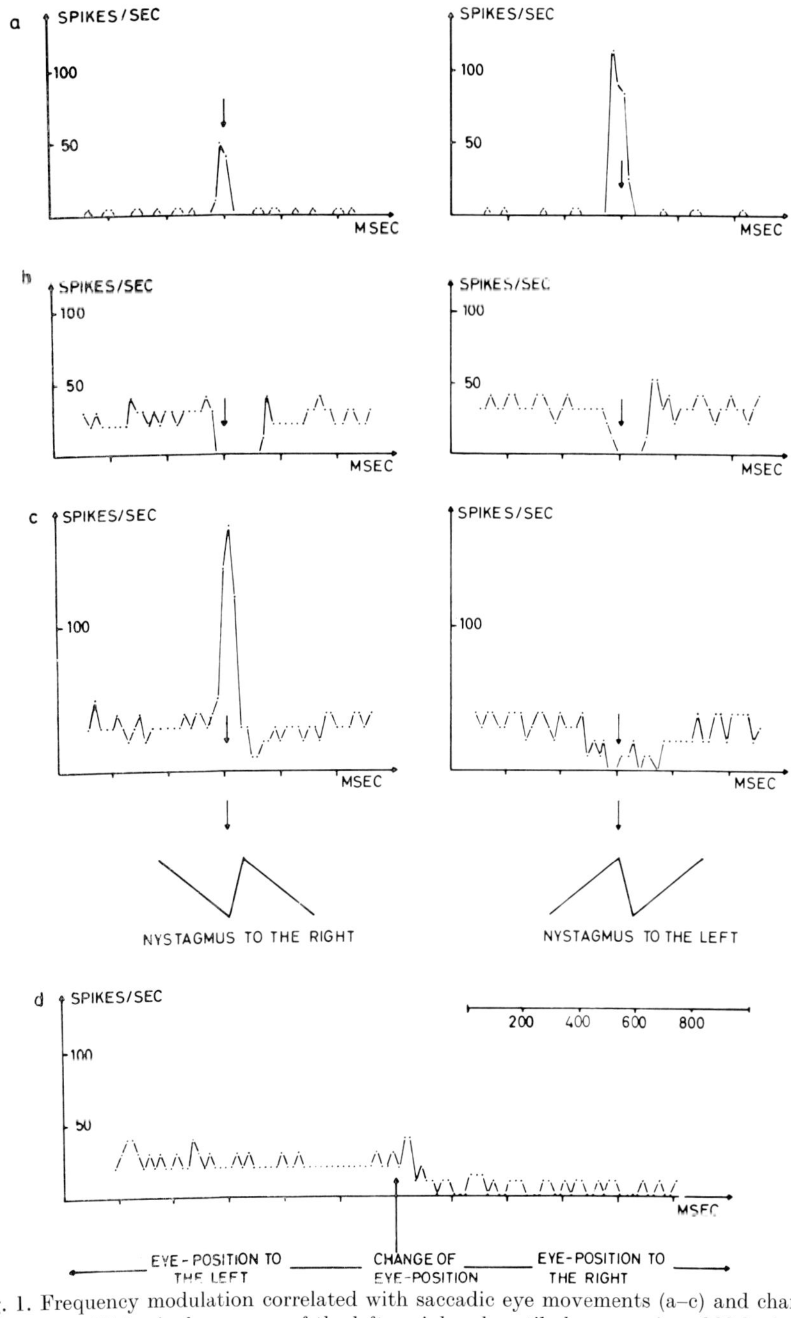

Fig. 1. Frequency modulation correlated with saccadic eye movements (a–c) and changes of eye position (d) in single neurons of the left peripheral vestibular nerve in goldfish. Averaged neuronal activity during 10 beats of nystagmus to the right and to the left as a function of time before and after saccade onset (a–c) or change of position of the eye (d). The dots represent the mean number of spikes per second over successive 50-msec periods. (a) bidirectionally activated neuron, (b) bidirectionally inhibited neuron, (c) directionally specific type d neuron; it is important to note that in neurons a to c the saccadic frequency modulation always starts *before* the onset of saccade, and (d) position-sensitive neuron. About 100 msec after change of eye position from left to right the neuron is tonically inhibited (By courtesy of Dr. DICHGANS)

thresholds were less than 3°/sec^2 (Fig. 2C and D). Higher accelerations, about 15°/sec^2 generate efferent activity in most cases. Thus it can be stated that in general a significant *difference in threshold* for frequency increase exists between primary *afferent* fibers (about 0.5°/sec^2) as determined in frog by PRECHT and LLINÁS (1969b) and PRECHT et al. (1971) and the *efferent* fiber system. The shortest latencies measured from the onset of acceleration to the appearance of the first efferent action potential seem to be about 200 msec in frog (GLEISNER and HENRIKSSON, 1963).

It has recently been shown that in goldfish, identified efferent vestibular nerve fibers projecting to the horizontal semicircular canal change their firing frequencies in relation to rapid eye movements (SCHMIDT et al., 1972). As shown in Fig. 1a, some efferent fibers increase their firing rate with fast phases of nystagmus both to the left and to the right, while others (Fig. 1b) are inhibited with saccades in either direction. Besides these bidirectionally sensitive units a third type has been found, which was inhibited during the rapid phase of nystagmus when its direction was ipsilateral and activated when its direction was contralateral to the side of the recording electrode. It is important to note that in all three types of units activation and inhibition started 9–100 msec *prior* to the saccade. Finally, a fourth type of neuron can be recorded from the VIII nerve, which was activated in relation to eye position (Fig. 1d). In this class of efferent neurons, frequency modulation began up to 100 msec *after* a position change. The activity of neurons recorded from otolith branches of the VIII nerve was not influenced by eye movements.

III. Central Location of Efferent Neurons

Various attempts have been made to localize the central sites of origin of efferent fibers. Thus it has been found that electrical stimulation of the *lateral vestibular nucleus* of cat evokes action potentials in the *contralateral* vestibular nerve that have a latency of about 20–30 msec (SALA, 1965) and might be efferent in nature. Similarly, electrical stimulation of the ipsilateral and contralateral lateral vestibular nucleus in guinea pig causes activation of efferent vestibular fibers (TRINCKER, 1968). These findings might suggest that the somata of efferent neurons are located in the lateral vestibular nucleus, but a direct demonstration is still outstanding since the stimulus might excite fibers that only pass through the lateral nucleus and originate somewhere else. Recently it has been shown that in *frog*, efferent neurons are located in the vestibular nucleus. Vestibular neurons were found to be antidromically excited after stimulation of the ipsilateral VIII nerve (PRECHT et al., 1974). The same neurons as were activated antidromically were also driven synaptically by stimulation of the ipsi- and contralateral VIII nerves, suggesting that both labyrinths converge on efferent neurons (OZAWA et al., 1974). This finding is completely consistent with previous data on the activity recorded from efferent fibers in response to horizontal angular acceleration (PRECHT et al., 1971), showing that many efferent fibers increase their discharge rate on rotation in either direction (type III response). Two examples of type III units are shown in Fig. 2. Neurons giving rise to efferent axons are located in the rostrolateral part of the frog vestibular nucleus.

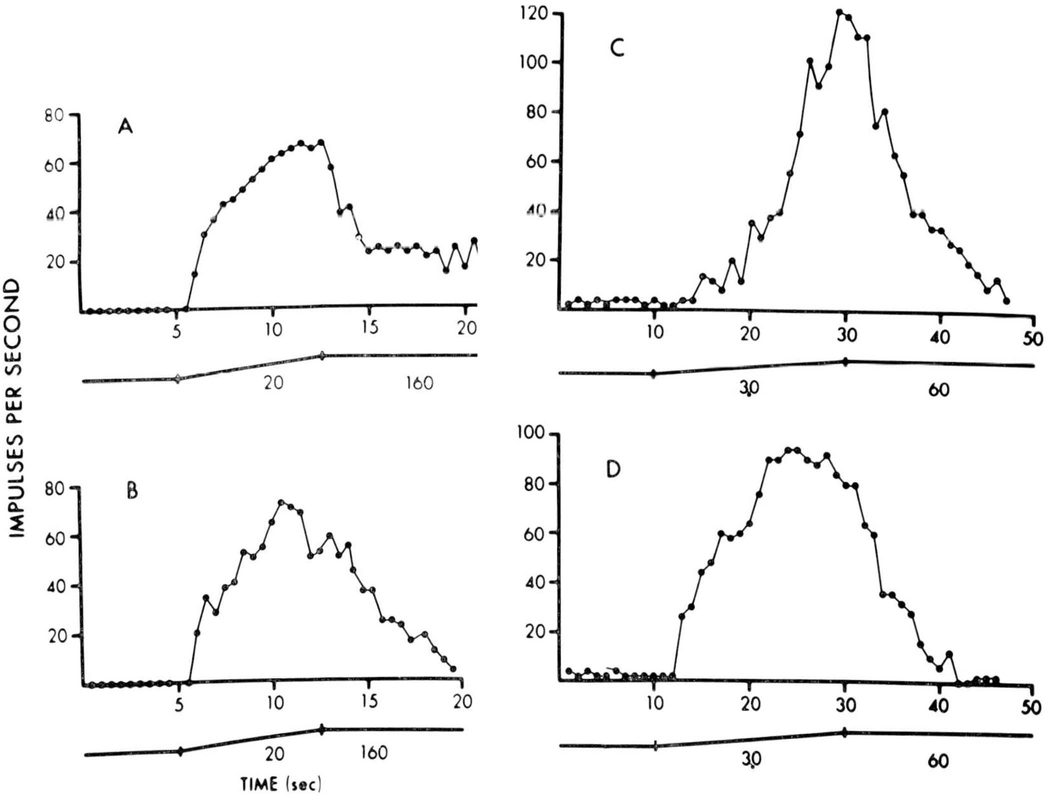

Fig. 2. Frequency diagrams of efferent fibers in response to angular acceleration. (A) and (B), responses of same fiber to ipsi- and contralateral horizontal angular acceleration respectively. (C) and (D), responses of a low-threshold efferent fiber to ipsi- and contralateral horizontal angular acceleration. Ordinate represents spikes per second of single unit discharges measured in each half-second. Abscissa gives time in seconds. The line below each frequency diagram indicates velocity of rotation. The left-hand number in each diagram indicates the acceleration rate (arc degree/sec^2), and the right-hand number the velocity of constant rotation (arc degree/sec) (From PRECHT et al., 1971)

When the vestibular nerve of frog is stimulated electrically at the peripheral branches detached from the receptors, efferent action potentials can be recorded proximally in the same nerve with latencies as short as 3 msec (LLINÁS et al., 1968). This also suggests a short pathway from the VIII nerve to the central system and back to the nerve, involving very few synapses. As described above, part of this central pathway may involve the vestibular nucleus, and as will be shown below the cerebellar Purkinje cells too, since cells in both these regions can be antidromically activated following VIII nerve stimulation. The long latencies found with adequate stimulation in frog imply that a considerable temporal and spatial summation is required in order to activate silent efferent neurons. This assumption is supported by the fact that acceleration of higher magnitude produces shorter and more constant latencies. Long latencies have also been observed in spontaneously inactive second-order vestibular neurons in cat following angular acceleration (SHIMAZU and PRECHT, 1965), although electrical stimulation of the vestibular nerve monosynaptically excited these neurons (PRECHT and SHIMAZU, 1965).

IV. Mode of Action of Efferent Fibers

In an attempt to study the function of the efferent system in cat, SALA (1962, 1965) first observed a *decrease* of the spontaneous activity of single *afferent* nerve fibers as a consequence of tetanic stimulation of the area of the contralateral *Deiters' nucleus*. In some cases, however, single shock stimulation of the vestibular nucleus evoked action potentials in the contralateral vestibular nerve. The nature of these action potentials is not clear; they may belong to either afferent or efferent fibers. Since it is known that primary vestibular fibers do not cross the midline (SHIMAZU and PRECHT, 1966; LADPLI and BRODAL, 1968) the activation of these spike potentials cannot be due to direct excitation of vestibular afferents. The long latencies of activation also exclude this possibility. If it were assumed that these evoked spike potentials are recorded from afferent fibers, two mechanisms could explain the finding. Firstly, the effect could be mediated by excitatory efferent fibers being triggered by the stimulation of the lateral nucleus, and secondly activation could be caused by inhibition of a tonically active inhibitory efferent system (disinhibition). In view of the fact that natural stimulation of the contralateral labyrinth activates units proved to be efferent (see above), the alternative explanation would be that these units that are activated by stimulation of the contralateral Deiters' nucleus belong to the efferent system. Using anatomical techniques, PETROFF (1955) has described *crossing* efferent fibers originating in the vestibular nuclei. *Uncrossed* efferent fibers have been reported by RASMUSSEN and GACEK (1958), GACEK (1960), and ROSSI and CORTESINA (1962, 1965). At this point, it may tentatively be assumed that the *decrease* of the afferent vestibular discharge following tetanic stimulation of the contralateral Deiters' nucleus of cat is caused by the activation of *inhibitory efferent fibers* and

Fig. 3. (A) Diagram of frog brainstem, labyrinth, and experimental arrangement; *BC*, bipolar ganglion cells; *CER*, cerebellum; *CF*, climbing fiber; *GC*, granule cell; *ME*, recording microelectrode; *MF*, mossy fiber; *OL*, optic lobe; *PC*, Purkinje cell; *RC*, receptor cell; *S*, peripheral nerve stimulating electrode; *V*, trigeminal nerve; *VII*, facial nerve; *VIII*, stato-acoustic nerve; *PB*, posterior branch; arrows indicate the direction of impulse conduction. (B–F) Antidromic extracellular action potentials from Purkinje cells in the auricular lobe, recorded at a depth of 250 μm and evoked by stimulation of the VIII nerve. (B and C) All-or-none spike responses at threshold intensity from two different Purkinje cells. (D–F) Purkinje cell action potentials evoked by activation of VIII nerve at 1.3 times the threshold. (D) Control. (E) Refractory period for antidromic invasion of the Purkinje cell after double shocks with a short interval between stimuli. (F) As in E, but with longer interval between stimuli, showing second Purkinje spike. (G and H) Extracellular record. (H and I) Intracellular records of the same cell showing the antidromically excited action potential and an excitatory postsynaptic potential. (J) At slightly higher stimulus intensity the Purkinje cell shows also a transsynaptic response. (K) Latency histogram of the early spike responses after stimulation of VIII nerve. Abscissa, time in msec. Ordinate, number of Purkinje cells recorded. The arrows in B–J indicate stimulus artifact location. Time and voltage calibration as indicated. The polarity is expressed by the positive and negative signs on the amplitude calibrating bar (From LLINÁS et al., 1967)

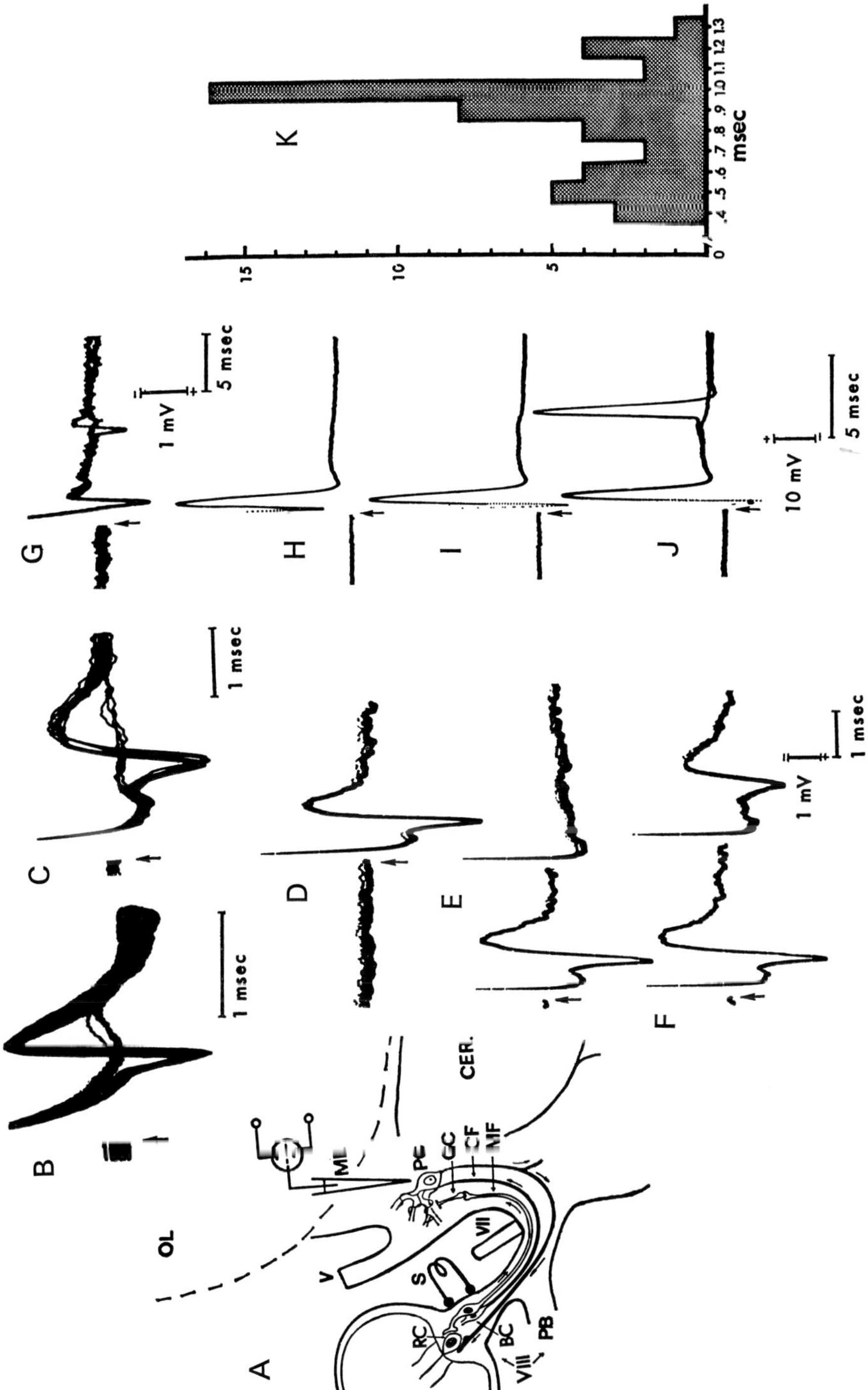
A
B
C
D
E
F
G
H
I
J
K
OL
V
S
RC
BC
VIII
PB
VII
PE
GC
CF
MF
ML
CER.
1 msec
1 msec
1 mV
1 msec
1 mV
5 msec
10 mV
5 msec
0
5
10
15
.4 .5 .6 .7 .8 .9 1.0 1.1 1.2 1.3
msec

Fig. 3

that the efferent vestibular system as such is inhibitory in nature. This hypothesis would imply that excitatory effects on the afferent vestibular input following central stimulation are caused by inhibition of the tonically active inhibitory efferent neurons. Depending on the requirements of the physiological situation, the efferent path could thus increase or decrease the excitability of the vestibular receptor cells.

This hypothesis is further supported by recent studies of the efferent vestibular system of bullfrog (LLINÁS et al., 1968; LLINÁS and PRECHT, 1969). These authors have demonstrated that cerebellar *Purkinje cells* located in the *auricular lobe* (flocculus) of the cerebellum of *frog* are activated antidromically by electrical activation of the ipsilateral vestibular nerve (Fig. 3). As shown in Fig. 3K, there appear to be two groups of action potentials activated by stimulation of the VIII nerve. The first group has its peak at 0.5 msec, whereas the second has a peak at about 1.0 msec. The cell shown in Fig. 3B is an example of a cell with an action potential of short latency (about 0.5 msec) and the neuron shown in Fig. 3C has a latency of about 0.9 msec. This difference in latency of antidromic activation may reflect the presence of two groups of Purkinje cell axons with different fiber diameters causing differences in conduction velocity. Fig. 3G to J show extra- and intracellular recordings from a Purkinje cell after stimulation of the VIII nerve. As the stimulus strength increases a subthreshold excitatory postsynaptic potential is seen to follow the antidromic action potential. In Fig. 3J a further slight increase in stimulus intensity generated an action potential synaptically. This record shows that the same *Purkinje* cell receives *synaptic* input from the *vestibular nerve* and sends its *axon* or an axon collateral to the *peripheral receptor* organ. Not all Purkinje cells found in the flocculus participate in the efferent projection; some cells receive only synaptic vestibular input (LLINÁS and PRECHT, 1969; PRECHT and LLINÁS, 1969a, b), others show no relation at all to the vestibular system. On the basis of these data, it is concluded that some Purkinje cells from the auricular lobe project directly onto the peripheral vestibular organ, thus participating in the efferent vestibular system.

Light- and electron-microscope studies have confirmed the existence of a cerebellar pathway to the labyrinth in bullfrog by showing that section of the VIII nerve extracranially produces degeneration of both climbing and mossy fibers (synaptic input) as well as characteristic, *retrograde* changes in the somas of Purkinje cells (LLINÁS et al., 1967a, b). Furthermore, if the cerebellar cortex is removed, *degenerating synaptic boutons* (Fig. 4) can be demonstrated in contact with the peripheral vestibular receptor cells (HILLMAN, 1969). The receptor cells of the maculae and cristae are normally contacted by vesicle-filled boutons which terminate synaptically in relation to a submembranous sac within the receptor cell. Following lesions at different sites of the central nervous system of frog it was found that there are several areas that might give rise to efferent fibers. Most of the centrifugal fibers degenerated when the brainstem was hemisected above the level of the vestibular nerve. Brainstem sectioning above the V nerve produced degeneration of 35% of the efferent boutons. Cerebellar lesions caused degeneration of about 20% of the boutons. Nauta studies showed that the cerebello-

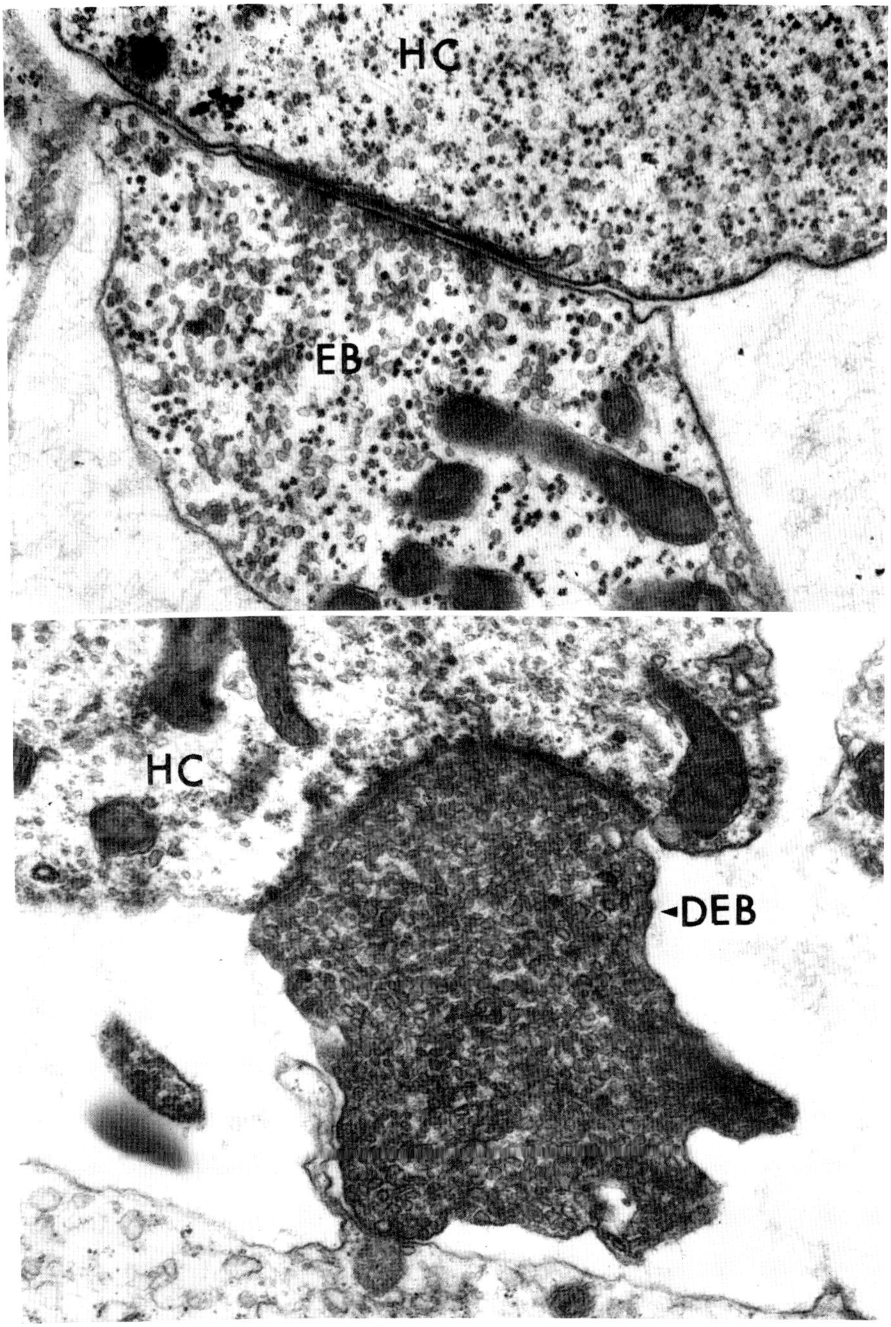

Fig. 4. Efferent synaptic terminals in the sensory epithelium of frog utriculus. (A) Normal efferent boutons (EB) synapsing on a utricular hair cell (HC) (32,000 ×). (B) Degenerated efferent boutons (DEB) contacting on a utricular hair cell (HC) 4 days after section of the ipsilateral cerebellar peduncle, (31,000 ×) (Hillman, unpublished results)

labyrinthine fibers form a small bundle located in the ventrocaudal side of the VIII nerve. Following sectioning of the whole vestibular nerve all efferent boutons were found to be degenerated. From this we conclude that the vestibular efferent system in frog has different sites of origin in the central nervous system, one of them being located in the auricular lobe of the cerebellum.

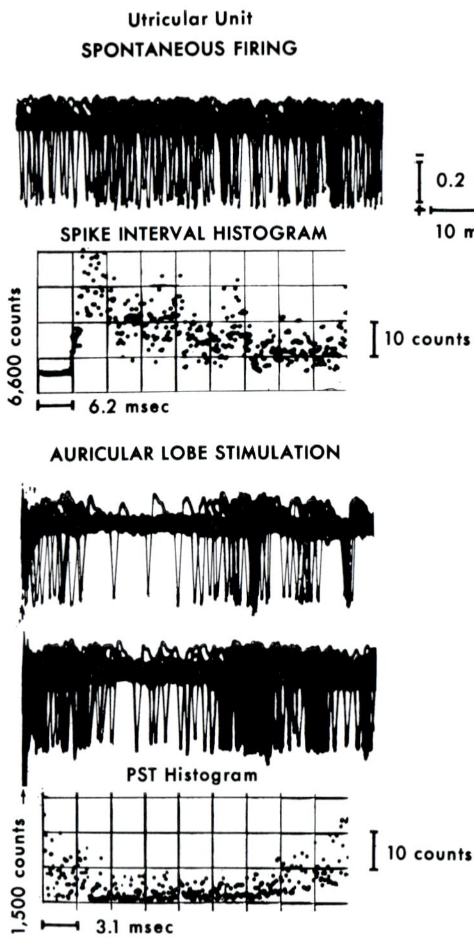

Fig. 5. Effect of stimulation of frog cerebellum (auricular lobe) on the activity of primary vestibular afferents. The uppermost record shows the spontaneous discharge of the utricular unit (30 sweeps superimposed). A spike interval histogram of the same unit was obtained before the stimulation. The effect of auricular lobe stimulation at a rate of 10/sec is exemplified by two records, the upper one being composed of 30 superimposed sweeps and the lower one consisting of 60 superimposed sweeps (stimulus artifact is indicated by an arrow). Time and amplitude calibrations are the same as for the uppermost record (polarity as indicated). The lowest diagram shows the post-stimulus histogram of the same units. Note the different time scales for the post-stimulus histogram and spike records (From Llinás and Precht, 1969)

Recent physiological studies have shown that the cerebellar *Purkinje cells* are *inhibitory in nature* (ITO and YOSHIDA, 1964; ITO et al., 1964; ECCLES et al., 1966; LLINÁS and AYALA, 1967). It is reasonable to assume that Purkinje cells projecting onto the vestibular sensory epithelium are also inhibitory in nature. This hypothesis has been tested by observing the effect of electrical stimulation of the cerebellar auricular lobe on the spontaneous discharge of vestibular nerve fibers identified as primary afferent fibers. It has been shown that a number of spontaneously firing primary *afferent fibers* are *inhibited* (Fig. 5) by repetitive stimulation of the *auricular lobe* (LLINÁS and PRECHT, 1969). Similarly, stimulation of the vestibular nerve during recording from primary vestibular fibers caused depression of their spontaneous discharge. Activation of afferent discharge was not observed under these conditions. In some cases, however, a relative increase in afferent discharge frequency might be expected following stimulation of central structures that are inhibitory on the efferent neurons or by inhibition of structures that are excitatory on them. In the case of a tonically active Purkinje cell that projected to the labyrinth, LLINÁS and PRECHT (1969) observed a long-lasting depression of tonic discharge that followed direct excitation of the Purkinje axon by stimulation of the cerebellar surface. Since no inhibitory neurons are known in the cerebellum of frog (LLINÁS and BLOEDEL, 1967) the depression of the tonic activity has been explained by a temporary withdrawal of the excitatory background to the Purkinje cell originating in the brainstem. This latter effect could be caused by excitation of many Purkinje cells via parallel fibers and their inhibitory action on brainstem neurons.

On polarizing stimulation of brainstem centers, TRINCKER (1968) observed tonic activity in previously silent *afferent* vestibular fibers. This effect could be due to a decrease in activity of a tonic inhibitory efferent system (disinhibition) caused by stimulation of inhibitory neurons converging on efferent neurons directly or on neurons that are responsible for their tonic activity (disfacilitation). In recording directly from *efferent* fibers while polarizing brainstem nuclei, TRINCKER (1968) found increased or decreased discharge frequency, depending on the polarity of stimulation.

It is known from studies by TRINCKER (1957) that utriculopetal deflection of the cupula of the horizontal canal causes a *negative* DC potential shift recorded extracellularly in the crista ampullaris while utriculofugal deflection leads to a *positive* potential change. Throughout the negative deflection the impulse frequency of the primary afferent neurons increases while the opposite is the case when the potential moves in the positive direction. Attempts have been made to record DC potential changes from the sensory epithelium in response to stimulation of the vestibular efferent system. Studies by SALA (1962, 1965) did in fact demonstrate that tetanic stimulation of the cat's brainstem in the area of the vestibular nuclei causes *positive DC shift* at the vestibular organ after a delay of about 10 msec. This effect can be observed regardless of the initial state of the labyrinth prior to the electrical stimulation, i.e. whether the DC potential was shifted by means of hot water (negative deflection) or cold water irrigation (positive deflection) before the electrical stimulation was applied. Furthermore, effects on the DC potential level have been observed by TRINCKER (1968) on polarizing stimulation of the ipsilateral and contralateral vestibular nuclei. The direction of the DC potential shift depended on the polarity of brainstem stimulation. Generally, the amplitude of the potential shift was larger in the positive direction (up to 14 mV) as compared to changes found in the negative direction (up to 8 mV).

It is well known that caloric stimulation of the inner ear causes endolymph movements that in turn lead to deflection of the cupula. The direction of the cupula deviation depends upon the temperature of the water used for irrigation (for details see Chapter D.II.).

In his study on the efferent vestibular system, SALA (1965) made use of the *caloric* stimuli by applying them to one ear while recording DC potential changes from the ipsilateral and contralateral labyrinths. While warm-water irrigation causes a negative potential shift on the stimulated side, the opposite, a positive potential shift, is observed in the contralateral labyrinth. Cold-water irrigation has the opposite effect, i.e. positive potential shifts occur in the ipsilateral labyrinth and negative changes are observed in the contralateral labyrinth. These results seem to be consistent with the findings obtained with single-unit analysis that showed that the efferent system can be influenced by the contralateral labyrinth. Of particular interest is the negative potential shift occurring in the contralateral labyrinth while the ipsilateral side is subjected to cold-water stimulation. Cold-water irrigation would cause simultaneously a decrease of the frequency of afferent discharge on the same side. This decrease of afferent discharge may lead to a *disfacilitation* of the otherwise tonic efferent neurons projecting to the contralateral receptors and consequently to *disinhibition* of the receptor cells. The negative DC potential shift observed during irrigation could be related to this disinhibitory effect. On the other hand, positive DC potential shifts could be related to the activation of the inhibitory efferent system and their hyperpolarizing action on peripheral structures. The decrease of spontaneous discharge of afferent fibers following caloric stimulation of the contralateral labyrinth (LEDOUX, 1958) may be explained by this hyperpolarizing effect.

Finally, it is worthwhile mentioning that the positive potential change recorded on stimulation of the efferent vestibular system was reduced or abolished when the animal was treated with subconvulsant doses of *strychnine sulfate* (SALA, 1965). A similar effect of strychnine was observed by DESMEDT and MONACO (1960, 1961) in studying the effects produced by electrical stimulation of the olivocochlear bundle on cochlear potentials.

In summary, the data so far obtained in regard to the vestibular efferent system demonstrate its presence beyond doubt in various species, both by anatomical and by physiological means. As far as its mode of action is concerned, the system seems to be inhibitory in nature. Similarly, inhibitory actions have been postulated and demonstrated for efferent paths to the cochlea and to the lateral-line organs that are closely related to the vestibular receptors*. It has been pointed

* Note added on proof: Recent intracellular recordings from lateral line organs demonstrated inhibitory postsynaptic potentials (IPSPs) that were evoked by electrical stimulation of efferent fibers to the hair cells (FLOCK, RUSSEL, Nature New Biol. **243**, 89—91 (1973)).

out that a tonic efferent system that is inhibitory in nature does allow for the possibility that primary afferent fibers show both decrease or increase of their frequencies of discharge following stimulation of central structures. Reduction of the tonic firing of the efferent neurons resulting from central stimulation could lead to disinhibition of the peripheral organs and hence to an increase of afferent discharge.

As for the functional significance of the efferent system, little can be said at present. A few possibilities will be discussed here. As described above, some of the efferent fibers were activated by utriculopetal stimulation of the contralateral horizontal semicircular canal and other fibers showed activation following stimulating of the contralateral utriculus. If these efferent fibers were to project onto the corresponding receptor organs on their side, they might aid in the decrease of frequency of discharge of afferent units in the ipsilateral nerve occurring during contralateral stimulation. Similarly, decrease of this crossed tonic efferent inhibitory influence on ipsilateral receptors that occurs on adequate stimulation of the ipsilateral side (e.g. ipsilateral horizontal rotation) could cause an increase of the excitability of the ipsilateral receptors. Furthermore, efferent activity caused by stimulation of the contralateral canal system might affect the otolith organs or vice versa. Such an interaction between different receptors may function so as to sharpen certain vestibular inputs related to head movement in space.

In addition, it has been shown that a short feedback pathway does exist from a group of receptors to themselves, i.e. a negative feedback to a vestibular receptor organ from itself is quite possible. Such an efferent pathway may provide an inhibitory control mechanism thrown into action in case of strong sensory stimulation. The higher threshold for frequency increase of efferent neurons supports this view. Furthermore, frequency adaptation of primary vestibular fibers may be caused partly by the efferent system (PRECHT et al., 1971).

One puzzling observation in regard to the efferent system to the vestibular apparatus is the fact that various extralabyrinthine sources are able to influence its activity. It appears that effective stimuli are generally those that tend to make the animal move the body or the eyes. In all these cases efferent activity changes *precede* the movements – meaning that frequency modulation is not caused by proprioceptive feedback but rather by motor centers. Therefore, it is permissible to assume that during active head or body movements vestibular activity arising from the labyrinthine receptors which would cause movements opposite to the active ones is counterbalanced by the action of the efferent system as far peripheral as the receptor level. It should be kept in mind, however, that the effect of the efferent system on the afferent system is rather weak (KLINKE, 1970; RUSSEL and ROBERTS, 1971; PRECHT et al., 1971; SCHMIDT et al., 1972) and may, therefore, by itself not be sufficient for the compensation of the vestibular input during active movements. Similar compensatory changes may occur in higher order vestibular neurons which would then add to the direct effect on the receptors. It is clear that we are only just beginning to understand the functional role of the efferent system and that further investigation of its properties is needed for a more complete understanding.

References

BERTRAND, R.A., VEENHOF, V.B.: Efferent vestibular potentials by canalicular and otolithic stimulations in the rabbit. Acta oto-laryng. (Stockh.) **58**, 515–524 (1964).

DESMEDT, J.E., MONACO, P.: Suppression par la strychnine de l'effet inhibiteur centrifuge éxcercé par le faisceau olivo-cochleaire. Arch. int. Pharmacodyn. **129**, 244–248 (1960).

DESMEDT, J.E., MONACO, P.: Mode of action of the efferent olivo-cochlear bundle on the inner ear. Nature (Lond.) **192**, 1263 (1961).

ECCLES, J.C., LLINÁS, R., SASAKI, K.: The action of antidromic impulses on the cerebellar Purkinje cells. J. Physiol. (Lond.) **182**, 316–345 (1966).

FEX, J.: Augmentation of cochlear microphonics by stimulation of efferent fibers to the cochlea. Acta oto-laryng. (Stockh.) **50**, 540–541 (1959).

FEX, J.: Auditory activity in centrifugal and centripetal cochlear fibres in cat (a study of a feedback system). Acta physiol. scand. 55, Suppl. **189**, 1–68 (1962).

GACEK, R.R.: Efferent component of the vestibular nerve. In: Neural Mechanisms of the Auditory and Vestibular System. Springfield Ill.: Ch. C. Thomas 1960.

GALAMBOS, R.: Suppression of the auditory nerve activity by stimulation of efferent fibres to the cochlea. J. Neurophysiol. **19**, 424–437 (1956).

GLEISSNER, L., HENRIKSSON, N.G.: Efferent and afferent activity pattern in the vestibular nerve of the frog. Acta oto-laryng. (Stockh.) **58**, Suppl. 192, 90–103 (1963).

GRANIT, R.: Receptors and Sensory Perception. Yale University Press 1955.

HAGBARTH, K.E.: Centrifugal mechanisms of sensory control. Ergebn. Biol. **22**, 47–66 (1960).

HERNÁNDEZ-PÉON, R.: Central mechanisms controlling conduction along central sensory pathways. Acta neurol. lat.-amer. **1**, 256–264 (1955).

HILLMAN, D.: Light and electron microscopical study of the relationships between the cerebellum and the vestibular organ of the frog. Exp. Brain Res. **9**, 1–15 (1969).

ITO, M., YOSHIDA, M.: The cerebellar-evoked monosynaptic inhibition of Deiters' neurones. Experientia (Basel) **20**, 515–516 (1964).

ITO, M., YOSHIDA, M., OBATA, K.: Monosynaptic inhibition of the intracerebellar nuclei induced from the cerebellar cortex. Experientia (Basel) **20**, 575–576 (1964).

KERR, D.I.B., HAGBARTH, K.E.: An investigation of olfactory centrifugal fibre system. J. Neurophysiol. **18**, 362–374 (1955).

KLINKE, R.: Efferent influence on the vestibular organ during active movements of the body. Pflügers Arch. **318**, 325–332 (1970).

KLINKE, R., SCHMIDT, C.L.: Efferente Impulse im nervus vestibularis bei Reizung des kontralateralen Otolithenorgans. Pflügers Arch. **304**, 183–188 (1968).

LADPLI, R., BRODAL, A.: Experimental studies of commissural and reticular formation projections from the vestibular nuclei in the cat. Brain Res. **8**, 65–96 (1968).

LEDOUX, A.: Les canaux semi-circulaires. Acta oto-rhino-laryng. belg. **12**, 111–346 (1958).

LLINÁS, R., AYALA, J.F.: Purkinje axon collateral action upon interneurones in the cerebellar cortex, Neurophysiological Basis of Normal and Abnormal Motor Activities. Hewlett (N.Y.): Raven Press 1967.

LLINÁS, R., BLOEDEL, J.: Frog cerebellum: Absence of long-term inhibition upon Purkinje cells. Science **155**, 601–603 (1967).

LLINÁS, R., PRECHT, W.: The inhibitory vestibular efferent system and its relation to the cerebellum in the frog. Exp. Brain Res. **9**, 16–29 (1969).

Llinás, R., Precht, W., Bracchi, F., Huertas, J.: The inhibitory cerebello-vestibular system in the frog. Proc. int. Union physiolog. Sci. 7, Abst. 806, 269 (1968).

Llinás, R., Precht, W., Clarke, M.: Cerebellar Purkinje cell responses to physiological stimulation of the vestibular system in the frog. Exp. Brain Res. **13**, 408–431 (1971).

Llinás, R., Precht, W., Kitai, S.T.: Climbing fibre activation of Purkinje cell following primary vestibular afferent stimulation in the frog. Brain Res. **6**, 371–375 (1967a).

Llinás, R., Precht, W., Kitai, S.T.: Cerebellar Purkinje cell projection to the peripheral vestibular organ in the frog. Science **158**, 1328–1330 (1967b).

Lowenstein, O., Sand, A.: The mechanism of the semicircular canal. A study of the responses of single-fibre preparations to angular accelerations and to rotation at constant speed. Proc. roy. Soc. B **129**, 256–275 (1940).

Ozawa, S., Precht, W., Shimazu, H.: Crossed effects on central vestibular neurons in the horizontal canal system of the frog. Exp. Brain Res. **19**, 394–405 (1974).

Petroff, A.E.: An experimental investigation of the origin of efferent fibre projections to the vestibular neuro-epithelium. Anat. Rec. **121**, 352–353 (1955).

Precht, W., Llinás, R.: Functional organization of the vestibular afferents to the cerebellar cortex of frog and cat. Exp. Brain Res. **9**, 30–52 (1969a).

Precht, W., Llinás, R.: Comparative aspects of the vestibular input to the cerebellum. In: Neurobiology of Cerebellar Evolution and Development. R. Llinás, Ed. Chicago: Amer. med. Ass. Educ. and Res. Fdn. 1969b.

Precht, W., Llinás, R., Clarke, M.: Physiological responses of frog vestibular fibers to horizontal angular rotation. Exp. Brain Res. **13**, 378–407 (1971).

Precht, W., Ozawa, S., Richter, A. and Shimazu, H.: Intracellular study of frog's vestibular neurons in relation to the labyrinth and spinal cord. Exp. Brain Res. **19**, 377–393 (1974).

Precht, W., Shimazu, H.: Functional connections of tonic and kinetic vestibular neurones with primary vestibular afferents. J. Neurophysiol. **28**, 1014–1028 (1965).

Rasmussen, G.L., Gacek, R.R.: Concerning the question of the efferent fibre component of the vestibular nerve of the cat. Anat. Rec. **130**, 361 (1958).

Rossi, G., Cortesina, G.: The efferent innervation of the inner ear. Panminerva med. **4**, 478–500 (1962).

Rossi, G., Cortesina, G.: The efferent cochlear and vestibular system in Lepus cuniculus L. Acta anat. (Basel) **60**, 362–381 (1965).

Rossi, G.F., Zanchetti, A.: The brain stem reticular formation. Anatomy and physiology. Arch. ital. Biol. **95**, 199–435 (1957).

Russel, I.J.: Influence of efferent fibres on a receptor. Nature (Lond.) **219**, 177–178 (1968).

Russel, I.J., Roberts, B.L.: Efferent innervation of a mechanoreceptor. Proc. of the Int. Union of Physiol. Sciences, XXV Int. Congress Munich, Vol. IX, No. 1442, p. 485 (1971).

Sala, O.: Modificazioni dell'attivita del nervo vestibolare a seguito della stimulazione del sistema vestibolare efferente. Boll. Soc. ital. Biol. sper. **38**, 1048 (1962).

Sala, O.: The efferent vestibular system. Acta oto-laryng. (Stockh.) Suppl. **197**, 1–34 (1965).

Schmidt, R.F.: Frog labyrinthine efferent impulses. Acta oto-laryng. (Stockh.) **56**, 51–64 (1963).

Schmidt, C.L., Wist, E.R., Dichgans, J.: Efferent frequency modulation in the vestibular nerve of goldfish correlated with saccadic eye movements. Exp. Brain Res. **15**, 1–14 (1972).

Shimazu, H., Precht, W.: Tonic and kinetic responses of cat's vestibular neurones to horizontal angular acceleration. J. Neurophysiol. **28**, 991–1013 (1965).

Shimazu, H., Precht, W.: Inhibition of central vestibular neurones from the contralateral labyrinth and its mediating pathway. J. Neurophysiol. **29**, 467–492 (1966).

Trincker, D.: Bestandspotentiale im Bogengangssystem des Meerschweinchens und ihre Änderungen bei experimentellen Cupula-Ablenkungen. Pflügers Arch. ges. Physiol. **264**, 351–382 (1957).

Trincker, D.: Analyse des afferenten Informationsflusses von Labyrinthreceptoren, seiner Stabilisierung durch Rückkoppelung und der Kriterien für Konstanz der Raum- und Zeitkoordinaten zentraler Datenverarbeitung. In: BioKybernetik. H. Drischel, N. Tiedt, Hrsg. Leipzig: Karl-Marx-Universität 1968.

D. Central Mechanisms

Chapter I.

Anatomy of the Vestibular Nuclei and their Connections

By

A. Brodal, Oslo (Norway)

With 45 Figures

Contents

I. Introduction

The great majority of afferent fibers from the receptor areas of the vestibular organs terminate in the vestibular nuclei. Before the nervous impulses relayed to the nuclei can be transmitted further, they have to pass at least one synapse, and may accordingly be subject to modifications by impulses entering the nuclei in afferent fibers from many sources. The vestibular nuclei thus occupy a strategic position among the structures related to vestibular function.

Anatomical and physiological studies in recent years bear witness to the existence of an extreme complexity in the organization of the vestibular nuclei. Within this nuclear complex a number of minor units, territories or subdivisions can be distinguished, which differ structurally in cellular composition, fiber connections and other respects. The presence of structural differences of these kinds strongly suggests that there must be corresponding functional differences. As far as this assumption has been subjected to experimental tests, it has, in fact, turned out to be valid, and careful physiological studies by critical workers steadily bring forth new data in support of it. It is encouraging that the results of these studies are consistent with the anatomical data and that satisfactory correlations between structure and function are possible where in both fields of research attention has been paid to the minutest details in the organization. So far only a few of the "units" of the vestibular complex have been subjected to detailed functional analyses. Many units identified anatomically and known in some detail structurally are still virgin territory in physiological research. The functional properties of these will have to be explored in future in physiological studies where the points stimulated or recorded from are precisely indicated. The time has long passed when it was permissible to state that recordings were made "from the nucleus of Deiters," or that "the vestibular nuclei were destroyed on the left side."

The term "vestibular nuclei" is often used rather loosely. (Occasionally authors even speak of "the vestibular nucleus"!) Generally the term is used to cover the four classic vestibular nuclei: the superior, the lateral, the medial and the descending (or inferior) vestibular nucleus. As will be described below, several small cell groups are closely associated topographically with the main nuclei and should be included as parts of the vestibular nuclear complex, although some of the small groups, like certain regions within the four main nuclei, do not receive primary vestibular fibers. These regions and cell groups could therefore be excluded from the concept "vestibular nuclei" if this is taken in the strict sense. It is deemed practical, however, to retain the traditional collective name of "vestibular nuclei" for the entire complex.

This chapter gives a survey of our present knowledge of the structural organization of the vestibular nuclei, including their connections. Some correlations with physiological data will be attempted. No exhaustive review of the relevant literature will be given. Readers interested in references to older papers should consult the original papers cited. Some aspects of the subject have been treated in previous reviews (Brodal, 1960, 1964a, 1964b, 1966, 1967a) and in a monograph (Brodal et al., 1962).

II. Structure of the Vestibular Nuclei

The vestibular nuclei are phylogenetically relatively old parts of the brain, but they differ among vertebrates in details. The comparative anatomy of the vestibular nuclear complex will not be considered here (for a review see KAPPERS et al., 1936). Since most recent experimental work on these nuclei has been made in the cat, the account given will center on the nuclei in this species. This seems permissible because in all essentials the vestibular nuclei of most mammals, including man, appear to be organized like those of the cat.

As mentioned in the introduction *the vestibular nuclear complex may be subdivided into a number of cell groups*. The maps shown in Figs. 1 and 2 were constructed by BRODAL and POMPEIANO (1957) on the basis of a systematic analysis of series of Nissl-stained sections through the vestibular region of the brain stem in cats and kittens. The subdivision of the vestibular nuclear complex arrived at on the basis of its cytoarchitecture in transverse sections can also be recognized in sections prepared with silver impregnation methods and the Golgi method, and in the horizontal and sagittal planes (Figs. 3 and 4) as well as in the transverse plane. Experimental studies of afferent and efferent connections of the nuclear complex lend support to the subdivision employed, as will be apparent from the account of these subjects given later.

The borders between the subdivisions as outlined in cell or fiber stained preparations are not uniformly sharp. Where a border is indistinct it is not possible to allot a particular cell to one of two neighboring subdivisions. The fact that dendrites of the cells of one subdivision often extend into an adjacent one (see section on Intrinsic Organization) is a further indication that borders between regions should not be conceived of as being sharp. *The lines used in drawings to illustrate the subdivisions of a nuclear complex virtually represent transition zones where elements belonging functionally to one or the other subdivision are intermingled.* This explains why scattered units with particular functional properties are quite often found in an area (for example the descending vestibular nucleus) adjacent to a subdivision containing a large number of units with the same properties (for example the medial vestibular nucleus) in physiological studies. In anatomical studies scattered cells (or fibers) of this kind cannot usually be identified, and even if they can, they are difficult to indicate in the diagrams usually employed to represent the findings. This should be borne in mind in order to avoid unnecessary misinterpretations of apparent inconsistencies between anatomical and physiological findings.

In the analysis of physiological as well as experimental anatomical observations on the vestibular nuclei (as on other nuclei) it is important to know their structural organization in as much detail as possible. Misleading conclusions may be drawn if such features as the presence of fibers passing through the region which is stimulated or destroyed (see also below, p. 262) are not taken into account. In physiological studies of afferent impulses to a region, it is essential not to overlook the presence of possible other afferents. In the future, knowledge of the kinds, patterns and regional distributions of synaptic contacts will probably become increasingly important. In the presentation in this chapter considerable attention will therefore be directed to many minor features of the structure of the vestibular nuclei, which will have to be taken into consideration in future physiological studies as well as in chemical and histochemical investigations of the nuclei.

It follows from the complexity of the vestibular nuclei that in physiological studies precise identification of sites recorded from or stimulated is necessary if reliable results are to be obtained. For this reason no references to Horsley-Clarke stereotaxic

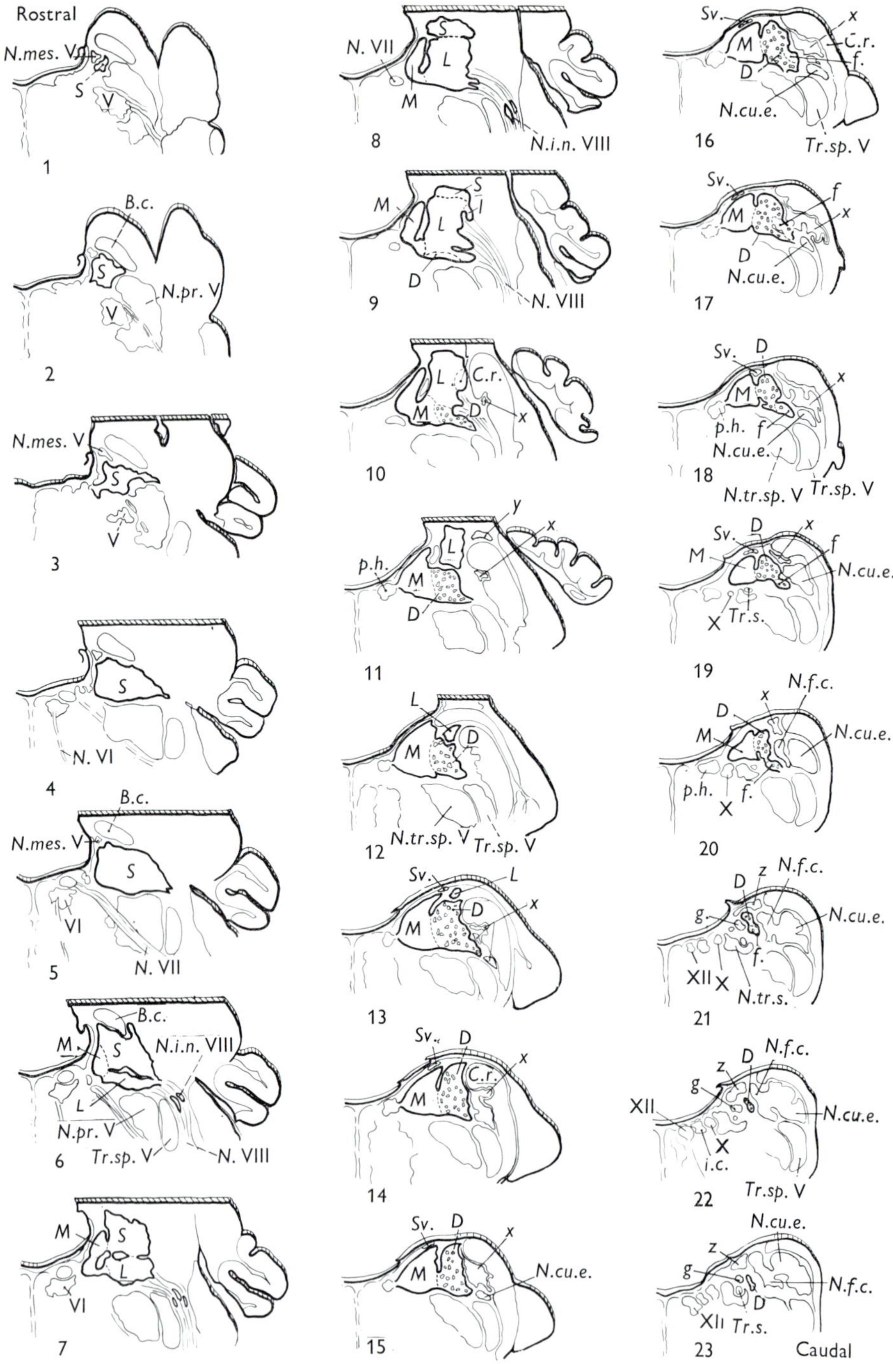

Fig. 1. A series of equally spaced camera lucida drawings of transverse Thionine stained sections through the brain stem of the cat, to show the topography and subdivisions of the vestibular nuclear complex. The rings in the descending nucleus represent the longitudinally running fibre bundles within this. From Brodal and Pompeiano (1957). For abbreviations see list on p. 340

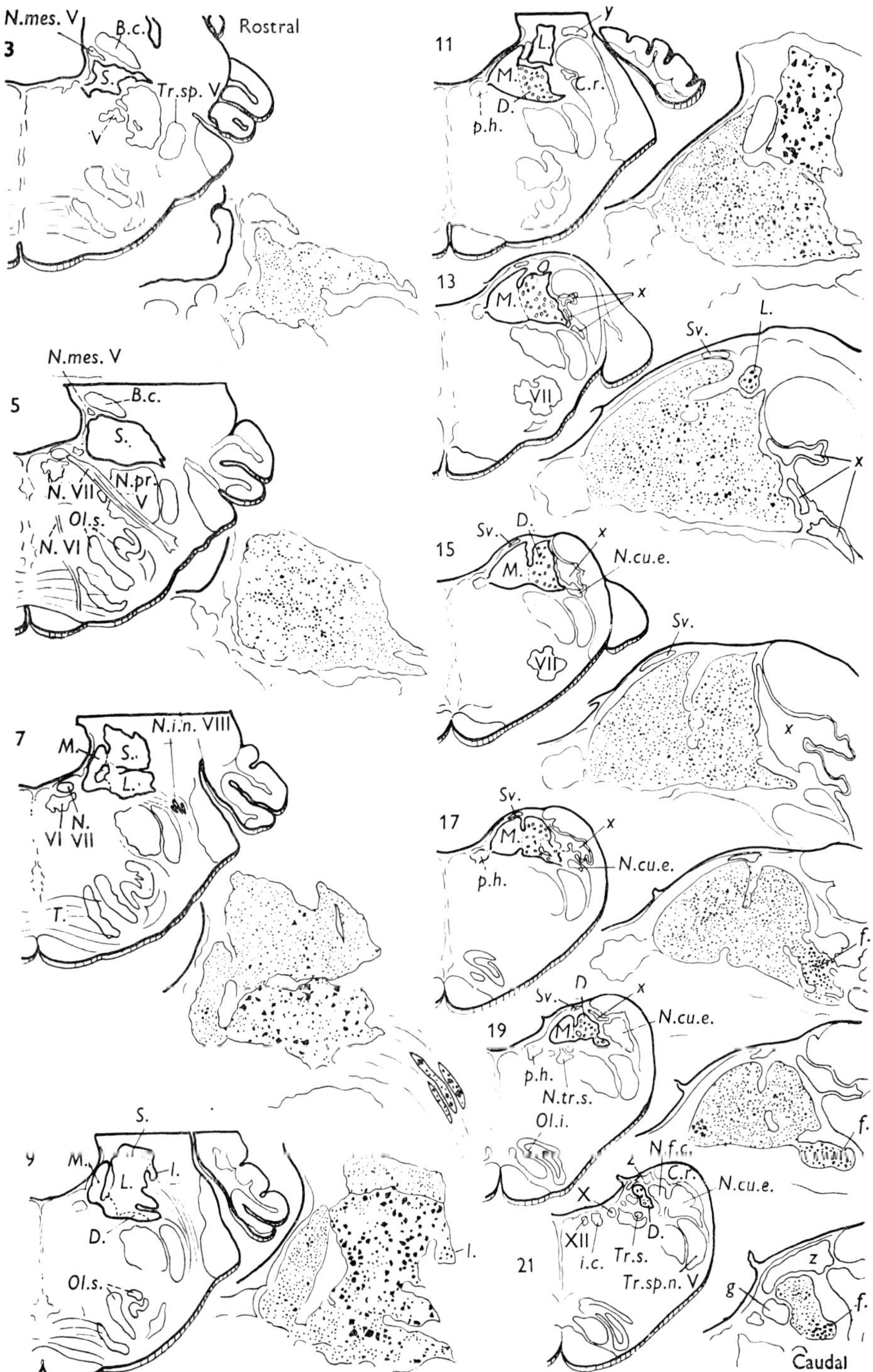

Fig. 2. A map showing the topography and cytoarchitecture of the vestibular nuclear complex in the cat as seen in transverse sections. The numbers of the sections reproduced correspond to those in Fig. 1. From BRODAL and POMPEIANO (1957). For abbreviations see list on p. 340

16*

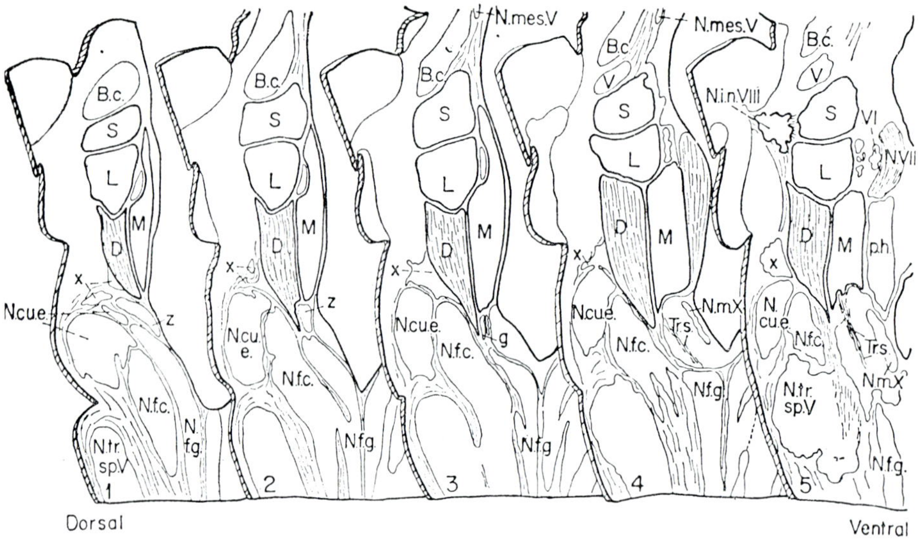

Fig. 3. A series of drawings, taken with equal intervals, of horizontal silver impregnated sections through the vestibular nuclear complex of the cat. The topographical relations of the small cell groups x and z, which may be mistaken to be parts of the descending vestibular nucleus, are clearer than in transverse sections. From BRODAL and POMPEIANO (1957). For abbreviations see list on p. 340

coordinates will be included. These can never be more than approximations. It is not permissible to indicate the placement of an electrode with reference to Horsley-Clarke coordinates on the assumption that the electrode tip has been in the place suggested in some or other atlas. Unfortunately, this is still sometimes done and has resulted in much unnecessary confusion and many conflicting statements.

All essentials of the topographical relations between the various cell groups of the vestibular nuclei and their relations to other brain stem structures can be seen from the drawings in Figs. 1–4. These relations will therefore not be systematically described. Attention will be focused on the structural features characteristic of the individual cell groups or nuclei of the vestibular complex. Altogether the following cell groups can be distinguished:

The superior nucleus
The medial nucleus
The lateral nucleus
The descending nucleus
The interstitial nucleus of the vestibular nerve
The group f
The group l
The group x
The group y
The group z
The nucleus supravestibularis

A small group g and the nucleus parasolitarius are quite closely related to some of the others and might perhaps be considered as parts of the complex.

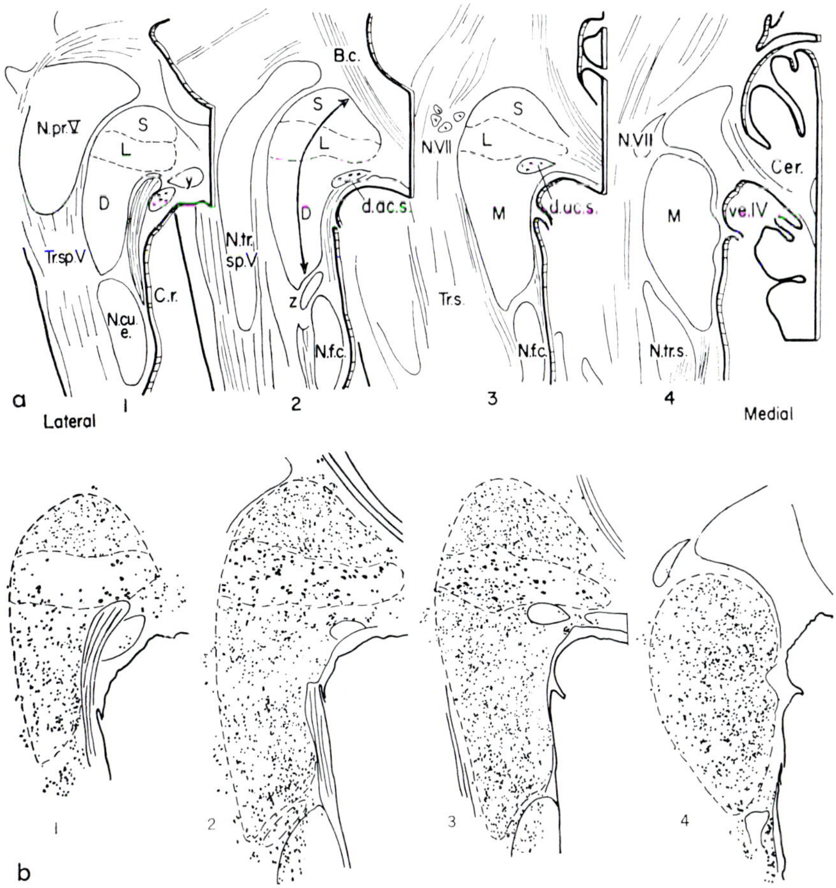

Fig. 4. A map showing the topography and cytoarchitecture of the vestibular nuclei as seen in sagittal sections through the brain stem of a 5-day old kitten. Above (a) a series of drawings from silver impregnated sections (Bodian method). Below (b) a series of drawings from Thionine stained sections corresponding to those in a, showing the cytoarchitecture of the nuclei. In the cell-free area in the lateral nucleus in drawing 1 the primary vestibular fibres arrive. The interval between drawings 1 and 2 is half the interval between drawings 2, 3 and 4. From HAUGLIE-HANSSEN (1968). For abbreviation see list on p. 340

A. The Superior Vestibular Nucleus

(Angular Nucleus, Nucleus of Bechterew)

The superior nucleus extends from a level a little rostral to the caudal pole of the motor trigeminal nucleus (drawings 1–3 in Figs. 1, 2) to a level slightly caudal to the nucleus of the abducent nerve (drawing 9).

Along its entire rostrocaudal extent the superior vestibular nucleus is capped dorsally by the superior cerebellar peduncle. Medially the nucleus comes close to the floor of the fourth ventricle, except at the most caudal point. Ventral to the caudal half of the superior nucleus is the lateral nucleus of Deiters. Their different cytoarchitecture makes the border between the two nuclei fairly distinct except

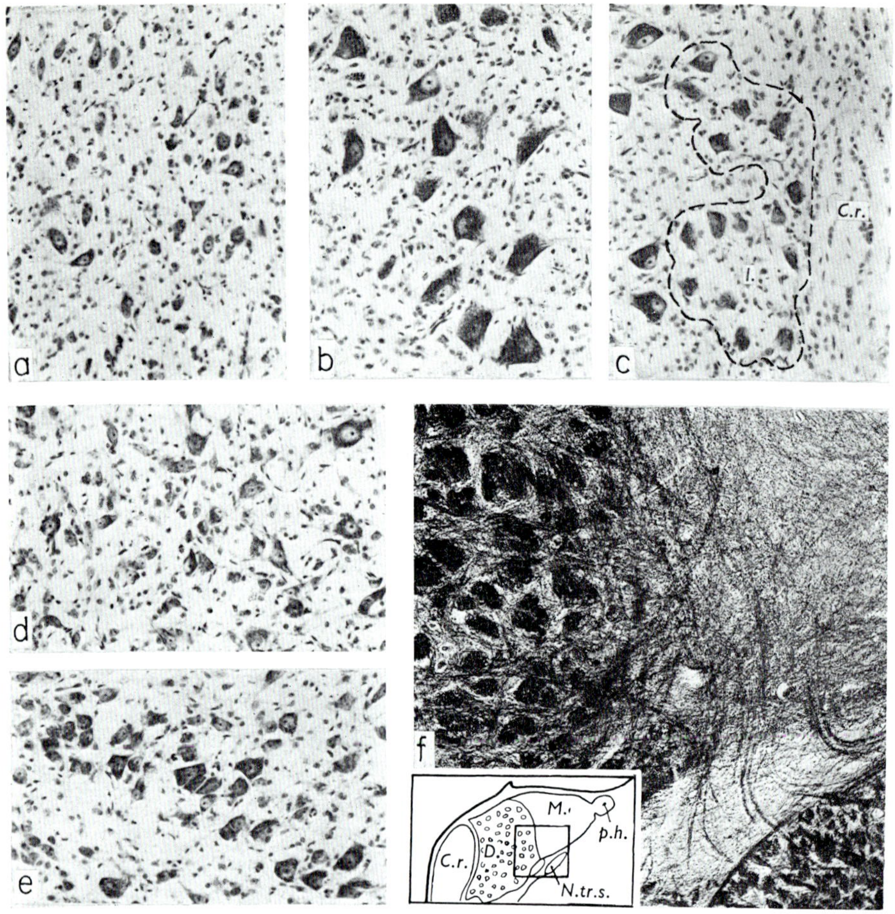

Fig. 5. Photomicrographs from the vestibular nuclei in the cat. a–e: Thionine stained transverse sections (× 70). *a:* From the superior vestibular nucleus. *b:* From the caudal part of the lateral nucleus. Note presence of some small cells. *c:* The group l of medium sized cells (within the broken lines) on the lateral aspect of the lateral nucleus. C. r.: fibres of the restiform body. *d:* From the rostral part of the descending nucleus. Cells of varying sizes, loosely arranged between the descending fibres. One of the scattered large cells above to the right. *e:* Part of the rather compact cell group f, situated ventrolaterally in the caudal part of the descending nucleus. *f:* A Weil stained section from an adult cat showing the difference in fibre pattern between the medial and descending vestibular nucleus (× 70). From Brodal and Pompeiano (1957)

rostrally, because there are relatively few giant cells in the most rostral part of the lateral nucleus. The rostral half of the superior nucleus is indistinctly separated from the principal trigeminal nucleus, which comes into contact with its ventral border.

The superior vestibular nucleus is composed of rather loosely scattered medium-sized and small cells (Fig. 5a). The medium-sized cells are multipolar or spindle- or pearshaped. In the central portion of the nucleus there are some clusters of somewhat larger multipolar cells (drawing 5 in Fig. 2). The cells tend to be arranged in groups elongated from dorsomedial to ventrolateral (see drawing 5 in Fig. 2), due to the presence of fiber bundles with this course.

In Golgi preparations (Fig. 6a) the presence of somewhat larger cells in the central part of the nucleus is confirmed. The cells give off straight dendrites with few or no branches. The dendrites radiate in different directions. A fair number of dendrites are directed dorsomedially and ventrolaterally. In the peripheral regions of the nucleus the dendrites tend to be arranged tangentially to the nuclear border. Ventrally some dendrites extend into the adjacent reticular formation and into the principal trigeminal nucleus. HAUGLIE-HANSSEN (1968) traced some axons for some distance medioventrally and rostrally, approaching the area of the medial longitudinal fasciculus.

In fiber preparations (Fig. 7a) the fiber bundles mentioned above, coursing from dorsomedial to ventrolateral, are distinct. Many of the fibers are myelinated. As will be realized, the direction of these fibers is parallel to the prevalent orientation of the dendrites of the cells. Most of these fibers are found chiefly laterally in the nucleus (Fig. 7a). Some of them are primary vestibular fibers (Fig. 26), some of which continue into the cerebellum; others belong to the hook bundle, derived from the contralateral fastigial nucleus.

By virtue of its uniform cytoarchitecture and relatively distinct borders, the superior vestibular nucleus is fairly unanimously delimited as in this study by most authors (CAJAL, 1909, in mouse; MEESSEN and OLSZEWSKI, 1949, in rabbit; WINKLER and POTTER, 1914, in cat; SABIN, 1897; JACOBSOHN, 1909; MARBURG, 1910; and OLSZEWSKI and BAXTER, 1954, in man). In a recent study of the vestibular nuclei in man (SADJADPOUR and BRODAL, 1968) the cytoarchitecture and fiber pattern of the superior nucleus were found to be in all essentials as in cat. In the literature, references are found to some small cell groups, usually labeled as nuclei, which have been distinguished at levels where the superior nucleus is present. LEWANDOWSKI (1904), describing work in cat, refers to a cell group which he calls "nucleus supremus acustici." FUSE (1912) speaks of a "nucleus of ONUFROWICZ" and a "nucleus of KOHNSTAMM". The justification for considering these small cell groups as separate nuclei is not clear from the descriptions given. What is known of the architecture, dendrite patterns and fiber connections of the superior nucleus (to be described later) suggests that these small groups are most likely integral parts of the superior nucleus as outlined here.

The structural differences between the central and peripheral parts of the superior vestibular nucleus described above are related to other features. As will be seen later, the central parts are supplied by primary vestibular fibers and fibers from the flocculus, the peripheral parts by fibers from the fastigial nucleus and the uvula and nodulus. The nucleus does not give off fibers to the spinal cord. Most of its efferents ascend in the medial longitudinal fasciculus.

B. The Lateral Vestibular Nucleus, Nucleus of Deiters

(großzelliger Vestibulariskern, noyau à grandes cellules de l'acoustique)

The name lateral vestibular nucleus has been used very inconsistently (see below), and considerable confusion has been created in this way. In agreement with SABIN (1897), CAJAL (1896, 1909), KAPPERS et al. (1936) and others, we use the term here for the part of the vestibular nuclear complex that contains the giant cells of Deiters. The lateral vestibular nucleus has been studied more thoroughly than any other part of the complex and is the part of it which is best known.

When followed in a series of transverse sections the lateral nucleus begins rostrally at the level of the middle of the superior nucleus (drawing 6 in Fig. 1). Its caudal end is found caudal to the nucleus of the abducent nerve (drawing 13 in Figs. 1 and 2). The caudal part of the nucleus borders dorsally on the white matter of the cerebellum ventral to the nucleus interpositus. Ventrolaterally the rostral part of the lateral nucleus approaches the trigeminal principal sensory nucleus and the spinal trigeminal tract. Ventral to the caudal third of the lateral nucleus the descending nucleus is interposed between it and the spinal trigeminal nucleus (drawings 9–11 in Figs. 1 and 2). Caudally it borders medially on the medial vestibular nucleus. It can be clearly distinguished from this by its content of giant cells, and more dorsally by a bundle of fibers almost free from nerve cells (d.ac.s. in Fig. 7b). Lateral to the lateral nucleus is the restiform body.

Examination of Nissl-stained sections reveals that *in addition to the giant cells of Deiters there are numerous smaller cells in the nucleus.* The giant cells are multipolar and have coarse Nissl granules arranged concentrically around the nucleus, which is most commonly fairly centrally placed (Fig. 5b). They vary considerably in size, having in 2- to 3-week-old kittens a maximum diameter across the perikarya of approximately 30–45 μm. The smaller cells, which outnumber the giant cells, are of various sizes and shapes, and range from fairly large to very small in size. The variations among the cells in the nucleus are more clearly evident in Golgi preparations (Fig. 8), which also show that the dendritic pattern varies among cell types. From the large and multipolar perikarya of the giant cells of Deiters dendrites radiate in almost all directions and divide several times. Dendrites of giant cells have a fairly constant length, averaging about 450 μm. Occasionally very long dendrites can be observed on some of the larger cells, extending for some 600–700 μm (HAUGLIE-HANSSEN, 1968).

Although there is a gradual transition in size from the giant cells to the smallest ones, *the distribution of the different cell types is not uniform throughout the nucleus.* On the contrary, there are clear regional differences. The giant cells are relatively more numerous and in general somewhat larger in the dorsocaudal part of the nucleus than in its rostroventral part (drawings 7–11 in Fig. 2, Fig. 4b). The number of smaller cells is definitely lower in the former part. Furthermore, giant cells located in the two parts of Deiters' nucleus may differ in their dendritic pattern. Most giant cells in the dorsocaudal part of the nucleus (Figs. 6b and 8) have more numerous dendrites than giant cells in the rostroventral part, and cells in the former region have more richly branched dendrites which are distributed more evenly in various directions than have the cells in the rostroventral part (Fig. 8). The latter cells have somewhat more slender dendrites. Most of these are usually oriented in certain directions. Some dendrites extend mainly rostroventrally and somewhat medially, others caudodorsally and somewhat laterally.

There is no sharp border between the rostroventral and the dorsocaudal part of the nucleus of Deiters, but the differences mentioned strongly indicate that the two parts are functionally dissimilar. This assumption is indeed supported by other data, for example the observation that primary vestibular fibers terminate only in the rostroventral part (see later). It may be mentioned that there appear to be differences in the content of cholinesterases in the two regions of the nucleus (see Figs. 5 and 6, Pl. 1 in GEREBTZOFF, 1959).

The *fiber pattern of the lateral vestibular nucleus is dominated by the entering primary vestibular fibers (Fig. 26).* They enter the nucleus from its lateral aspect. In transverse fiber-stained sections the fibers are seen to radiate in a fan-like pattern within the territory of the nucleus (Fig. 7b), frequently producing a separation of its cells into minor aggregations (Fig. 4b). In transverse sections through the ventrolateral part of the nucleus, bundles of cross-sectioned fibers are seen between the bundles of primary vestibular fibers. Fairly heavy bundles of myelinated fibers enter the nucleus from its dorsal aspect (Fig. 7b). Most of these

Fig. 6. Drawings which illustrate the main regional differences in cell size and dendrite patterns in the vestibular nuclear complex as seen in transverse sections (150 μ, Golgi-Cox method) from a 7-day old kitten. a: Note presence of medium-sized and small cells and the tendency of orientation of dendrites in dorsomedial and ventrolateral directions in the superior nucleus. b: In the lateral nucleus giant cells only are seen in this drawing. Note the aggregation of small cells ventrolaterally in the descending nucleus. One cell (arrow) at the border against the nucleus of the spinal trigeminal tract extends rather long dendrites into this nucleus as well as into the descending vestibular nucleus. c: Note some larger cells in the medial part of the descending nucleus. Each drawing is made from one section. Impregnation was deficient in the areas near the floor of the fourth ventricle. From HAUGLIE-HANSSEN (1968). For abbreviations see list on p. 340

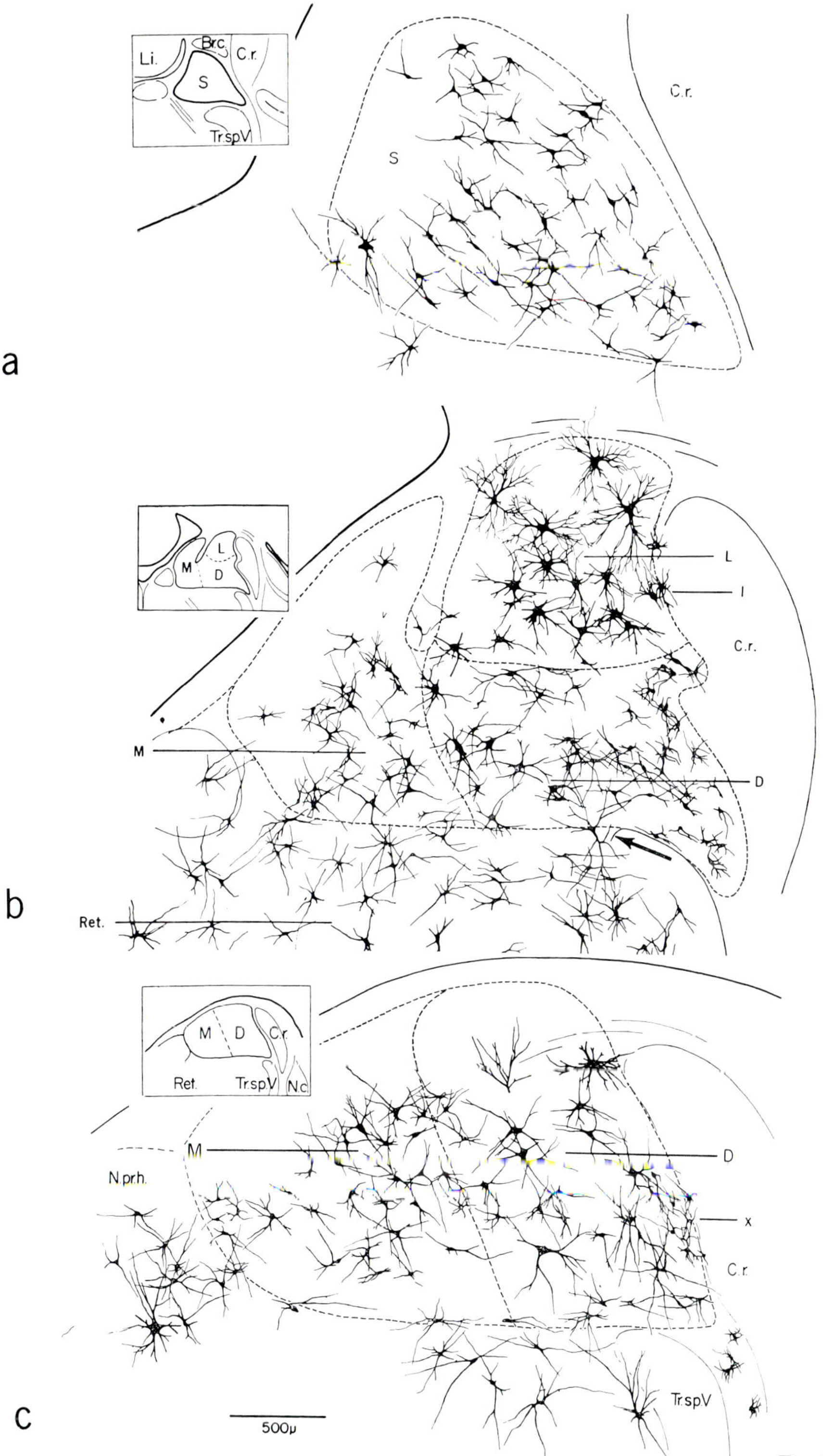

a
Li.
Brc.
C.r.
S
Tr.spV
C.r.
S
b
L
M
D
L
I
C.r.
M
D
Ret.
c
M
D
C.r.
Ret.
Tr.spV
Nc
M
D
N.pr.h.
x
C.r.
Tr.spV
500μ

Fig. 6

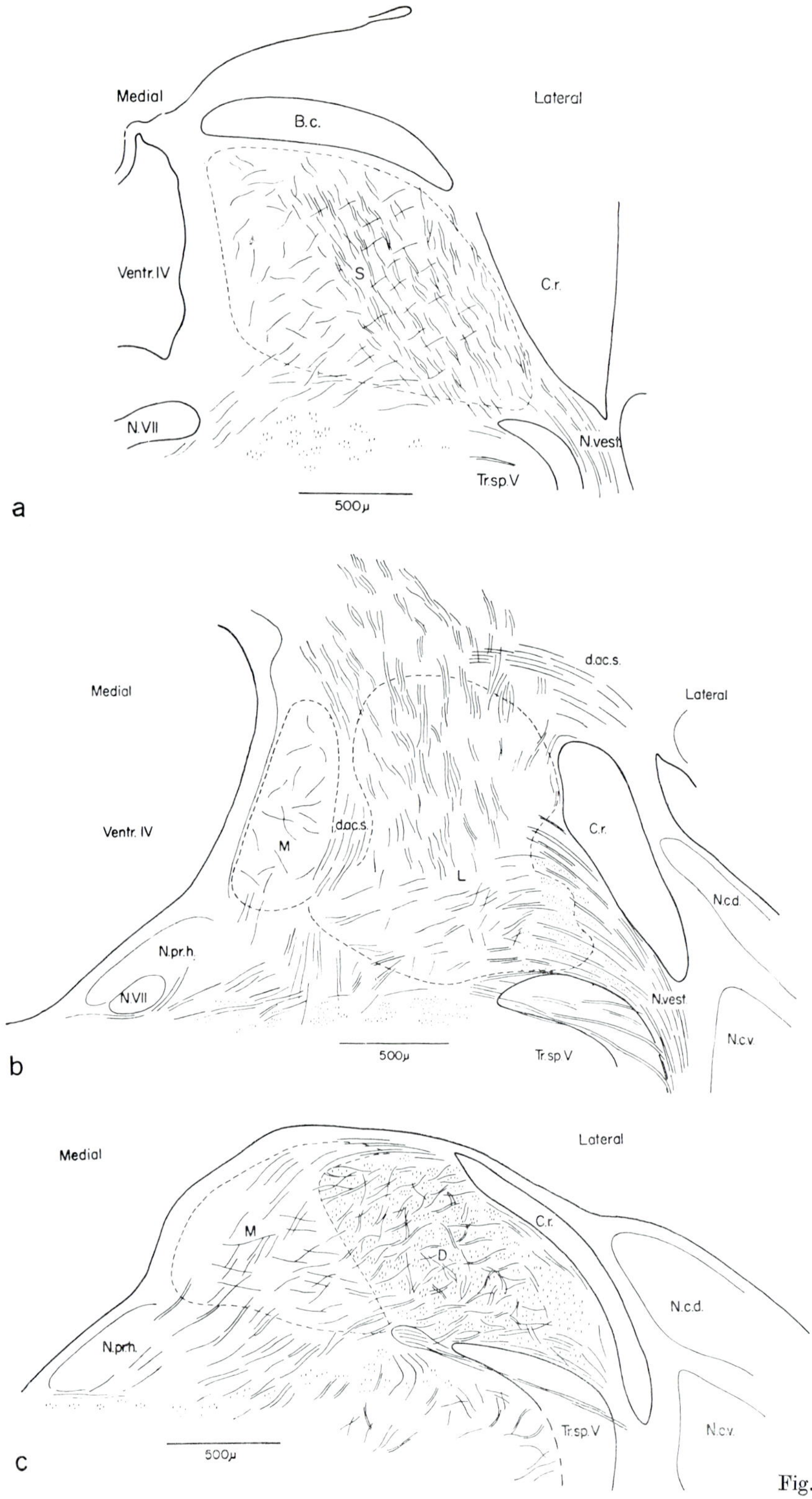
Medial
Lateral
B.c.
Ventr. IV
S
C.r.
N.VII
N.vest.
Tr.sp.V
500μ
a
d.ac.s.
Medial
Lateral
Ventr. IV
M
d.ac.s.
C.r.
L
N.c.d.
N.pr.h.
N.VII
N.vest.
500μ
Tr.sp.V
N.c.v.
b
Medial
Lateral
M
C.r.
D
N.c.d.
N.pr.h.
Tr.sp.V
N.c.v.
500μ
c

Fig. 7

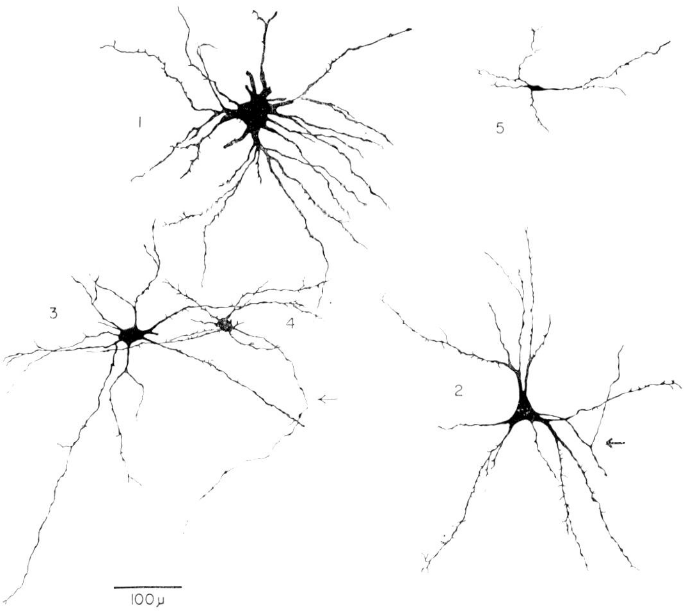

Fig. 8. Drawings to illustrate nerve cells of different sizes in the lateral vestibular nucleus, as seen in Golgi preparations from 3–4-day old kittens. 1: Giant cell from the dorsocaudal part of the nucleus. Note the multipolar cell body. 2: Large cell from the rostroventral part of the nucleus. Note the axon (arrow) with a short part of a collateral. 3: A middle-sized cell from the middle part of the nucleus, with long and sparsely branched dendrites. 4: A small cell from the middle part of the nucleus with an axon (arrow). 5: A small cell from the ventral part of the nucleus. From HAUGLIE-HANSSEN (1968)

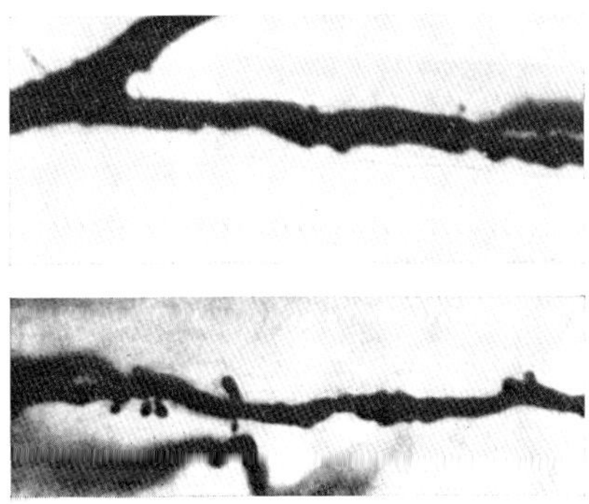

Fig. 9. Photomicrographs of Golgi sections (100 μ, Golgi-Kopsch method) through the lateral vestibular nucleus in a 5-week old kitten showing dendritic spines. Above some spines and "bulgings" on the first part of a secondary dendritic branch, below spines from the middle segment of a dendrite. From HAUGLIE-HANSSEN (1968)

Fig. 7. Drawings to illustrate the main features of the fibre architecture in the vestibular nuclear complex as seen in transverse silver stained sections from a 5-day old kitten. Note the difference in the fibre patterns in the medial and lateral parts of the superior nucleus (S), in the ventral (rostroventral) and dorsal (dorsocaudal) parts of the lateral nucleus (L), and between the medial (M) and descending (D) nuclei. From HAUGLIE-HANSSEN (1968). For abbreviations see list on p. 340

are certainly cerebellovestibular afferents. There are certain differences in the fiber pattern between the rostroventral and dorsocaudal part (see HAUGLIE-HANSSEN, 1968).

Electron microscopy of the lateral vestibular nucleus in cat (MUGNAINI, WALBERG and HAUGLIE-HANSSEN, 1967) and rat (SOTELO and PALAY, 1968, 1970) has increased our knowledge of the ultrastructure of the nucleus and supplemented information obtained with the Golgi method. As found with the latter method, spines regularly occur on proximal and distal dendrites (Fig. 9), and some are present even on the perikarya of small nerve cells as well as large ones. Both the spines and the smooth parts of dendrites and soma are contacted by a large number of terminal boutons, establishing synaptic contacts (Fig. 10). The vast majority of afferent fibers in the lateral vestibular nucleus are myelinated. They lose their myelin sheath only just before giving off the terminal bouton. Afferent fibers often "climb" along soma and dendrites for some distance, and may establish numerous synaptic contacts with a dendrite (Fig. 11). The synaptic relationships will be discussed more fully in a later section.

In contrast to large cells in some other parts of the nervous system, the giant and large cells in Deiters' nucleus have numerous boutons on their soma, up to two-thirds of their surface being covered by boutons establishing synaptic contacts. The rest of the protoplasmic layer surrounding the soma is made up of astroglial sheaths and processes (Fig. 12). In contrast, the small cells have only few boutons on their soma, which is chiefly in contact with myelinated fibers and oligodendrocytes. These differences between large and small cells, which have been observed both in cat and in rat, are presumably of functional importance, as are other ultrastructural differences. For example, the large cells have nuclei with smooth surfaces, while the

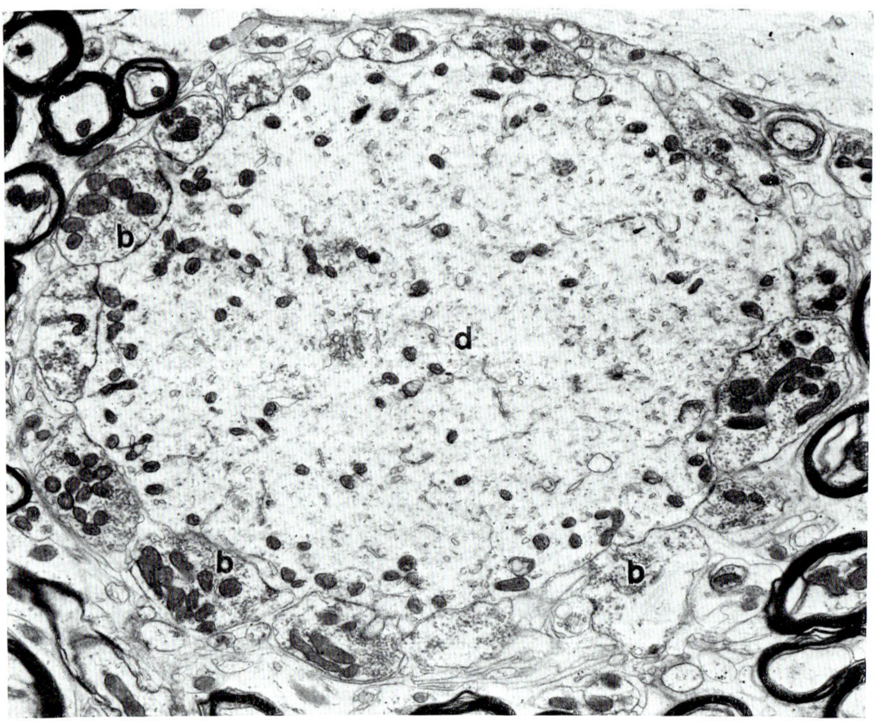

Fig. 10. Electron micrograph from the lateral vestibular nucleus of the cat. A large proximal dendrite (d) is densely beset with terminal boutons (b) with mitochondria and synaptic vesicles. × 9500. From MUGNAINI, WALBERG and HAUGLIE-HANSSEN (1967)

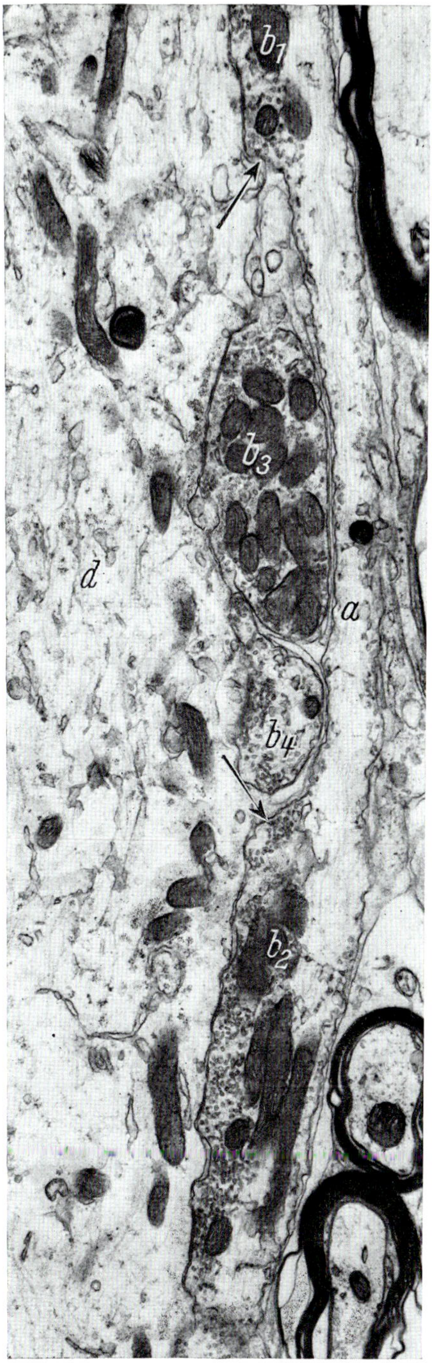

Fig. 11. Electron micrograph from the lateral vestibular nucleus in the cat. A "climbing fibre" (a) has boutons en passage (b_1 and b_2) which establish synaptic contact with a large dendrite (d). The part of the axon connecting the boutons b_1 and b_2 is separated from the dendrite by other boutons (b_3 and b_4). × 15400. From MUGNAINI, WALBERG and HAUGLIE-HANSSEN (1967)

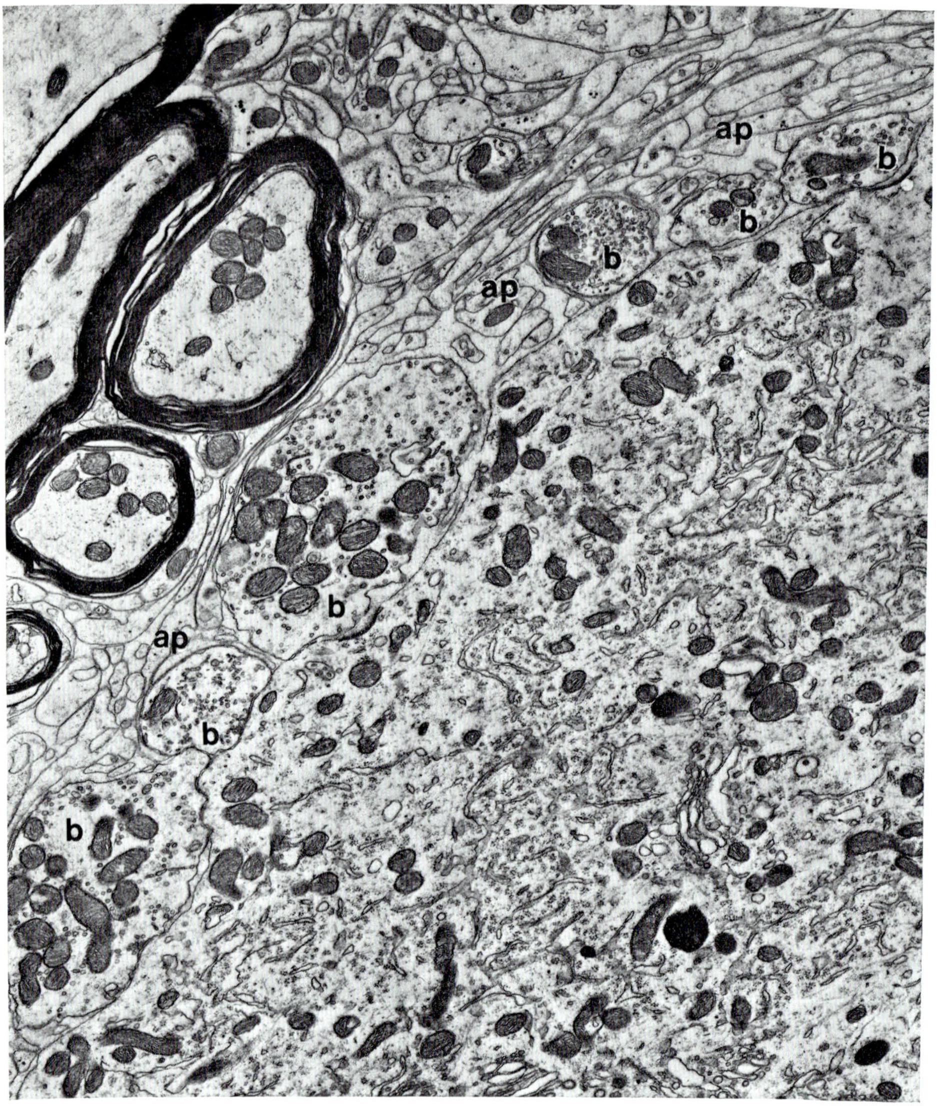

Fig. 12. Electron micrograph showing portion of a giant cell from the nucleus of Deiters (cat) with the surrounding protoplasmic layer. This is made up of many boutons (b) and some astrocytic processes (ap). Above to the left some myelinated fibres. × 13500. From Mugnaini, Walberg and Hauglie-Hanssen (1967)

small ones have nuclei with numerous indentations and also have other peculiarities. Possible functional correlates of these differences have been discussed by Mugnaini et al. (1967)[1].

1 The observation that oligodendrocytes are not satellites of giant cells is of relevance for the theories of functional relations between nervous and glial cells (see Hydén, 1960), as discussed by Mugnaini et al. (1967) and Sotelo and Palay (1968).

Sotelo and Palay (1970) have recently described further details observed in rat. In the nucleus of Deiters they found three different kinds of axon terminals, large, slender (boutons en passage) and small. Three types of contacts occur: "active zones," assumed to be sites of chemical transmission; "gap junctions," interpreted as sites of low electrical resistance between the apposed cells; and "small attachment plaques," considered to be simply adhesive contacts. All three types of contacts can occur at the same synaptic interface.

The name "lateral vestibular nucleus of Deiters" has been used very inconsistently. While von Monakow (1883, and later) considered as the nucleus of Deiters the part of the vestibular nuclear complex in which the giant nerve cells undergo chromatolysis following lesions at rostral levels of the cord, other anatomists have defined the nucleus of Deiters as including extensive parts of the entire vestibular complex. Fuse (1912), for example, distinguished seven subgroups, only four of which appear to belong to the nucleus of Deiters as defined here. Other authors have also used the term nucleus of Deiters to cover rather extensive (and not the same) areas of the vestibular nuclear complex (for some data see Brodal and Pompeiano, 1957). Meessen and Olszewski (1949) present a rather confusing description of what they refer to as the nucleus of Deiters in rabbit.

As judged from the cytoarchitecture and from the position of the groups labeled by Meessen and Olszewski only groups (subnuclei) Dtγ on Plates IX and X, and Dtα on Plates X and XI belong to the nucleus of Deiters proper. On Plates VIII and IX the group labeled Dtα clearly differs in its cytoarchitecture from the group carrying the same name on Plates X–XI. There is little doubt that group Dtα on their Plates VIII and IX as well as group Dtβ on Plate IX belong to the descending nucleus. It is seen from the photographs that, contrary to what is said in the text, the group Dtγ does not consist exclusively of giant cells. The reasons for its separation are not entirely clear.

Voogd (1964), in the cat, and van Rossum (1969), in the rabbit, use the name lateral vestibular nucleus in a more restricted sense. They label what most authors consider to be the ventral part of the nucleus of Deiters as part of the medial vestibular nucleus.

As mentioned above *the term lateral nucleus of Deiters is used here* (in agreement with Kappers, Huber and Crosby, 1936, and others) *for that part of the vestibular complex in which the multipolar giant cells of Deiters form a characteristic cytoarchitectonic element*, even if there are even more cells of other types within its territory. It is true that a few large cells, some of them attaining the size of the giant cells of Deiters, commonly occur in what is here called the descending nucleus, and occasionally in the regions of the medial nucleus bordering on the lateral nucleus. However, the architecture of the lateral nucleus proper (Figs. 2 and 5b) is characteristic enough to justify its distinction as a separate nucleus, and the scattered giant cells found elsewhere are probably to be considered as displaced specimens. Support for this delimitation of the nucleus of Deiters is derived from the results of experimental studies, since following lesions of the spinal cord at high cervical levels not only the giant cells, but the other cells of the lateral nucleus (as defined here) as well, are affected with retrograde cellular changes (Pompeiano and Brodal 1957a), while no changes occur in other vestibular nuclei. Furthermore, all descending fibers from the lateral nucleus appear to course in the vestibulospinal tract. According to Vraa-Jensen (1956), in the chicken the cells of the nucleus of Deiters are derived from the medial part of the matrix in the basal lamina and not, like the other vestibular nuclei, from the dorsal part of the alar lamina.

The findings mentioned indicate that *the nucleus of Deiters* as outlined here *forms a particular unit of the vestibular nuclear complex.*[2] *However, this unit may be subdivided into two major regions, a rostroventral and dorsocaudal part.* This is

2 The small group 1 (see below) should probably be considered to be closely related to the nucleus of Deiters on account of its similar fiber connections.

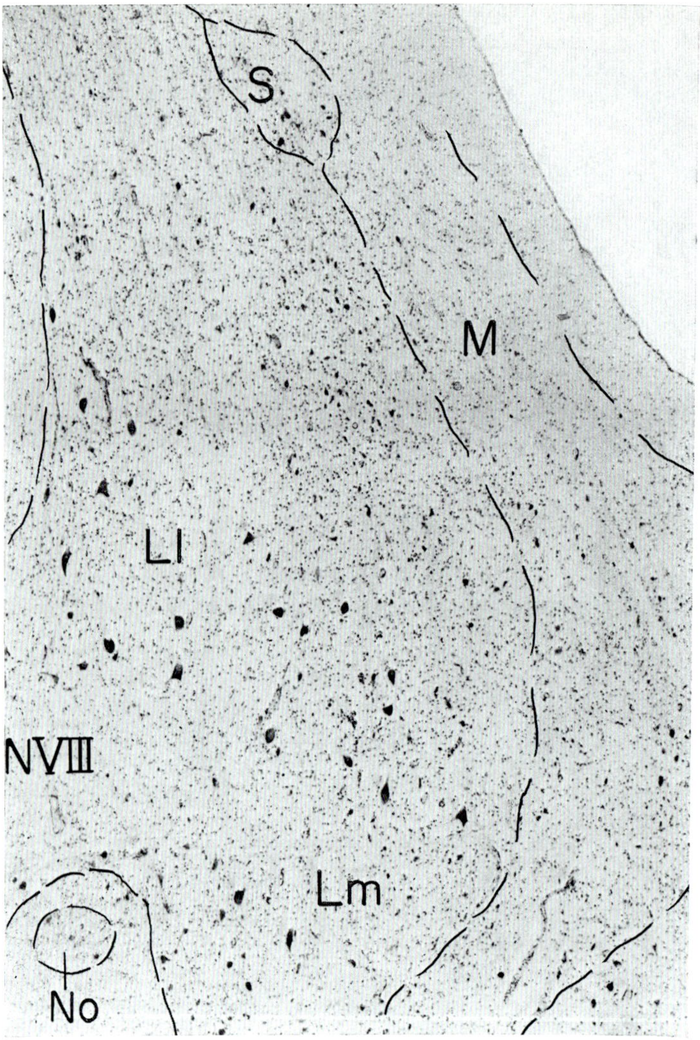

Fig. 13. Photomicrograph from a transverse Nissl stained section through the lateral vestibular nucleus in man. Note the numerous small cells in the medial part (Lm) and that the giant cells present are generally smaller than in the lateral part of the nucleus (Ll). × 27. From SADJADPOUR and BRODAL (1968)

shown not only by the differences between the two parts in cyto- and fibroarchitecture described above, but also by certain differences in the distribution of some afferent fiber contingents (to be described later). A corresponding architectonic difference is found in the lateral vestibular nucleus of man (SADJADPOUR and BRODAL, 1968), but there appears to be some change in the mutual orientation of the two regions: The dorsocaudal part, containing the most numerous large cells and the largest cells, is situated more laterally than in cat, the rostroventral part is displaced somewhat medially (Ll and Lm, respectively, in Fig. 13). This was also noted by OLSZEWSKI and BAXTER (1954).

C. The Medial Vestibular Nucleus

(Dorsal Vestibular Nucleus, Triangular Nucleus, Principal Vestibular Nucleus, Nucleus of Schwalbe)

In the cat the rostral end of the medial vestibular nucleus is found approximately at the same level as the rostral pole of the lateral nucleus (drawing 6 in Fig. 1). Throughout its extent to its caudal extremity at the level of the rostral pole of the hypoglossal nucleus, the nucleus is situated just underneath the floor of the fourth ventricle. The caudal end of the nucleus (see also Fig. 3) is found a little rostral to the caudal disappearance of the descending nucleus. Rostrally the medial nucleus is not clearly separated from the superior nucleus (drawings 6 and 7 in Figs. 1 and 2). Ventrally is has indistinct borders towards the reticular formation, and medially it is connected by cell strands with the nucleus praepositus hypoglossi (drawings 11–18 in Figs. 1 and 2). The lateral border of the medial vestibular nucleus is easily recognized at rostral levels, where a fiber bundle (the dorsal acoustic stria) separates it from the lateral vestibular nucleus (Figs. 1, 2, 6b, d.ac.s. in Fig. 7b). More caudally the ventral part of the nucleus fuses laterally with the descending nucleus (drawings 9–20 in Figs. 1, 2, Fig. 7c), while its dorsal part is separated by a narrow cell-free zone from the latter.

The medial vestibular nucleus is made up of cells of different sizes, the majority being medium-sized, triangular, or multiform with rather fine Nissl granules. Smaller cells occur in between the medium-sized ones and are round or pear-shaped in Nissl-stained sections. The cells of the medial nucleus lie rather close together. Particularly dorsolaterally towards the descending nucleus, there are some more of the largest elements (drawings 11, 13 and 17 in Fig. 2). In many animals a tiny group of larger cells may be seen in the most medial corner of the nucleus dorsal to the dorsal motor vagal nucleus (drawing 19 in Fig. 2).

In Golgi sections the dendrites of the nerve cells in the medial nucleus are found to be relatively long and slender, with few or no branches. They radiate in all directions with no definite orientation. Dendrites were found by Hauglie-Hanssen (1968) to extend into the superior nucleus, and there is a particularly dense dendritic overlap with the nucleus praepositus hypoglossi and with the descending nucleus where this borders on the medial nucleus. Axons can be traced in a ventromedial direction, some of them into the area of the medial longitudinal fasciculus. Some axons emerge in a dorsolateral direction and may be secondary vestibulocerebellar fibers.

The fiber pattern of the medial vestibular nucleus is a fine meshwork (Figs. 7b–c). Fine fibers are seen to course in all directions within the medial nucleus. More compact strands of fibers occur only in its most lateral region. These fibers run in a ventral direction to the ventrolateral angle of the nucleus, where they turn medially and course closely ventral to the nucleus. As in Golgi sections, the fibers can be traced to the nucleus praepositus hypoglossi and to the area of the medial longitudinal fasciculus. The border between the medial and the descending nucleus is clearly seen in fiber preparations, particularly with myelin-sheath staining (Fig. 5f), on account of the large number of longitudinal fibers in the descending nucleus.

The medial vestibular nucleus as outlined here corresponds to the nucleus as described for example by Sabin (1897), Cajal (1909), Ferraro et al. (1940) and Meessen and Olszewski (1949). As far as the medial delimitation of the medial nucleus is concerned, the descriptions in the literature largely conform, and it is generally agreed that the medial nucleus is situated beneath the floor of the fourth ventricle. Concerning the lateral borders of the nucleus, however, there are conflicting views (see Brodal and Pompeiano, 1957). As mentioned above, some authors include part of it in the concept of the lateral nucleus, while others have apparently considered the nucleus praepositus hypoglossi as part of the medial nucleus (see Brodal, 1952). The ventral border may be difficult to outline in cell preparations since it fuses with the reticular formation. The lateral border against the descending nucleus can be identified by the presence of the numerous longitudinal fibers in the latter. These fibers can also be identified in cell-stained sections. In a recent study the medial vestibular nucleus of man was found to be structured essentially as that of cat (Sadjadpour and Brodal, 1968). *Studies of the fiber connections of the medial nucleus, to be considered later, show that it is not a uniform structure.*

D. The Descending Vestibular Nucleus

(Nucleus of the Descending Vestibular Root, Inferior or Spinal Vestibular Nucleus)

This is the most difficult part of the vestibular complex to outline. As defined here (Figs. 1–4), it is a rather large nuclear group. It begins rostrally at the level where the caudal vestibular root fibers enter the vestibular complex (drawing 9 in Fig. 1) as a transversely extended zone of cells immediately ventral to the lateral nucleus. A little further caudally (drawing 11 in Figs. 1 and 2) bundles of longitudinally running fibers, some belonging to the spinal vestibular root, intrude between the two nuclei. The delimitation of the nucleus medially, where it more or less fuses with the medial nucleus, was mentioned above (Fig. 5f). At the caudal levels the cytoarchitectonic differences between these two nuclei are less distinct than more rostrally (see drawings 11–19 in Fig. 2). Lateral to the descending nucleus are the restiform body rostrally, and the group x caudally (see below), the external cuneate and the cuneate nucleus (Fig. 3). At some places the nucleus almost fuses with the group x. Its caudal extremity lies immediately ventral to the group labeled z (drawings 21–23 in Figs. 1 and 2). On its medial side is a group of glial cells (g). It should be noticed that the descending nucleus extends dorsally to the surface of the rhombencephalon along its rostrocaudal extent, except for its caudal extremity and its most rostral part.

The cytoarchitecture of the descending nucleus is not completely uniform. In addition to small and medium-sized cells resembling those of the medial nucleus, the descending nucleus contains a certain number of larger cells (drawings 11–15 in Fig. 1 and Fig. 5d). Some of these are multipolar and almost approach the giant cells of the lateral nucleus in size. Such large cells occur throughout the nucleus, but are particularly abundant in its rostral part (drawings 11–13 in Fig. 2). Ventrolaterally in its most caudal part (drawings 17–21 in Fig. 2) numerous fairly large cells are so densely packed (Fig. 5e) that it appears justified to consider this region as a particular subdivision. It is called *group f* in this paper and will be considered below. Apart from the region of this group f, the descending nucleus is characterized by the scattering of its cells, due to the presence within it of the numerous longitudinal fibers (shown as rings in the drawings in Figs. 1 and 2).

The cells in the descending nucleus, like those in the medial nucleus, have long and straight dendrites which are rather sparsely branched. The dendrites tend to be oriented transversely. The dendrites in the regions of the nucleus bordering the medial nucleus extend into the neighboring part of the latter. Ventrolaterally the dendrites are often oriented dorsolaterally as well as ventromedially. Yet others run tangential to the ventral border of the nucleus.

In Golgi preparations no definite border is found between the descending nucleus and the rostroventral part of the lateral nucleus. The dendrite spheres of the neighboring parts of the two nuclei seem to overlap to some extent (see Fig. 43). Dendrites of cells in the descending nucleus extend into the group x, while no extension of dendrites into the neighboring external cuneate nucleus is observed (Hauglie-Hanssen, 1968).

In fiber preparations, the descending nucleus, as mentioned above, *is characterized by numerous longitudinal fiber bundles* (Figs. 5f and 7c). Strands of fibers continue caudally below the caudal end of the nucleus of the solitary tract (Fig. 3).[3]

3 It is important to be aware that the medial part of the external cuneate nucleus is frequently broken up into minor clusters of cells which are very close to the lateral border of the descending nucleus. The presence between these two nuclei of the small-celled zone x (see Figs. 1–3) may facilitate the distinction between the descending vestibular nucleus and the external cuneate nucleus.

As in other vestibular nuclei, afferents from different sources have their particular regions of termination within the nucleus (see below). In man the descending nucleus is essentially similar to that in cat (SADJADPOUR and BRODAL, 1968).

When our definition is used, the descending nucleus is a quantitatively important part of the vestibular nuclear complex. The main criterion for its delimitation is the presence of the bundles of longitudinal fibers, which can be seen in fiber-stained as well as Golgi preparations. Authors using this criterion (for example CAJAL, 1909, SABIN, 1897) define the nucleus as we have done, while authors who have restricted their studies to cell-stained sections have considered parts of the nucleus as belonging to the medial nucleus, and in particular do not extend the territory of the nucleus as far caudally as we have done (e. g. JACOBSOHN, 1909; OLSZEWSKI and BAXTER, 1954).

E. The Small Cell Groups of the Vestibular Nuclear Complex

These cell groups were primarily separated from the main nuclei on account of special cytoarchitectonic features. The fact that in many cases their fiber connections have been found to differ from those of neighboring vestibular nuclei justifies their treatment as particular units of the complex.

The interstitial nucleus of the vestibular nerve. This consists of small groups or strands of cells interspersed between the root fibers of the vestibular nerve (noyaux interstitiels du nerf vestibulaire of CAJAL, 1909). The cells (drawings 6–8 in Figs. 1 and 2) are medium-sized and commonly elongated, with their long axis oriented along the vestibular root fibers. Occasionally the nucleus contains scattered giant cells like those in the nucleus of Deiters, which may be connected with the interstitial nucleus by a strand of cells. Other strands may form a connection with the descending nucleus, and scattered cells may extend towards the superior nucleus. The cells of the nucleus have numerous, richly branching dendrites. Most of them curl up within the territory of the group. The nucleus can be seen in the illustrations of the vestibular nuclei of many authors, but some of them have not paid attention to it, or have given it special names (see SADJADPOUR and BRODAL, 1968, for references). It is present in man, and is possibly better developed than in the cat. In its fiber connections is resembles the lateral vestibular nucleus in many respects. It may perhaps be considered as an aberrant part of this, as maintained by CAJAL (1909) and FUSE (1912).

The group f was mentioned in the description of the descending vestibular nucleus as a collection of rather densely packed, relatively large cells (drawings 17–21 in Fig. 2, Fig. 5e). Ventrolaterally it approaches the spinal trigeminal tract and its nucleus. It shows some variations in shape between different animals and frequently forms a longitudinal column which is, however, sometimes interrupted. In Golgi sections the dendrites of its cells are more richly branched than those of the cells in the descending nucleus but they do not extend as far from the perikarya (HAUGLIE HANSSEN, 1968). The group f was described by MEESSEN and OLSZEWSKI (1949) in rabbit, and can also be recognized in man in a situation corresponding to that in cat and rabbit (SADJADPOUR and BRODAL, 1968). In contrast to the adjoining areas of the descending nucleus the group f receives massive hook bundle afferents, but not primary vestibular fibers, and it gives off fibers to the cerebellum. These clear-cut differences in fiber connections justify its being *considered as a particular group of the vestibular nuclear complex.*

Group l was mentioned above. It appears as a group of medium-sized cells on the lateral aspect of the lateral vestibular nucleus at its middle levels (drawings 9–10 in Figs. 1 and 2, Fig. 5c). The cells have richly branched dendrites which appear to be oriented mainly parallel to the fiber bundles of the restiform body. The dendrites extend only for a very short distance into the lateral nucleus (HAUGLIE-HANSSEN, 1968). In man a similar group is present, although in a somewhat different situation (SADJADPOUR and BRODAL, 1968). Like the lateral vestibular nuclei, the group l sends its fibers to the spinal cord, chiefly to levels below Th_1 (POMPEIANO and BRODAL, 1957a). It can be considered a particular part of the lateral nucleus.

Group x is another fairly well-characterized small cell group (Figs. 1–3). It is situated lateral to the caudal part of the descending nucleus, surrounded by this, the restiform body and the external cuneate nucleus (Fig. 3). Its cells are relatively small and have rather short, branching dendrites radiating in many directions. The dendrites tend to be confined to the territory of the group. On account of its close contact with the descending nucleus, group x might be considered as part of this, and it has probably been interpreted in this way by some authors. However, no degeneration is found in this group following lesions of the VIII nerve, while the descending nucleus is full of degenerating particles. Nor does group x belong to the external cuneate nucleus, since lesions of the dorsal funiculi do not produce degeneration in it (POMPEIANO and BRODAL, 1957b) while it produces extensive degeneration in the external cuneate nucleus. On the other hand, zone x receives a heavy influx of spinal afferents ascending in the lateral funiculus of the cord and a heavy projection from the contralateral fastigial nucleus. These findings on the afferents to *group x* strongly suggest that it *represents a separate unit*, even if its efferent connections appear to be similar to those of the adjoining regions of the descending vestibular nucleus (see below). The fact that the external cuneate nucleus projects onto different regions of the cerebellum than group x furnishes additional evidence that the group is not related to the external cuneate nucleus.

Group x can best be distinguished from the adjoining nuclei in horizontal silver-impregnated sections (see Fig. 3). There appear to be no specific references to this group in the literature. It appears also to be present in the rabbit, judging from MEESSEN and OLSZEWSKI's (1949) atlas. Their Plate VII shows that the most lateral part of the area outlined as the N.Rd. VIII (descending nucleus) has smaller, less densely packed cells than the medial part. It is possible that the group x is what some authors refer to as the nucleus (proprius) corporis restiformis. Cell strands can frequently be followed laterally from the group into the area of the restiform body. (There is a great deal of confusion in the literature about the so-called nucleus corporis restiformis, which has sometimes even been confused with the external cuneate nucleus.) A group x can be identified in man, but it appears to be less well-developed than in the cat (SADJADPOUR and BRODAL, 1968).

Group y is a small-celled group situated dorsocaudal to the restiform body where this begins to fan out into the cerebellar white matter (Figs. 1 and 2). In transverse sections it is seen to cap the restiform body dorsally. It is situated immediately lateral to the caudal part of the nucleus of Deiters, and ventrolaterally it is practically in contact with the dorsal cochlear nucleus. From the dorsal aspect of this group, scattered cells form strands extending to the most ventral part of the dentate nucleus. Cells of group y are occasionally impregnated in Golgi sections. The cells have thin, sparsely branched dendrites (HAUGLIE-HANSSEN, 1968). The group cannot be identified with certainty in man (SADJADPOUR and BRODAL, 1968). Its smallness makes studies of its connections difficult. The fact that it receives primary vestibular fibers (BRODAL and HØIVIK, 1964; GACEK, 1969) shows that it should be considered as part of the vestibular nuclear complex.

The literature includes descriptions of group y by some authors. It is drawn but not labeled by WINKLER and POTTER (1914, Plate XXV), and it was noticed by FUSE (1912) who shows it in his Fig. 27; his findings correspond precisely to ours. It may perhaps correspond to what CAJAL called the nucleus cerebello-acusticus (1896, p. 66). The position of the group Dtθ on Plate X in MEESSEN and OLSZEWSKI's (1949) atlas suggests that it may be group y in the rabbit.

Group z. This is a small collection of cells found immediately rostral to the rostral end of the nucleus gracilis (drawings 21–23 in Figs. 1 and 2, see also Fig. 3). It is situated just underneath the dorsal surface of the medulla oblongata, dorsal to the caudal end of the descending vestibular nucleus and group g (see below). Its cells are medium-sized, and ovoid to polygonal in shape. Caudally the group is usually separated from the dorsal end of the nucleus gracilis by a narrow cell-free interval. Its cytology is rather reminiscent of that of the latter nucleus, which makes it difficult to keep the two apart in cell-stained sections. In horizontal silver-stained sections (see drawings 1–2 in Fig. 3) group z clearly differs from the nucleus gracilis in its fiber pattern. It is also different from group x. In Golgi sections its cells are seen to have rather sparsely branched dendrites which do not appear to extend far beyond the nuclear borders. A tendency to longitudinal orientation of the dendrites is noted (HAUGLIE-HANSSEN, 1968). This group does not appear to receive primary vestibular fibers, but some spinal afferents terminate in it. In these respects it is similar to group x, but its other connections are not known. Group z can be identified in man but appears to be relatively less well developed than in cat (SADJADPOUR and BRODAL, 1968). Some earlier authors noted a cell group which appears to correspond to group z (see BRODAL and POMPEIANO, 1957). (See ref. to GRANT et al. in Addendum).

The nucleus supravestibularis is found immediately beneath the dorsal surface of the medulla oblongata at levels between the caudal end of the nucleus of Deiters and the rostral pole of the external cuneate nucleus (drawings 13–19 in Figs. 1 and 2). It is separated ventrally from the most lateral part of the medial vestibular nucleus by some transverse fibers. It may consist of a rostral and a caudal portion, and has more or less spindle-shaped cells with their longitudinal axis oriented along the surface of the medulla. This group probably corresponds to the nucleus supravestibularis described in man by OLSZEWSKI and BAXTER (1954) and was also observed in the human brain by SADJADPOUR and BRODAL (1968). Primary vestibular fibers have not been traced experimentally to this group.

Group g is a dense accumulation of glia cells with a few nerve cells (g in Figs. 1–3) situated below the caudal end of the medial nucleus which continues caudally between the nucleus of the solitary tract, the descending vestibular nucleus and the group z. Medial to group g there is a slender column of relatively big multipolar cells. These cells may be a caudal prolongation of the medial vestibular nucleus, which, as noted above, frequently contains some larger cells medially in its most caudal part. A group with a similar situation and architecture is present in man (SADJADPOUR and BRODAL, 1968). It is also described by OLSZEWSKI and BAXTER (1954), who label it nucleus parvocellularis compactus.

The nucleus parasolitarius deserves mention since it is sometimes confused with the nucleus of the solitary tract. It is a slender longitudinal column of small, densely packed cells, situated immediately lateral to the nucleus of the solitary tract and caudal to the descending vestibular nucleus (see Fig. 40, not indicated in Figs. 1, 2 and 3). Its rostral end is found a little caudal to the rostral end of the nucleus of the solitary tract, which it accompanies along almost its entire rostrocaudal extent. The nucleus is difficult to identify in cell-stained sections.Between the nucleus of the solitary tract and the cuneate nucleus there is a fiber bundle (the parasolitary tract) where fibers enter the nucleus parasolitarius, and when these fibers degenerate (following lesions of the contralateral fastigial nucleus) the nucleus stands out very clearly from its surroundings owing to the dense degeneration within it (Fig. 14). Primary vestibular fibers have not been traced to the nucleus parasolitarius. It is present in man in a similar situation and with a similar architecture to that in the cat (SADJADPOUR and BRODAL, 1968). It was described by KOHNSTAMM and WOLFSTEIN (1907) and by ALLEN (1923), but appears to have been frequently overlooked by later authors. OLSZEWSKI and BAXTER (1954) illustrate the nucleus (their Plates XII–XIII) but erroneously label it as part of the external cuneate nucleus.

The small cell groups described above have been dealt with in some detail, because if they are overlooked in experimental anatomical and physiological studies erroneous conclusions are apt to be drawn. Some small strands of cells found in relation to the vestibular nuclei in some places should finally be mentioned. The most frequent are loosely structured strands of cells that extend dorsally into the white matter of the cerebellum, where they approach the nucleus fastigii and the ventrolateral part of the nucleus interpositus. Other cell strands have also been described, especially in the human brain (see SADJADPOUR and BRODAL, 1968).

III. Fiber Connections of the Vestibular Nuclei. General Remarks

The fiber connections of the vestibular nuclei have turned out to be extremely complex, but in general it may be said that the vestibular nuclei give off fibers to the same parts of the brain from which they receive their afferents: the vestibular apparatus, the spinal cord, the cerebellum, the reticular formation and certain nuclei in the rostral brainstem. There is, however, no simple relationship between the afferent and efferent components within the various reciprocal connections. Although systematic fiber counts have not been made, it appears that of the efferent connections, those passing to the spinal cord are quantitatively the most important. On the afferent side the fibers from the cerebellum outnumber those from any of the other sources of afferents. These data are morphological indications that the vestibular nuclei are of particular importance as links in the mediation of cerebellar influences on the spinal cord.

Before discussing the various *fiber connections* it may be appropriate to consider briefly *the methods used in their study and the limitations of these methods.* A short survey of these subjects may be useful as a guide for the neurophysiologist in his evaluation of discordant anatomical reports of connections of the vestibular (and other) nuclei. As in other fields of research, inconclusive and uncritically evaluated findings can be found in the relevant literature.

While examination of fiber-stained sections of normal material and of Golgi preparations may give some information on fiber connections, experimental studies are essential if more complete and specific mapping is to be possible. For the *determination of the sites of origin of efferent fibers* from the vestibular nuclei two approaches are possible:

1: Lesions can be made in the vestibular nuclei and the efferent fibers degenerating as a consequence of these may be traced along their course to their destination with the aid of one of the many silver-impregnation methods. An obvious (but sometimes disregarded) source of error with this approach is the risk of transecting fibers passing through the nucleus damaged and coming from other regions, for example the cerebellum. If conclusions on the origin of efferent fibres from a particular subdivision of the vestibular nuclei are to be drawn, the possibility of concomitant injury to fibers coming from other subdivisions and running through the damaged one must be considered. This necessitates mapping of these fiber connections as a preliminary step, which may sometimes be extremely difficult. A close microscopical scrutiny of the lesion is essential in all cases. Not only may the lesion not be exactly as planned (quite a common occurrence), but secondary damage may have been caused in the neighborhood of the lesion on account of circulatory disturbances. These difficulties are all avoided with the second approach, which, however, has other sources of error.

2: The origin of efferent fibers can be determined by a study of retrograde cellular changes in a nucleus following interruption of its efferent fibers. When marked, the early changes in the cells (chromatolysis, peripheral displacement of the nucleus, which is often flattened, and usually swelling of the cell) may be unequivocal and easy to recognize. Unfortunately, the different cells in a nucleus do not all react to transection of their axons at the same speed. Accordingly all cells affected will never be at the same stage of changes. Depending on the survival period, the animal species, the nucleus studied and on other, largely unknown factors, a greater or lesser proportion of the affected cells will show either no changes or changes which are very slight and which cannot be distinguished from the rather wide variations which normally occur among cells in a nucleus. Many faulty conclusions have been made because subtle changes have been considered significant without sufficient reason. Retrograde cellular changes are especially difficult to recognize in small cells. The occurrence of shrunken cells in an area has sometimes been taken as evidence of acute retrograde changes, but at least in most instances such cells ("dark neurons") are to be considered as artificially changed (Cammermeyer, 1960).

In recent years increasing attention has been devoted to the *risk of misinterpreting transneuronal cell changes as retrograde*. Contrary to what was formerly generally believed, transneuronal cell changes can occur quite early in some nuclei. This may cause confusion if the pathway transected contains efferent as well as afferent fibers of the nucleus under study, even if in general the cytological alterations are not identical in early retrograde and transneuronal cellular reactions. A knowledge of the direction of fiber connections, derived from studies with other methods, may help to resolve doubts in such cases.

In animals which are only a few days old, cells whose axons have been cut react more rapidly with retrograde changes than do cells in adult animals, and often the cellular alterations are more marked. The damaged cells usually disintegrate within a few days. For these reasons *the acute retrograde changes (see Fig. 19) are easier to evaluate in newborn than in adult animals*. This fact is exploited in the modified Gudden method (BRODAL, 1940a). This method has made it possible to obtain more precise information on the origin of fibers from a number of nuclei than when adult animals are used.

In any study of acute retrograde changes it is essential that only unequivocally changed cells are taken into account. The cells recorded as pathologic will therefore always represent only a minor proportion of all cells that have actually suffered transection of their axons. While the method thus permits precise determination of the site of origin of a transected fiber tract, quantitative estimates are difficult and insecure. The modified Gudden method is better in this respect on account of the more clear-cut cellular changes.

On account of the difficulties encountered in studying acute cellular changes, in some studies the *late retrograde changes* have been examined. If the experimental animals are kept for weeks or months there is usually a cell loss in the area whose efferent fibers have been transected, due to the disappearance of some of the affected cells. In almost all instances this cell loss is only partial and it may be difficult to ascertain, especially when the corresponding region on the other side is also affected. These difficulties in the evaluation of retrograde cell loss are further increased by the secondary shrinkage of the affected area. It can be said in general that *if reliable conclusions are to be drawn on the basis of the occurrence of cell loss, this has to be very marked*.

The *determination of the sites of termination* of a fiber tract meets with other problems. While formerly the Marchi method was almost the only method available, different silver-impregnation methods are now in use. All of them demonstrate not only myelinated but also unmyelinated fibers. When degenerating, the fibers appear as rows of globular, spindle-shaped or more irregular fragments, and with several methods they stand out because of their dark color against a lighter background (see Figs. 14 and 33). With many of these methods, degenerating terminal boutons are impregnated as well and appear as irregular dark globules. Such degenerating particles are often seen closely attached to the surface of the soma and thicker dendrites which are quite easily recognized, while contacts with thin dendrites are usually difficult or impossible to see. Combined electron microscope and silver-impregnation studies have shown that degenerating terminal boutons can indeed be impregnated with silver methods, even with the NAUTA (1957) method, which is the most commonly used and was formerly often held not

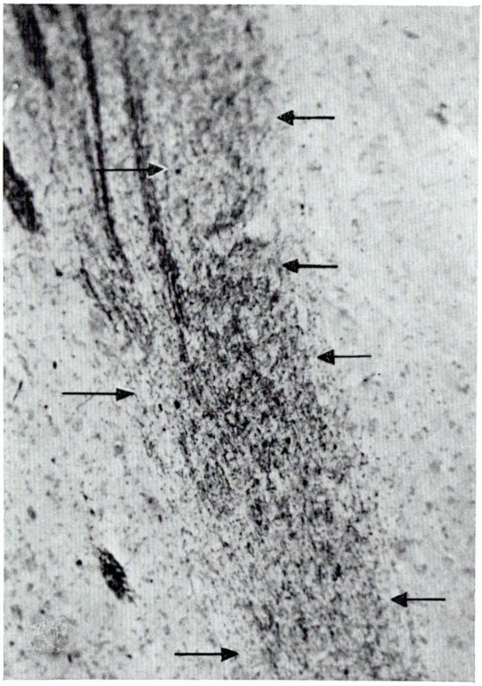

Fig. 14. Photomicrograph of a horizontal Nauta impregnated section through the brain stem of a cat with a total lesion of the left fastigial nucleus. The right nucleus parasolitarius (arrows) is filled with degenerating fine fibres and can easily be outlined. × 120. From Walberg, Pompeiano, Brodal and Jansen (1962)

to impregnate degenerating boutons. These studies have made clear some other important points. Structures appearing as degenerating boutons in silver-impregnated preparations and situated close to a cell surface may be separated from this by an interposed glial sheeth. Often series of impregnated particles are seen lying along cell surfaces. They are usually interpreted as fragments of degenerating fibers taking part in so called pericellular basket formations. While this may be so in some cases some of these particles may actually be boutons "en passage".

It follows from this that *no final conclusions as to the existence of synaptic contacts can be made from silver-impregnated material, although suggestive evidence for the presence of contacts may be obtained.* Decisive proof of synaptic relations between the cells of a nucleus and a particular contingent of afferents can only be obtained in experimental electron microscope studies, where degenerating boutons can be identified following interruption of afferents. Before such studies can be performed it is necessary first to map the area of termination of a fiber contingent within the nucleus precisely by light-microscope methods. In the vestibular nuclei the synaptic relations of the primary vestibular and corticocerebellar afferents have been studied in this way, as will be described later.

A number of silver-impregnation methods are currently available for the mapping of fiber tracts and their sites of termination. They differ in some respects. (This subject will not be discussed here.) If used critically, these methods may yield important and reliable information. When evaluating the reliability of findings reported, however, it is important to be aware of certain facts. In the first place there are wide variations in fiber tracts and in different animal species in the speed at which the fibers degenerate. Furthermore, fibers with different calibers do not degenerate with the same speed. For these reasons a negative finding may be due to the use of a survival period inappropriate to the connection under study.

Another source of false-negative findings is the use of processes intended to reduce or suppress the concomitant impregnation of normal fibers in some methods. The presence of normal fibers will make the interpretation of degenerating ones difficult. If the process of suppression is carried too far, even degenerating fibers will not be impregnated.

On the other hand, false-positive evidence may be inferred if the evaluation of degeneration is uncritical. Early stages in the degeneration of fibers, when they are still continuous and not broken up into fragments, are difficult to distinguish from normally occurring slighter irregularities in the caliber of fibers. Artificial granular silver deposits may be falsely interpreted as degenerating boutons. Much depends on careful work in the preparation of the sections, and erroneous conclusions are apt to be drawn if attention is not paid to the sources of error mentioned above.

If used critically the silver-impregnation methods can yield valuable and precise information of the sites of ending of fiber tracts. It must be realized, however, that *when an area of degeneration is found, its borders are almost never quite sharp*. There is usually a transition zone between the area showing marked changes and the normal surroundings. In this transition zone scattered degenerating fibers are found, and when the findings are to be presented in drawings or diagrams, it is to some extent arbitrary where the lines indicating the borders of the "area of degeneration" are drawn. This should be recalled in attempts to correlate anatomical and physiological findings. For example, responses to stimulation of afferents may well be picked up from isolated single cells in the peripheral zone showing only sparse degeneration. The fact that dendrites often extend for considerable distances from the perikaryon further explains that responses may be picked up in a field outside that mapped anatomically as being the site of termination of the fibers stimulated. The absence of distinct borders between areas of termination of afferent fibers from different sources is consistent with the lack of clear-cut borders between cytoarchitectonically different regions referred to above.

The difficulties in outlining precise borders between areas of termination of afferents increase proportionally as the number of fibers transected and degenerating is reduced. If, for example, the degeneration in the nucleus of Deiters following small lesions of adjacent regions of the cerebellar anterior lobe are compared, the overlap between the fields of degeneration may obscure possible topical differences (especially as findings made in different animals usually have to be compared). If the lesions are very small the ensuing degeneration will be too scanty to be assessed with any degree of certainty. However, if rather larger lesions are produced, the principal pattern in the organization of the terminations of a fiber system may be made clear. It is important to be aware that *as concerns topical patterns within areas of termination of fiber systems anatomical methods do not allow the demonstration of a strict point-to-point relation. The same applies to studies of the origin of fibers when the retrograde cellular changes are mapped.* However, this does not exclude that the topical relations between two regions are far more precise than is apparent from the degeneration found in the experiments. Physiological mechanisms, such as lateral inhibition, may help to increase precision. In many instances where anatomical investigations have clarified only the principal patterns, single-unit recordings have shown a remarkably sharp functional topical relation between two regions. For example a Deiters' cell may respond to stimulation of one folium of the anterior lobe, but not of the neighboring folium (Pompeiano and Cotti, 1959).

IV. Efferent Connections of the Vestibular Nuclei

As is apparent from the preceding section, precise mapping of the sites of origin of efferent connections of a nucleus usually meets with greater difficulties than mapping of its afferents. This explains why the detailed organization of the efferent connections of the vestibular nuclei are less well known than those of the afferents. Nevertheless, on many points the sites of origin of the various contingents of efferent fibers can be indicated fairly precisely. Where this is the case, differences in efferent projections can be correlated with architectonic differences among nuclear regions and subdivisions of the vestibular complex. Electrophysiological studies of efferent projections based on the recording of antidromic potentials in the cells of origin have generally confirmed anatomical findings. When critically used this method may give information on details of the structural organization which cannot be achieved with the same exactness with current anatomical methods.

Efferent fibers from the vestibular nuclear complex pass to many other regions: the spinal cord, the cerebellum, higher levels of the brainstem, especially the nuclei of the motor ocular nerves, the reticular formation, the contralateral vestibular nuclei, and the vestibular receptor organs. Minor contingents have been traced to some other nuclei in the brainstem.

A. Efferent Connections to the Spinal Cord

These connections have been studied by numerous authors using various methods. Inconsistencies in the nomenclature of the vestibular nuclei and the use of too large lesions in many studies has made the evaluation of many reports in the literature, especially the older ones, difficult. Many conflicting opinions have been expressed, especially on the basis of studies of fiber degenerations following lesions of the nuclei. More agreement is found among authors who used the method of mapping retrograde cellular changes. No review of the pertinent literature will be given here (for some references see Pompeiano and Brodal, 1957a). The account below is based largely on the most recent studies. According to these the opinion held by some early authors has turned out to be correct: *there are two separate pathways from the vestibular nuclei to the cord, the classic vestibulospinal tract and fibers descending in the medial longitudinal fasciculus*. Following a suggestion by Nyberg-Hansen (1966) the latter fibers will here be referred to as the *medial vestibulospinal tract*, while the classic tract is called the *lateral vestibulospinal tract*.

1. The Lateral Vestibulospinal Tract

This was discovered by the early anatomists who used the Marchi method for impregnation of degenerating myelinated fibers following lesions of the vestibular nuclei. After leaving the vestibular nuclei the fibers proceed ventrally and somewhat medially. Turning gradually in a caudal direction they are situated dorsomedial to the nucleus of the facial nerve and further caudally dorsal to the lateral reticular nucleus, dorsolateral to the inferior olive and lateral to the hypoglossal nerve. From the caudal part of the medulla the fibers continue into the spinal cord where most of them are found in the ventral half of the lateral funiculus, while others pass in the lateral part of the ventral funiculus. Almost all authors found the fibers descended throughout the cord and were entirely ipsilateral. Confirming the early observations of von MONAKOW (1883), KOHNSTAMM (1899) and LLOYD (1899), several authors reported tigrolysis in the giant cells of the nucleus of Deiters following lesions of the cord in various animal species (for references see POMPEIANO and BRODAL, 1957a). Only a few workers comment upon retrograde cellular changes in the small cells of the nucleus of Deiters. Whether other vestibular nuclei contribute fibers to the lateral vestibulospinal tract has been a matter of much dispute.

In an attempt to obtain more precise information on the origin and organization of the tract an experimental study was undertaken in the cat by POMPEIANO and BRODAL (1957a). They used the modified Gudden method (BRODAL, 1940a) and searched the vestibular nuclei for acute retrograde cellular changes following lesions at various levels of the cord in very young kittens. It was found that *not only large and giant cells but also small cells in the ipsilateral nucleus of Deiters*

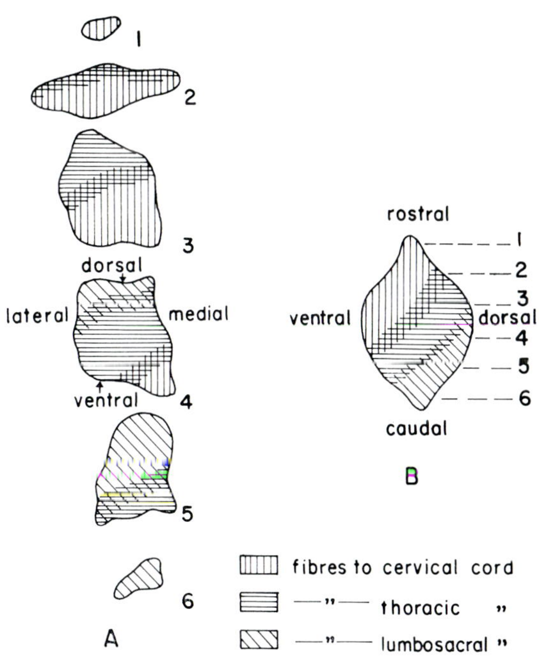

Fig. 15. Diagrams to show the somatotopic arrangement of the origin within the lateral vestibular nucleus of fibres passing to different levels of the cord. To the left (A) the pattern is shown as seen in transverse sections, to the right (B) as it appears when projected on a sagittal reconstruction of the lateral vestibular nucleus. From POMPEIANO and BRODAL (1957a)

present clearcut retrograde changes, i.e. send fibers to the cord, as do also cells in the small group l (see Figs. 1 and 2). Assuming that the general notion that small cells have thin axons and large cells thick axons is correct, this is consistent with the fact that the lateral vestibular tract contains fibers of different calibers and with the conclusions drawn from physiological studies of the conduction velocities in the lateral vestibulospinal fibers, which have been found to vary between 24 and 140 m/sec (ITO et al., 1964; WILSON et al., 1965). No convincing retrograde cellular changes were found in the other vestibular nuclei.

Another finding of interest was the *demonstration of a somatotopical pattern in the Deiterospinal projection*. After lesions at high cervical levels the cellular changes are distributed throughout the entire nucleus. With lesions placed at successively more caudal levels of the cord the areas containing changed cells are restricted to successively more dorsocaudal regions of the nucleus of Deiters. Accordingly, *a rostroventrally situated neck and forelimb region, a trunk region and a dorsocaudal hindlimb region can be distinguished within the nucleus of Deiters*, as shown in Fig. 15.[4] This localization has been confirmed in anatomical studies of the distribution of degenerating fibers following small lesions of the nucleus of Deiters (NYBERG-HANSEN and MASCITTI, 1964) and in physiological studies following circumscribed stimulation of various parts of the nucleus (POMPEIANO, 1960) and in studies recording antidromic potentials following stimulation of vestibulospinal fibers (ITO et al., 1964; WILSON et al., 1965; see also the chapters by POMPEIANO and by PRECHT et al., this Handbook).

It will be seen that the hindlimb region of the nucleus of Deiters covers the part of the nucleus which contains the largest cells (see Fig. 2), while the forelimb region coincides with the part where giant cells are less large and smaller cells are predominant. It is conceivable that this might be related to the length of the vestibulospinal fibers to the lumbosacral and cervical cord. It is also unknown whether cells of different sizes are involved in the influence exerted on spinal alpha and gamma motoneurons. It is of interest in this connection that the gamma motoneurons discharge at a lower strength of stimulation of the nucleus than do the alpha motoneurons (see POMPEIANO, this Handbook).

The studies mentioned demonstrate the principle of somatotopical organization in the nucleus of Deiters. But *the borders between the somatotopical regions are not sharp*. This is learned from the anatomical findings and is even more clearly demonstrated in physiological studies, since in the rostroventral part some units can be activated antidromically from lumbar levels (Precht et al., 1967; WILSON et al., 1967).

In the anatomical study by POMPEIANO and BRODAL (1957a) all cells in the nucleus of Deiters were never altered following lesions of the spinal cord.[5] For reasons mentioned in the introduction to this section, this does not exclude the possibility that all cells give off axons to the cord, but it is only permissible to assume that *most* of the cells behave in this way. According to CAJAL (1896, 1909), many cells of the nucleus of Deiters have a dichotomizing axon, one branch

---

4 It should be noted, however, that group l, consisting of medium-sized cells (200–350 cells in all) sends most of its fibers to levels below Th_1 (POMPEIANO and BRODAL, 1957a).

5 The most rostroventral pole is only partially affected even with lesions at the level of C_2–C_3. This may be explained by the assumption that these cells supply the uppermost cervical segments, but the preserved cells may also project onto nuclei in the brainstem.

ascending in the brainstem and the other descending. In keeping with this, retrograde cellular changes occur in cells of the lateral vestibular nucleus following lesions of the brainstem involving the ascending medial longitudinal fasciculus (BRODAL and POMPEIANO, 1958; see also section F below). Some axons from the lateral nucleus also end in — or give off collaterals to — the lateral reticular nucleus (see section D below). The absence of retrograde changes in the other vestibular nuclei following cord lesions does not exclude the possibility that some of these cells contribute to the lateral vestibulospinal tract, but there appears to be no positive evidence in favor of this (for a discussion see POMPEIANO and BRODAL, 1957a). Nor is there any support for the assumption made by some authors that fibers from the nucleus of Deiters join the descending medial longitudinal fasciculus (CARPENTER, 1960a; NYBERG-HANSEN and MASCITTI, 1964).

The somatotopical pattern in the Deiterospinal projection was probably not discovered earlier because it was not searched for. HASHIMOTO (1928), however, comments upon the different distribution of tigrolytic cells following lesions at various levels of the cord in the rabbit. From an illustration in a paper by FOERSTER and GAGEL (1932) it appears that the Deiterospinal projection in man is somatotopically organized, and this is supported by a study of a human case of spinal cord lesion (LØKEN and BRODAL, 1970).

The *termination of the fibers of the lateral vestibulospinal tract* has been studied by several workers. While SCHIMERT (1938) found the fibers ended on motoneurons in the medial groups supplying the axial musculature, others have claimed terminations in the "intermediate zone" of the spinal gray matter (for references see NYBERG-HANSEN and MASCITTI, 1964). REXED's map of the spinal cord (1952, 1954) was used to indicate the sites of termination more precisely in a recent study by NYBERG-HANSEN and MASCITTI (1964) with the NAUTA (1957) method. After the production of small lesions restricted to the lateral vestibular nucleus the degenerating fibers were traced throughout the cord. During their descent their position changes (see below). Degeneration was found in the ipsilateral lamina VIII and the ventral and central parts of lamina VII (Fig. 16c), while only very few fibers could be traced to lamina IX, which contains the alpha as well as the gamma motoneurons (ECCLES et al., 1960; NYBERG-HANSEN, 1965). ERULKAR et al. (1966) and PETRAS (1967) likewise found only few fibers in lamina IX. The fact that many of the cells in lamina VIII send their axons across the midline (see SCHEIBEL and SCHEIBEL, 1966) may be of relevance to the explanation for the bilateral effects observed after stimulation of the lateral vestibular nucleus. (It is also possible that vestibulo-reticulo-spinal connections are involved see p. 284.) No final conclusions as to synaptic contacts can be drawn from silver impregnation studies (see p. 264), but it appears likely that some of the vestibulospinal fibers contact thick dendrites (NYBERG-HANSEN and MASCITTI, 1964).

The anatomical findings are not entirely compatible with the results of physiological studies which indicate that vestibulospinal fibers exert a *monosynaptic* excitatory influence on most extensor alpha motoneurons (LUND and POMPEIANO, 1965, and others). It appears that the static gamma motoneurons in extensor muscles are monosynaptically activated from the nucleus of Deiters (see POMPEIANO, this volume). These discrepancies between anatomical and physiological findings might be explained on the assumption that the vestibulospinal fibers contact dendrites of motoneurons extending into laminae VIII and VII. Such dendrites have been observed by several workers (CAJAL, 1909; AITKEN and BRIDGER, 1961; SPRAGUE and HA, 1964, and others.). However, according to the recent Golgi studies of SCHEIBEL and SCHEIBEL

(1966) and Sterling and Kuypers (1967), the majority of the dendrites of motoneurons are oriented longitudinally within lamina IX. Experimental electron-microscope studies of the terminations of the vestibulospinal fibers are needed to determine the synaptic relations of the lateral vestibulospinal fibers.

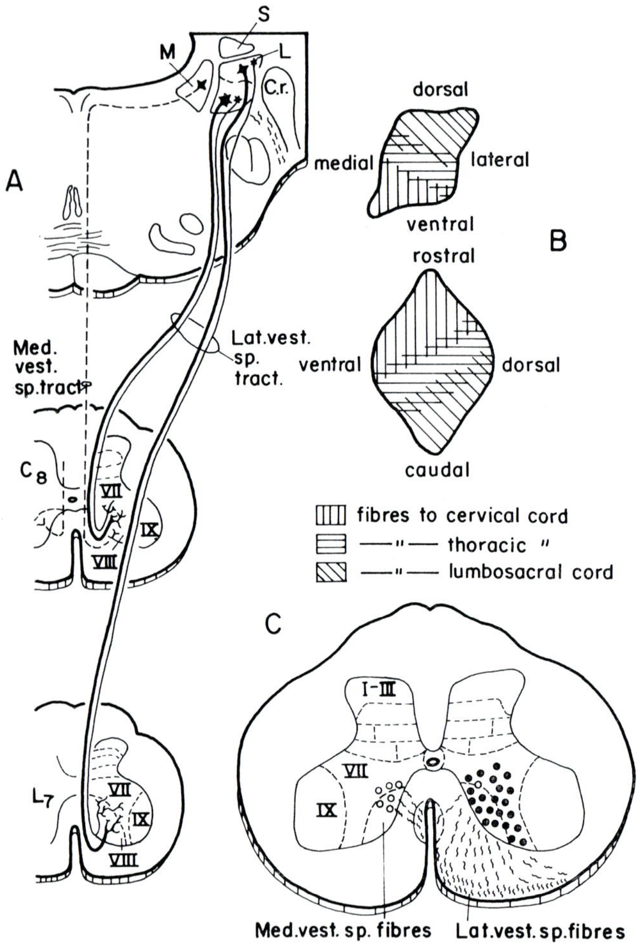

Fig. 16. A diagram summarizing some data on the organization of the vestibulospinal pathways in the cat as determined experimentally. *A* shows the sites of origin and the course of the two vestibulospinal tracts. Small as well as large cells of the lateral vestibular nucleus (L) give rise to the classical lateral vestibulospinal tract which descends ipsilaterally throughout the cord. The medial vestibular nucleus (M) gives rise to the medial vestibulospinal tract, descending in the area of the medial longitudinal fasciculus to upper thoracic levels. A few fibres are crossed. C. r.: restiform body. S: superior vestibular nucleus. Based on studies of Nyberg-Hansen and Mascitti (1964) and Nyberg Hansen (1964). *B* shows the somatotopic organization in the lateral vestibular nucleus, above as seen in a transverse section, below in a sagittal reconstruction of the nucleus (cf. Fig. 15). Based on observations of Pompeiano and Brodal (1957a). *C* shows the sites of termination in the gray matter of the cord of the two vestibulospinal pathways. Roman numerals refer to Rexed's zones. Based on observations of Nyberg-Hansen and Mascitti (1964) and Nyberg-Hansen (1964). From Brodal (1967a)

The *polysynaptic* actions of the lateral vestibular nucleus on extensor and flexor motoneurons may be mediated via internuncials in laminae VII and VIII, where the majority of the lateral vestibulospinal fibers terminate. This is supported by physiological findings (ERULKAR et al., 1966). For a discussion of the influence of the nucleus of Deiters on the cord see POMPEIANO, this volume.

2. The Medial Vestibulospinal Tract

This is quantitatively far less impressive than the lateral tract. Its fibers pass to the cord in the descending medial longitudinal fasciculus, but it should be noted that this bundle also contains other fibers, for example fibers of the interstitiospinal tract (see p. 325) and some reticulospinal fibers. After leaving the vestibular nuclear complex the fibers assemble immediately lateral to the midline and proceed caudally in this position until at the level of the pyramidal decussation they are pushed lateral to this. They then continue in the ventral funiculus of the cord to mid-thoracic levels.

There have been divergent opinions on the *origin of the fibers of the medial vestibulospinal tract* (for reviews of the literature see POMPEIANO and BRODAL, 1957a; NYBERG-HANSEN, 1964), but practically all students agree that the superior vestibular nucleus does not project onto the cord. From an analysis of the available literature POMPEIANO and BRODAL (1957a) concluded that there was convincing evidence that the medial vestibular nucleus contributes fibers to the tract, that evidence for a contribution from the descending nucleus was rather meager, and that the lateral nucleus, as mentioned above, does not participate. The discrepancies found in the literature appear to be due largely to the difficulties discussed previously in evaluating retrograde cellular changes and in obtaining small lesions of individual vestibular nuclei.

As mentioned previously, POMPEIANO and BRODAL (1957a), in contrast to some previous authors, did not find convincing retrograde cellular changes in other vestibular nuclei than the lateral following lesions of the cord. This, however, does not exclude a spinal projection from these nuclei. The lack of changes may be explained by the fact that the spinal projection is made up of descending branches of the axons of cells in the medial and descending nuclei, which send another branch rostrally. Such axons have been seen in Golgi preparations (CAJAL and others). According to the physiological study of WILSON et al. (1968a), however, only few of the cells in the medial nucleus which project to the cord appear to have long ascending branches.

Recent studies have clarified the situation. CARPENTER (1960a), CARPENTER et al. (1960) and NYBERG-HANSEN (1964) found no degenerating fibers passing to the spinal cord following lesions restricted to the descending vestibular nucleus in cat. Lesions involving the medial vestibular nucleus, however, have been reported by several authors, for example RASMUSSEN (1932), to give rise to degeneration in the descending medial longitudinal fasciculus. Most of the fibers are uncrossed, and some descend on the contralateral side. In a recent study, where lesions were restricted to separate vestibular nuclei in cat, NYBERG-HANSEN (1964) found that *only the medial vestibular nucleus gives off fibers to the descending medial longitudinal fasciculus* (Fig. 16). The fibers could be traced only to mid-thoracic levels and are on the whole thinner than those of the lateral vestibulospinal tract.

It is important to notice the *topographical relation between the two vestibulospinal tracts in the cord.* The lateral vestibulospinal tract alters its position during its descent (Nyberg-Hansen and Mascitti, 1964). In the cervical cord it is situated peripherally in the ventrolateral funiculus. It extends laterally to the most lateral emerging ventral root fibers but does not extend into the dorsal three-fourth of the ventral funiculus where the medial longitudinal fasciculus is situated (Fig. 16C). During its descent in the thoracic cord the lateral vestibulospinal tract is gradually displaced mediodorsally, and in the lumbosacral enlargement it is situated medially in the ventral funiculus along the anterior median fissura. It follows from this that the only place where vestibular fibers descending in the cord in the medial longitudinal fasciculus (sometimes called the sulcomarginal fasciculus) can be identified, is the area allotted to the fasciculus in the *cervical* cord. This shift of the position of the tract may explain some erroneous conclusions on the origin of the fibers of the medial longitudinal fasciculus in the literature and should be taken into consideration in physiological studies.

The method used in the anatomical studies mentioned is not suited to decide if the spinal projection of the medial nucleus arises in certain parts of it only. By antidromic stimulation of the cells in the medial nucleus Wilson et al. (1968a) found that the cells projecting caudally are located chiefly in the rostral half of the nucleus, but they are not concentrated in particular areas. (It is of some interest that only a few units were found in the caudal part from which fibers pass to the cerebellum; see next section.) The authors confirm the anatomical findings that the spinal projection of the medial nucleus is modest. In another study, Wilson et al. (1967) used the same method, and identified some cells in the descending vestibular nucleus which project onto the cord. These are probably so few that damage to them in the experimental anatomical studies has not given rise to detectable fiber degeneration. Most of them are situated close to the medial nucleus and may functionally belong to this (cf. pp. 241 and 261ff.).

The *sites of termination of the fibers of the medial vestibulospinal tract* have been mapped precisely by Nyberg-Hansen (1964). The majority end in the cervical cord. They enter the gray matter at the dorsomedial aspect of lamina VIII and end in the dorsal half of this and in the immediately adjoining regions of lamina VII (Fig. 16C) within the somewhat wider terminal area of the lateral vestibulospinal tract. No fibers were found to end in lamina IX (nor do fibers enter the intermediolateral cell column or the column of Clarke).

The medial vestibulospinal tract is presumably mainly concerned in activation of the motor apparatus of the cervical cord (neck and forelimb muscles). Many of its cells of origin are influenced from the labyrinth, in part monosynaptically (Wilson et al., 1967, 1968b). This, as well as the restriction of primary vestibular fibers to the forelimb region of the nucleus of Deiters, shows that the forelimb and neck muscles are under vestibular control to a greater extent than are the hindlimb muscles. This conclusion receives support from the recent neurophysiological studies of Wilson and Yoshida (1969a, 1969b).

B. Efferent Connections to the Cerebellum

The cerebellum receives a relatively small number of fibers from the vestibular nuclei. These secondary vestibular fibers are supplemented by some primary vestibulocerebellar fibers which bypass the vestibular nuclei. It is appropriate to include the latter in this account, while the primary vestibular afferents ending in the vestibular nuclei will be considered in a later section (p. 296).

Primary vestibulocerebellar fibers have been described in normal material of reptiles, birds and mammals, for example, in the opossum and the bat by LARSELL (1936a, 1936b) who traced such fibers to the flocculonodular lobe and to the nucleus fastigii, confirming the observations of CAJAL (1896, 1909–1911) with the Golgi method. LORENTE DE NÓ (1924), however, who used the same method, denies the existence of direct vestibulocerebellar fibers.

In most experimental studies of the primary vestibular fibers the Marchi method has been used. Fibers were traced to the ipsilateral flocculus, the nodulus and the adjoining folia of the uvula and the nucleus fastigii by INGVAR (1918) in a cat and by DOW (1936) in cats and rats. LEIDLER (1914) noticed fibers to the ipsilateral intracerebellar nuclei in the rabbit, but not to the cerebellar cortex. According to DOW (1936) all primary vestibular fibers end in the homolateral half of the cerebellum, while INGVAR found fibers to both fastigial nuclei. In Nauta preparations of cat and monkey, CARPENTER (1960b) briefly describes the fibers as ending in the nodulus, in the cortical area ventral to the fastigial nucleus, the flocculus and the fastigial nucleus. Some authors maintain that the primary vestibulocerebellar fibres end as mossy fibers while others are convinced that they terminate as climbing fibers. (For a review see JANSEN and BRODAL, 1958.)

In an experimental study in cat with the Nauta method, BRODAL and HØIVIK (1964) confirmed *the termination of primary vestibulocerebellar fibers in the flocculus*

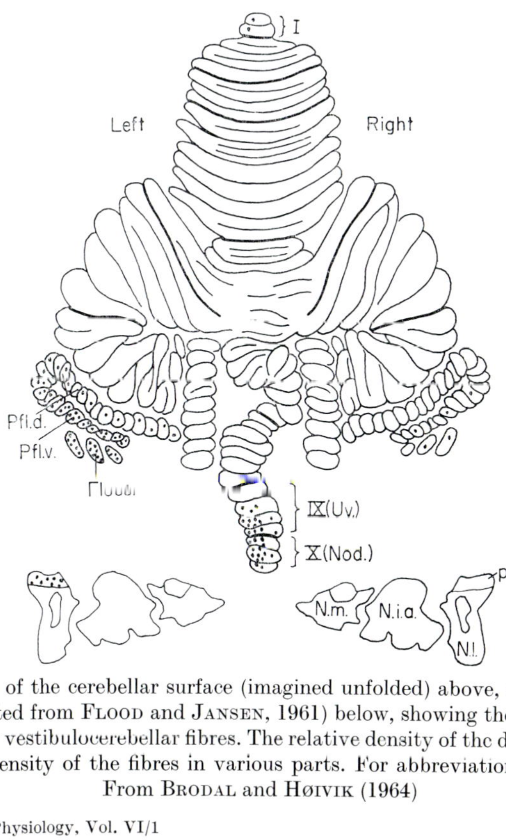

Fig. 17. A diagram of the cerebellar surface (imagined unfolded) above, and of the intracerebellar nuclei (adapted from FLOOD and JANSEN, 1961) below, showing the sites of termination (dotted) of primary vestibulocerebellar fibres. The relative density of the dots serves to indicate the approximate density of the fibres in various parts. For abbreviations see list on p. 340. From BRODAL and HØIVIK (1964)

and nodulus, and also the predominantly ipsilateral course of the fibers. Precise mapping shows that in addition to the flocculus, *the ventral paraflocculus receives primary vestibular fibers* and some pass to the dorsal paraflocculus (Fig. 17). The terminal area in the vermis covers the nodulus and *the caudal folia of the uvula*. A few fibers end in the lingula. In spite of a careful search Brodal and Høivik could not convince themselves that fibers end in the fastigial nucleus even if many fibers pass through it. However, a conspicuous but restricted area of termination was found in the ventralmost part of the lateral (dentate) nucleus in the small-celled part (p in Fig. 17) described by Flood and Jansen (1961).[6]

The *course of the primary vestibulocerebellar fibers* may be of some importance in physiological studies, because erroneous interpretations may result if they are not taken into account. For a detailed mapping the reader is referred to Brodal

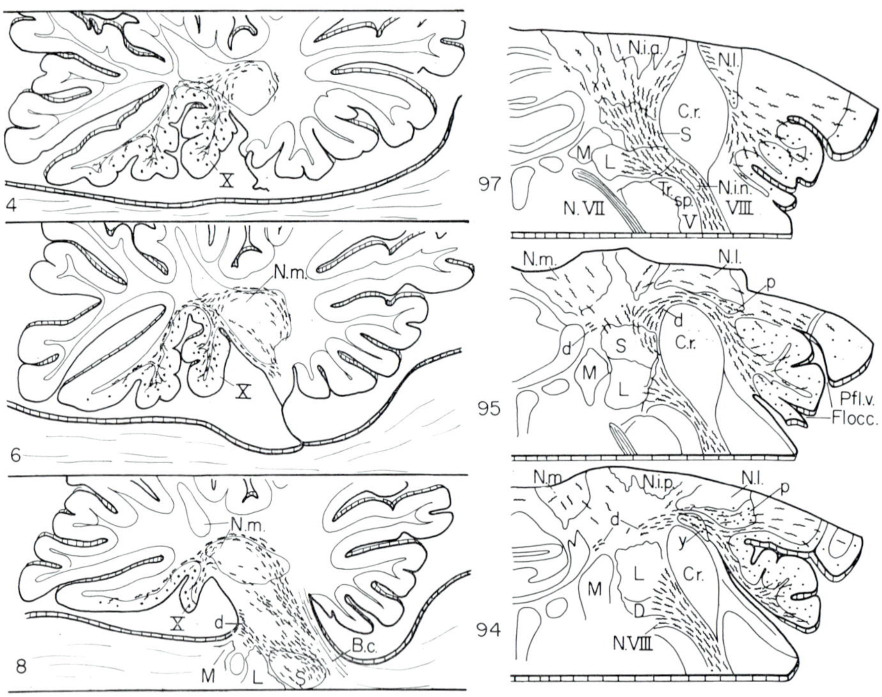

Fig. 18. Drawings showing some features in the course of primary vestibulocerebellar fibres as determined experimentally in the cat (for further illustrations see Brodal and Høivik, 1964). To the left three sagittal sections. Note fibres passing through the fastigial nucleus (N. m.) to enter the nodulus (X) and ventral part of the uvula. To the right three transverse sections. Note fibres running in the ventral part of the lateral nucleus (N. l) towards the ventral paraflocculus-flocculus and terminations in the small-celled part p. For other abbreviations see list on p. 340. From Brodal and Høivik (1964)

6 It has been suggested (Korneliussen, 1967) that the fibers traced by Brodal and Høivik (1964) may be cochlear fibers, since in their experiments the cochlear nerve was transected in addition to the vestibular. However, in an experimental study in which only the cochlear ganglion was injured Osen (1970) found no fibres passing to the cerebellum.

and HØIVIK (1964). Only a few points will be mentioned in this paper. Numerous primary vestibular fibers destined for the cerebellum penetrate the superior vestibular nucleus. Dorsal to the superior nucleus they are aggregated in well-defined bundles (Fig. 18), but gradually they spread out fan-like in a dorsal direction. In their further course they can be grouped into a medial, an intermediate and a lateral component, but these are not clearly separated from each other.

The *medial group of fibers* passes dorsally and in part through the rostral part of the medial (fastigial) nucleus (Fig. 18, left). The fibers curve along or run embedded in the rostrodorsal parts of the nucleus, and many of them then bend ventrally and enter it. Some continue ventrally and emerge at the ventral aspect of the nucleus and enter the nodulus and uvula. The smaller *intermediate group of fibers* passes through the rostral part of the nucleus interpositus anterior (Fig. 18, right) or between this and the nucleus medialis. The *lateral group* consists of fibers with a slight lateral, dorsally directed bend, turning caudal to the restiform body (Fig. 18). When emerging on the lateral side of this some fibers pass laterally and lateroventrally. Some of these fibers run through the ventral part of the nucleus lateralis (dentatus), while others pass ventral to it. The lateral group of fibers supplies the flocculus and paraflocculus.

The course of the primary vestibulocerebellar fibers described above makes it extremely difficult to decide on the basis of light-microscope studies whether they establish synaptic contacts with cells in the intracerebellar nuclei. The solution of this problem will require experimental electron microscope investigations.

The observations of BRODAL and HØIVIK (1964) leave no doubt that *the primary vestibulocerebellar fibers end as mossy fibers*, as suggested by SNIDER (1936). Evidence of degenerating climbing fibers was never found. The degenerating mossy fiber terminals resemble those seen following transection of spinocerebellar fibers (described by BRODAL and GRANT, 1962), but minor differences can be noticed. This may be related to the fact that in normal animals most of the mossy fibers in the "vestibular part" of the cerebellum differ in some respects from those of the classic type found, for example, in the anterior lobe (BRODAL and DRABLØS, 1963).

The diagram in Fig. 17 shows that primary vestibular fibers end in more extensive cerebellar regions than the "vestibulocerebellum" of comparative anatomy represented by the flocculonodular lobe. If defined on the basis of vestibular afferents the "vestibulocerebellum" consists in addition of the ventral (caudal) folia of the uvula, the ventral paraflocculus, to some extent the dorsal paraflocculus, and the small-celled ventral part of the lateral (dentate) nucleus. The cerebellar cortical areas receiving primary vestibular fibers differ in some respects from other parts of the cortex as concerns details in their structure (see BRODAL, 1967b, for some data).

Secondary vestibulocerebellar fibers originating in the vestibular nuclei might be expected to end in the same cerebellar regions as the primary fibers. It is not known, however, whether the terminal areas of the two kinds of fibers are in fact the same. The termination of the secondary fibers can be studied only by tracing degenerating fibers into the cerebellum following lesions of the vestibular nuclei. The difficulties involved in damaging these without affecting, for example primary vestibulocerebellar fibers or fibers entering the restiform body are considerable. According to the Marchi studies of DOW (1936) secondary vestibulocerebellar fibers end ipsilaterally in the nodulus, the adjoining folia of the uvula, the flocculus and the fastigial nucleus. Some fibers supply the corresponding contralateral regions. Secondary fibers appear to be somewhat more abundant than primary vestibular fibers. The same distribution of secondary vestibular fibers was described by CARPENTER et al. (1959) and CARPENTER (1960a). Following lesions of the descending nucleus (CARPENTER, 1960a) the number of fibers to the fastigial nucleus was found to be scanty.

The *sites of origin of secondary vestibulocerebellar fibers* are difficult to establish in studies where lesions are made in the vestibular nuclei. While DOW (1936), using this approach did not venture conclusions on the subject, CARPENTER (1960a), as just mentioned, found evidence for an origin in the descending vestibular nucleus. More decisive results might be expected from studies of the retrograde changes in the nuclei following lesions of the cerebellum. In material of this

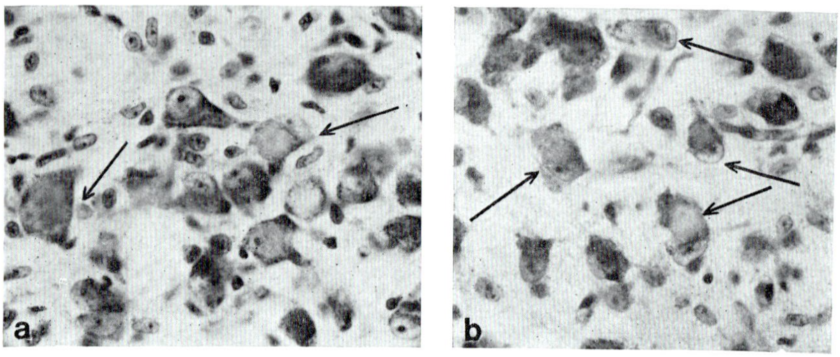

Fig. 19. Photomicrographs from Nissl-stained sections, showing retrograde cellular changes in some cells (arrows) in the ventrolateral part of the descending nucleus (a) and the group f (b) in kittens 8–9 days old, subjected to cerebellar lesions involving the nodulus-uvula. × 360. From BRODAL and TORVIK (1957)

kind some early authors reported changes in the nucleus of Deiters or the superior vestibular nucleus (for references see BRODAL and TORVIK, 1957), but their findings are not convincing. In an attempt to obtain more reliable information on this question BRODAL and TORVIK (1957) undertook a study in kittens, using the modified Gudden method. By taking into account only unequivocally retrograde changed cells (Fig. 19) they determined that the sites of origin were as follows. Most of the fibres come from the ventrolateral areas of the caudal part of the descending vestibular nucleus including group f; a more modest contingent comes from the ventral parts of the medial nucleus, and finally there are fibers from group x (Fig. 20). The areas of origin of fibers to the nodulus-uvula and to the flocculus are not entirely identical (see BRODAL and TORVIK, 1957). No changes were found in the nucleus of Deiters or in the superior nucleus, in agreement with CAJAL's (1896, 1909–1911) Golgi studies. As discussed previously the mapping of retrograde cellular changes brings out a minimum only of the cells which may contribute to a fiber projection. The number of secondary vestibulocerebellar fibers may, therefore, be greater and their area of origin somewhat more extensive than indicated in the diagram in Fig. 20.

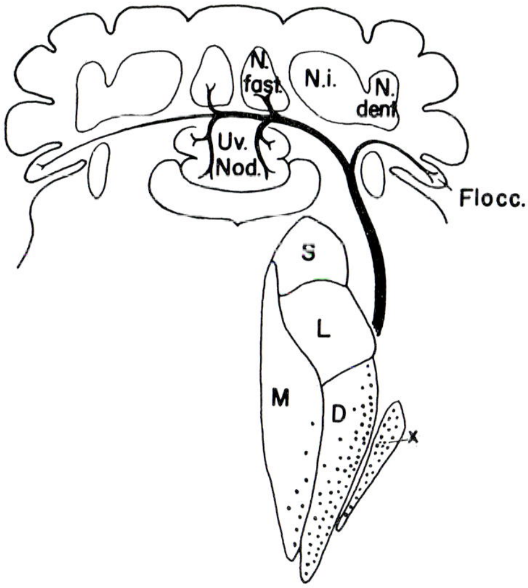

Fig. 20. Diagram showing the sites of origin (dots) of secondary vestibulocerebellar fibres as determined by a study of the occurrence of retrograde cellular changes (see Fig. 19) following cerebellar lesions in kittens (modified Gudden method). The group f (not indicated in the drawing) in the descending nucleus (D) takes part in the projection. The sites of termination of the vestibulocerebellar fibres are indicated according to Dow (1936). From Brodal and Torvik (1957)

Retrograde changes in the regions shown in Fig. 20 were found only following lesions involving the "vestibular parts" of the cerebellum. Since the lesions in most cases were not restricted to particular subdivisions (flocculus only, nodulus only etc.) no conclusions on the precise sites of termination of secondary vestibulocerebellar fibers can be drawn from the findings of Brodal and Torvik (1957). This should be especially emphasized as concerns the fastigial nucleus, since lesions of this always in addition encroached upon the uvula-nodulus.

From a functional point of view it is of interest that the areas giving rise to secondary vestibulocerebellar fibers do not appear to receive primary vestibular fibers, but some of them, especially the caudal part of the descending nucleus and group x, are supplied by spinal afferents. *The secondary vestibulocerebellar fibers may therefore be concerned chiefly in mediating spinal impulses to the vestibular areas of the cerebellum* and bear only a remote relation to the vestibular apparatus. Physiological studies of this problem have apparently not yet been made.

C. Efferent Connections to the Vestibular Receptor Organs

Like other sensory organs, the vestibular receptors are under the influence of the central nervous system (for some references see Kornhuber, 1966). The central transmission of vestibular impulses may be influenced in the vestibular nuclei by afferent fibers to this from other structures. While it is still difficult to identify particular fiber contingents as responsible for these effects, the anatomical substratum of the effect exerted on the receptor organs is fairly well known. This takes place via *fibers originating in the vestibular nuclear complex and passing centrifugally in the vestibular nerve.* (For a more complete account, see GACEK, this Handbook.)

As early as 1914, LEIDLER observed degenerating fibers in the ipsilateral vestibular nerve in Marchi preparations following lesions of the medulla in the vicinity of the genu of the facial nerve. RASMUSSEN and GACEK (1958) and GACEK (1960) gave experimental definitions of fine myelinated fibers running centrifugally in the vestibular nerve. The fibers were traced into the individual peripheral branches of the nerve (GACEK, 1960). In the central part of the nerve these fibers run together with the olivocochlear bundle of RASMUSSEN. In silver-impregnated material the fibers can be traced almost to the vestibular epithelia, but their synaptic relations cannot be established. In electron-microscope studies (WERSÄLL, 1956; SMITH, 1956, and others) small terminal boutons provided with synaptic vesicles are found in contact with the receptor cells or with the chalyces of sensory endings surrounding hair cells of type I. These boutons have been interpreted as belonging to the efferent vestibular fibers, an assumption which receives some support from electron-microscope observations which indicate that they degenerate following transection of vestibular nerve fibers (SMITH and RASMUSSEN, 1968). Indirect support for the existence of an efferent innervation of the vestibular receptors comes from the histochemical demonstration of cholinesterase in relation to receptor cells (DOHLMAN et al., 1958, and others).

The number of efferent vestibular fibers appears to be modest. According to GACEK, (1960, p. 353 in "Neural Mechanisms of the Auditory and Vestibular Systems") there are some 200 of these fibers in cat, as against a total of some 12,000 in the entire vestibular nerve.

Several authors have concluded that *the site of origin of the efferent fibers in the vestibular nerve* is the nucleus of Deiters, since some fibers in the vestibular nerve have been found to degenerate following lesions of this nucleus (RASMUSSEN and GACEK, 1958; GACEK, 1960; CARPENTER, 1960a). Attempts to define the origin of the fibers more precisely by means of a study of retrograde cellular changes in the nuclei following extirpation of the labyrinth were made in cat by CARPENTER et al. (1959). These authors reported bilateral cellular changes and cell loss in the descending, medial and superior vestibular nucleus, in the interstitial nucleus of the vestibular nerve and in the fastigial nucleus, while no changes were found in the nucleus of Deiters. The extensive alterations described by these authors are difficult to correlate with the small number of efferent fibers, and the cellular changes described and illustrated can scarcely be considered retrograde. Following extirpation of the labyrinth in the guinea pig (1962) and in the rabbit (1965), ROSSI and CORTESINA found retrograde changes in a small caudally situated cell group of Deiters' nucleus and in a group which they call the "interposed vestibular nucleus" (not identified as a particular group by BRODAL and POMPEIANO, 1957) and in some cells in the reticular formation. Their "interposed vestibular nucleus" contains some 120–150 nerve cells.

D. Efferent Connections to the Reticular Formation

Advances in our understanding of the functional role of the reticular formation of the brainstem have prompted studies on the precise organization of its fiber connections. The vestibular nuclear complex is one of many structures which send fibers to the reticular formation.

The data to be found in the literature on the projections of the vestibular nuclei onto the reticular formation are relatively scanty. Based on Golgi studies CAJAL (1909), LORENTE DE NÓ (1933b), and SCHEIBEL and SCHEIBEL (1958) concluded that axonal branches and collaterals of the cells of all four main vestibular nuclei (superior, lateral, medial and descending) are distributed to the pontomedullary reticular formation, chiefly to its medial two thirds, but specific sites of origin and termination are not given. CAJAL (1909) and HELD (1923) mention specifically that the fibers of the vestibulospinal tract give off collaterals to the reticular formation, and VALVERDE (1961a) followed axons from the lateral vestibular nucleus to the nucleus reticularis parvicellularis. Experimental studies of the fiber degeneration following lesions in the vestibular nuclear complex have been made by several workers, most of whom have used the Marchi method (GRAY, 1926; RASMUSSEN, 1932; BUCHANAN, 1937; FERRARO et al., 1940; MATANO et al., 1964a, and others). Some reference is made to the fibers to the reticular formation, but most of the lesions were rather large and often involved other structures as well as the vestibular nuclei. Using silver-impregnation methods, SZENTÁGOTHAI (1943) found numerous degenerating fibers to the ipsilateral pontine and contralateral mesencephalic reticular formation following unspecified lesions of the vestibular nuclear complex in cat. CARPENTER (1960a), working with cats, found bilateral degeneration, more ipsilaterally, in the caudal reticular formation of the pons following lesions in the descending and lateral vestibular nuclei. MCMASTERS et al. (1966), in a study in the monkey of the efferent projections of the four main vestibular nuclei to the nuclei of the extraocular muscles, refer only briefly to fibers to the reticular formation (see also TARLOV, 1969).

In view of the specific patterns found in the arrangement of other vestibular fiber connections, and since the reticular formation is composed of more or less distinctive regions, it would be of interest to know the organization of the vestibuloreticular projection in more detail. LADPLI and BRODAL (1968) therefore undertook an experimental study in the cat, in which the fiber degenerations following small lesions restricted to each of the four main vestibular nuclei were studied in Nauta preparations. In order to avoid misinterpretations, the course of fibers from other sources passing through the vestibular nuclei was first mapped. (A few primary vestibular fibers end in the reticular formation, but only close to the vestibular nuclei.) Of particular importance is a precise knowledge of the fastigioreticular fibers, which, when interrupted, may lead to erroneous conclusions. (A map of these fibres can be found in Fig. 1 of LADPLI and BRODAL, 1968.) On account of the course of these fibers and since efferent fibers from one vestibular nucleus may pass through other parts of the vestibular complex, complete mapping of the vestibuloreticular projections has not been possible. Nevertheless, several points have been clarified. It turned out that *the four main vestibular nuclei differ in their projections to the reticular formation* (as in many other respects).

In a study of this kind it is essential to indicate the sites of termination of the fibers as precisely as possible. This was done with reference to the various cytoarchitectonic subdivisions which can be distinguished in the reticular formation (for a survey see BRODAL, 1957). The nuclear groups of the pons and medulla oblongata which are of relevance to the observations can be mentioned. In the pons the *nucleus reticularis tegmenti pontis of Bechterew* is located dorsal to the pontine nuclei near the midline. Rostrally and laterally to this nucleus is the *nucleus reticularis pontis oralis* and caudally and dorsally the *nucleus reticularis pontis caudalis.* The border between the two last nuclei is indistinct. The first nucleus contains scattered giant cells only in its caudal part while the nucleus reticularis pontis caudalis contains numerous giant cells in cat. The *nucleus reticularis ventralis* forms a continuation of the nucleus reticularis pontis caudalis and extends caudally in the medulla oblongata ventromedial to the *nucleus reticularis parvicellularis,* which contains mostly small cells. The *nucleus reticularis gigantocellularis,* so named because of the content of giant cells scattered among large, medium-sized and small cells is situated dorsal to the rostral half of the inferior olive. The *nucleus reticularis lateralis* (nucleus of the lateral funiculus) is found lateral to the inferior olive.

The main findings are summarized in Table 1, but a brief description and illustrations of the projections from the superior and lateral vestibular nuclei to the reticular formation will be presented to give a better impression of the complexity of the vestibuloreticular projections and also of their rather specific pattern. This may be of interest in physiological studies (Table 1).

Table 1. *Summary of the main locations of terminal degeneration in the reticular formation following lesions in various vestibular nuclei.* Symbols: +, degeneration; ++, heavy degeneration; ?, degeneration present, but may come from other vestibular nuclei as well; blanc, no degeneration. From LADPLI and BRODAL (1968)

	Vestibular nuclei							
	Superior		Lateral		Medial		Descending	
	Ipsi	Contra	Ipsi	Contra	Ipsi	Contra	Ipsi	Contra
Retic. pontis oralis		+						
Retic. pontis caudalis	+	+	+	+			+	
Retic. parvocell.	+		+		?	?	?	++
Retic. gigantocell.	+		+		?	?	?	++
Retic. ventralis							?	
Nucl. retic. tegmenti		++		+				
Nucl. retic. later.			++					

From *the superior vestibular nucleus* two streams of degenerating fibers can be traced into the reticular formation (Fig. 21). The first group (labeled *a* in Fig. 21) leaves the nucleus rostromedially. Soon after this the fibers of bundle *a* separate into several contingents. Relatively numerous fibers pass through the dorsal part of the pontine reticular formation and proceed towards the midline, most of them crossing to the other side. Some end in the contralateral vestibular nuclei (see following section), while another group of crossing fibers turns ventrally. Some of these fibers terminate in the contralateral nuclei reticularis pontis caudalis and oralis, but a greater number proceed ventrally and end throughout the contralateral nucleus reticularis tegmenti pontis, but chiefly ventrally (drawings 53–57 in Fig. 21). Some fibers of bundle *a* do not cross but leave it just before it reaches the midline and ascend close to the latter. Other ipsilateral fibers in the bundle pass ventrally and terminate in the ipsilateral nucleus reticularis pontis caudalis and in the rostral part of the nucleus reticularis gigantocellularis. Finally a less massive contingent of efferents from the superior nucleus (labeled β in drawing 4 in Fig. 21) descends in the lateral and ventral parts of the lateral vestibular nucleus, and some fibers continue into the ventral part of the descending and medial nuclei. Some fibers appear to end in these nuclei, but a fair number of them can be traced to the reticular formation, where they terminate dorsomedially in the rostral part of the nuclei reticularis gigantocellularis and parvicellularis.

From the *lateral vestibular nucleus* some fibers pass to the contralateral vestibular nuclei (see following section). Among the fibers reaching the reticular formation (Fig. 22) several groups can be distinguished. Some fine fibers pass through the ventral part of the superior nucleus and can be traced ventromedially to the ipsilateral nucleus reticularis pontis caudalis.

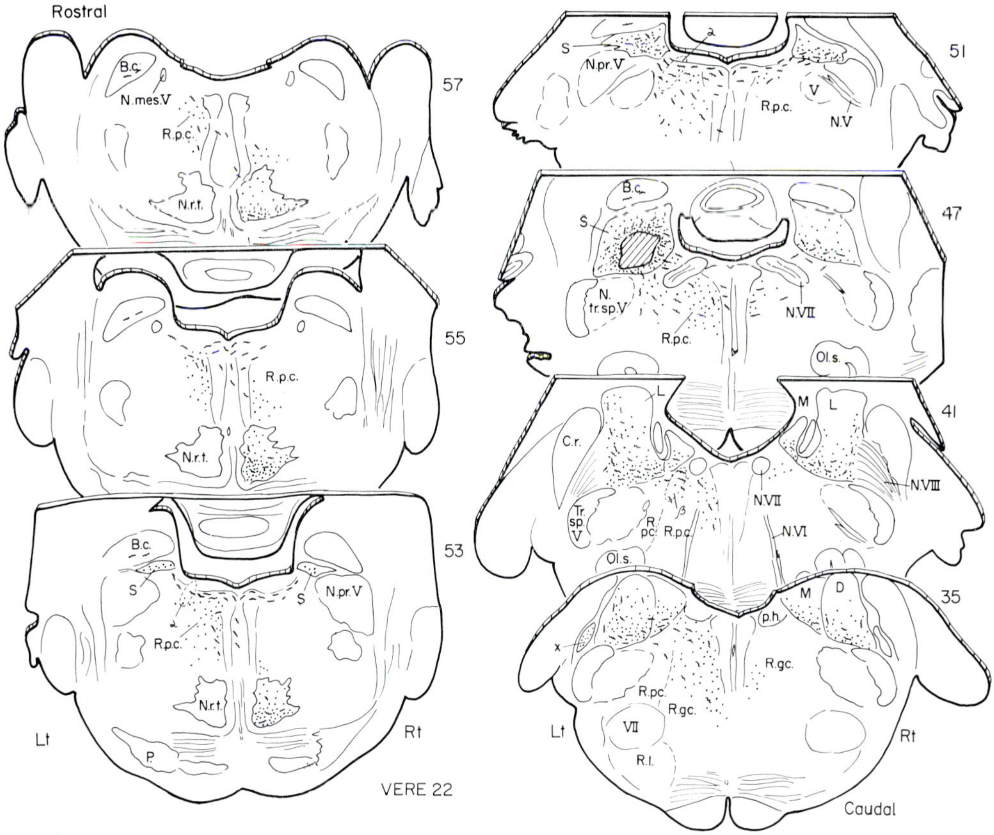

Fig. 21. Diagram showing the course and distribution of fibres from the superior vestibular nucleus to the reticular formation and to the contralateral vestibular nuclei, as seen in a series of transverse sections from a particular case. Terminal areas of fibres are shown dotted. Cp. text and Table 1. From LADPLI and BRODAL (1968)

The majority of fibers passing to the reticular formation leave the lateral vestibular nucleus at its ventromedial aspect and pass ventromedially towards the midline (somewhat ventral to bundle *a* which degenerates following lesions in the superior vestibular nucleus). After they have crossed the midline, some of the fibers can be traced to the contralateral nucleus reticularis pontis caudalis, especially its caudal part. The remaining fibers pass to the contralateral nucleus reticularis tegmenti pontis, where they terminate in its ventral part, chiefly caudally (drawings 27 and 29 in Fig. 22). Some fine fibers emerge from the ventral surface of the lateral nucleus and pass into the ipsilateral nucleus reticularis pontis caudalis, where they terminate, chiefly in its dorsal region, overlapping with the fibers to this nucleus mentioned above. A main group of fibers to the reticular formation runs caudally and medially through the ventral parts of the descending and medial vestibular nuclei. From the ventral surface of these two nuclei the fibers spread out ventrally in the medial half of the nuclei reticularis parvicellularis and gigantocellularis, where some of them terminate. The remaining fibers continue laterally and caudally, and finally enter the ipsilateral lateral reticular nucleus (nucleus of the lateral funiculus), where they terminate throughout its medial half (drawings 17–22 in Fig. 22) right to its caudal end.

Since a number of efferent fibers from the descending nucleus and some from the lateral and superior nuclei pass through the *medial vestibular nucleus*, no definite conclusions concern-

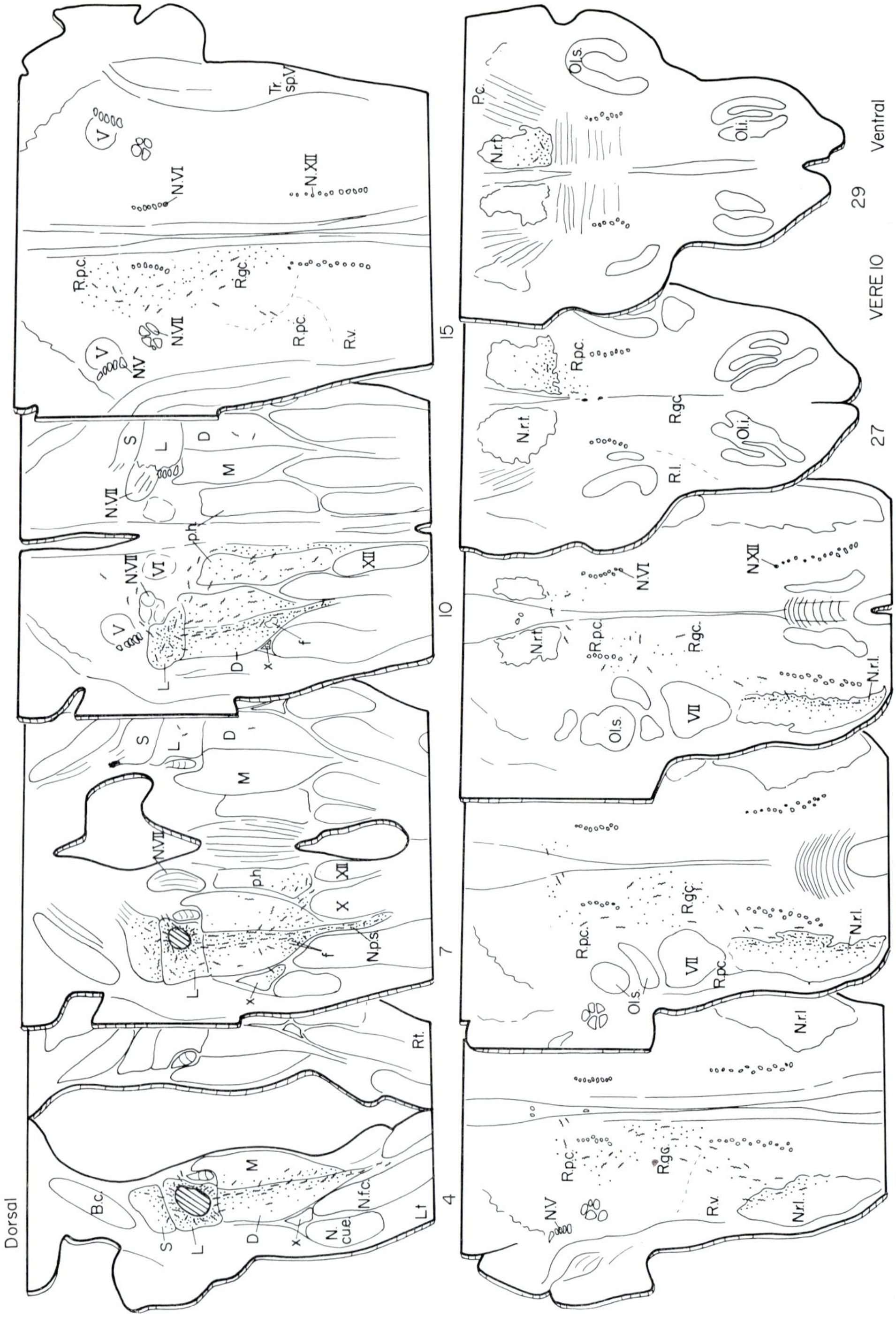

Fig. 22. Diagram showing the course and distribution of fibres from the lateral vestibular nucleus to the reticular formation and to the contralateral vestibular nuclei as seen in a series of horizontal sections from a particular case. Cp. text and Table 1. From Ladpli and Brodal (1968)

ing its projections onto the reticular formation are possible. The only possible conclusion concerning its projection (if there is one, as appears likely) is that it must be restricted to the reticularis gigantocellularis and parvicellularis.

The efferent connections of the *descending vestibular nucleus* to the reticular formation cannot be completely analyzed since some fibers from the superior and lateral vestibular nuclei pass through it as well as fastigioreticular fibers. Only regions which show degeneration following lesions restricted to the descending nucleus but not following lesions of the superior and lateral vestibular nuclei or the fastigial nucleus can be concluded to be projection areas of the descending nucleus. With this qualification the contralateral reticularis gigantocellularis and parvicellularis can be identified as receiving projections from the descending vestibular nucleus (see Table I). It may well be that the same nuclei receive fibers from the ipsilateral descending nucleus, as maintained by Carpenter (1960a), but no actual proof of this has been brought forward.

It should be noted that in a study like that of Ladpli and Brodal (1968) *it is not possible to decide if the fibers ending in a nucleus are true terminal fibers or collaterals of fibers passing to other sites.* The latter may be true in the case of the projection from the lateral vestibular nucleus onto the lateral reticular nucleus, since in Golgi preparations collaterals of lateral vestibulospinal fibers to the nucleus have been observed. Further support for this view is found in the fact that following high spinal cord lesions the majority of cells in the nucleus of Deiters show retrograde changes (Pompeiano and Brodal, 1957a).

Even if the picture given above is incomplete, the findings leave no doubt that *the various vestibular nuclei are not identical in their projection onto the reticular formation.* There is indeed some evidence that even different parts of a main nucleus may differ in this respect. For example, a lesion restricted to the dorsolateral part of the lateral nucleus did not result in degeneration in the contralateral nucleus reticularis tegmenti pontis, while lesions situated centrally and medially were positive in this respect (Ladpli and Brodal, 1968, p. 82–83). It may well be that this is another reflection of differences between the dorsocaudal and rostroventral parts of the lateral vestibular nucleus (see p. 248 and p. 268). Correspondingly, the projections described for the other nuclei cannot be taken as representative of the entire territory of the particular nucleus.

Further evidence for a quite *specific pattern within the vestibuloreticular projections is found when the sites of termination are considered.* Thus the lateral reticular nucleus is supplied by vestibular fibers from the ipsilateral lateral vestibular nucleus only, the nucleus reticularis tegmenti pontis from the contralateral superior and lateral vestibular nuclei only. Within the nucleus reticularis tegmenti pontis there is further evidence for a differentiation, since the afferents from the lateral vestibular nucleus end chiefly ventrally and caudally, while those from the superior vestibular nucleus supply the entire nucleus.[7]

From a functional point of view it is of interest that only the lateral and superior vestibular nuclei give off fibers to the reticular nuclei projecting onto the cerebellum (the lateral reticular nucleus and the nucleus reticularis tegmenti pontis). Both the lateral and superior vestibular nucleus receive abundant fibers

7 The terminal area of the vestibular afferents in the lateral reticular nucleus occupies the medial region throughout its rostrocaudal extent. Other contingents of afferents to the nucleus (spinal, cerebrocortical, rubral and fastigial) have other preferential sites of endings within it (P. Brodal et al., 1967). This arrangement is presumably of functional importance.

from the cerebellum, as will be described later. They are, therefore, links in vermal cerebello-vestibulo-reticulo-cerebellar circuits.

On the other hand, the regions of the reticular formation which give rise to long fibers passing to the spinal cord (TORVIK and BRODAL, 1957) or to levels above the mesencephalon (BRODAL and ROSSI, 1955), chiefly the nuclei reticularis gigantocellularis and pontis caudalis, receive fibers from the superior, lateral, and descending (and possibly the medial) vestibular nuclei, even if the projections from the different nuclei are not identical (see Table 1). Obviously all the three former vestibular nuclei may thus influence ascending as well as descending actions of the reticular formation, just as do the fastigioreticular fibers (WALBERG et al., 1962). The vestibuloreticular projections appear to be an important supplement to the fastigioreticular projections as pathways for cerebellar influences on the reticular formation.

Stimulation of the vestibular nerve has been shown to activate extensive areas of the reticular formation (GERNANDT et al., 1959, etc; for further references see PRECHT, this volume), but this has not been related to particular subdivisions. Since primary vestibular fibers to the reticular formation are scanty and have a very restricted distribution (see p. 300), the effect is presumably mediated via the vestibular nuclei. In this connection it is of interest to note that not only do the patterns of reticular projections of the individual vestibular nuclei differ, but the primary vestibular afferents from the various vestibular receptor epithelia are not diffusely and uniformly distributed within the vestibular nuclear complex (see p. 300). These facts make it appear extremely likely that the effect on the reticular formation and the area of this activated may differ according to the particular receptor organ stimulated (utricle, horizontal canal, etc.). Some workers have recorded action potentials from the reticular formation following stimulation of the labyrinth in movements of the head (see DUENSING and SCHAEFER, 1960), but the sites of the responses have not been mapped in detail. The problem of the influences exerted by the vestibular nuclei on the reticular formation is obviously a very complex one and will require meticulous physiological studies. For a discussion see PRECHT, this volume.

E. Efferent Connections to the Contralateral Vestibular Nuclei (Commissural Connections)

There is abundant clinical and experimental physiological evidence that the vestibular nuclei of the two sides collaborate in an intimate manner. Much of this collaboration has been assumed to occur by way of commissural connections, and recent refined physiological investigations have fully confirmed this (see PRECHT, this volume). In anatomical studies with the Golgi method some authors have concluded that commissural connections exist. Thus axons of cells in the medial nucleus have been described as crossing the midline, but it has not been possible to decide whether they reach the contralateral vestibular nuclei (CAJAL, 1909; LORENTE DE NÓ, 1933a; HAUGLIE-HANSSEN, 1968). Specific information as to the sites of ending of possible commissural fibres is difficult to obtain in Golgi studies. In experimental studies GRAY (1926) and MCMASTERS et al. (1966) found commissural connections between the two superior vestibular nuclei. Interconnections between the two lateral vestibular nuclei were described for example by GRAY (1926), CARPENTER (1960a) and MCMASTERS et al. (1966). It should be noted that in most cases of these studies the lesions encroached upon the descending nucleus, which has been shown to give off commissural fibers (CARPENTER, 1960a; MCMASTERS et al., 1966).

In experimental studies of the commissural connections the same difficulties are encountered as when the projections of the vestibular nuclei to other regions are to be determined: the possibility of damaging nonvestibular fibers as well as fibers from other vestibular nuclei than the damaged one. If the course of such fibers is taken into account some features of the commissural connections may be clarified while on others no reliable information can be obtained. (Primary vestibular fibers do not appear to reach the contralateral vestibular nuclei.) In a recent study of this kind with the Nauta method LADPLI and BRODAL (1968) succeeded in mapping the pattern of the vestibular connections in some detail. Their findings are summarized in the diagram of Fig. 23. Although the diagram is self-explanatory, some comments are appropriate. (See also Figs. 21 and 22.)

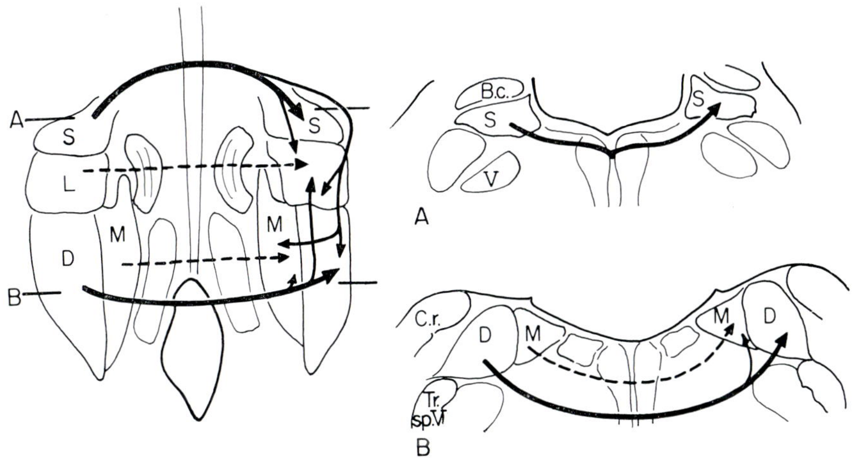

Fig. 23. To the left a diagram summarizing the main commissural connections between the vestibular nuclei as determined experimentally. A and B represent transverse sections at the levels indicated. Broken lines indicate commissural connections which are either scanty or whose origin has not been definitely established. See text for particulars. From LADPLI and BRODAL (1968)

The *superior vestibular nucleus* appears to be the part of the vestibular complex which *gives off the largest contingent of commissural fibers*. The fibers pass closely beneath the floor of the fourth ventricle in the most rostral part of the pontine reticular formation (Figs. 21 and 23) and enter the contralateral superior nucleus. The entire nucleus appears to receive such fibers, but their number is somewhat larger in the ventral and central regions. Some fibers pass around the lateral border of the superior nucleus and enter the lateral vestibular nucleus in its lateral part. Some of the fibers end here while others continue into the descending nucleus, where they curve medially and end in the ventral parts of the descending and medial nucleus.

Following lesions restricted to the *lateral vestibular nucleus* (Fig. 22) only a few fibers could be traced to the contralateral vestibular nuclei. They end in the lateral and descending nucleus (Fig. 23).

Lesions restricted to the *descending vestibular nucleus* are followed by degeneration in fibers which cross the midline more caudally than the commissural connections between the superior nuclei and are also situated somewhat deeper (Fig. 23). Some of the fibers pass through the contralateral nucleus of the spinal trigeminal tract. Within the contralateral vestibular complex most of the fibers end in the ventral and lateral parts of the descending nucleus, some end ventrally in the medial and the lateral nucleus and a few in the superior nucleus (not shown in Fig. 23).

Since commissural fibers from the descending nucleus pass through the *medial nucleus*, direct information on the contralateral projections of the latter could not be obtained. The degeneration following lesions of the medial nucleus is similar to that seen after lesions of the descending nucleus. If the former has commissural connections, as appears likely, they probably correspond to those of the descending nucleus. The findings made by Tarlov (1969) in macaques, baboon and chimpanzee following lesions affecting large parts of the vestibular nuclei are in agreement with the findings described above.

It appears from the study of Ladpli and Brodal (1968) that *there is a certain pattern in the commissural connections of the vestibular nuclei*. For example, in the lateral, descending, and medial nuclei it is chiefly the ventral parts that receive commissural afferents, while the distribution in the superior nucleus covers its entire territory. The commissural afferents to the superior nucleus come almost exclusively from its partner on the other side. The two superior nuclei are thus more specifically and more heavily interconnected than any of the other four main nuclei. In contrast, the two lateral vestibular nuclei have only scanty interconnections, suggesting a modest degree of cooperation between them.

Physiological studies on the commissural connections are in good accord with the anatomical findings described above. Neurons of the lateral vestibular nucleus were first shown by Devito et al. (1956) to be influenced by the contralateral labyrinth. In further studies Shimazu and Precht (1966) found that stimulation of the vestibular nerve gave inhibition of type I neurons and excitation of type II neurons in the contralateral vestibular nuclei (both types of neurons respond to stimulation of the horizontal canal). The neurons were located mainly in the ventral part of the medial nucleus and the ventromedial part of the superior nucleus. The contralateral responses were abolished following midline incisions of the brainstem about 2 mm deep, and were assumed to be mediated via commissural connections. These results are in agreement with the anatomical patterns within these connections (see Fig. 23), even if, as described above, no positive evidence of commissural connections between the two medial nuclei can be produced. Inhibitory commissural cells in the medial nucleus activated by primary vestibular fibers might explain the contralateral inhibition of the type I neurons, and on direct stimulation of the medial nucleus evidence in support of the presence of direct inhibitory commissural fibers was obtained by Mano et al. (1968). It appears from physiological studies (Shimazu and Precht, 1966; Wilson et al., 1968b) that more complex mechanisms may be involved as well. Furthermore, the contralateral vestibular nuclei may be influenced via vestibuloreticular and reticulovestibular pathways. (For an account of the physiology of the commissural connections see Precht, this volume.)

F. Ascending Connections from the Vestibular Nuclei

On account of the diagnostic importance of nystagmus in clinical neurology, the ascending projections of the vestibular nuclei have probably attracted more interest than any other contingent of their connections. The close correlation between the direction of nystagmus and the planes of movement of the head in space shows that the connections between the vestibular receptors and the motoneurons supplying the extrinsic ocular muscles must indeed be very precisely organized. In spite of much research, anatomical, physiological and clinical, our understanding of the organization of the vestibulo-ocular pathways is still fragmentary, even if some main features are known. Considering that not only the cristae but also the maculae influence nystagmus and considering the complex mechanics of the ocular movements, this is not astonishing. Care should be taken that the relevant problems are not oversimplified.

It is obvious that the several extrinsic ocular muscles cooperate in a finely coordinated pattern when a conjugate eye movement is elicited. *It follows from the anatomical arrangement of the muscles that no movement of an eye is likely to be produced by contraction of one muscle only and relaxation of its antagonist.* STARLING's well-known diagram of the actions of the extrinsic ocular muscles, reproduced in many textbooks, illustrates this. The insertion point of a muscle on the eyeball is important in determining its action. Since the axis of a muscle in relation to the axis of the eyeball will change during movements of the eyes, the action of a muscle varies according to the position of the eye. Abduction of the eye is often taken to be produced by contraction of the lateral rectus only. However, the inferior and superior oblique muscles, on account of their insertion lateral to the axis of the eyeball and behind its equator may also take part in abduction movements. The change in the mechanical effect of a particular muscle according to changes in the position of the eyeball can be illustrated with reference to the superior rectus muscle. This will function as a pure elevator of the bulb only when the eye is slightly abducted, since only in this position is the axis of the muscle parallel to the longitudinal axis of the bulb. Another example is the superior oblique, which has its attachment to the bulb behind its equator. The superior oblique will depress the eyeball when the eye is adducted, while it will act as a lateral mover and rotator of the eyeball in all laterally directed positions of the eye, until in maximal abduction of the eye it will act as a pure rotator, when the axis of the tendon is in the equatorial plane (for a recent analysis of the superior oblique see TOKUMASU et al., 1965). This fits in well with the demonstration by COHEN et al. (1964) that "every eye muscle was either activated or inhibited during stimulation of any single canal nerve in the cat."

The functional aspects of eye movements elicited from the labyrinth are treated in other chapters of this volume. The account below is restricted to data on the anatomical structures involved. Fibers ascending from the vestibular nuclei pass to the nuclei of the extrinsic ocular muscles, but also to other regions in the upper brainstem and above. The ascending fibers from the vestibular nuclei are generally said to pass in the distinct fiber bundle called the *medial longitudinal fasciculus*, situated closely beneath the floor of the 4th ventricle and the aqueduct. The bundle continues caudally in the spinal cord. This part is often referred to as the *descending* medial longitudinal fasciculus or the sulcomarginal fasciculus (cf. p. 272), while the part rostral to the vestibular nuclei is called the *ascending* medial longitudinal fasciculus. Since the latter contains some descending fibers (for example from the interstitial nucleus of Cajal in the mesencephalon (see p. 323) the designation is not quite appropriate.

A number of authors have examined the rostral projections of the vestibular nuclei experimentally. The earlier literature has been reviewed by BRODAL and POMPEIANO (1958) and will not be considered in detail. Most authors, traced the ascending fibers with the Marchi method after lesions of the nuclei. Only rarely were the lesions restricted to particular vestibular nuclei, and the descriptions and illustrations given often do not permit any opinion on whether the conclusions drawn are justified. Some claims of terminations of ascending vestibular fibres, for example in the colliculi, the medial geniculate body or the red nucleus, are presumably due to concomitant damage of nonvestibular fibers. The proportions and origins of crossed and uncrossed fibers described vary widely from author to author. Authors studying the retrograde cellular changes in the vestibular nuclei following lesions of the ascending medial longitudinal fasciculus also reported diverging findings, but changes have been described to occur in all four main nuclei. This method, as mentioned previously (p. 263), is well suited to investigation of the origin of transected fibers but less useful for determining their sites of ending.

In an attempt to decide the *origin of the ascending vestibular fibers* more precisely, BRODAL and POMPEIANO (1958) undertook an experimental study in kittens, using the modified Gudden method (BRODAL, 1940a). Characteristically changed cells were found in *all four main nuclei*. In addition *the interstitial nucleus of the vestibular nerve and group x give off ascending fibers*, since some of their cells are changed following transection of the medial longitudinal fasciculus in the lower mesencephalon. In the nucleus of Deiters the changes affect large as well as small cells (just as after lesions of the spinal cord). This is explicable on the basis that many cells of the nucleus of Deiters give off dichotomizing axons, with one descending and one ascending branch (CAJAL, 1896, 1909–1911). Little information was obtained as to whether the ascending fibers arise predominantly from specific regions of the main nuclei. It appears that as suggested by FERRARO et al. (1940), in the medial nucleus a greater number of ascending fibers come from its dorsomedial than from its ventrolateral region (the latter projects mainly to the cerebellum; BRODAL and TORVIK, 1957). Lesions above the oculomotor nucleus are followed by some cellular changes in the vestibular nuclei, indicating that a considerable number of ascending fibers pass beyond these nuclei, as found with other methods.

CARPENTER and MCMASTERS (1963; see also CARPENTER and STROMINGER, 1965) following lesions of the medial longitudinal fasciculus found retrograde changes in all four main nuclei in monkey; they were located chiefly as follows: ventrally in the nucleus of Deiters; centrally in the superior nucleus; laterally, mainly rostrally, in the medial nucleus; rostrally in the descending nucleus. The authors draw attention to the fact that on the whole these regions correspond to those which receive primary vestibular fibers (see p. 299).

It appears from the literature that *the ascending fibers from the superior nucleus ascend entirely ipsilaterally, while the other main nuclei give off crossed as well as uncrossed ascending fibers* (for reviews see BRODAL and POMPEIANO, 1958; MCMASTERS et al., 1966). Several authors have discussed the relative positions in the medial longitudinal fasciculus of fibers from the different nuclei, but there is no unanimity among the authors (for some references see BRODAL and POMPEIANO, 1958). It appears settled, however, that the fibres from the superior nucleus occupy the lateral winglike process of the medial longitudinal fasciculus, while those from the medial nucleus are found in the medial portions of the contralateral fasciculus (see Tarlov, 1970). It appears that all long ascending fibers from the vestibular nuclei to the nuclei of the extrinsic ocular muscles are in the ascending medial longitudinal fasciculus (see MCMASTERS et al., 1966).

Among *the sites of terminations of the ascending secondary vestibular fibers* the nuclei of the extrinsic ocular muscles have been most intensively studied. There is no doubt that *the abducent, the trochlear and the somatic efferent divisions of the oculomotor nucleus receive fibers from the vestibular nuclei*. Different subdivisions of the oculomotor nucleus supply particular extrinsic ocular muscles as has been found in anatomical studies by WARWICK (1953) in monkey, and in cat in studies based on antidromic stimulation by BIENFANG (1968). Several attempts have been made to decide the precise relations between particular vestibular nuclei and specific oculomotor nuclear groups. SZENTÁGOTHAI (1943, 1952, 1964) concludes from studies of the degeneration observed in the oculomotor nuclei following lesions of the vestibular nuclei that "the direct connection between vestibular nuclei and the motor cell groups serving innervation of individual ocular muscles displays an amazing degree of somatotopic patterning" (1964, p. 210). Six of the extrinsic muscles seem to be innervated preponderantly from one labyrinth, and the other six preponderantly from the other labyrinth. Two recent studies are particularly valuable in providing important new information. Following lesions restricted to individual vestibular nuclei the distribution of degeneration in the various parts of the oculomotor nucleus and in the abducent and trochlear nuclei was studied in monkey by MCMASTERS et al. (1966) and in the cat by TARLOV (1970). There are some minor discrepancies between the results of the two studies. This, at least in part, may reflect species differences. Thus in the monkey fibers were traced from all four vestibular nuclei, although very few from the descending,

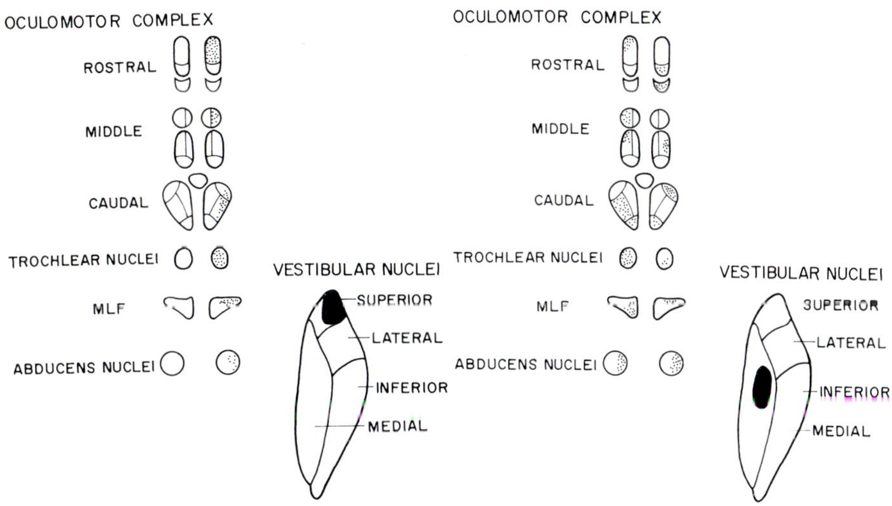

Fig. 24a. Diagram showing the sites of termination (dots) of ascending fibres from the medial and superior vestibular nuclei within the different subdivisions of the oculomotor nucleus (cf. WARWICK, 1953) and the trochlear and abducens nuclei in the monkey. The oculomotor nucleus is shown in transverse sections at three levels. (The "visceral nuclei" of the oculomotor complex are omitted.) The areas of the lesions are shown in black in a diagram of the vestibular nuclei as seen in horizontal sections of the brain stem. Note the largely different localization of degeneration following lesions of the superior and the medial vestibular nuclei. Cf. text. From MCMASTERS, WEISS and CARPENTER (1966)

while in the cat TARLOV (1970) found the contribution from the lateral as well as the descending nucleus to be negligible. For particulars the original papers should be consulted, but some major points deserve mention.

According to MCMASTERS et al. (1966), *in monkey the projection of the superior vestibular nucleus onto the oculomotor nuclear groups differs in some respects from the projections of the three others.* In the first place it is strictly *ipsilateral.* Secondly, it appears largely to supply regions of the oculomotor nuclear groups which do not receive fibers from the other vestibular nuclei (see Fig. 24a). The scanty ascending projection from the descending nucleus appears to come chiefly from its rostral part. In the lateral nucleus only its ventral part, receiving primary vestibular fibres (see Fig. 27) gives off ascending fibers. It is further apparent that *in general the projections from the bilaterally projecting nuclei (the medial, lateral and descending nucleus) are asymmetrical, i.e. portions of the oculomotor nuclei receiving ascending projections on one side have none on the other side* (see Fig. 24a).

Correlations with WARWICK'S (1953) pattern of the oculomotor innervation in monkey suggest some specific relations. For example, the projections of the superior vestibular nucleus appears to influence chiefly motor cell groups innervating both lateral recti (there is an asymmetrical innervation of the two abducens nuclei, see Fig. 24a), the ipsilateral superior oblique (contralateral trochlear nucleus), ipsilateral medial rectus, and the contralateral inferior oblique. To a lesser extent, the ipsilateral inferior oblique, the contralateral medial rectus and both inferior recti will be influenced from the superior nucleus. The projection to the abducent nuclei is scanty. Considering the physiological findings of inhibitory actions of some of the ascending fibers from the superior vestibular nucleus (COHEN et al., 1964) it appears that "ascending fibers from the superior vestibular nucleus may provide controlling influences for muscles involved primarily in vertical or rotatory eye movements" (MCMASTERS et al., 1966, p. 178). Analogies can be drawn for the projections from the other main vestibular nuclei. Thus fibers from the medial and lateral vestibular nuclei appear to be most abundant to oculomotor nuclei which innervate muscles whose primary functions concern horizontal and rotatory eye movements.

In *cat* TARLOV (1970) likewise found that *fibers from the superior nucleus ascend only ipsilaterally, but that cat differs from monkey in that these fibers supply nuclei on both sides* (except for the abducent nucleus). This occurs by fibers leaving the medial longitudinal fasciculus and crossing at the level of the oculomotor nucleus (see Fig. 24b). Furthermore, the separation between areas supplied by the superior and the medial nucleus appears less clear-cut than in the monkey. The two nuclei "have widely overlapping as well as apparently separate projection fields." (For diagrams illustrating the relations see TARLOV, 1970.)

MCMASTERS et al. (1966) draw attention to the fact that the regions of the vestibular nuclei that give off fibers to the oculomotor nuclei all appear to be within the regions which receive primary vestibular fibers according to WALBERG et al. (1958). The same is stressed by TARLOV (1970). This author, furthermore, provides some evidence that certain regions within the oculomotor nucleus receive preferential projections from certain areas within the superior vestibular nucleus and the rostral part of the medial nucleus. This is of interest in view of the findings of STEIN and CARPENTER (1967) on the distribution of primary vestibular afferents from different receptor organs of the labyrinth. These indicate that the various receptors do not have entirely separate representations in the vestibular nuclei (see Fig. 29). For example, afferents from all three semicircular ducts appear to

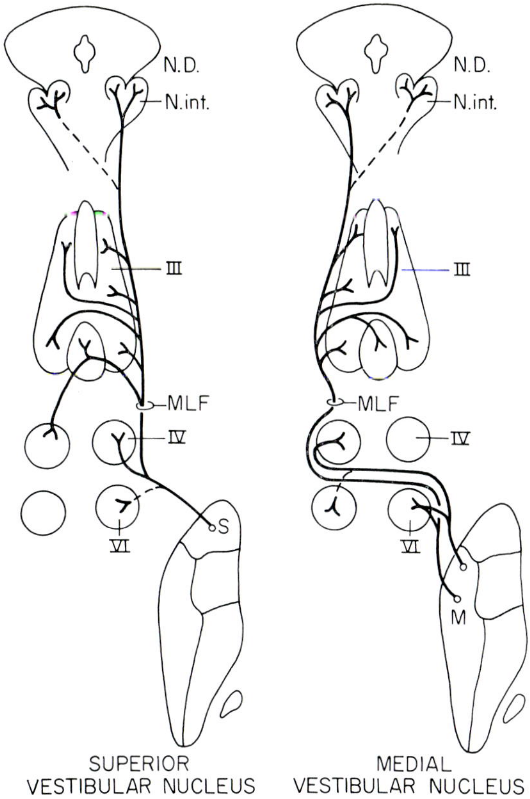

Fig. 24b. Diagrams showing the course of the ascending vestibular fibres to the nuclei of the extrinsic ocular muscles and the interstitial nucleus of Cajal and the nucleus of Darkschewitsch in the cat. The fibres from the superior vestibular nucleus ascend ipsilaterally in the medial longitudinal fasciculus, those from the rostral part of the medial vestibular nucleus ascend in the contralateral fasciculus. Both components give off fibres to most nuclear groups on both sides. From Tarlov (1970)

end in the superior and the medial nucleus and to a lesser extent in the descending nucleus. Nevertheless, while fibers from the three ducts appear to share a common area rostrally in the medial nucleus, in the superior nucleus they seem to be distributed in a definite pattern to distinctive regions. This seems to be the case in cat as well (Gacek, 1969).

It appears that the anatomical organization provides possibilities for point-to-point as well as for diverging and converging conduction of nervous impulses from the particular vestibular receptor organs to the motoneuron groups which supply the various extrinsic ocular muscles. The anatomical data support the opinion expressed by Szentágothai (1950, 1952) among others that the *elementary vestibulo-ocular reflex arc* is a three-neuron arc, where the second link is made up of neurons in the vestibular nuclei projecting upon the nuclei of the extrinsic eye muscles. Further confirmation is provided by physiological observations. Thus, in the medial nucleus, Wilson et al. (1968b) identified cells with axons ascending in the medial longitudinal fasciculus which were monosynaptically excited from the labyrinth.

Many particulars in the pattern of the projection of the different subdivisions of the labyrinth onto the vestibular nuclei remain to be established, and our knowledge of the ascending projections from the minor divisions receiving the various contingents of primary afferents is still not complete. The data of CARPENTER et al., of GACEK, and of TARLOV make it clear that the pathways from one receptor organ to particular oculomotor nuclear divisions cannot be organized in a simple manner. This is, in fact, only what might be expected from data on the integrated action of the extraocular muscles and the complexities in the anatomy and physiology of the receptor organs, but it does not invalidate the assumption that there must be a high degree of order in the anatomical organization of the pathways from the receptor organs to the nuclei of the extrinsic ocular muscles.

In addition to the elementary vestibulo-ocular reflex arc, considered above, there are other pathways for influences from the vestibular apparatus on the eye muscle nuclei. More complex vestibulo-ocular reactions appear to be mediated via the *reticular formation* (e.g. LORENTE DE NÓ, 1933a; SZENTÁGOTHAI, 1950). The anatomy of these connections is imperfectly known, even if the vestibuloreticular projections have recently been mapped in some detail as discussed in a previous section (see Figs. 21 and 22). Ascending fibers from the reticular formation have been found to give off collaterals to the oculomotor, trochlear and abducens nuclei in Golgi studies (SCHEIBEL and SCHEIBEL, 1958). NAUTA and KUYPERS (1958) describe ascending reticular formation fibers to the interstitial nucleus of CAJAL. Some authors have claimed that fibers from the vestibular nuclei to the eye muscle nuclei ascend in the reticular formation, but according to the findings of McMASTERS et al. (1966) in cases with isolated lesions of the vestibular nuclei this is not the case, even if it appears that not all ascending fibers from the vestibular nuclei pass in the medial longitudinal fasciculus.

From a functional point of view it is of interest that in Golgi preparations *the afferent fibers entering the nuclei of the oculomotor nerves are of two types* (SZENTÁGOTHAI, 1964). Fibers of type A have rather large presynaptic terminals which are distributed within a well-circumscribed area of the nucleus and appear to establish contacts with the body or proximal dendrites of a few neighboring motoneurons (Fig. 25). Fibers of type B are of smaller caliber and their terminal branches are distributed over a wide area. From experimental studies SZENTÁGOTHAI (1964) concludes that the type A fibers belong to secondary vestibular neurons, while type B fibers appear to come from the interstitial nucleus of CAJAL in the mesencephalon and from the reticular formation. Some fibers from the medial vestibular nucleus appear to be of this type. The type A fiber appears to be well suited to the establishment of a powerful and precisely localized activation of motoneurons by cells of the vestibular nuclei. These findings are of interest for the analysis of the various influences exerted by vestibular impulses on the motoneurons of the oculomotor nuclei (see PRECHT, this volume). Further anatomical studies, especially experimental electron microscope studies, are needed, however, and can be expected to give valuable information for the interpretation of recent electrophysiological observations. Much remains to be done with regard to the anatomy of the pathways concerned in the influences exerted by the reticular formation on the oculomotor nuclei also. The pathways responsible for the cerebellar influences

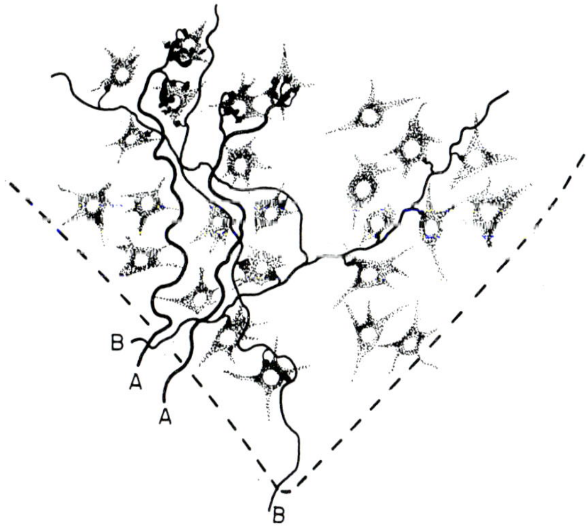

Fig. 25. Schematic drawing to illustrate the two types of afferent fibres to the oculomotor nuclei. Fibres (collaterals) of type A, relatively thick, end with dense terminal arborizations around a few motor cells. Fibres (collaterals) of type B are thin and distributed over wide areas. They give off short terminal branches along their course and end with individual terminal boutons. From SZENTÁGOTHAI (1964)

are also imperfectly known, but they will not be considered here. For some anatomical data see POMPEIANO (this volume).

Mention was made previously of *ascending fibers from the vestibular nuclei to other destinations than the nuclei of the motor ocular nerves*. The literature on this subject is quite extensive and contains many conflicting statements. This literature will not be reviewed here (references can be found in BRODAL and POMPEIANO, 1958; BRODAL et al., 1962; CARPENTER and HANNA, 1962; and in other publications of CARPENTER and collaborators; see also TARLOV, 1969). In general there seems to be fairly good agreement on the vestibular projections to nuclei in the mesencephalon, while projections to more rostral regions of the brain are disputed.

After interruption of the ascending medial longitudinal fasciculus in monkey CARPENTER and STROMINGER (1965, see also CARPENTER and MCMASTERS, 1963) found degenerating fibers in the mesencephalon in *the interstitial nucleus of* CAJAL, *the nucleus of the posterior commissure, the nucleus of Darkschewitsch* and the ventrolateral portions of *the periaqueductal gray*. (For some comments on these nuclei see p. 323.) Most of the fibers end in the interstitial nucleus of CAJAL. Largely corresponding findings were made in cat by CARPENTER and HANNA (1962) and in macaque, baboon and chimpanzee by TARLOV (1969).

Whether the ascending vestibular fibers ending in different nuclei in the mesencephalon arise from the same or from different parts of the vestibular nuclei is still largely unknown. It appears from the observations of MCMASTERS et al. (1966) and TARLOV (1970) that the interstitial nucleus of CAJAL and the nucleus of Darkschewitsch receive fibers from the superior nucleus and rostral parts of the medial vestibular nucleus. The former are mainly uncrossed while the latter are predominantly crossed. In addition there seems to be a very sparse projection from the ipsilateral lateral and descending vestibular nuclei.

Several authors have claimed the existence of fibers ascending from the vestibular nuclei to certain *thalamic nuclei*, and some have described a particular "vestibulothalamic tract." The literature on this subject is difficult to analyze, especially since most lesions were not restricted to the vestibular nuclei. Many authors did not find such fibers, and there may have been confusion with the "dorsal trigeminothalamic tract" (for a brief discussion see BRODAL et al., 1962, p. 47ff.). Following discrete lesions of the medial longitudinal fasciculus a relatively small number of degenerating fibers was traced into the ipsilateral half of the diencephalon in the monkey by CARPENTER and STROMINGER (1965), to the ventral posterior inferior nucleus and to ventrolateral parts of the ventral posterior medial nucleus. (Some fibers were found in the parafascicular, centromedian and reticular nuclei.) Following similar lesions in cat, CARPENTER and HANNA (1962) found degeneration in portions of the posteroventral medial thalamic nucleus and the centromedian nucleus. Largely corresponding sites of endings have been reported by HASSLER (1948, 1956), but the fibers described by HASSLER follow a different course than those found by CARPENTER and collaborators when the medial longitudinal fasciculus was transected, and their origin from the vestibular nuclei cannot be convincingly proved.

In a recent study in macaques, baboons and a chimpanzee TARLOV (1969) found no evidence that fibers from the vestibular nuclei project to the thalamus. By using sections in three planes he was able to follow the degenerating fibers in each case in detail. In cases where degeneration was found in the thalamus there was always concomitant injury of the dorsal column nuclei or the superior cerebellar peduncle. No vestibular fibers appear to ascend beyond the level of the posterior commissure. The observations of CARPENTER and STROMINGER (1965), mentioned above, of direct vestibulothalamic connections, appear to rest on inconclusive evidence.

Finally it should be mentioned that some authors have advocated the existence of fibers from the vestibular nuclei to the *hypothalamus*. Following lesions of the medial longitudinal fasciculus rostral to the abducens nuclei a distinct bundle of degenerating fibers was found by CARPENTER and HANNA (1962) and CARPENTER and STROMINGER (1965) to continue into the hypothalamus. It is thought, however, that these fibers probably do not arise from the vestibular nuclei but from the reticular formation.

On the basis of electrophysiological and clinical evidence (see, for example, BRODAL et al., 1962; KORNHUBER, 1966, for reviews) some authors have claimed that vestibular impulses reach the acoustic regions of the cortex and are transmitted along fibers which follow the ascending auditory pathway. Other authors have placed *the cortical vestibular area* elsewhere. Some studies (see KORNHUBER, 1966; FREDRICKSON et al., 1966) suggest that the cortical vestibular area in the monkey is situated in the postcentral gyrus, between the first and the second somatosensory cortex, and appears to belong to Brodmann's cytoarchitectonic cortical area 2 (see also LANDGREN et al., 1967, in the cat).[8] The convergence of vestibular impulses from joint and deep tissue receptors in this cortical area is

8 A second vestibular cortical area has been defined in the motor cortex of the cat and monkey (see KORNHUBER, 1966). The latencies for responses of vestibular origin are usually longer in this area than in the area in the postcentral gyrus.

probably of functional importance (see Kornhuber, 1966). According to Le Gros Clark and Powell (1953) there is a topical pattern in the projection to cortical areas 3, 1 and 2 from the thalamic nucleus ventralis posterior. It appears likely that vestibular impulses reaching the cortex are relayed, at least in part, through this nucleus. (For some comments on this question see Tarlov, 1969.) Since the evidence for fibers from the vestibular nuclei to the thalamus is inconclusive, *it must be assumed that vestibular impulses probably reach the thalamus via indirect routes*. The vestibular (primary and secondary) projections onto the cerebellum are modest and do not appear to reach regions which give off impulses to the thalamus. Most likely the vestibulothalamic route involves projections from the vestibular nuclei to the reticular formation and reticulothalamic fibers. Further studies of indirect vestibulothalamic connections are needed.

G. Some Minor Efferent Fiber Contingents from the Vestibular Nuclei

In the literature scattered references can be found to efferents from the vestibular nuclei to many neighboring structures of the brainstem. No attempt will be made to list these data. Usually the fiber contingents are described as scanty. On account of the difficulties in making isolated lesions of the vestibular nuclei, some of the reported connections cannot be considered established. In addition, damage inflicted to efferents from the intracerebellar nuclei, especially the fastigial nucleus, may give rise to erroneous interpretations. Brodal and Gogstad (1957) found some fibers to the paramedian reticular nucleus following lesions in the vestibular nuclei. These may possibly be fastigial efferents, since the fastigial nucleus gives rise to such fibers (Brodal and Gogstad, 1957; Walberg and Pompeiano, 1960) particularly since in a later study where this possibility was taken into account (Ladpli and Brodal, 1968) no convincing evidence of a projection to the paramedian reticular nucleus was found.

Some authors, for example Muskens (1934), suggest the existence of fibers to the inferior olive from the vestibular nuclei. Since there is no reliable evidence that cerebellofugal fibers pass to the olive*, concomitant lesions of efferent cerebellar fibers cannot explain these observations. Other authors have not observed vestibulo-olivary fibers (Walberg, 1956; Weiss et al., 1964). Possible vestibulo-olivary fibers were not searched for in the study of Ladpli and Brodal (1968) in their material with isolated lesions of separate vestibular nuclei. An examination of this material discloses the presence of a scanty vestibulo-olivary projection, but closer mapping has still not been done.

After lesions of the medial longitudinal fasciculus rostral to the abducent nucleus, Carpenter and Hanna (1962) in cat and Carpenter and McMasters (1963) in monkey found degenerating fibers to the rostral and medial portions of the medial accessory olive and the ventrolateral outgrowth of the olive. Corresponding findings have been reported by some other authors (see Carpenter and Hanna, 1962, for references). The fibres may arise mainly from the interstitial nucleus of Cajal in the mesencephalon.

* Note added in proof: See, however, the paper by Graybiel et al., Brain Res. **58**, 205–211 (1973).

V. Afferent Connections of the Vestibular Nuclei

As mentioned previously, greater precision is generally possible in the anatomical determination of the sites of termination of afferents to a nucleus than in determination of the sites of origin of its efferent projections. The distributions of the various contingents of afferents within the nuclear complex are quite well known in the case of the vestibular nuclei. Careful mapping shows that *each contingent of afferents has its particular sites of termination.* Some contingents may be restricted to only one or two of the main nuclei, and often they supply only part of the individual nuclei. *Within one nucleus, afferents from various sources often have their preferential sites of ending.* Some of the afferents are organized in a topical pattern. In addition, afferent contingents differ in their patterns of terminal branching and modes of synaptic contacts. In many instances the regional differences in the termination of afferents can be correlated with architectonic differences and with the sites of origin of efferents. The main afferent contingents are the following: primary vestibular fibers; three main groups of afferents from the cerebellum; spinovestibular fibers; fibers from the mesencephalon; reticulovestibular fibers; fibers from the contralateral vestibular nuclei; some minor contingents from other sources.

A. Primary Vestibular Fibers

The primary vestibular fibers have their bipolar perikarya in the vestibular ganglion in the bottom of the internal acoustic meatus. In cat there are more than 12000 vestibular ganglion cells altogether (Gacek, 1969). Their peripheral branches contact the receptor cells of the maculae and cristae, while the central branches enter the brainstem at the border between the pons and medulla. The vestibular ganglion may be separated into a superior and an inferior ganglion. Fibers with their perikarya in the superior ganglion supply the crista of the anterior and the horizontal (or lateral) canal and the macula utriculi. Branches from the inferior ganglion pass to the crista of the posterior canal and the macula sacculi. This has been studied by Stein and Carpenter (1967) in monkey and by Gacek (1969) in cat. In the main the situation appears to correspond to that found in mouse by Lorente de Nó (1931, 1933b). The myelinated primary vestibular fibers are of different calibers (Engström and Rexed, 1940, in man; Wersäll, 1956, in guinea pig; Gacek and Rasmussen, 1961, in guinea pig, cat and monkey), but some 66% of them are between 3–5 μm (Wersäll, 1956). In cat the thickest axons have a diameter of 11 μm according to Gacek (1969). Gacek further noted that most of the utricular fibers are small, and that there are caliber differences between the fibers supplying the crests and those supplying the slopes of the cristae. The latter fibers are almost exclusively very small.

Early students of Golgi preparations (Koelliker, 1891; Held, 1892; Cajal, 1896, 1909) demonstrated that *most if not all primary vestibular fibers dichotomize into an ascending and a descending branch* when they enter the vestibular nuclear complex. This has repeatedly been confirmed (Lorente de Nó, 1933b; Hauglie-Hanssen, 1968; and others). In general the ascending branches are somewhat thinner than the descending ones (Fig. 26). The branches give off numerous collaterals, mainly directed medially and provided with side branches (see below).

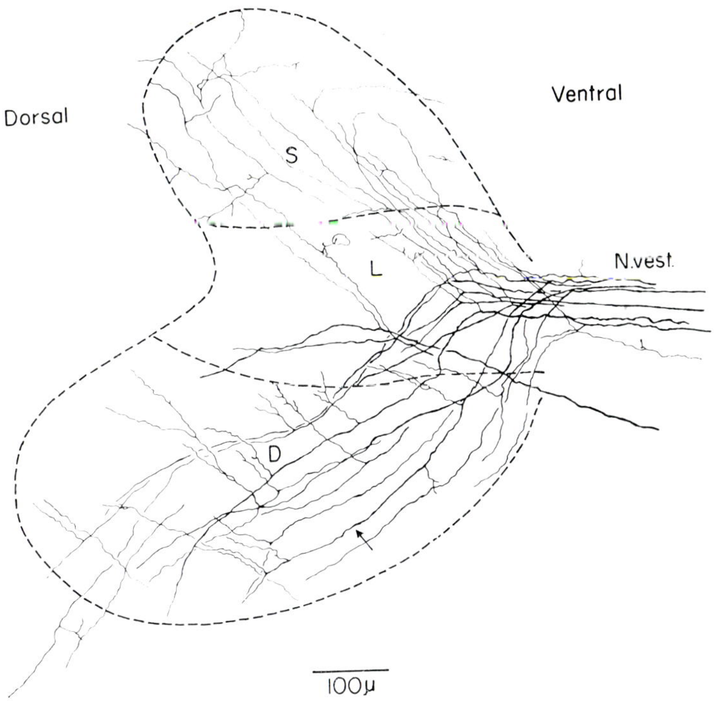

Fig. 26. Drawing to illustrate the division of the primary vestibular fibres as seen in a nearly sagittal section (Golgi rapid method) from a newborn rat. The ascending branches are usually the thinner. Collaterals are seen on some of the branches, emanating at nearly right angles from the parent fibres. One descending branch (arrow) has four collaterals. The approximate borders of the vestibular nuclei are indicated. From HAUGLIE-HANSSEN (1968)

In Golgi preparations the ascending fibers have been found to supply the superior vestibular nucleus and the superior part of the lateral nucleus, while the descending branches give off collaterals ending in the descending and medial vestibular nucleus. Just before the parent fibers enter the vestibular nuclei some of them give off collaterals to the interstitial nucleus of the vestibular nerve (Fig. 27). A few primary vestibular fibers end in the dorsolateral reticular formation (see below).

In most textbooks the *distribution of the primary vestibular fibers within the vestibular nuclei* is described as covering the entire territory. This is an undue oversimplification, presumably based on studies in which the problem of a differential distribution was not considered (for references see WALBERG et al., 1958). LEIDLER (1914) in a Marchi study in rabbit, however, noted that after transection of the vestibular nerve degeneration is found only ventromedially in the descending nucleus, and he also noted that what appears to correspond to Deiter's nucleus is free from degeneration dorsally. A closer study of the distribution of primary vestibular fibers by means of the NAUTA (1957) and GLEES (1946) methods (WALBERG et al., 1958) confirmed these observations and in addition brought forward other data.

Figure 27 shows a map of the distribution of terminal degeneration in the vestibular nuclei as seen in a series of horizontal sections following transection of

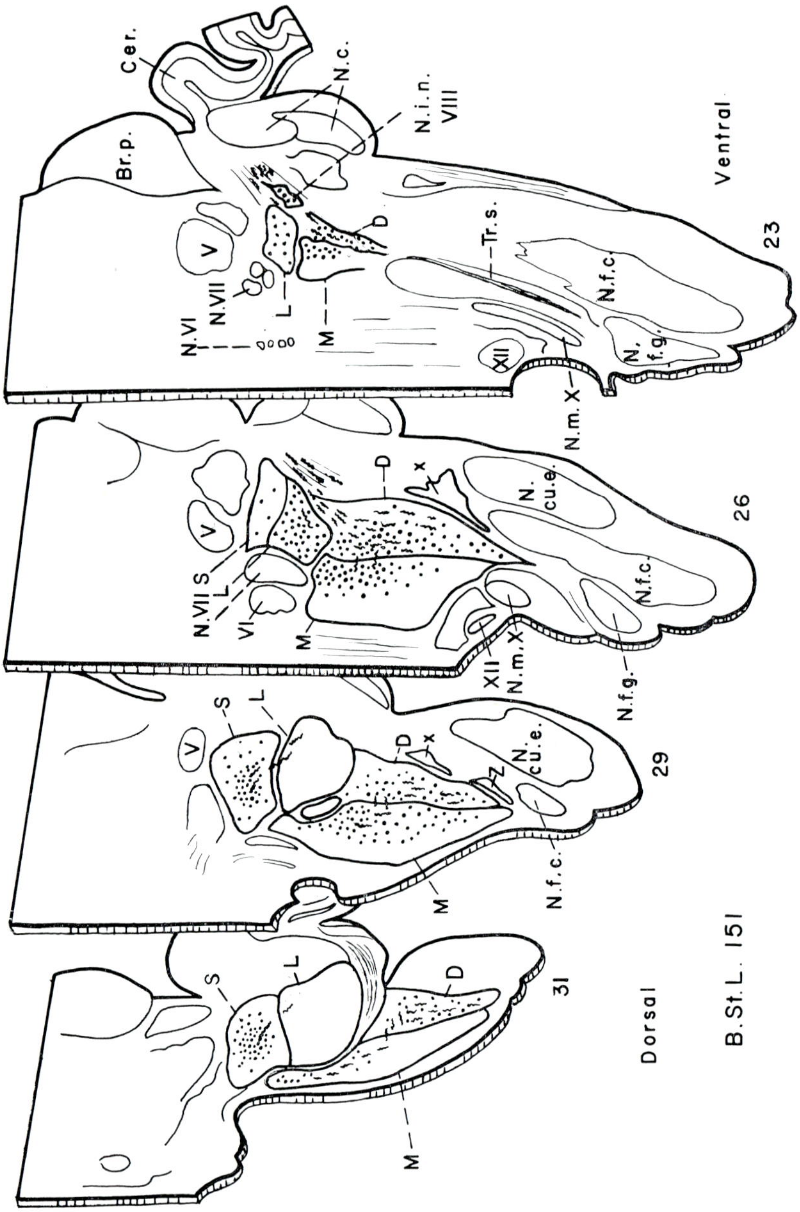

Fig. 27. Diagrammatic representation of the sites of termination (dots) of primary vestibular fibres as seen in a series of horizontal sections through the vestibular nuclei from a cat in which the vestibular nerve had been transected 10 days before sacrifice. Degenerating fibres of passage are shown as wavy lines. The group f (not shown in the diagram) in the descending nucleus is free from degeneration. For abbreviations see list on p. 340. (For a diagram of the distribution as seen in transverse sections see the original paper.) From WALBERG, BOWSHER and BRODAL (1958)

the vestibular nerve in cat. As will be seen, *there are regions that do not receive primary vestibular fibers within all four main nuclei*. In the superior nucleus the fibers supply the central region, in the lateral nucleus the ventral part, chiefly rostrally, in the medial nucleus they end chiefly laterally (and are less abundant caudally than rostrally). In the descending nucleus degeneration is widespread, but it is less intense at the most rostrolateral point and less intense ventrolaterally than dorsomedially throughout the nucleus. The small group f (see Figs. 1–2) within the descending nucleus is free from degeneration, in spite of the occurrence of degeneration in its immediate surroundings. Primary vestibular fibers end in the interstitial nucleus of Cajal (N. i.n. VIII in drawing 23, Fig. 27), while groups x and z are free. In a later study (Brodal and Høivik, 1964) the small group y (see Figs. 1 and 2) was found to receive primary vestibular fibers. Even if the borders between regions receiving primary vestibular fibers and those not receiving such fibers are not sharp, the preferential distribution is obvious. This is most clearly recognized in transverse sections (Fig. 28). It should be noted that in the lateral vestibular nucleus the primary vestibular fibers supply chiefly the forelimb region.

The restricted distribution of primary vestibular fibers described above has in the main been confirmed by Carpenter (1960b) and Gacek (1969) in cat, van Rossum (1969) in rabbit, and by Carpenter (1960b) and Stein and Carpenter (1967) in monkey. In this animal, however, the number of fibers to the lateral nucleus was found to be surprisingly modest. Observations in Golgi material (Lorente de Nó, 1933b; Hauglie-Hanssen, 1968) are in agreement with the experimental data, even if they do not permit correspondingly precise mapping.

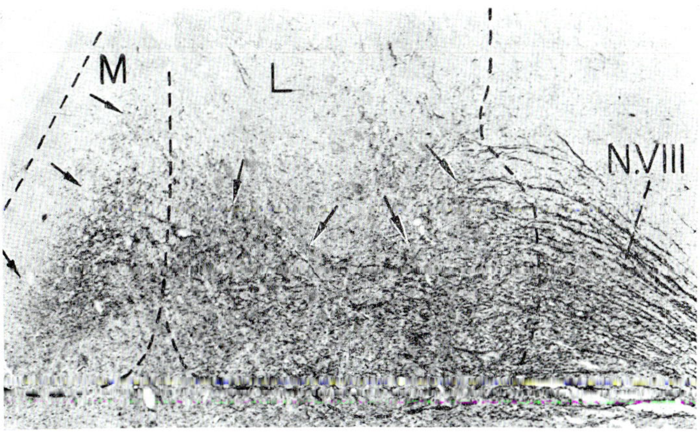

Fig. 28. A photomicrograph (× 35) of a transverse section through the brain stem of a cat following complete destruction of the vestibular nerve (Nauta method) showing distribution of degeneration in vestibular nuclei. Borders of nuclei are indicated by broken lines. Arrows point to the transitions between areas showing degeneration and areas free from degeneration. In the medial vestibular nucleus (M), degeneration at the level shown is restricted to the lateral regions. In the lateral nucleus (L), a relatively sharp border (arrows) is seen between the ventral regions, showing degeneration, and the dorsal regions. Particularly in the latter, some perikarya of Deiter's cells are visible. To the right, degenerating fibres entering in the vestibular nerve (N. VIII). From Walberg, Bowsher and Brodal (1958)

Primary vestibular fibers crossing the midline to enter the contralateral vestibular nuclei have been described by some authors following lesions of the nerve. Presumably these findings (for example by LEIDLER, 1914, and INGVAR, 1918, using the Marchi method) can be explained as consequences of inadvertent damage to the vestibular nuclei. In spite of a careful search, no such fibers were found in our study (WALBERG et al., 1958), nor did CARPENTER (1960b) find any. This is consistent with previous observations in the Marchi material examined by RASMUSSEN (1932). Following stimulation of the vestibular nerve, SHIMAZU and PRECHT (1966) found no evidence for impulse transmission via primary fibers to the contralateral vestibular nuclei.

Collaterals of primary vestibular fibers to the reticular formation have been observed in Golgi material (LORENTE DE NÓ, 1933b; HAUGLIE-HANSSEN, 1968). They appear to be very scanty and to be restricted to the most dorsolateral part of the reticular formation. In an experimental study in cat CARPENTER (1960b) saw a few fibers of this kind. He also describes some fibers passing ventromedially "into and around the solitary fasciculus and its nucleus". In corresponding experiments in monkeys, CARPENTER (1960b) noted degeneration in the solitary fasciculus, and suggests that this may be due to interruption of fibers in the intermediate nerve. This may perhaps explain his findings in the cat. WALBERG et al. (1958) did not find any of these fibers, nor did they trace primary vestibular fibers to the sensory trigeminal nuclei, the abducent nucleus or the perihypoglossal nuclei (nucleus praepositus hypoglossi etc.). Primary vestibular fibers do not appear to ascend in the medial longitudinal fasciculus (CARPENTER, 1960b).

It follows from the anatomical distribution of primary vestibular fibers that *impulses from the labyrinth cannot activate all parts of the vestibular nuclear complex monosynaptically*. We shall come back to the anatomical possibilities for an activation of the non-vestibular regions later. Before discussing this, it is appropriate to consider some other important issues.

The first of these is the question *whether fibers from the individual cristae and maculae have separate projection areas within the vestibular nuclei*. A further problem is whether the different kinds of receptor cells found in the sensory epithelia of the labyrinth (the flask-shaped type I cells and the cylindrical type II cells, see WERSÄLL, this volume) differ with regard to the distribution or types of endings of their central fibers. While at present nothing can be said about this, some information relevant to the first question is available.

LORENTE DE NÓ (1931) gave a detailed description of the bundles arising from the individual cristae and maculae and determined the topography of the associated ganglion cells, and in a subsequent paper he (LORENTE DE NÓ, 1933b) analyzed the distribution within the vestibular nuclei of the fibers arising from the various parts of the ganglion (Golgi preparations of the mouse). He distinguished 5 groups of such fibers. If the findings in the two studies are combined it appears that even if the fibers from the maculae and the cristae have some different central representations there is no clear selective distribution. Although the interpretation of LORENTE DE NÓ's findings in mouse meets with some difficulties (on account of differences in delimitations of nuclei and nomenclature), it appears that fibers from the cristae terminate in the superior vestibular nucleus, the most lateral parts of the descending nucleus and in what appears to be the medial nucleus but not the lateral (Deiters') nucleus. This receives fibers to its ventral regions from the utricular macula. Fibers from this also supply the descending nucleus, which also receives fibers from the saccular macula.

The results of the first experimental study of this kind performed by STEIN and CARPENTER (1967) in monkey are in general agreement with the above pattern. The authors traced the central distribution of the fibers degenerating as a consequence of small lesions of the different parts of the vestibular ganglia. Figure 29 shows their summarizing diagram. The fibers from the three cristae appear to terminate largely in the same regions, even if those from the crista of the posterior

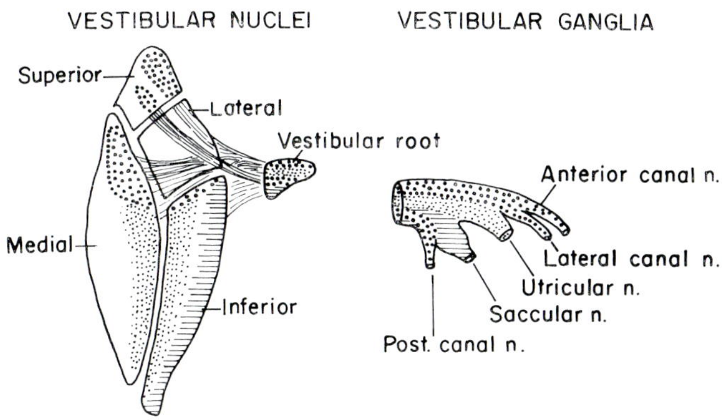

Fig. 29. Diagrammatic representation of relationships between portions of the vestibular ganglia and central projecting fibres within the vestibular nuclear complex. The vestibular ganglia and peripheral branches are shown on the right. The canal nerves and portions of the ganglia innervating the canal nerves are shown with coarse dots; the utricular part of the superior vestibular ganglion is shown with fine dots, while the saccular ganglion is shown with hatchings. On the left the vestibular nuclei and root are shown as they would appear in a horizontal section of the brain stem. Only the principal central projections of distinctive parts of the vestibular ganglia are shown. Portions of the vestibular ganglia innervating the cristae of the semicircular canals project primarily to the superior vestibular nucleus and rostral parts of the medial vestibular nucleus. Portions of the vestibular ganglia innervating the macula of the utricle project primarily to parts of the medial and descending vestibular nuclei. Central fibres from the saccular ganglion project mainly to dorsolateral parts of the descending vestibular nucleus. From STEIN and CARPENTER (1967)

canal travel in a different branch of the nerve than the fibers from the two other canals. The terminations of the main components are described in the legend to Fig. 29. The diagram does not show the partially different distribution of fibers from the three canals within their total area, especially in the superior nucleus, which was mentioned in the discussion of the ascending projections from the vestibular nuclei (p. 291, see also the illustrations in the original paper). It will be noted that there are no symbols in the lateral nucleus, but according to the authors some fibers from the utricle give off collaterals to the ventral part of the nucleus. The authors state that the lesions of the utricular part of the ganglion were the most difficult to produce, and it may be that this explains the scanty projection to the lateral nucleus, especially since in a previous study CARPENTER (1960b) found that medial fibers of the root projected to the medial and ventral part of the lateral vestibular nuclei. It is, however, possible that the utricular projection to the lateral nucleus is more sparse in monkey than in cat.[9] This assumption receives support from Gacek's experimental study (1969) in cat. Following small lesions of the utricular part of the vestibular ganglion, degenerating fibers were found to terminate on cells in the ventral part of the lateral vestibular nucleus (as well as in the rostral part of the medial nucleus and parts of the descending but not in the superior nucleus). On the whole, Gacek's (1969) findings correspond to those made by Stein and Carpenter (1967) in monkey. Concerning Gacek's (1969) findings of a differential distribution of canal fibers within the superior nucleus, the reader is referred to the original paper. Of particular interest is his observation that the group y of Brodal and Pompeiano (1957) receives vestibular afferents only from the saccule. Scanty fibers from the saccule pass to the rostral part of the descending and a few to the ventral part of the lateral nucleus.

Physiological studies (for details see Precht, this Handbook) are quite compatible with anatomical studies as far as the distribution of primary vestibular fibers is concerned. For example, units responding to horizontal, angular acceleration have been observed in the medial vestibular nucleus in the rabbit (Eckel, 1954; and others). In cat electrical stimulation of the labyrinth excites cells in the medial nucleus, mainly in its rostral part, monosynaptically (Wilson et al., 1968b), where a fair number of primary vestibular afferents end (cp. Figs. 27 and 29). These neurons belong to type I kinetic neurons, activated from the horizontal canal (Precht and Shimazu, 1965), while the tonic type I units are apparently activated multisynaptically. Type I neurons responding to angular horizontal acceleration also occur in the superior nucleus (Precht and Shimazu, 1965; Shimazu and Precht, 1965), a few also in the descending and lateral nucleus. Units activated from the vertical canals are likewise found mainly in the superior and medial vestibular nuclei (Markham, 1968).

In the lateral vestibular nucleus units responding monosynaptically to vestibular nerve stimulation were found in the rostroventral part (Wilson et al., 1967) in agreement with the distribution of primary vestibular fibers (Fig. 27). Adrian (1943) first observed responses to changes in the position of the head in space in the caudal regions of vestibular nuclei in the cat. Peterson (1967) performed a systematic analysis and found single units activated by tilting (and presumably arising from stimulation of the receptor cells in the utricle) in all of the four main nuclei, but with the highest ratio in the descending and lateral nucleus. In the latter the most responsive cells were found chiefly in its ventral part. The majority of the highly responsive cells were found to be activated monosynaptically.

Even if particular receptor organs thus appear to effect monosynaptic activation of cells in different regions of the total area of the vestibular nuclei which receives primary vestibular fibers, there is no complete segregation. Physiological studies have shown (see Precht, this volume) that many neurons in the nuclei are activated by impulses from different receptor organs, while others derive their input from one organ only. There is even convergence of impulses on single units from otolith organs and semicircular canal organs, which is of interest from a clinical point of view. The basis for the convergence must be sought in the anatomical arrangements of the primary vestibular fibers, more specifically the course and length of their dichotomizing branches.

9 According to Stein and Carpenter (1967) all five receptor regions appear to project onto the interstitial nucleus of the vestibular nerve, but to different parts of it. In cat, Gacek (1969) found no fibers from the maculae (utricle and sacculus) ending in the interstitial nucleus. The fibers from the superior and horizontal canal end in the rostral part of the nucleus, those from the posterior canal in its caudal part.

It must be assumed from the experimental studies of Stein and Carpenter (1967) that the length and distribution of the ascending and descending branches of primary fibers from different receptor organs are not identical. Impulses from various receptor organs may converge by way of collaterals of fibers running in parallel (for example fibers from the three canals in the superior nucleus), or the convergence may be explained if some of the fibers from a receptor organ are assumed not to behave in the same way as the majority but to join fibers from another receptor organ; for example, some fibers from the utricle may send an ascending branch to the superior nucleus. Other mechanisms can also be imagined, but the slender evidence for purely internuncial cells in the vestibular nuclei (see p. 330) should be recalled in attempts to explain the anatomical basis of the convergence established physiologically.

The problems of convergence within the vestibular nuclei of impulses from the receptor organs lead us to a consideration of another subject: the *patterns of terminal arborizations of primary vestibular fibers and their synaptic contacts.* When studying the degeneration within the vestibular nuclei following transection of the vestibular nerve in the cat Walberg et al. (1958) noted that following incomplete lesions of the nerve the degenerating terminals are aggregated in small clusters, often lying rather far apart. This was taken to suggest that a single axon may give rise to such a group of terminals, *i.e.* that the spatial distribution of a single axon is rather restricted. This fits in with the results in Golgi preparations (Hauglie-Hanssen, 1968). The ascending and descending branches of the primary vestibular fibers (Fig. 26) deliver collaterals directed medially, which give off numerous short side-branches along their course. Some of the branches are simple, while others show a small number of sub-branches making up small clusters. Each side-branch

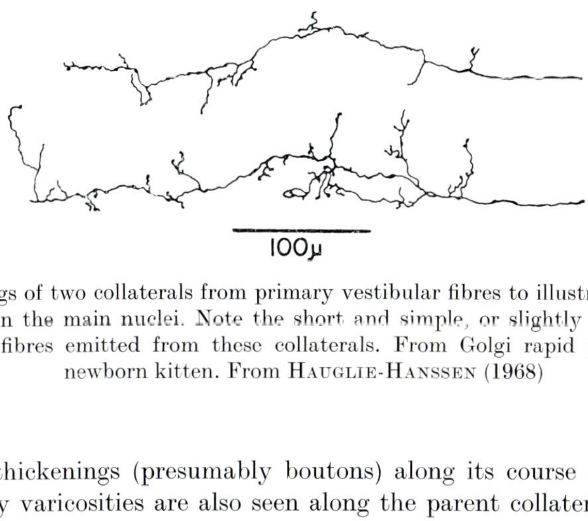

Fig. 30. Drawings of two collaterals from primary vestibular fibres to illustrate their mode of branching within the main nuclei. Note the short and simple, or slightly branched, preterminal-terminal fibres emitted from these collaterals. From Golgi rapid preparations of a newborn kitten. From Hauglie-Hanssen (1968)

shows small thickenings (presumably boutons) along its course and at its ends (Fig. 30). Tiny varicosities are also seen along the parent collaterals. Due to the parallel course of the collaterals and the small side-branches, the terminal field covered by the collaterals of each descending branch is a rather narrow zone extending from lateral to medial (Fig. 31b). In spite of some overlapping this arrangement appears to favor a spatially precise transmission of impulses from the vestibular receptors through the vestibular nuclei.

A closer analysis of the terminal and preterminal branches of the axons of afferent fibers to the vestibular nuclei shows that they differ morphologically (see

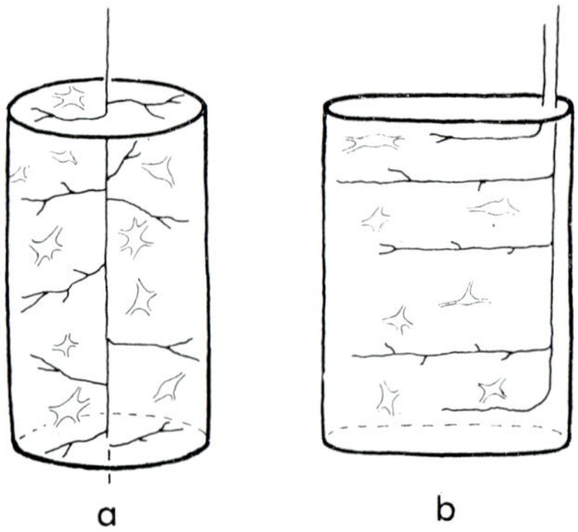

Fig. 31. Schematic drawing to illustrate principal features concerning the distribution of collaterals and terminals from individual stem fibres as found on ipsilateral cerebellovestibular afferents (a) and on primary vestibular fibres and crossed fastigiovestibular afferents (b). The collateral and terminal fibres from each ipsilateral, probably cortical, cerebellovestibular stem fibre are found within an area represented by a cylinder around the fibre. Collaterals from the primary vestibular fibres and the fastigial collaterals are found within narrow lamellae, mainly oriented medially and ventromedially, respectively. From Hauglie-Hanssen (1968)

also section on intrinsic organization). Hauglie-Hanssen (1968) distinguishes three types (see Fig. 32).[10] Fibers of his types 2 and 3 often "climb" along soma and dendrites of the nerve cells. It was not possible to find evidence that a particular contingent of afferents is provided with only one type of terminals. Cajal (1896, 1909) held that the "pericellular baskets" found in the nucleus of Deiters are formed by collaterals of primary vestibular fibers. This view is scarcely tenable, since Hauglie-Hanssen (1968) found other afferents, particularly the cerebellovestibular fibers, to participate in the formation of such baskets. According to Hauglie-Hanssen (1968, p. 92) "it is obvious that the pericellular baskets seen in Golgi preparations represent a generalized mode of organization of terminal

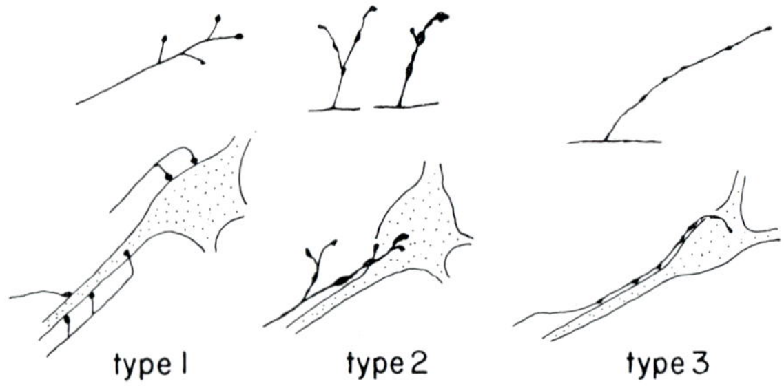

Fig. 32. Schematic drawing to indicate the general features of the three main types of terminal fibres distinguished in Golgi material from the vestibular nuclear complex in kittens (cp. text). From Hauglie-Hanssen (1968)

10 Mugnaini, Walberg and Hauglie-Hanssen (1967) undertake a further differentiation into five types.

axonal arborizations related to the proximal (or primary) dendrites and the somata and that these baskets are composed of terminal fibers of various types and, most probably, from various sources." This conclusion is supported by electron-microscope studies of the degeneration following transection of the vestibular nerve (MUGNAINI et al., 1967). So far these are limited to the lateral vestibular nuclei.

In silver-impregnated sections of the lateral vestibular nucleus following lesions of the vestibular nerve, "baskets" of degenerating fibers are often seen around cells in the rostroventral part of the nucleus of Deiters (Fig. 33). From a study of material of this kind WALBERG et al. (1958) concluded that primary vestibular fibers establish contact with somata and proximal dendrites of nerve cells in the lateral vestibular nucleus (its rostroventral part). The presence of

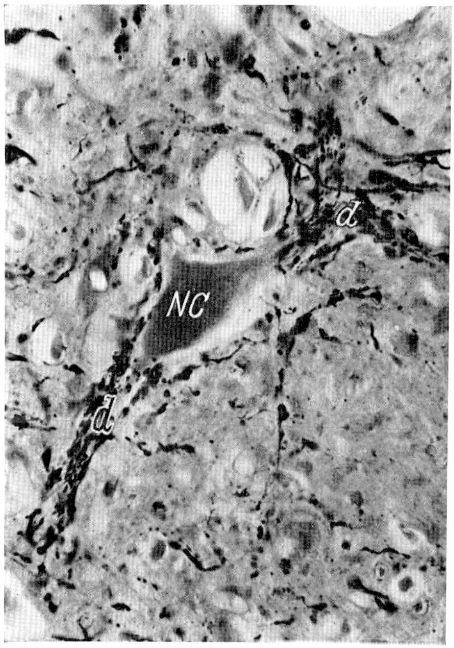

Fig. 33. Light micrograph of a Nauta section from the nucleus of Deiters in a cat killed 5 days after a lesion of the eighth nerve. Note the degenerating fibres and fragments along the dendrites (d) and the soma (NC) of a small cell. Degenerating fragments are present also in the neuropil. In addition many small granules are present in the section, but the exact nature of these can not be established. × 270. From MUGNAINI, WALBERG and BRODAL (1967)

degenerating fragments in the neuropil (Fig. 33) suggests that contacts may be established also with thin, distal dendrites. The authors further noted that while contacts with small cells were easily found, practically all giant cells were free from contact with degenerating fibers. As mentioned previously, final conclusions cannot be drawn concerning synaptic relationships from findings in silver-impregnated sections. The study of degenerating boutons with the electron microscope

(MUGNAINI et al., 1967) has, however, confirmed that *primary vestibular fibers contact somata, as well as thick and thin dendrites in the rostroventral part of the nucleus of Deiters*. The constant presence of a number of normal boutons on the cells contacted by degenerating ones shows that the cells are contacted by other afferents than primary vestibular fibers, as mentioned above. These must belong to other fibers known to end in this part of the nucleus of Deiters, as has been demonstrated by WALBERG and MUGNAINI (1969). In the electron-microscope studies synaptic contacts were occasionally seen also with giant cells. This is compatible with the results of the physiological study of WILSON et al. (1967).

The degenerating boutons can be recognized as early as two days after transection of the vestibular nerve. They appear as dark, often irregularly shaped bodies, with a finely granular appearance of the matrix, mitochondrial changes and changes in the synaptic vesicles. The changes proceed very rapidly, and after 9–11 days practically no degenerating boutons are left. It appears that astroglia takes part in the process of removal, but other factors may also be involved (see MUGNAINI et al., 1967, for particulars). The rapidity of the process contrasts with the slower speed of degeneration of the cerebellovestibular fibers. The degenerating boutons appear to be of the rounded type seen in normal material (MUGNAINI et al., 1967).

As we have seen, the area of termination of primary vestibular fibers in the nucleus of Deiters covers its "forelimb region" only. A correlation of the regions supplied by primary fibers in the other subdivisions of the nuclear complex with the sites of termination and origin of other connections of these nuclei is of some functional interest. The subject will be considered in the final section of the present chapter.

B. Spinal Afferents to the Vestibular Nuclei

While the efferent projections of the vestibular nuclei to the spinal cord are rather massive, direct pathways from the cord to the vestibular nuclear complex are modest. It appears that most of the influences exerted by the cord on the vestibular nuclei must occur via indirect spinovestibular pathways (see below).

Early authors such as THIELE and HORSLEY (1901) and COLLIER and BUZZARD (1903) worked with Marchi preparations of human material and described spinovestibular fibers arising largely in the lumbar cord.

Fairly similar findings were reported by McNALTY and HORSLEY (1909) and by HASHIMOTO (1928). Some of these authors indicate the nucleus of Deiters as the main site of termination of spinovestibular fibers. COLLIER and BUZZARD (1903) advocated that the fibers ascend with, or are collaterals of, fibers of the ventral spinocerebellar tract, but most authors found them to pass with the dorsal spinocerebellar fibers. According to LORENTE DE NÓ's (1924) Golgi studies in the mouse all or practically all fibers of the dorsal spinocerebellar tract give off one, two or three collaterals to the vestibular nuclei. The area of termination is restricted to the ventrocaudal part of the descending nucleus and the ventrolateral part of the medial nucleus. HAUGLIE-HANSSEN (1968), in his Golgi studies, also noted fibers to the caudal part of the lateral nucleus and the group x of BRODAL and POMPEIANO (1957).

Experimental studies are necessary to obtain more precise data on the spinovestibular projection. Using the GLEES (1946) method, POMPEIANO and BRODAL (1957b) mapped the degeneration occurring in the vestibular nuclei of the cat

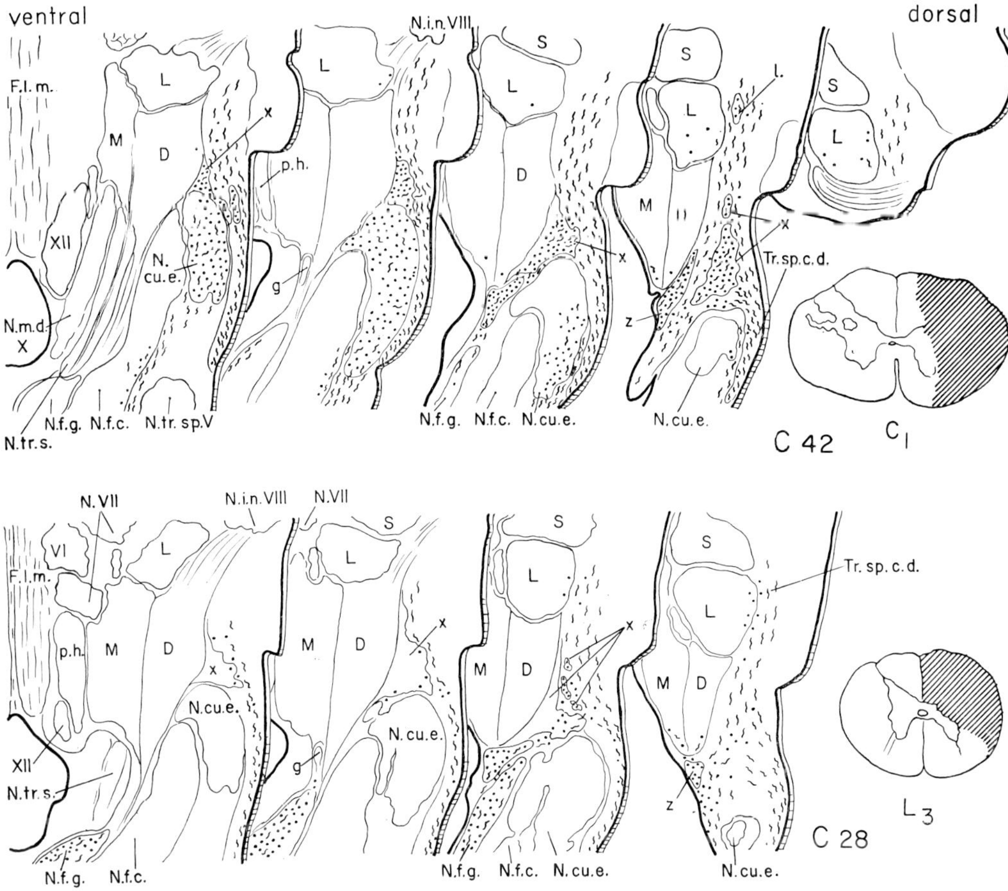

Fig. 34. Diagrams showing the sites of terminations of spinovestibular fibres (dots) as seen in series of horizontal sections of two cats subjected to spinal cord lesion at C_1 and L_3, respectively. (The degeneration in the external cuneate nucleus and dorsal column nuclei is due to concomitant lesion of the dorsal columns.) Note abundant degeneration in groups x and z following a lesion at C_1 and restriction of degeneration to the dorsal part of group x with a lesion at L_3. From Pompeiano and Brodal (1957b)

following lesions at various levels of the cord and involving different parts of its cross-sectional area. As a control a corresponding study was made later with the Nauta (1957) method (Brodal and Angaut, 1967). The results of the two studies were concordant. *The direct spinovestibular projection in cat was found to be very modest* (Fig. 34) *and entirely ipsilateral*. The fibers ascend in the dorsal half of the lateral funiculus. In agreement with Lorente de Nó (1924) some degeneration was found in *the most caudal part of the descending and medial nuclei*, and the observations of some authors of fibers to the lateral vestibular nucleus were confirmed. Degeneration within *the lateral nucleus* is slight and is confined to its dorsal and caudal parts. The only parts of the vestibular nuclear complex which show ample degeneration following spinal cord lesions are *groups x* and *z* (Fig. 34). In group x the fibers end in a somatotopical pattern, fibers from caudal segments ending most dorsocaudally (POMPEIANO and BRODAL, 1957b).

A comparison of the findings in different cases shows that *a large proportion of the direct spinovestibular fibers comes from low levels of the cord.* Even following a lesion at L_5 there is clear-cut degeneration in the nuclei (BRODAL and ANGAUT, 1967). LORENTE DE NÓ (1924) appears to have included group x in the descending nucleus and to have traced abundant spinal afferents to it. This is of interest in relation to the question whether the spinovestibular afferents are collaterals of dorsal spinocerebellar fibers or are independent fibers, even if they run together in the cord and in the restiform body. It appears that *at least many of the spinovestibular afferents are not collaterals of fibers of the dorsal spinocerebellar tract,* since there is clear-cut degeneration in the nuclei following lesions of the cord below levels of the caudal end of the column of Clarke (L_4 in the cat). Furthermore, some of the fibers are so coarse that they are unlikely to be collaterals.[11] Final conclusions as to synaptic contacts cannot be made, but there is suggestive evidence of contacts with dendrites, since most degenerating particles in Nauta sections are found in the neuropil (BRODAL and ANGAUT, 1967). In Glees sections (POMPEIANO and BRODAL, 1957b) degenerating terminal boutons are occasionally seen on the surfaces of perikarya.

Observations on spinovestibular fibers have been made in studies with the Nauta method in monkey by MEHLER, FEFERMAN and NAUTA (1960), who in their Fig. 2B indicate terminations in the lateral vestibular nucleus, but no details are given. In man, BOWSHER (1962) found the spinal afferents to the nucleus of Deiters to be restricted to its dorsal part and in addition found terminations in a group which appears to be group x in man (see SADJADPOUR and BRODAL, 1968).

As will be seen, *the direct spinovestibular fibers are distributed only to parts of the vestibular nuclear complex which do not receive primary vestibular afferents.* Of particular interest is the termination in the dorsocaudal part only of the nucleus of Deiters, its hindlimb region, since at least most of the spinovestibular fibers come from lower levels of the cord. The ample terminations in the group x, which projects onto the cerebellum (see Fig. 20), points to the presence of a spinocerebellar pathway via the vestibular nuclei to which little interest has yet been devoted.

In view of the scanty number of spinal afferents it might be assumed that spinal impulses are of little relevance for the function of the vestibular nuclei, an assumption which seems somewhat strange. In fact, it has been conclusively demonstrated by WILSON et al. (1966, 1967; see also PRECHT, this volume) that the cells in Deiters' nucleus, in both its forelimb region and its hindlimb region, are markedly influenced (facilitated) by spinal impulses, and according to ITO et al. (1964) they can be monosynaptically activated from the cervical cord. Cells in the medial nucleus, especially ventrally, can also be synaptically activated from the spinal cord (WILSON et al., 1968b). It appears from the careful experiments of Wilson et al. (1966), however, that the direct spinovestibular fibers are involved only to a slight extent in the facilitation by spinal impulses if at all. According to these authors the most likely pathways are spinal afferents to the reticular formation and collaterals or axons of cells in this which reach the vestibular nuclei, among them the nucleus of Deiters. ITO et al. (1966) maintain that impulses from the spinal cord entering the inferior olive are propagated via colla-

11 It cannot be entirely excluded that some fibers to groups x and z ascend in the dorsal funiculus.

terals of olivocerebellar fibers to Deiters' nucleus where they produce (probably monosynaptic) EPSPs. Since the olivocerebellar fibers are assumed to end as climbing fibers on Purkinje cells, the impulses ascending via the olive will further produce inhibitory potentials in the cells in Deiters' nucleus by way of Purkinje cell axons. Conclusive anatomical evidence for collaterals of olivocerebellar fibers to the vestibular nuclei appears so far not to have been brought forward, but LORENTE DE NÓ (1924) considers it likely that such collaterals exist (see also p. 327). An influence of spinal impulses on the vestibular nuclei via the cerebellum may also occur via other relays (for example group x, as mentioned above). Since the observations of WILSON et al. (1966) were made in decerebellated cats, it is clear, however, that the cerebellum is at least not essential for the mediation of spinal influences on the nucleus of Deiters. For a further discussion of the physiology of the spinovestibular relations the reader is referred to other chapters of this volume. For a review of possible anatomical pathways see BRODAL (1967a).

C. Fibers from the Cerebellum to the Vestibular Nuclei

As mentioned previously, the largest contingent of afferents to the vestibular nuclei comes from the cerebellum. However, it is scarcely correct to consider the cerebellar afferents as belonging to one contingent. Some fibers come from the "vestibular part" of the cerebellum, others from its "spinal part". Among the latter some fibers pass directly from the cerebellar cortex to the vestibular nuclei, while others have a relay in the fastigial nucleus. It will be appropriate to discuss the three groups of cerebellovestibular projections separately.

1. The Projection of the "Vestibulocerebellum" onto the Vestibular Nuclei

As mentioned previously, the "vestibulocerebellum" is generally said to correspond to the flocculus and nodulus (the flocculonodular lobe). According to the distribution of primary vestibular fibers to the cerebellum, however, the concept should be extended to comprise the caudal (ventral) part of the uvula, the ventral paraflocculus and the ventralmost, small-celled part of the lateral cerebellar nucleus (see Fig. 19 and BRODAL and HØIVIK, 1964).

Experimental studies on the efferent projections of these cerebellar subdivisions are scanty, and such studies involve considerable technical difficulties. Some early authors who claimed to have made lesions in the flocculus in the rabbit obviously referred to the lobulus petrosus by this term, which represents the paraflocculus in this animal (see BRODAL, 1940c, for comments). The first systematic studies of the projections are those of DOW (1936, 1938a), who used the Marchi method in cat and rat (1936) and in monkey (1938a) and succeeded in making small lesions.

DOW described two fiber bundles passing from the flocculus to the brainstem: a dorsal one becomes mixed up with fibers of the brachium conjunctivum and ends in the homolateral superior vestibular nucleus. A second, more ventral bundle arches around the restiform body, and most of its fibers end in the lateral part of the lateral vestibular nucleus, some in the superior nucleus. Fibers from the flocculus to the nucleus fastigii and the nucleus dentatus were not found, and no fibers from the paraflocculus were seen to pass to the vestibular nuclei. GEREBTZOFF (1941), who worked with rabbit, largely confirmed DOW's findings.

As far as the "vermal" part of the "vestibulocerebellum", the nodulus and uvula, is concerned, DOW, although he did not achieve isolated lesions of either the nodulus or the uvula, was able to conclude from his cases that both lobules send fibers to all four main vestibular nuclei on the homolateral side as well as to the nucleus fastigii. The pyramis does not give off fibers to the vestibular nuclei. Observation supporting the conclusions of DOW have been made by JANSEN and BRODAL (1940, 1942) in Marchi studies in rabbit, cat and monkey. VOOGD

(1964), who used both the Häggqvist and the Nauta method, traced projections from both parts of the "vestibulocerebellum" to the superior, descending and medial nuclei, while the lateral vestibular nucleus, as defined by him, is devoid of such fibers. Within the former nuclei the two contingents of fibers have in part different sites of ending.

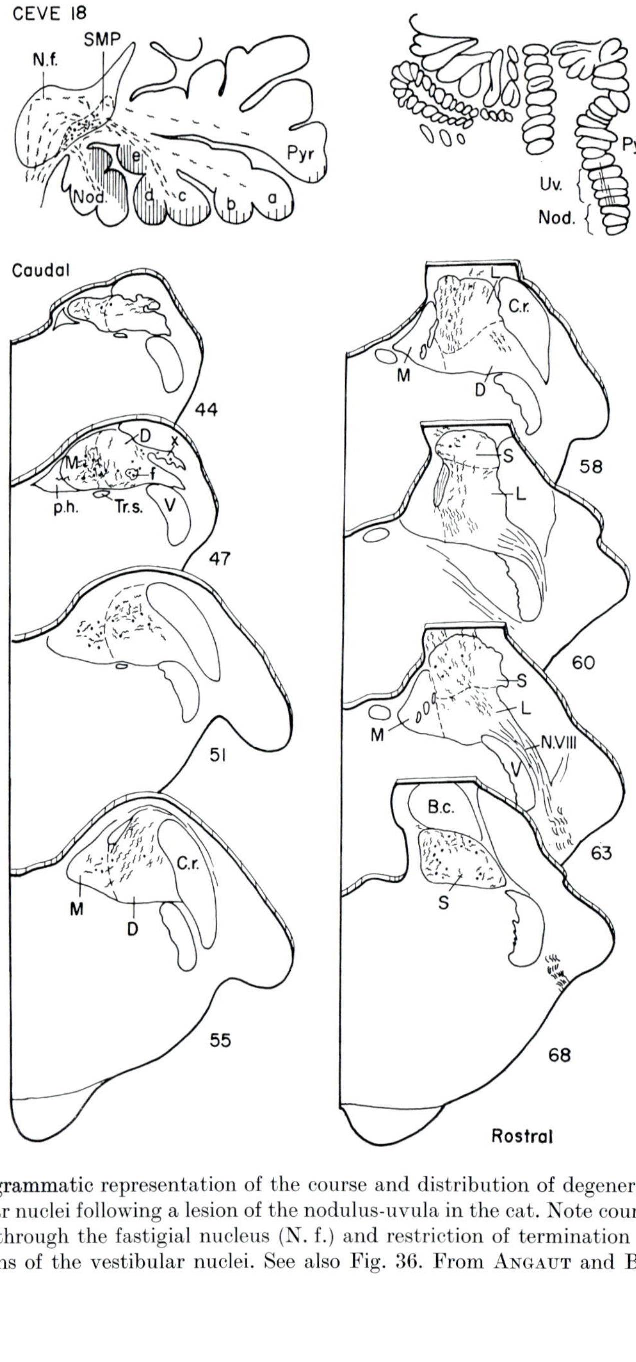

Fig. 35. Diagrammatic representation of the course and distribution of degenerating fibres in the vestibular nuclei following a lesion of the nodulus-uvula in the cat. Note course of degenerating fibres through the fastigial nucleus (N. f.) and restriction of termination (dots) to particular regions of the vestibular nuclei. See also Fig. 36. From Angaut and Brodal (1967)

In view of the very specific sites of termination within the vestibular nuclear complex of other afferent contingents established in recent studies, it was deemed to be of interest to make an attempt to see if a corresponding specific pattern is present in the termination of the afferents from the "vestibulocerebellum". In an experimental study in cat with the Nauta method (ANGAUT and BRODAL, 1967) it was found that this is indeed the case. The findings, which add to those made by previous workers on several points, are summarized below.

From the *flocculus*, two fiber bundles pass to the ipsilateral vestibular nuclear complex. A smaller bundle, corresponding to LÖWY's "*angular bundle*", spreads out in a rostrocaudal direction and *supplies the superior and the medial nucleus*, the latter only in its small rostral expansion. *A second bundle*, passing ventrally in a more lateral position than the angular bundle, *gives off fibers to all four main vestibular nuclei and group f in the descending vestibular nucleus*. Caudally some fibers enter the solitary tract and its nucleus, while others pass medially and supply the *nucleus praepositus hypoglossi*. In all main vestibular nuclei the fibers from the flocculus terminate in rather circumscribed regions, as can be seen in the summarizing diagram of Fig. 36. In most of the cases there was some injury to the paraflocculus, and it may be that some of the fibers to the solitary tract are derived from this. Lesions restricted to the paraflocculus did not give rise to degeneration in the vestibular nuclei, confirming the conclusion of most previous workers that *the paraflocculus does not project onto the vestibular nuclei*.

The *nodulus and uvula* differ to some extent from the flocculus in their vestibular projection. It was impossible to damage the nodulus without some concomitant damage to the uvula, while the uvula could be injured separately. However, a comparison of several cases permitted a fairly precise analysis of the projection of the two lobules. They turned out to differ in some respects. *Both projections appear to be ipsilateral only*. Figure 35 shows the findings in one of the cases. It should be noted that many efferent fibers of both lobules pass through the fastigial nucleus, most of them in its caudoventral part (where some fibers end), while others follow a dorsally curved course through the nucleus (for particulars see ANGAUT and BRODAL, 1967). Some fibers pass through the most medial part of the nucleus interpositus (as delimited by COURVILLE and BRODAL, 1966). They all leave in the inferior cerebellar peduncle. The uvular fibers to the vestibular nuclei appear to be derived mainly from its ventral (caudal) part. No fibers were traced from the pyramis to the vestibular nuclei.

The *uvula sends fibers to the superior vestibular nucleus*, chiefly to its peripheral part, *to group x*, and *to the descending nucleus*, particularly its caudal half. No uvular fibers end in the medial nucleus. There is some doubt about the *lateral nucleus*, but it appears extremely likely that it receives some uvular fibers.

The *nodulus gives off fibers to the superior nucleus*, chiefly peripherally, *to the medial nucleus*, chiefly caudally and medially, *to the descending nucleus*, chiefly ventrocaudally, *to group f*, and *to group x*. A few fibers pass to the caudodorsal part of the *lateral nucleus* and to the *nucleus praepositus hypoglossi*.

Most of the fibers from the vestibulocerebellum are rather thin. Only rarely have degenerating fiber fragments been found closely attached to the perikarya or to thick dendrites of cells in the vestibular nuclei. Most fragments were found

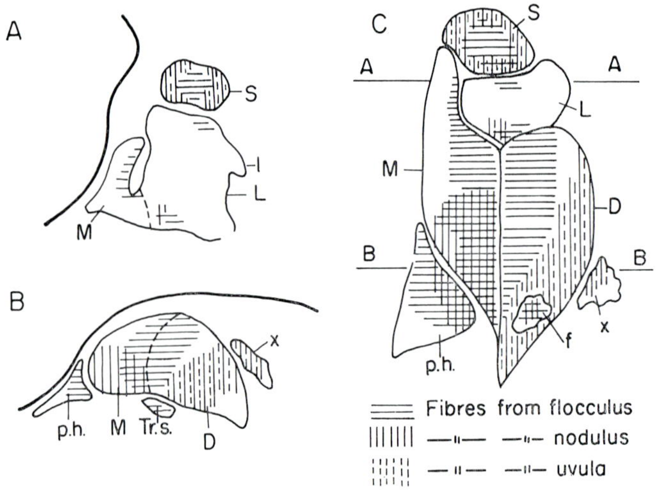

Fig. 36. Diagrams summarizing the projections of different parts of the vestibulocerebellum onto the vestibular nuclei in the cat. The distributions within the vestibular nuclei of afferents from the flocculus, the nodulus and the uvula are shown by different symbols (see key below). *A* and *B*, from transverse sections at two levels, rostral and caudal, respectively. *C*, from a horizontal section. The levels of drawings *A* and *B* are indicated. Differences in density of terminations are not shown. Note that the contingents of fibres from the vermal and hemispheral parts of the "vestibulocerebellum" largely have their particular fields of termination within the individual nuclei, although there is considerably more overlapping than appears from the schematic drawings. For abbreviations see list on p. 340. From Angaut and Brodal (1967)

in the neuropil. This suggests, but does not prove, that most of the fibers establish synaptic contact with thin dendrites.

The diagram of Fig. 36 summarizes the distribution of the afferents to the vestibular nuclei from the "vestibulocerebellum". (The projections to the nucleus praepositus hypoglossi and the nucleus of the solitary tract are included.) As will be seen, among the four large vestibular nuclei the lateral nucleus appears to be the one that is least well supplied from the "vestibulocerebellum". Within the projections to the other main nuclei there is a clear-cut organization. *Even if there is a certain overlapping between the terminal regions of the afferents from the flocculus and the nodulus-uvula, the two groups of afferents are generally distributed to different areas within each of the nuclei. Furthermore, the terminal areas of the fibers from the uvula (its ventral part) are not entirely the same as those of the nodular fibers.*[12] These anatomical features show that the influence of the various lobules of the "vestibulocerebellum" on the vestibular nuclei cannot be identical, and suggest that there must be functional dissimilarities between the lobules.

Voogd (1964) and van Rossum (1969) studied the vestibular projections of the nodulus and uvula in cat and rabbit respectively. Their findings of the distribution

12 No information is available as to whether the vestibular nuclei receive fibers from the small-celled part of the lateral (dentate) cerebellar nucleus, presumably belonging to the "vestibulocerebellum", though there are occasional references in the literature to fibers from the dentate to the vestibular nuclei.

of fibers within the vestibular nuclei, though less detailed, appear to correspond with those of Angaut and Brodal (1967). In addition they found that these vestibular fibers are derived only from one of the longitudinal zones of the cerebellum, the zone B of Voogd (1964). Van Rossum (1969) maintains that three subzones of the zone B in the nodulus-uvula project (from medial to lateral) specifically to the descending, the superior and the medial nucleus, respectively.

The preferential distribution of afferents from the flocculus and the nodulus-uvula is further evidence indicating a far-reaching differentiation within the vestibular nuclear complex. Comparison of the pattern with that of other connections of the nuclei reveals that in the medial, the superior and the descending nucleus, afferents from the flocculus end preferentially in areas which receive primary vestibular fibers, while the afferents from the nodulus-uvula cover territories supplied from the contralateral fastigial nucleus. Even if the distributions of the fiber contingents which end in particular regions of the nuclei are not exactly identical, the convergence indicates that there must be possibilities for a close functional cooperation between the impulses carried by the afferents from different sources to a particular nuclear region.

The relatively scarce physiological studies of the "vestibulocerebellum" have been devoted chiefly to studies of the nodulus-uvula. It appears that these two lobules both exert an inhibitory action on the vestibular nuclei (Dow, 1938b; Fernandéz and Fredrickson, 1964; Grant et al., 1964, etc.). The fact that unilateral lesion or stimulation of the nodulus-uvula results in clearly asymmetrical reactions may be correlated with the almost exclusively ipsilateral projections of these lobules. According to Grant et al. (1964), lesions of the nodulus and of the uvula provoke positional nystagmus in opposite directions (in rabbit). The authors suggest that this is related to the function of the fastigial nucleus as a link in the efferent path from the uvula but not in that from the nodulus. An alternative or supplementary explanation might be that the two lobules differ in their projections onto the vestibular nuclei. Thus the nodulus but not the uvula projects onto the medial vestibular nucleus. The available physiological data appear to be too scanty to permit any conclusions as to whether the different projections of the nodulus-uvula and the flocculus are reflected functionally. Single unit studies of the vestibular afferents from the "vestibulocerebellum" might be rewarding.

2. The Direct Projections from the "Spinal" Parts of the Cerebellum to the Vestibular Nuclei

Fibers passing from the vermis of the cerebellum to the vestibular nuclei have been known since the early experimental Marchi studies of Allen (1924), Hohman (1929) and others (for references see Brodal et al., 1962). Most of the relevant observations were made in studies primarily devoted to the cerebellar cortical projections to the intracerebellar nuclei, and they were undertaken at a time when the functional subdivision of the cerebellum was poorly understood and the complexity of the vestibular nuclei was not known. Accordingly, little information can be gathered from these studies, although most of them agree that the fibers are entirely ipsilateral and reach the vestibular nuclei via the inferior cerebellar peduncle.

In recent years some workers have investigated the direct corticocerebellar projections to the vestibular nuclei more closely with silver-impregnation methods. Walberg and Jansen (1961) found that rather abundant fibers arose from the vermis of the anterior lobe in cat, some from the posterior vermis (chiefly the pyramis and rostral part of the uvula), while the middle parts of the vermis, especially Larsell's lobulus VI, appear to give off few, if any, fibers to the vestibular nuclei. Fibers from the different regions end within the same territory of the ipsilateral vestibular nuclei, but *the sites of termination are restricted to the dorsorostral part of the descending nucleus and the dorsal part of the lateral nucleus.* There are a few fibers to the superior nucleus (see also VOOGD, 1964), but none could be traced to the medial nucleus or to the smaller cell groups. The projections onto the nucleus of Deiters

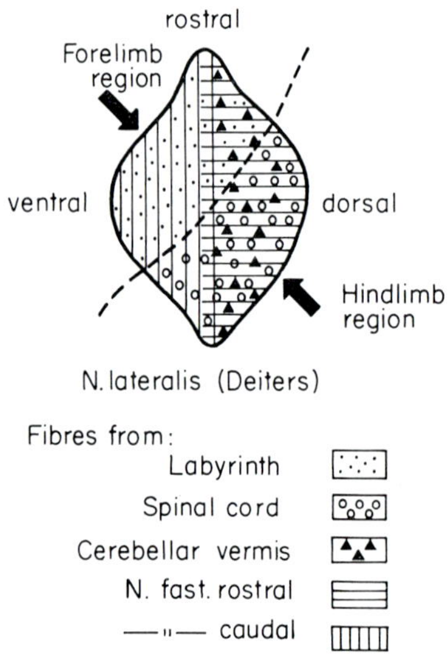

Fig. 37. Diagram of a sagittal reconstruction of the lateral vestibular nucleus of Deiters showing the sites of termination of some of its afferents (see key below) and their relations to the somatotopic subdivisions of the nucleus. Varying densities of terminations are not shown. Cf. text. From BRODAL (1967a)

is of particular interest for two reasons. Its restriction to the dorsal half only (see Figs. 37 and 39) means that it covers neither the entire "forelimb" nor the whole "hindlimb" region of the nucleus (cf. Fig. 15), since the ventral border of the terminal area runs across the border between the somatotopical regions (Fig. 37). Accordingly, parts only of both these regions receive fibers from the cerebellar vermis. Secondly, the experiments of WALBERG and JANSEN (1961) show that *the projection from the vermis of the anterior lobe to the nucleus of Deiters is somatotopically arranged.* Figure 38 shows one of their cases with a lesion involving chiefly the "forelimb" region of the anterior lobe. As will be seen, the dorsocaudal part of the nucleus (its "hindlimb" region) is almost free from degeneration. Lesions extending further anteriorly in the anterior lobe vermis result in degeneration extending also to the dorsocaudal part of the nucleus. The pattern of the projection is shown in the diagram of Fig. 39 (on the left). Less clear-cut findings have been reported by EAGER (1963) and VOOGD (1964). Whether the projection from the posterior vermis is somatotopically organized was not established. As mentioned previously, it should be realized that anatomical studies such as those

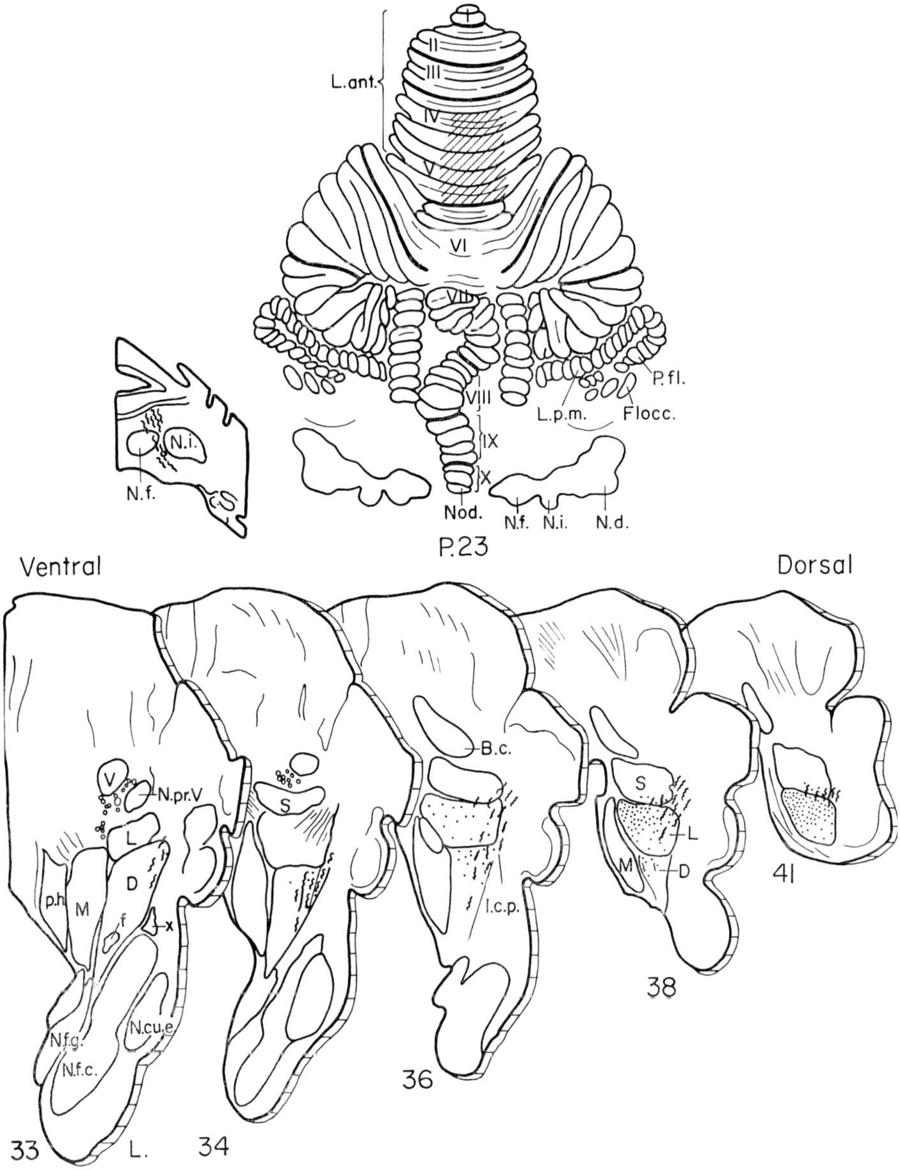

Fig. 38. Drawing showing the distribution of degeneration (dots) in the vestibular nuclei as seen in a series of horizontal sections from a cat in which a lesion (hatchings) had been made in the posterior part of the anterior lobe vermis. Note restriction of degeneration in the nucleus of Deiters (L) chiefly to its rostrodorsal part. Inset shows the relations of cerebello-cortico-vestibular fibres to the fastigial nucleus. From WALBERG and JANSEN (1961)

mentioned can only establish the main pattern in the somatotopical projection onto the nucleus of Deiters. The physiological studies of POMPEIANO and COTTI (1959; see also POMPEIANO, this volume) demonstrate that the localization is indeed sharp, since single units in the nucleus of Deiters may be influenced from one folium of the cortex, but not from the immediately neighboring ones.

VAN ROSSUM (1969), in rabbit, found a topical pattern which appears to agree with that described by WALBERG and JANSEN (1961). Concerning the origin of the fibers his findings differ somewhat from those of the latter authors. He also finds some fibers coming from Larsell's lobules VI, VII and VIII, as maintained also by EAGER (1963) and VOOGD (1964) in the cat. Of greater interest are the observations of VOOGD (1964) and VAN ROSSUM (1969) that the fibers from the cerebellar vermis to the nucleus of Deiters originate from only one of the longitudinal cerebellar zones of VOOGD (1964), zone B. These authors give evidence supporting the view of HOHMAN (1929) that the different contingents of cortical efferents arise as separate bundles from particular longitudinal zones, at least in the anterior lobe. A medial zone A sends fibers to the fastigial nucleus, then follows a zone B, projecting to the nucleus of Deiters, and more laterally a zone C, corresponding to the intermediate part of the cortex, which projects to the nucleus interpositus anterior. These observations are of considerable interest with regard to the longitudinal subdivision of the cerebellum established in physiological and other anatomical studies in recent years. (For some data see BRODAL, 1967b).

The course followed by the fibers is of some importance in experimental studies of the fastigial nucleus. As emphasized by WALBERG and JANSEN (1961) the cerebellar corticovestibular fibers are topographically closely related to the nucleus fastigii. The fibers from the anterior lobe pass rostral to or through the rostrolateral part of the fastigial nucleus (see inset in Fig. 38). The fibers from the caudal vermis largely pass ventral to the nucleus, but some fibers pursue a course dorsal to it. It follows from this that in experimental studies of the fastigial nucleus (recording of potentials, effects of stimulation, consequences of lesions) erroneous results may be obtained if the presence of cortico-cerebellovestibular fibers (as well as primary vestibulocerebellar fibers and fibers from the nodulus-uvula to the vestibular nuclei) passing through the fastigial nucleus is not taken into account.

In view of physiological demonstrations of a monosynaptic inhibitory action of the Purkinje cells on the neurons of the nucleus of Deiters (ITO and YOSHIDA, 1964, etc.) *the synaptic relationships between the cerebellocortical fibers and the cells in the nucleus of Deiters* are of interest. From their silver-impregnated sections WALBERG and JANSEN (1961) concluded that the majority of contacts are established with giant cells. Degenerating fragments were seen especially along proximal dendrites of such cells. In a corresponding experimental electron-microscope study, MUGNAINI and WALBERG (1967) brought forward more precise information by studying degenerating boutons in the nucleus of Deiters following lesions of the anterior lobe.[13] Synaptic contacts were found with cells of all sizes, and with soma, proximal and distal parts of dendrites and spine-like dendritic projections. Some of the degenerating boutons appear to belong to thin fibers seen in Golgi sections to end with small swellings, while others appear to represent degenerating specimens of the large, rounded or sausage-like boutons seen in normal material (MUGNAINI et al., 1967). These findings suggest that not all Purkinje axons

13 The cerebellar afferents differ from the primary vestibular fibers in their speed and pattern of degeneration (see MUGNAINI and WALBERG, 1967; MUGNAINI et al., 1967).

establish synaptic contacts of the same kind. This and the occurrence of synaptic contacts on all parts of the neuron are of physiological interest, particularly with regard to the question of whether the Purkinje cells are all inhibitory or not. (For a discussion see POMPEIANO, this Handbook.)

3. The Indirect Projections from the "Spinal" Parts of the Cerebellum to the Vestibular Nuclei

These pathways for cerebellar impulses to the vestibular nuclei have a *relay in the fastigial nucleus*. Some authors have claimed that the nucleus interpositus, or part of it, is involved as well, but so far decisive evidence in favor of this view has not been produced (for some data see FLOOD and JANSEN, 1966). Only the cerebellovestibular pathway via the fastigial nucleus will be considered below.

This pathway consists of two links: Purkinje cell axons to the fastigial nucleus and axons of cells in this nucleus passing to the vestibular nuclei. The pathways are not yet completely known anatomically. It is clear from physiological studies, especially of MORUZZI and POMPEIANO and their collaborators, that they must be very complex. This is true especially for the efferent projections from the fastigial nucleus, since there is evidence of functional differences not only between the rostral and caudal parts of the fastigial nucleus but also between lateral and medial regions within each of these parts (see POMPEIANO, this volume, for particulars).

The first link, the cerebello-fastigial projection, appears in principle to be fairly simply organized. JANSEN and BRODAL (1940, 1942) concluded from experimental Marchi studies in rabbit, cat and monkey, that *only the vermis proper of the cerebellar cortex projects onto the fastigial nucleus*, while the intermediate part projects onto the nucleus interpositus (anterior and posterior) and the hemispheres onto the lateral (dentate) nucleus. Thus a rather schematic longitudinal subdivision of the cerebellum was postulated. The general correctness of this idea has been substantiated in later anatomical and physiological studies, though the pattern is less simple than originally assumed (see BRODAL, 1967b, for some data), especially in the projection of the hemispheres (see VOOGD, 1964). JANSEN and BRODAL (1940, 1942) further advocated *a fan-like arrangement within the longitudinal zones of the corticonuclear projection*. Thus anterior parts of the vermis send fibers to the anterior regions of the fastigial nucleus, posterior parts to the posterior regions. Subsequent studies by others with silver-impregnation methods (VACHANANDA, 1959; EAGER, 1963, 1966; GOODMAN et al., 1963; WALBERG and JANSEN, 1964; VOOGD, 1964; VAN ROSSUM, 1969) have confirmed these general principles for the projection onto the fastigial nucleus, even if some authors advocate that the longitudinal arrangement is less precise than held by JANSEN and BRODAL (1940, 1942). This may be due to the difficulties in obtaining sufficiently circumscribed lesions. The finding of even considerable overlap of the terminal areas of fibers from neighboring regions of the extremely foliated cerebellar cortex is only what is to be expected and does not invalidate the conclusion that the basic principle is one of a rather precise localization (cf. WALBERG and JANSEN, 1964). As mentioned previously, VOOGD (1964) in cat and VAN ROSSUM (1969) in rabbit found that the fibers to the fastigial nucleus take origin only from VOOGD's longitudinal zone A, the most medial part of the vermis. Single unit studies of cells in the fastigial nucleus following stimulation at different sites of the cerebellar vermis would be of interest.

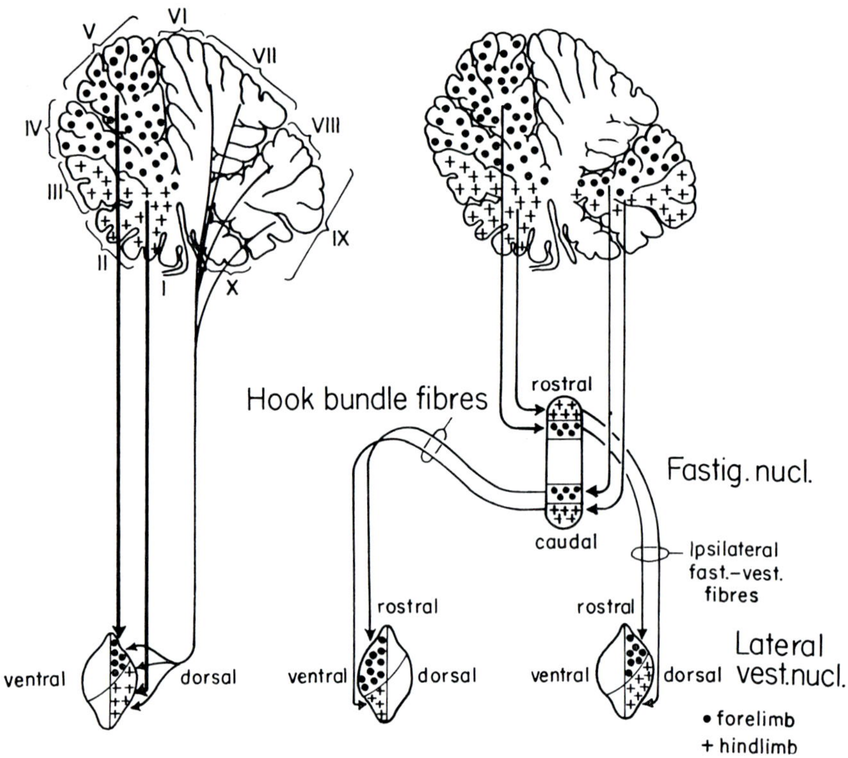

Fig. 39. Diagram illustrating major features in the projections from the cerebellar cortex onto the nucleus of Deiters (to the left) and (to the right) in the projections from the cerebellar cortex onto the fastigial nucleus and from this to the lateral vestibular nuclei. Note that the direct cerebellovestibular fibres and the projection from the rostral part of the fastigial nucleus end in the dorsal half of the ipsilateral lateral vestibular nucleus, while the fibres from the caudal part of the fastigial nucleus via the hook bundle supply the ventral half of the contralateral lateral vestibular nucleus. Within each of these projections there is a somatotopic localization. See text. (Slightly altered from Brodal, Pompeiano and Walberg, 1962)

From silver-impregnation studies it appears that the cerebellar corticonuclear fibers end on soma and dendrites of large as well as small cells in the intracerebellar nuclei (Walberg and Jansen, 1964; Eager, 1966). Electron-microscope studies have shown that the synaptic relationships correspond to those in the lateral vestibular nucleus (Mugnaini and Walberg, 1967).

The second link of the pathway, the *fastigiovestibular projection*, has been studied by a number of authors (for a review see Brodal et al., 1962). Following the demonstration of a very specific pattern in the organization of several other fiber connections of the vestibular nuclei, it was deemed of interest to try to determine in greater detail than done by previous authors the fastigiovestibular projection. As repeatedly mentioned, this involves considerable difficulties.

Not only do direct cerebellocortical fibers to the vestibular nuclei pass through the rostrolateral part of the fastigial nucleus, but complications are also caused by the course taken by the fastigiofugal fibers. While one contingent passes in the ipsilateral inferior cerebellar peduncle, other fibers cross the midline in the cerebellum and leave it on the contralateral side in the hook bundle (fasciculus uncinatus) curving around the superior cerebellar peduncle. Some of these fibers ascend within the fastigial nucleus in which they originate, especially ventrally, before they cross the midline.

Several authors tracing the degeneration of efferent fibers following lesions of the fastigial nucleus (ALLEN, 1924; RASMUSSEN, 1933; JANSEN, 1956; THOMAS et al., 1956; COHEN et al., 1958; CARPENTER et al., 1958; VOOGD, 1964) concluded that most of the crossing fibers of the hook bundle come from the caudal part of the fastigial nucleus, the majority of the ipsilateral ones from the rostral part.[14] This has been confirmed in studies of the retrograde cellular changes (modified Gudden method) in the cerebellar nuclei following transection of the cerebellar peduncles. JANSEN and JANSEN JR. (1955) and FLOOD and JANSEN (1966) found that about equal proportions of fibers leave along the two routes, and that *the ipsilateral fastigiovestibular fibers are derived predominantly from the rostral half of the nucleus, while all or at least the vast majority of the crossing fibers come from its caudal two-thirds.*

On account of the course of the efferent fastigial fibers described above, decisive conclusions cannot be obtained concerning certain details in the fastigiovestibular projection. However, by comparing the findings in several cats where stereotactic lesions were produced in different parts of the fastigial nucleus by introducing the electrode through folium VI (which gives off few, if any, fibers to the vestibular nuclei; see above) it has been possible to establish some essential points (WALBERG et al., 1962) and to extend the observations made by some previous authors. Only a brief account of the main findings will be given here. For particulars the reader should consult the original paper or the monograph by BRODAL et al. (1962).

The total distribution of the crossed fastigiovestibular fibers can be determined in cases where a lesion is restricted to one fastigial nucleus, and the ensuing degeneration is mapped in the contralateral vestibular nuclei. A case of this kind is shown in Fig. 40. The degenerating crossed fastigiovestibular fibers, emanating from the left fastigial nucleus, end in circumscribed regions in the right vestibular nuclei (dotted areas in the left half of a series of horizontal sections through the brainstem). *The distribution of the crossed fastigiovestibular fibers* is as follows: *the peripheral zone in the superior nucleus; the most ventral part of the medial nucleus; the ventral half of the lateral nucleus; the ventrolateral part of the descending nucleus; group f and group x*. In addition there is heavy degeneration in the *nucleus parasolitarius* (see Fig. 14). Fibers continuing through the vestibular nuclei pass to the perihypoglossal nuclei and the lateral reticular nucleus and to other divisions of the reticular formation. In agreement with the findings of other authors, it follows from the findings in cases with lesions restricted to the caudal or rostral parts of the fastigial nucleus that the majority of the crossed fibers are derived from the caudal part of the fastigial nucleus. The projections to group x, however, appear to be derived

14 In the above account and in the following the various parts of the fastigial nucleus are loosely referred to as rostral, middle and caudal, although cytoarchitectonic features suggest a more refined subdivision (see FLOOD and JANSEN, 1961). Since these minor parts cannot be damaged in isolation without affecting also fibers from other parts, it would be futile to attempt more specific indications of the site of the lesion.

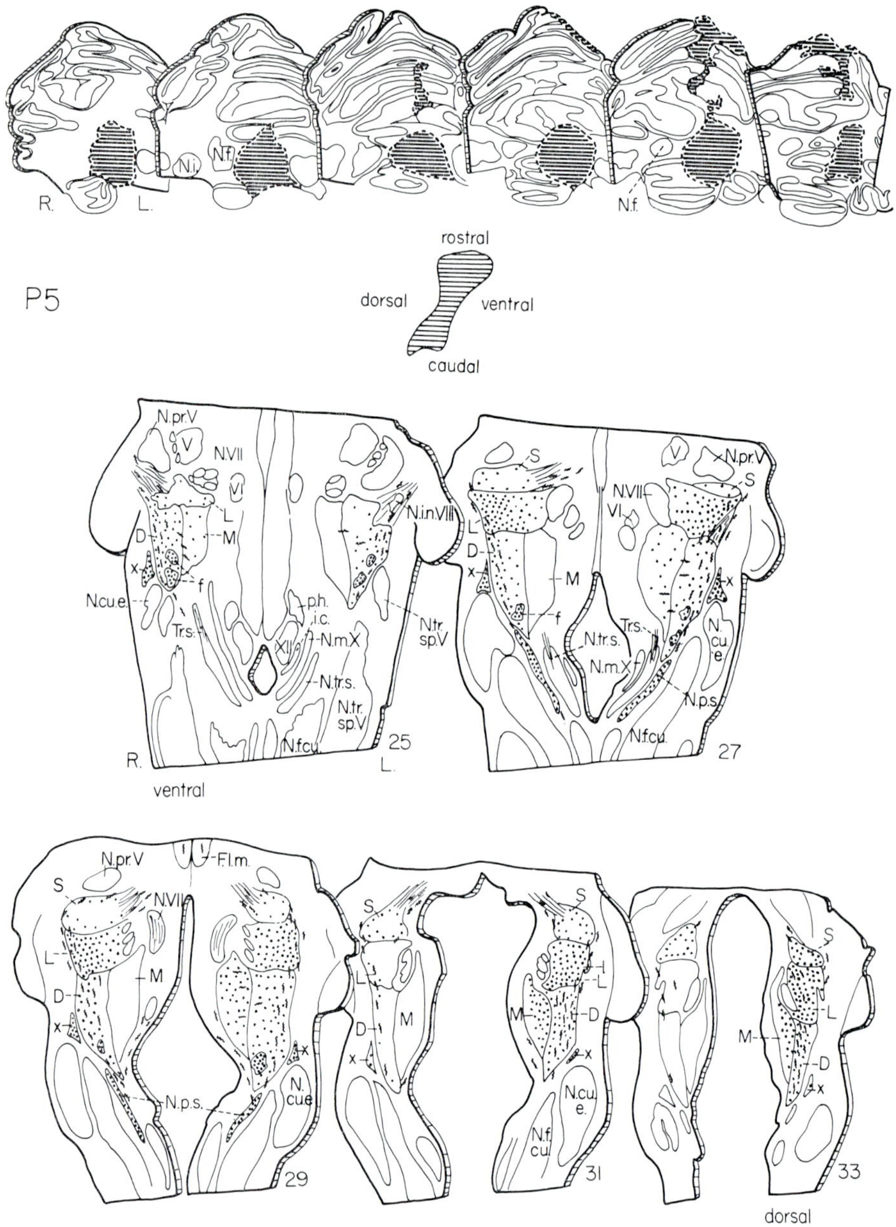

Fig. 40. Diagrammatic presentation of the sites of termination (dotted areas) in the vestibular nuclear complexes of the cat (seen in a series of horizontal drawings below) following a lesion of the left fastigial nucleus (above). The degeneration in the right half of the brain stem (to the left in the drawings) shows the terminal areas of the crossed fastigiovestibular fibres. The degeneration in the left half is due to involvement of crossed as well as uncrossed fibres (cp. text). From Walberg, Pompeiano, Brodal and Jansen (1962)

chiefly from middle levels of the fastigial nucleus. The restriction of the terminations in the lateral vestibular nucleus to its ventral part has also been noted by others, for example THOMAS et al. (1956) and CARPENTER et al. (1958). No terminations were established in the nucleus of the solitary tract as maintained by THOMAS et al. (1956), who apparently have not differentiated this nucleus from the neighboring nucleus parasolitarius (see Fig. 40).

An analysis of the *ipsilateral fastigiovestibular projection* is complicated by the fact that lesions of the fastigial nucleus will interrupt crossing fibers from the nucleus on the other side and, if situated laterally (see inset in Fig. 38), also direct cerebellocorticovestibular fibers. A comparison of the distribution of degeneration in the vestibular nuclei of the two sides in cases as that shown in Fig. 40 allows some conclusions. If the areas of the nuclei known to receive fibers directly from the cerebellar vermis (see above and Fig. 38) and the areas shown to receive crossed fibers (to the left in Fig. 40) are subtracted from the total area showing degeneration on the side of the lesion (to the right in the drawings of Fig. 40) it can be concluded that *ipsilateral fastigial efferents supply most of the medial vestibular nucleus, except its most ventral strip*. Concerning the projection to the other nuclei it is necessary to include studies of cases with differently placed lesions, involving only parts of the fastigial nucleus. On the basis of findings in 18 cats in which successful lesions of this kind were obtained, WALBERG et al. (1962; for particulars see the original paper) venture the following conclusions: *ipsilateral fastigiovestibular fibers end in the peripheral regions of the superior vestibular nucleus* (being somewhat more numerous than the crossed fibers to the same part); *the dorsal half of the lateral nucleus* (sharing this area with the direct corticovestibular fibers); *the large dorsomedial parts of the descending nucleus and the medial nucleus except its ventralmost region*. It appears that groups x and f and the nucleus parasolitarius receive only, or at least chiefly, crossed fibers. The uncrossed fibers arise almost exclusively from the rostral part of the fastigial nucleus, in agreement with the findings of other authors.

It is seen from the above that *the ipsilateral fastigiovestibular fibers* (from the rostral part of the fastigial nucleus) *and crossed fibers* (from the caudal part of the fastigial nucleus) *supply different regions within the lateral, medial and descending vestibular nuclei. Only in the superior nucleus do they have a common territory.*[15] Considering that the rostral part of the fastigial nucleus receives fibers from the vermis of the anterior lobe, the caudal part from the posterior vermis, the differential distribution of fastigial fibers to the vestibular nuclei provides morphological evidence for the existence of functional differences between the anterior and posterior vermis (see POMPEIANO, this volume). Further indications can be derived from a comparison of the distribution of the two contingents of fastigiovestibular fibers with other fiber connections of the vestibular nuclei. For example, second-

15 It may be objected that some of the degeneration in cases with lesions of the fastigial nucleus may be due to damage to fibres from the nodulus-uvula which pass through the fastigial nucleus (see ANGAUT and BRODAL, 1967). This factor will, however, not invalidate the conclusions concerning the crossed fastigiovestibular projection. Nor can it explain the ipsilateral degeneration in the lateral, medial and descending nucleus. Only in the fibers to the superior nucleus are the terminal territories of fastigial and nodulus-uvula fibers identical. The far more abundant degeneration following fastigial lesions suggests, however, that the fastigial nucleus gives off ipsilateral fibers to the superior nucleus.

ary vestibulocerebellar fibers come from areas of the medial and descending vestibular nuclei (Brodal and Torvik, 1957) which receive crossed fastigial fibers only.

Of particular interest is the differential distribution of the fastigial fibers to the lateral vestibular nucleus. Its ventral half receives fibers from the contralateral fastigial nucleus (caudal part), its dorsal half from the rostral part of the ipsilateral nucleus (see Fig. 37 and Fig. 39, to the right). The dorsal half, as seen above, receives direct fibers from the anterior lobe vermis in addition. This, therefore, has two routes, a direct and an indirect, to the dorsal half of the lateral vestibular nucleus. Both contingents of fastigial fibers to the lateral nucleus supply the two main somatotopical regions of the nucleus, since the border between the two fastigial contingents crosses the border between forelimb and hindlimb regions (Figs. 37 and 39). As described in the preceding section, the direct cerebellovestibular route to the nucleus of Deiters is somatotopically organized. By comparing the distribution of degeneration in the lateral nucleus of Deiters following lesions involving different regions of the rostral and caudal parts of the fastigial nucleus, Walberg et al. (1962) adduced evidence for a topographical pattern within both components of the fastigiovestibular projection, as illustrated diagramatically in Fig. 39. (For particulars see the original paper.) Since there is an orderly pattern in the cerebellar corticofastigial projection, as described above, *both components of the cerebello-fastigio-vestibular projections appear to be somatotopically organized.* Accordingly, the dorsal part of the forelimb region in the nucleus of Deiters is acted upon from the forelimb region of the vermis of the anterior lobe (directly and via the fastigial nucleus), the ventral part from the posterior lobe via corresponding pathways. The same principle is valid for the hindlimb region.

It should be emphasized that the patterns brought out in the anatomical study of Walberg et al. (1962) can be no more than an indication of the principal organization of the pathways. Furthermore, it has not been possible so far to determine anatomical differences between the projections of the lateral and medial regions of the rostral and caudal parts of the fastigial nucleus. It appears extremely likely that such differences exist in view of the physiological differences established. These will not be discussed here (see Pompeiano, this volume, and Pompeiano, 1967), but like the available anatomical data, they bear witness to an extremely complex organization of the cerebellovestibular connections. As concerns major features, however, satisfactory correlations between anatomical and physiological findings can be made (see Pompeiano, this volume).

The modes of ending of fastigial fibers in the vestibular nuclei is not finally settled, since the subject has so far not been studied by experimental electron-microscope methods. The findings made in silver-impregnation studies are not conclusive, but they may be taken to suggest that synaptic contacts are probably established with cells of different sizes within all four vestibular nuclei. In the lateral nucleus relatively few fibers appear to end on large cells. (For some data see Walberg et al., 1962.)

The quantitatively important cerebellovestibular connections and their complex patterns indicate that of all afferent impulses reaching the vestibular nuclei, those coming from the cerebellum are probably the functionally most important ones.

D. Descending Connections to the Vestibular Nuclei

While a considerable number of efferents from the vestibular nuclei ascend in the brainstem, there appears to be only a modest projection in the reverse direction. At least most of these fibers pass in the medial longitudinal fasciculus. Their main source appears to be the interstitial nucleus of Cajal in the mesencephalon.

On account of some discrepancies in the nomenclature of the small nuclei in the vicinity of the oculomotor nucleus a brief comment is appropriate. (For particulars see POMPEIANO and WALBERG, 1957, or BRODAL et al., 1962.) The *interstitial nucleus* of CAJAL, the best characterized of the nuclei, is situated ventrolateral to, and partly in between, the fibers of the medial longitudinal fasciculus (Fig. 41) lying just ventrolateral to the oculomotor nucleus. Rostrally the interstitial nucleus extends a little beyond the oculomotor. The *nucleus of Darkschewitsch* is a rather indistinct cell group, situated dorsomedial to the middle part of the interstitial nucleus on which it borders. The nucleus is found internal to the lateral border of the periaqueductal gray (Fig. 41). The *nucleus of the posterior commissure*, like the interstitial nucleus, is situated outside the periaqueductal gray. It is found further rostrally than the nucleus of Darkschewitsch and is associated with the fibers of the posterior commissure (Fig. 41).

It is difficult to achieve lesions of the individual small nuclei in the vicinity of the oculomotor nucleus, and several uncritical conclusions have been drawn concerning projections of these nuclei. From a comparison of the findings in several cases POMPEIANO and WALBERG (1957), in an experimental study in cat with the Glees method, concluded that *fibers to the vestibular nuclei descending in the medial longitutinal fasciculus from the mesencephalon are derived only from the interstitial nucleus of Cajal.* This agrees with the opinion of several other students (for references see POMPEIANO and WALBERG, 1957). Some of these descending fibers

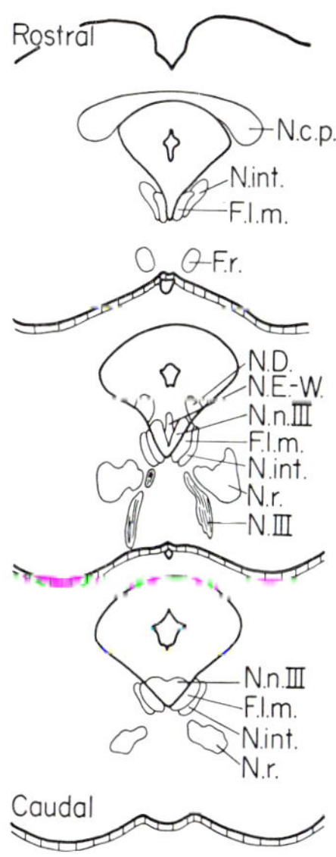

Fig. 41. A diagram showing the mutual positions of the nucleus interstitialis of Cajal (N. int.), the nucleus of Darkschewitsch (N. D.) and the nucleus of the posterior commissure (N. c. p.) as seen in three transverse sections through the mesencephalon of the cat. From POMPEIANO and WALBERG (1957)

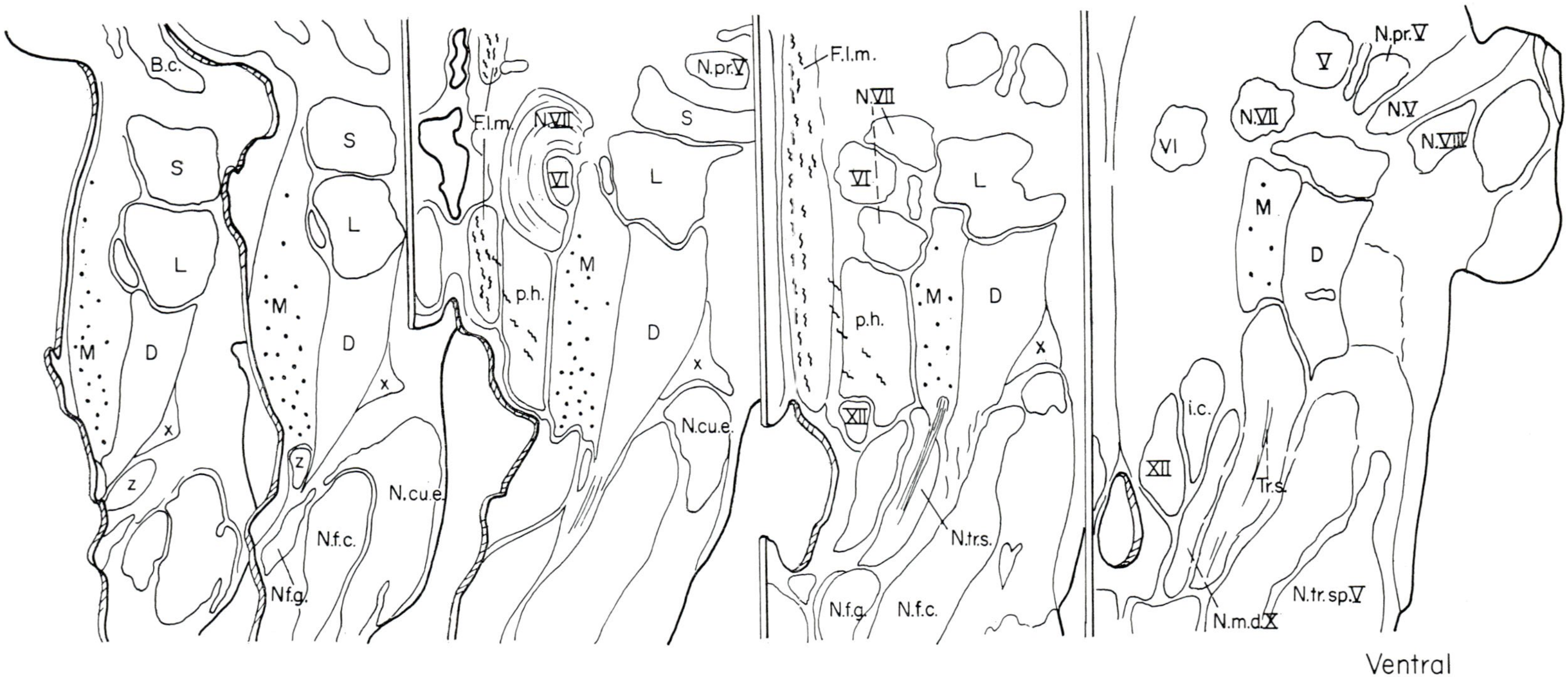

Fig. 42. Drawings of a series of horizontal sections through the brain stem of the cat, showing the sites of termination (dots) in the vestibular nuclei of fibres descending from the interstitial nucleus of Cajal. Note restriction of termination to the medial nucleus (M). From POMPEIANO and WALBERG (1957)

continue to the spinal cord as the interstitiospinal tract (NYBERG-HANSEN, 1966).[16] It should be noted that in the vestibular nuclei *the terminal area (Fig. 42) is restricted to the ipsilateral medial vestibular nucleus, chiefly its dorsal and caudal parts* (POMPEIANO and WALBERG, 1957). On their way to the nucleus many of the fibers traverse the nucleus praepositus hypoglossi (Fig. 42). The fact that most of the fibers to the medial vestibular nuclei are thin may indicate that they may be collaterals of interstitiospinal fibers. LORENTE DE NÓ (1933a), in a Golgi study in mouse, describes collaterals to the vestibular nuclei from the medial longitudinal fasciculus and in his Fig. 8 II illustrates fibers from the interstitial nucleus of CAJAL entering the vestibular nuclei. On stimulation of the ipsilateral interstitial nucleus of CAJAL, type I neurons of the horizontal canal were found to be inhibited, while type II neurons are excited, some probably monosynaptically (see MARKHAM et al., 1966; MARKHAM, 1968; PRECHT, this volume, for particulars). It appears that at least most of these units are located in the medial vestibular nucleus. Of neurons responding synaptically to stimulation of the medial longitudinal fasciculus the majority were found in the ventral part of the medial nucleus (WILSON et al., 1968b).

Other authors have suggested different descending fiber connections from those described above. For example, MATANO et al. (1964b), using the Marchi method in rabbits, describe terminations only in the superior and lateral vestibular nuclei. The few black particles shown in their photograph 1 scarcely allow this interpretation.

The interstitial nucleus of CAJAL is generally considered to be important for rotational movements of the head and for movements of the eye. As mentioned previously, it receives ascending fibers from the vestibular nuclei. By way of its descending connections it may influence the activity of these nuclei, even if its direct actions will be restricted to the medial vestibular nucleus. "Higher levels" of the brain can be assumed to influence the interstitial nucleus if connections from such structures exist. There are reports of fibers to the interstitial nucleus of CAJAL from the frontal cortex (SZENTÁGOTHAI, 1943; SZENTÁGOTHAI and RAJKOVITS, 1958), the occipital cortex (METTLER, 1935, to the periaqueductal grey; SZENTÁGOTHAI, 1943) and from the pallidum (WOODBURNE et al., 1946; JOHNSON and CLEMENTE, 1959). These, as well as other connections which have been reported (superior colliculus, ALTMAN and CARPENTER, 1961; MATANO et al., 1965), appear to be rather scanty (for additional references see POMPEIANO and WALBERG, 1957).

The possibility that "higher levels" may influence the vestibular nuclei indirectly without a relay in the interstitial nucleus is suggested by the observations of some authors of direct connections to the vestibular nuclei from, for example, the cerebral cortex (SZENTÁGOTHAI and RAJKOVITS, 1958, a few fibers to the descending and medial vestibular nuclei). POMPEIANO and WALBERG (1957) did not find such fibers, nor were they able to find degenerating fibers to the vestibular nuclei following lesions of the basal ganglia or ventral part of the mesencephalon. Even if it is admitted that with the GLEES (1946) method scanty degeneration

16 Some fibers descending in the medial longitudinal fasciculus have been found to end in the ipsilateral inferior olive (see p. 295).

may escape recognition, it appears permissible to conclude that there can scarcely be important direct descending connections to the vestibular nuclei arising in structures situated rostral to the interstitial nucleus of Cajal.

E. Afferent Connections from the Contralateral Vestibular Nuclei

The commissural connections between the vestibular nuclei have been dealt with in a previous section. Like other afferent connections of the vestibular nuclei, the commissural fibers present a rather specific pattern with regard to their sites of termination within the vestibular nuclei (see Figs. 21, 22 and 23, and p. 284ff.).

F. Afferents to the Vestibular Nuclei from the Reticular Formation

Just as the vestibular nuclei give off fibers to the reticular formation, the latter sends fibers back to the vestibular complex. The available data on these connections are scanty, and there is no specific information on which cell groups give off fibers to the vestibular nuclei or of their precise sites of termination. Experimental studies of the reticulovestibular connections meet with the difficulties that the lesions have to be precisely placed if reliable information is sought for, and that in certain areas there is a high risk of damaging nonreticular vestibular afferents. Most of our information comes from Golgi studies (Cajal, 1909–1911; Lorente de Nó, 1933a; Scheibel and Scheibel, 1958).

It appears that all reticular fibers to the vestibular nuclei come from the pontomedullary reticular formation. In agreement with this, following experimental lesions of the mesencephalic reticular formation Pompeiano and Walberg (1957) did not trace degenerating fibers (Nauta method) to the vestibular nuclei. According to Scheibel and Scheibel (1958), all axons of cells in the reticular formation "appear characterized by the frequent emission of collaterals during their entire trajectory" (loc. cit. p. 39). The fibers passing to the vestibular (as well as other cranial nerve) nuclei appear to be collaterals of axons projecting elsewhere. Lorente de Nó (1933a) found collaterals to the vestibular nuclei from fibers of the reticulospinal tract, the medial longitudinal fasciculus, the predorsal and vestibulospinal tracts. Scheibel and Scheibel (1958) picture (their Fig. 13) collaterals from long ascending fibers to the lateral vestibular nucleus. Hauglie-Hanssen (1968) also observed afferents to this nucleus.

At least the majority of cells in the medial two-thirds of the reticular formation have long axons, which ascend in the brainstem or descend to the spinal cord (see Brodal, 1957; Scheibel and Scheibel, 1958; Valverde, 1961a). Many reticular cells have dichotomizing axons, one branch taking an ascending and the other a descending course. The fibers passing to the cerebellum come from three fairly well circumscribed nuclei, the lateral reticular nucleus (nucleus of the lateral funiculus), the paramedian reticular nucleus and the nucleus reticularis tegmenti pontis (see Brodal, 1957, 1967b; Jansen and Brodal, 1958, for particulars).[17] *A priori* the cerebellar projecting reticular nuclei are more likely to supply the vestibular nuclei than is the remaining part of the reticular formation. The reticulo-cerebellar fibers pass

17 On the basis of electrophysiological studies Avanzino et al. (1966) conclude that some cells of the main reticular formation (nucl. retic. gigantocell.) also send axonal branches to the cerebellum. The electrodes were, however, not far from the paramedian reticular nucleus.

in the vicinity of the vestibular nuclei (most of them in the restiform body) and accordingly are favorably situated to give off collaterals to the vestibular nuclei. Some authors have described collaterals from fibers in the restiform body entering the vestibular nuclei, but the origin of the axons cannot be established.

The scanty data available concerning details in the reticulovestibular connections should not induce us to believe that these are not arranged in an orderly patterns, like all other vestibular afferent fiber projections so far been studied in sufficient detail. Since afferents from the spinal cord as well as from the cerebral cortex and other "higher" levels of the brain end in the reticular formation, the reticulovestibular connections cannot be disregarded as links in possible pathways for impulse transmission to the vestibular nuclei from the spinal cord, the cerebral cortex and certain other regions of the brain.

G. Some Minor Contingents of Afferents to the Vestibular Nuclei

In addition to the afferents described in the preceding sections, fibers have been traced to the vestibular nuclei from various other sources. In general the number of fibers in these contingents is modest, and for most of them the precise sites of termination have not been decided. Even if their scanty numbers preclude these fiber contingents from being considered of great functional importance, they should not be disregarded. Their occurrence serves as an additional reminder of the complexity of the organization of the vestibular nuclei.

The *inferior olive* appears to send some fibers to the vestibular nuclei. As mentioned previously, LORENTE DE NÓ (1924) considered it likely that some olivocerebellar fibers give off collaterals to the nucleus of Deiters. In an experimental study of the olivocerebellar projection in cat and rabbit (BRODAL, 1940b) it was found that the most caudal part of a particular small division of the inferior olive, the dorsal cap of Kooy, appears to project onto the vestibular nuclei. Whether the connection is established with one or more vestibular nuclei or with the scattered cells between these and the intracerebellar nuclei could not be decided.

Small contingents of fibers have been traced to the descending and superior vestibular nuclei from the *mandibular nerve* (TORVIK, 1956) and to the descending nucleus from the *vagoglossopharyngeal nerve* (CAJAL, 1909; KERR, 1962).

The *most cranial dorsal roots* have likewise been found to give off some fibers to the descending nucleus (CORBIN and HINSEY, 1935; YEE and CORBIN, 1939; ESCOLAR, 1948; and others). These fibers are few in number, and some have been traced to certain minor cell groups related to the vestibular nuclei (RANSON et al., 1932; ESCOLAR, 1948), but it is not quite clear to which cell groups reference is made. Many units in the medial and descending nuclei responding to galvanic stimulation of the vestibular nerve are influenced by neck movements, presumably by proprioceptive impulses entering in the upper dorsal roots (FREDRICKSON et al., 1965).

Fibers from the *nucleus gracilis* to the medial vestibular nucleus were described in rabbit by GEREBTZOFF (1940).

VI. Intrinsic Organization of the Vestibular Nuclear Complex

For a proper understanding of the mode of operation of the vestibular nuclei a knowledge of their intrinsic morphological organization is essential. Some problems to be solved are the following. Do afferent fibers from different sources differ with regard to their terminal patterns of branching and types of synaptic contacts established? Does each contingent of afferents have synaptic contacts, exclusively or preferentially, with nerve cells of a specific type? Is there convergence of afferents from different sources upon individual cells? Do axons of cells in the vestibular nuclei have collaterals distributed to other subdivisions of the complex? Do dendrites of cells of a particular subdivision extend into neighboring subdivisions? Do purely internuncial cells occur in the vestibular nuclei?

Final answers cannot yet be given to many of these questions. Information on the intrinsic organization can be obtained mainly by studies of Golgi preparations and in electron microscope studies of normal and experimental material. Investigations of the latter type have so far been published only insofar as they have some bearing on the lateral vestibular nucleus of Deiters. As described in preceding sections many differences have been found between the various vestibular nuclei and even between their minor subdivisions as regards architecture and efferent and afferent connections. It seems a likely assumption that differences are present also between subdivisions as concerns their intrinsic organization. It is not permissible, therefore, to assume that findings made, for example in the nucleus of Deiters, are valid for all subdivisions of the vestibular nuclear complex.

Some features of the intrinsic organization of the vestibular nuclei have been touched upon in other sections of this chapter. Some additional data will be considered below, in conjunction with those already mentioned. For an account of the cell types present in the various nuclei the description in the section of the structure of the vestibular nuclei should be consulted, where the orientation of dendrites and the fiber patterns have also been dealt with.

From a functional point of view a problem of particular interest is the following: *What are the anatomical possibilities for impulses from a particular source to act upon regions of the vestibular complex outside the area determined anatomically as the site of termination of the particular fiber contingents?* In the nucleus of Deiters primary vestibular fibers are distributed chiefly to the forelimb region, but in spite of this vestibular stimulation influences the hindlimb as well as the forelimb. The assumption that this occurs by way of a circuit through the cerebellum appears not to be tenable.

A priori *three arrangements may be suggested* to explain an activation of the hindlimb region of the nucleus of Deiters by primary vestibular afferents (leaving out of consideration influences via the scanty primary vestibular fibers to restricted areas of the reticular formation). 1) There may be internuncials in the forelimb region sending axons into the hindlimb region. 2) Axons of projecting cells in the forelimb region may give off collaterals to the hindlimb region. 3) Dendrites of cells in the hindlimb region may extend into the forelimb region.

Mannen (1965), in a Golgi study of the pattern and quantitative features of the dendritic arborizations of cells in the vestibular nuclei of cat, is inclined to deny the justification for a subdivision of the vestibular nuclei into minor groups (as outlined on the basis of cytoarchitecture and fiber connections), since he found dendrites of cells in a particular vestibular nuclear subdivision to extend into other subdivisions of the vestibular complex or into neighboring nuclei. This was observed also by HAUGLIE-HANSSEN (1968) and by LORENTE DE NÓ (1933a). In an extensive Golgi study of the vestibular nuclei HAUGLIE-HANSSEN (1968) directed attention particularly to these questions. By careful mapping the "dendrite spheres" of cells impregnated he found that *in general the dendrites of cells in a particular nucleus or subdivision tend to be restricted to this.* The cells which have dendrites extending into neighboring regions are almost only those situated at the zones of transition, and the majority of cells are not of this kind. (See comments on p. 241 concerning the drawing of borders between nuclei.) This is seen from Fig. 43, which shows one of HAUGLIE-HANSSEN's (1968) illustrations. Even if the lines interconnecting the distal ends of dendrites represent minima, it is unlikely that the true "dendrite fields" are appreciably larger. As to the nucleus of Deiters it is clear that most of the cells in the dorsal half of the nucleus do not extend their

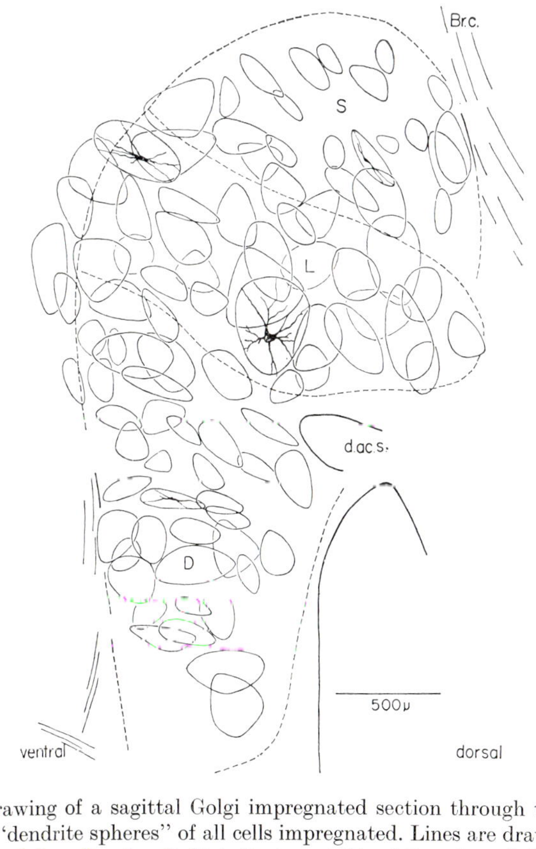

Fig. 43. On a drawing of a sagittal Golgi impregnated section through the vestibular nuclei are entered the "dendrite spheres" of all cells impregnated. Lines are drawn between the ends of the longest dendrites of each cell. Note that most "dendrite spheres" do not extend beyond the borders of the nucleus in which the soma is found. From HAUGLIE-HANSSEN (1968)

dendrites into the rostroventral half. The giant cells have a "dendrite sphere" of about 900 μm. Since the total dorsoventral diameter of the lateral nucleus is more than 2000 μm (measured in the Golgi-Cox preparations), a nerve cell situated in the middle of the dorsocaudal half of the nucleus, with a "dendrite sphere" of 900 μm, will extend some peripheral dendrite branches to the border zone between the dorsal and ventral halves, while cells located further dorsally do not extend dendrites into the ventral half of the nucleus. Furthermore, the "dendrite spheres" of the dorsally located giant cells are almost globular without any particular tendency to dendritic extension ventrally. Some observations of LORENTE DE NÓ (1927) are in agreement with these findings. Finally there are in the dorsocaudal half of the nucleus cells with "dendrite spheres" considerably smaller than those of the giant cells. When taken together these findings strongly suggest that most cells in the dorsocaudal part of the lateral nucleus probably do not receive direct information from the vestibular receptors by way of primary vestibular fibers.

In the other vestibular nuclei the "dendrite spheres" are likewise fairly restricted (see Fig. 43).[18] On the whole, therefore it *appears that the various contingents of afferents ending in fairly circumscribed regions of the vestibular complex will have only very restricted possibilities for influencing monosynaptically cells in other regions, except for cells situated in the border zones between regions or nuclei.*

In physiological studies (see PRECHT, this volume) evidence has been found for the presence of *internuncials* in some of the vestibular nuclei, especially the medial and superior. In his Golgi material HAUGLIE-HANSSEN (1968) did not find cells of the Golgi II type, provided with short axons branching heavily in the vicinity of the perikaryon. This agrees with previous observations of CAJAL (1896, 1909–1911) and LORENTE DE NÓ (1933a). It appears that the majority of cells in the vestibular nuclei have long axons. However, some cells of this type were found by HAUGLIE-HANSSEN (1968) to give off a few simple collaterals within the subdivision to which their perikarya belong, or to give rise to thin, relatively richly branched, collaterals distributed in the neighborhood of the parent cell. Cells of the latter type, which are always small, were found only in the medial and descending nucleus. Some representative specimens are shown in Fig. 44. It was rarely possible to follow the axons of these cells to their destinations, nor could it be decided whether the collaterals establish contact with cells in the neighborhood. It is, however, likely that they do so, and that therefore such cells, in addition to transmitting their impulses to more remote places, may also function as internuncials. Whether this assumption will explain the activation of the vestibulospinal projection to the lumbosacral cord on stimulation of the vestibular nerve is an open question, since cells with collaterals of the types discussed above were not found in the lateral vestibular nucleus (HAUGLIE-HANSSEN, 1968).

It is interesting to note that internuncial cells of the Golgi II type have not been found in the reticular formation (SCHEIBEL and SCHEIBEL, 1958), except for a few in the lateral small-celled part (VALVERDE, 1961b), and that the situation appears to be the same in the ventral horn of the spinal cord (SCHEIBEL and SCHEIBEL, 1966). All cells which give off collateral branches to the vicinity also have a long projecting axon. Presumably in these regions of the nervous system cells of this kind can function as internuncials.

18 The most marked overlapping occurs between the medial and the descending nucleus.

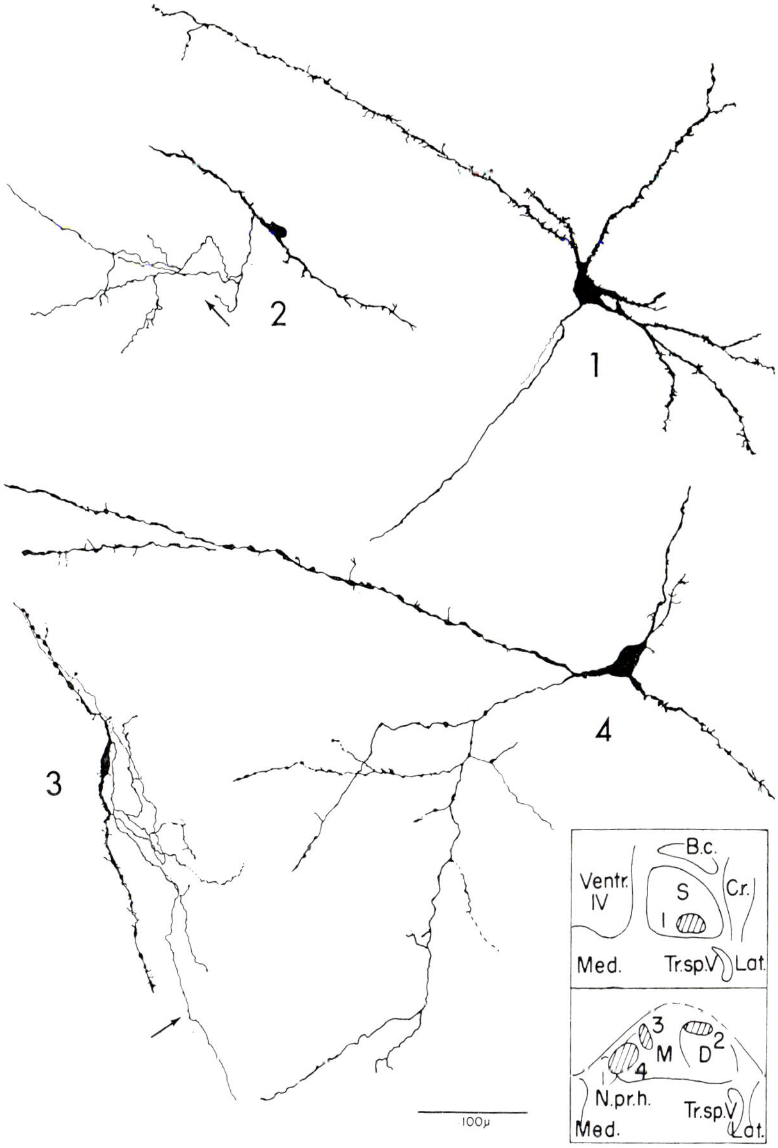

Fig. 44. Drawings of nerve cells in the vestibular nuclear complex showing various types of axonal collaterals as seen in transverse sections (100 μ, Golgi rapid method) from 3 days old kittens. The location of the cells and the distribution of their dendrites and axonal branches shown in the drawings, are indicated by the hatched areas in the inset figures. 1: A middle-sized cell in the superior nucleus with a short and thin collateral from the initial part of the axon. 2: A small cell in the dorsal part of the descending nucleus with a relatively richly branched axon. The arrow indicates the axonal branch assumed to represent the projecting part of the axon. 3: A small cell in the medial nucleus. A projecting axon (arrow) gives off three simply branched collaterals distributed in the immediate neighbourhood of the parent cell. Note the very simple dendrites on the cells 2 and 3. 4: A middle-sized cell in the ventromedial part of the medial nucleus, extending a branched axon towards the area of the nucleus praepositus hypoglossi. From HAUGLIE-HANSSEN (1968)

The *patterns of the axonal ramifications of afferent fibres within the vestibular nuclei* is another aspect of the intrinsic organization. The general tendency of afferent axons to pursue a course parallel to the dendritic orientation in their area of termination has already been mentioned, as have the different shapes of the territories within a nucleus which are supplied by single afferent fibers from different sources. According to Hauglie-Hanssen (1968) a descending branch of a primary vestibular fiber with its collaterals covers a rather narrow zone, extending in a mediolateral direction (see Fig. 31 b). Each collateral has short preterminal branches (see Fig. 30), and the terminal sub-branches are grouped into clusters. A corresponding pattern is found for the crossed fastigiovestibular fibers, coming (at least chiefly) from the caudal part of the fastigial nucleus (the orientation here is ventromedial to dorsolateral). The cerebellovestibular fibers coming from the cerebellar vermis, on the other hand, supply territories (in the dorsal half of the nucleus of Deiters and the rostral part of the descending nucleus) which have a cylindrical shape (Fig. 31 a). These fibers also have short collaterals. Even if there is some overlap between the territories of adjacent fibers, an arrangement of either type is well suited for mediating topically localized impulse transmissions. This is in complete agreement with the conclusions drawn from experimental anatomical and physiological studies of the afferents from the vestibular apparatus and the cerebellum. The patterns of branching of other contingents of afferents are so far not known in detail.

In Golgi preparations the final ramifications of terminal branches and collaterals of afferent fibers to the vestibular nuclei can be seen to differ morphologically. As mentioned previously, Hauglie-Hanssen (1968) distinguished the three types shown in Fig. 32. For particulars his paper should be consulted. The type I fibers have delicate branchlets with small round terminal boutons occurring singly or in clusters of three or four on each preterminal fiber. Types 2 and 3 have in common that in addition to terminal boutons they have swellings along their course. These are small on the type 3 fibers, much larger and often oval on the type 2 fibers (see Fig. 32). These swellings along the course of the terminal fibers are interpreted as boutons en passage. The correctness of this has been demonstrated in electron-microscope studies of the nucleus of Deiters by Mugnaini et al. (1967), where likewise two types of boutons en passage can be distinguished. One of these (see Fig. 11) is assumed to belong to the typical "climbing" fibers seen in Golgi sections and referred to here as type 3 fibers. Such "climbing fibers" are often found attached to the soma as well as the proximal dendrites. Occasionally the same fiber "climbs" even along dendritic branches of the third order (Cajal, 1896; Hauglie-Hanssen, 1968). The direction of these fibers is generally from the dendrites towards the perikaryon. Electron-microscope studies (Mugnaini et al., 1967; Sotelo and Palay, 1968) have further shown that in the lateral vestibular nuclei there is a wide variety of boutons which differ in their finer morphology.

The question may be raised whether the different kinds of terminal fibers and the different types of boutons belong to separate contingents of afferents. This is a difficult problem to solve, not least because any territory of the vestibular nuclei receives afferents from more than one source. Hauglie-Hanssen (1968) concluded from his observations that probably all main afferent contingents have terminal fibers of type 1 (see Fig. 32). The corticocerebellar fibers probably end partly with terminals of type 2 (provided with large boutons en passage), while some of the fastigiovestibular fibers end as fibers of type 3 ("climbing" fibres). Correspondingly, electron-microscope observations (Mugnaini and Walberg, 1967) suggest that many of the Purkinje cell axons are provided with round or sausage-like boutons (of type 2 above), while others may end with thin fibers with small boutons (type 1, above). The observations mentioned tend to show that the *fibers coming from one source may differ with regard to their patterns of termination and of the morphology of their synaptic contacts.* As concerns the primary vestibular fibers such differences may be assumed to be related to the two kinds of receptor cells in the sensory epithelia. As concerns the Purkinje cells the data may cast doubt on the assumption that all Purkinje cells are functionally similar (inhibitory).

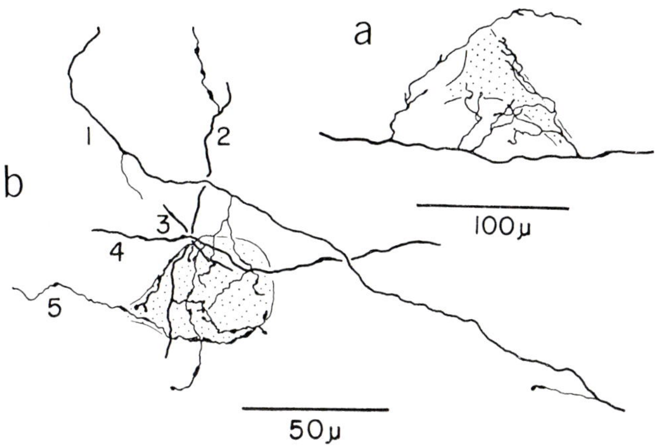

Fig. 45. Drawings illustrating convergence onto a nerve cell of collaterals from a single stem fibre (a) and from different sources (b). From Hauglie-Hanssen (1968)

Whether fibers coming from different sources establish synaptic contact with the same cells is difficult to decide anatomically. Golgi studies give suggestive evidence that this is the case (see Fig. 45b). As mentioned previously there is physiological evidence in some instances of convergence of impulses from different sources on the same cell in the vestibular nuclei. In experimental electron-microscope studies of the cerebellar cortical afferents to the lateral nucleus (Mugnaini and Walberg, 1967) and of the primary vestibular fibers (Mugnaini et al., 1967) a number of normal boutons were always found on those cells which were contacted by the degenerating fibers, suggesting the convergence of other afferents, but the source of the latter cannot be decided in this way. Since the time course of the degeneration of the two kinds of vestibular afferents and the appearance of the degenerating boutons differ, it is possible to study this convergence in cases where two operations are performed in the same animal. In a study of this kind suggestive evidence was found that some cells in the middle region of the nucleus of Deiters are contacted by primary vestibular as well as corticocerebellar fibers (Walberg and Mugnaini, 1969). Continued studies along this line would be of interest.

As briefly mentioned previously, electron microscopy of the normal nucleus of Deiters in cat (MUGNAINI et al., 1967) and rat (SOTELO and PALAY, 1968) have revealed a number of ultrastructural features, for example differences between cells of different types. For particulars the original papers should be consulted. Obviously such features as the relations of nerve cells to surrounding glial cells, nerve fibers and boutons are of relevance for functional aspects of the intrinsic organization of a nuclear complex, as are the types of boutons present and the patterns of synaptic contacts established. Much remains to be done in this field, but it appears to be essential for further progress in our understanding of the intrinsic organization of the vestibular nuclei that their ultrastructural features are known. Likewise, studies of possible chemical differences and peculiarities, not least with regard to transmitter substances, are important. Also here topical relations must be taken into account if information of value is to be obtained, and if fruitful correlations with anatomical and physiological findings are sought for.

VII. Concluding Remarks. Summary

The preceding account of the anatomy of the vestibular nuclear complex is far from complete. Attempts have been made to emphasize anatomical features which are of functional interest, and which are important in physiological studies. It is deemed to be of value in concluding this chapter to summarize briefly some principal features and to supplement the description with a summarizing statement of the anatomical characteristics of the various cell groups.

1. *The vestibular nuclear complex in the cat consists of several minor cell groups in addition to the four main nuclei (superior, lateral, medial and descending or inferior).* On the basis of their architecture and fiber connections the main nuclei may be subdivided into minor territories which differ in one or more respects from each other. The anatomical observations on the subdivisions of the nuclear complex are in general agreement with the results of detailed physiological studies where such studies have been performed. The evidence available strongly suggests that the general pattern and principles of organization of the vestibular nuclei determined in the cat are valid also for other mammals, including man.

2. *The characteristics of the various nuclei and cell groups may be summarized as follows:*[19]

a) *The superior vestibular nucleus.* A distinction can be made between a *peripheral zone and the central region.* The latter contains cells of somewhat greater dimensions than the peripheral zone.

Among the *afferent fibers* to the nucleus those from the vestibular receptors and the flocculus terminate chiefly in the central region. The primary vestibular fibers appear to be derived only from the cristae of the semicircular ducts, and to some extent the fibers from each crista appear to have their separate projection areas within the superior nucleus. Crossed as well as uncrossed fastigial fibers (derived mainly from the caudal and rostral halves of the fastigial nucleus, respectively) and fibers from the nodulus-uvula end chiefly in the peripheral zone. A few fibers from the vermis of the anterior lobe probably end in the superior nucleus.

19 Diagrammatic representations of some of the features summarized below can be found in BRODAL et al. (1962).

Commissural fibers end throughout the territory of the superior nucleus and appear to be derived from the contralateral superior nucleus only. Fibers from the spinal cord and fibers from the interstitial nucleus of CAJAL in the mesencephalon have not been convincingly shown to end in the superior nucleus. There are probably some afferents from the reticular formation.

The majority of the *efferent fibers* from the superior nucleus ascend in the ipsilateral medial longitudinal fasciculus. They appear to come from the entire territory of the nucleus, perhaps mainly from its central region, and end in certain regions of the nuclei of the motor ocular nerves. Some end in the interstitial nucleus of Cajal in the mesencephalon. Fibers continuing to the thalamus have been described by some authors but there is no good evidence for their existence. Other efferent fibers pass from the superior nucleus to the reticular formation where they supply certain regions of the main central region, some ipsilaterally, others contralaterally (see Table 1), and the contralateral nucleus reticularis tegmenti pontis. Commissural efferents pass mainly to the contralateral superior nucleus with some fibers to the other main vestibular nuclei. There is no evidence for efferents from the superior nucleus to the spinal cord or to the cerebellum.

Judging from its fiber connections, the superior vestibular nucleus appears to be particularly closely related to the oculomotor apparatus, and to serve the mediation of vestibular and cerebellar influences on these nuclei. These relations are rather specific (particular distribution of ascending fibers to specific parts of the oculomotor nuclei, differential termination of vestibular fibers in the superior nucleus). The vestibular influences appear to come mainly from the cristae. Possible relations of the superior nucleus with the spinal cord can only be indirect. The superior nucleus of one side must be functionally closed linked with its fellow on the other side.

b) *In the lateral vestibular nucleus of Deiters two subdivisions can be distinguished* (although without sharp borders): *a rostroventral and a dorsocaudal*. In addition to giant cells and large cells the nucleus contains numerous small cells. The number and density of cells are greater in the rostroventral than in the dorsocaudal part. Most of the giant cells and the largest ones are found in the dorsocaudal part. The dendrite patterns are different in the two parts of the nucleus.

The lateral nucleus gives off its *main efferents* to the spinal cord as the ipsilateral vestibulospinal tract which descends throughout the entire cord. Small as well as large and giant cells contribute to the tract, which is composed of fibers of varying diameters. Almost all lateral vestibulospinal fibers terminate on internuncial cells in Rexed's laminae VII–VIII. Conclusive anatomical demonstration of synaptic contacts with motoneurons in lamina IX is lacking. The *vestibulospinal projection is somatotopically organized*. Fibers to the cervical cord come from the rostroventral part of the nucleus, fibers to the lumbosacral cord from the dorsocaudal part (cf. above). An intermediate zone supplies the thoracic cord. Accordingly the two main regions of the nucleus can be referred to as forelimb and hindlimb region respectively.

The lateral nucleus contributes to the ascending medial longitudinal fasciculus bilaterally. The ascending fibers are probably not distributed to the various oculomotor nuclei. The nucleus does not give off fibers to the cerebellum but supplies certain regions of the main reticular formation, mainly ipsilaterally, and the ipsilateral lateral reticular nucleus (nucleus of the lateral funiculus) and the contralateral nucleus reticularis tegmentis pontis. Commissural efferents are scanty and pass to the contralateral lateral and descending vestibular nuclei. Efferent fibers in the vestibular nerve appear to be derived from certain minor parts of the lateral nucleus.

Afferent fibers to the lateral vestibular nucleus come from many sources, the most important being the cerebellum and the vestibular receptors. The primary vestibular fibers supply the rostroventral forelimb region (with some overlapping into the trunk region). The majority of these fibers appear to be derived from the utricular macula. Electron-microscope studies have shown that the primary vestibular fibers establish synaptic contacts with perikarya and proximal as well as distal dendrites, chiefly of small and medium-sized cells.

Cerebellar afferents to the lateral nucleus are numerous and consist of several contingents. Fibers from the vermis of the anterior lobe and from the posterior vermis pass to the ipsilateral nucleus of Deiters and end in its dorsal part. The projection from the anterior lobe is somatotopically organized. Other cerebellar afferents come from the fastigial nucleus. Those from the rostral part of the nucleus end in the dorsal half of the ipsilateral nucleus of Deiters, those from the caudal part pass in the hook bundle and terminate in the ventral half of the contralateral nucleus of Deiters. Both projections are somatotopically organized. By way of the topically arranged cerebellar corticonuclear projection onto the fastigial nucleus, somatotopically patterned disynaptic pathways are established from the anterior lobe vermis and the posterior vermis onto the dorsal and the ventral half respectively of the nucleus of Deiters. (The border between the two contingents of fastigial fibers crosses the border between the somatotopical subdivisions of the nucleus.) A few fibers from the "vestibulo-cerebellum" end in the lateral nucleus.

Compared with the fiber contingents from the cerebellum and the vestibular apparatus, the contingents from other sources are small. A few fibers from the spinal cord end in the most caudal part of the hindlimb region. There are some commissural afferents from the contralateral superior, lateral and descending nuclei. They appear to end mainly ventrally in the nucleus of Deiters. Some fibers from the reticular formation have been traced in Golgi preparations to the nucleus. No convincing evidence for afferents from the mesencephalon or other rostrally situated regions of the brain has been produced.

Judging from its fiber connections the lateral vestibular nucleus appears to be of primary importance as a station in pathways mediating cerebellar influences on the spinal cord. The pathways (except for the small contribution from the vestibulo-cerebellum) *all appear to be somatotopically organized and are presumably essential in the production of somatotopically localized effects on the spinal motor apparatus elicitable from the cerebellar vermis.* The preponderant contribution of primary vestibular afferents from the utricle to the nucleus, the restriction of these fibers to its forelimb region, and the contribution of small as well as large cells to the vestibulospinal tract are features of functional interest. The scanty commissural connections, the unilateral (chiefly ipsilateral, in part contralateral) course of the cerebellar pathways to the nucleus and the purely ipsilateral course of the lateral vestibulospinal tract are anatomical features which indicate a functional relative independence of the nuclei of the two sides.

c) *The medial vestibular nucleus* is not quite uniform in its cytoarchitecture but characteristic subdivisions cannot be recognized in cell- or fiber-stained preparations. However, the patterns of sites of origin of efferent fibers and particularly of the sites of terminations of afferents furnish anatomical evidence that *the nucleus is scarcely an entity from a functional point of view.*

Among the *afferent fibers*, primary vestibular fibers, apparently derived chiefly from the cristae, terminate dorsolaterally mainly at more rostral levels. The fibers from the rostral part of the ipsilateral fastigial nucleus supply the same region, as do also the fibers from the flocculus. The "nonvestibular," most ventral region of the medial nucleus is the main site of ending of cerebellar afferents from the caudal part of the contralateral fastigial nucleus and from the ipsilateral half of the nodulus. Descending fibers from the interstitial nucleus of Cajal in the mesencephalon supply mainly the dorsocaudal part, and some spinal afferents end in its most caudal part. The medial nucleus receives some commissural fibers from the contralateral superior and descending nuclei, perhaps also from the medial. The commissural afferents are restricted to the ventral part of the nucleus. Presumably there are some afferents from the reticular formation.

The *efferent connections* of the medial nucleus pass to several regions. Fibers reach the cervical and upper thoracic cord by way of the medial vestibulospinal tract running in the descending medial longitudinal fasciculus (sulcomarginal fasciculus), chiefly ipsilaterally. Like the fibers of the lateral vestibulospinal tract from the lateral nucleus the fibers end in laminae VII–VIII, but they do not extend below the upper thoracic segments. Ascending fibers, some of which may be ascending branches of bifurcating axons which send another branch to the spinal cord, pass via both ascending medial longitudinal fascicles to specific regions of the nuclei of the oculomotor nerves (different regions within each group are supplied by crossing and noncrossing fibers). These ascending fibers appear to come predominantly from the region of the nucleus which receives primary vestibular afferents. A small contingent of afferents from the medial vestibular nucleus pass to the cerebellum (chiefly at least, to the "vestibulocerebellum") and are derived from its ventrolateral, "nonvestibular", part, chiefly caudally. The medial nucleus probably gives off fibers to the reticular formation and commissural fibers, but conclusive experimental demonstrations of these projections are difficult because the nucleus is traversed by a number of fibers from the descending nucleus destined for the reticular formation and the contralateral vestibular nuclei.

Judging from its fiber connections, the medial vestibular nucleus appears to be organized in a less specific manner than the superior and lateral nuclei. Like the superior nucleus the medial appears to have its main task in the orderly transmission of impulses from the cristae to the motor nuclei of the ocular nerves. Its projection to the cervical cord suggests that the nucleus may be of functional importance for the integration of movements of the eyes and the neck.

d) *The descending (inferior) vestibular nucleus* is characterized by the presence of numerous longitudinally running fibers (mainly descending branches of primary vestibular fibers and cerebellar afferents from the fastigial nucleus). The nucleus is less uniform with regard to cytoarchitecture than the medial nucleus. Rostrally some large cells are present, and in the caudal part, ventrolaterally, is *group f* which differs from the rest of the nucleus with regard to its connections (see below). As in the medial nucleus clear-cut architectonic subdivisions cannot be made, but *the connections indicate functional differences between certain regions.*

The most abundant *afferent fibers* to the descending nucleus come from the vestibular apparatus and the cerebellum. Primary vestibular fibers (from the cristae, the utricle and the saccule) supply the largest part of the nucleus, except the dorsolateral part and the ventralmost strip. Cerebellar afferents from the anterior lobe and fibers from the rostral part of the fastigial nucleus end in approximately the dorsal half of the ipsilateral nucleus, while the caudal part of the fastigial nucleus sends fibers to the ventrolateral part of the contralateral medial vestibular nucleus. A few spinal afferents reach the most caudal part of the nucleus, while fibers from the mesencephalon appear to be absent. Commissural fibers come mainly from the descending nucleus of the other side, some also from the contralateral superior nucleus. The commissural fibers end only in the ventral part of the medial nucleus, receiving crossed fastigial fibers. In this region terminate also the afferents from the nodulus, while those from the flocculus (as in the superior and medial nucleus) end in the region receiving primary vestibular fibers (mainly dorsomedially). The distributions and origins of afferents from the reticular formation have not been clarified.

A small number of *efferent fibers* from the descending nucleus may ascend in the medial longitudinal fasciculus. Some cells (near the border to the medial nucleus) appear to send their axons to the spinal cord. Another sparse contingent of efferents (from the ventrolateral part, especially) caudally passes to the vestibulocerebellum. Commissural efferents are relatively numerous and supply the ventral regions of the contralateral descending, medial and lateral nuclei. The descending nucleus gives off fibers to the reticular formation, among these to the magnocellular nuclei on the contralateral side.

Judging from its fiber connections, the descending nucleus (excepting group f) in many respects resembles the medial, but it appears searcely to be concerned with vestibular influences on the ocular muscles. It must be subjected to a differentiated cerebellar control, and has ample possibilities for cooperation with the contralateral descending nucleus.

e) *The smaller groups of the vestibular nuclear complex* are not known in all particulars of their connections. It is clear, however, that they differ from each other as well as from the main vestibular nuclei.

The *group f*, mentioned above, is situated in the substance of the descending nucleus, from which it differs in many respects. Its relatively large and densely packed cells probably do not give off ascending fibers, but many axons pass to the cerebellum, presumably the "vestibulocerebellum". It does not receive primary vestibular fibers or spinal afferents, but is influenced from the cerebellum by fibers from the caudal part of the fastigial nucleus, the nodulus and the flocculus. *Group f thus appears to be especially related to the cerebellum.*

The *group x* is fairly well characterized by its position and connections. Its main afferents come from the spinal cord and end in a somatotopical pattern. Other afferents come from the cerebellum, some from the fastigial nucleus (probably mainly its middle parts), others from the nodulus-uvula. Group x does not receive primary vestibular fibers. The majority of its efferents pass to the cerebellum, mainly presumably to the "vestibulocerebellum." Some efferents probably ascend in the medial longitudinal fasciculus. The fiber connections suggest that *group x is mainly a relay in a spinocerebellar pathway.*

The *interstitial nucleus of the vestibular nerve* is a characteristic group consisting of densely packed, relatively large cells with abundant dendrite branches curled up around the cells. The nucleus receives primary vestibular fibers and may be the only group of the vestibular nuclear complex which receives afferents from all five receptor regions of the vestibular apparatus. The presence of fibers from the maculae, however, is disputed. Cerebellar connections appear to be absent. The nucleus gives off ascending fibers, presumably passing in the medial longitudinal fasciculus. *These connections suggest that the nucleus may be particularly related to vestibular influences on movements of the eyes.*

Knowledge of the connections of the other small groups is fragmentary. Group y appears to receive primary fibers from the sacculus only.

3. *The available anatomical observations furnish convincing evidence that the particular cell groups and subdivisions of the vestibular complex must be functionally dissimilar.* Each group has its own specific pattern with regard to cellular architecture and fiber connections. Furthermore, there are differences among afferent fiber contingents with regard to the patterns of branching and the types and arrangement of terminal boutons. Conclusive information about the morphological aspects of synaptic relations can only be obtained in electron-microscope studies of normal and experimental material. Data of this kind are so far available only for the lateral vestibular nucleus. Even if cerebellar cortical and primary vestibular afferents entering this nucleus both establish contact with perikarya and proximal and distal dendrites, the synaptic formations of the two kinds of afferents show certain differences. Convergence of primary vestibular fibers and of afferents from the cerebellar vermis have been demonstrated on cells in the nucleus of Deiters. Further studies of this kind may be expected to yield valuable additional information on structural differences between nuclear groups and between various afferent fiber contingents. There is reason to believe that histochemical studies may bring forth further evidence for a minute parcellation of the vestibular nuclear complex. Detailed physiological studies, especially of single units, are in agreement with the conclusions drawn from anatomical observations.

4. *The many different "units" (cell groups and territories) of the vestibular nuclear complex cannot be considered independent of each other.* There are several anatomical arrangements by which cooperation between "units" may take place. Fibers from one "unit" may pass to an extravestibular cell group or region which sends fibers back to another "unit" in the vestibular complex.[20] More immediate ways of cooperation between "units" may be established by local arrangements. Spread of dendrites of cells in one "unit" into the territory of another appears to offer very restricted possibilities for cooperation. Classic internuncial cells of the Golgi II type appear to be absent or at least exceedingly rare in the vestibular nuclear

20 For example the medial vestibular nucleus may be influenced from the superior, lateral and descending nuclei via the interstitial nucleus of Cajal in the mesencephalon, since this receives ascending fibers from the three latter nuclei but gives off descending fibers to the medial nucleus only. The cerebellum may be of relevance from this point of view for several "units".

complex. However, many cells provided with long axons passing to other regions give off collateral branches in the vicinity of the perikaryon. Such cells may well function as internuncials (cf. similar arrangements in the reticular formation and the ventral horns of the spinal cord).

The many specifically organized connections of the various components of the vestibular nuclei with other regions of the central nervous system should serve as reminders of the collaboration of the vestibular nuclei with other structures.

5. *A correlation of the territories receiving the various contingents of afferents and of territories giving rise to efferent projections to different destinations is of functional interest.* Particularly close cooperation and integration must be assumed in the case of impulses entering the same territory of a nucleus. From this point of view it is striking to notice that the cerebellar fibers from the flocculus supply the same regions in the superior, medial and descending nuclei as do the primary vestibular fibers, while most of the cerebellar afferents from the caudal part of the fastigial nucleus and the nodulus-uvula end in other parts of these nuclei. The fibers ascending in the medial longitudinal fasciculus appear to be derived chiefly from nuclear regions which receive primary vestibular afferents, and to be activated monosynaptically. Another feature of a similar kind is the restriction of primary vestibular fibers in the nucleus of Deiters to its forelimb region.

6. *In functional analyses and physiological studies it is necessary to take into consideration the data known on the structural organization of the vestibular subdivision under study.* On account of the differences in structure and especially in connections between the many "units" of the vestibular nuclear complex, precise indications of the sites recorded from or stimulated are essential if reliable conclusions are to be drawn concerning functional aspects. The presence of fibers passing through the region studied must be kept in mind. In attempts to correlate physiological and anatomical data it should be recalled that borders between regions shown by lines in drawings of the nuclei represent zones of transition and are not to be taken as indicating clearly demonstrated structural differences.

7. *In continued anatomical and physiological research of the vestibular nuclei* (as of other central nervous structures) *meticulous studies of minor features are essential.* In spite of a number of studies of this kind in recent years on the structural and functional organization of the various "units" of the vestibular nuclei, much remains to be done in both fields of research. The wealth of minutiae known at present may appear overwhelming and may be difficult to integrate into coherent pictures. Yet it is only by continued clarification of the finest structural and functional patterns of organization that we can hope to obtain a foundation for a better understanding of the working machinery of the vestibular mechanisms, peripheral and central.

Abbreviations used in Figures

B. c., Br. c.	Brachium conjunctivum
Cer.	Cerebellum
C. r.	Restiform body (Inferior cerebellar peduncle)
D	Descending (inferior) vestibular nucleus
d. ac. s.	Dorsal acoustic stria
f	Cell group f in the descending vestibular nucleus
F	Fastigial nucleus

F. l. m.	Medial longitudinal fasciculus
Flocc.	Flocculus
F. r.	Fasciculus retroflexus
g	Group rich in glia cells, caudal to the medial vestibular nucleus
H. b.	Hook bundle of Russell (Uncinate fasciculus)
i. c.	Nucleus intercalatus (Staderini)
L	Lateral vestibular nucleus (of Deiters)
l	Lateral group (middle-sized cells) of lateral vestibular nucleus
L. ant.	Lobus anterior cerebelli
Li	Lingula cerebelli
Ll and Lm	Lateral and medial parts of the lateral vestibular nucleus in man
L. p. m.	Lobulus paramedianus
M	Medial vestibular nucleus
N. c.	Cochlear nuclei
N. c. d.	Dorsal cochlear nucleus
N. c. p.	Nucleus of posterior commissure
N. c. v.	Ventral cochlear nucleus
N. cu. e.	External (accessory) cuneate nucleus
N. D.	Nucleus of Darkschewitsch
N. dent.	Dentate nucleus
N. E.-W.	Edinger-Westphal nucleus
N. fast.	Fastigial nucleus
N. f. c.	Cuneate nucleus
N. f. g.	Gracile nucleus
N. i.	Nucleus interpositus cerebelli
N. i. a.	Nucleus interpositus anterior
N. i. n. VIII	Interstitial nucleus of vestibular nerve
N. int.	Interstitial nucleus of Cajal in mesencephalon
N. l.	Nucleus lateralis cerebelli (dentatus)
N. m.	Nucleus medialis cerebelli (fastigii)
N. m. X	Dorsal motor (parasympathetic) nucleus of vagus
N. m. XII	Motor nucleus of hypoglossal nerve
N. mes. V	Mesencephalic nucleus of trigeminal nerve
N. n. III	Oculomotor nucleus
No	Nucleus ovalis
Nod.	Nodulus
N. p. s.	Nucleus parasolitarius
N. pr. V	Principal sensory nucleus of trigeminal nerve
N. pr. h.	Nucleus praepositus hypoglossi
N. r.	Red nucleus
N. r. l.	Nucleus reticularis lateralis
N. r. t.	Nucleus reticularis tegmenti pontis
N. tr. s.	Nucleus of solitary tract
N. tr. sp. V	Nucleus of spinal tract of trigeminal nerve
N. vest.	Vestibular nerve
N. V, VII, VIII, IX, XII	Cranial nerves V, VII, VIII, IX, XII
Ol. i.	Inferior olive
Ol. s.	Superior olive
p	Small-celled part of dentate nucleus
P.	Pontine nuclei
Pfl. d. and Pfl. v.	Paraflocculus dorsalis and ventralis
p. h.	Nucleus praepositus hypoglossi
Pyr.	Pyramis
Ret.	Reticular formation
R. gc.	Nucleus reticularis gigantocellularis
R. p. c.	Nucleus reticularis pontis caudalis

R. pc.	Nucleus reticularis parvicellularis
R. v.	Nucleus reticularis ventralis
S	Superior vestibular nucleus (of Bechterew)
SMP	Small-celled part of fastigial nucleus
Sv	Supravestibular nucleus
Tr. s.	Solitary tract
Tr. sp. c. d.	Dorsal spinocerebellar tract
Tr. sp. V, Tr. sp. n. V.	Spinal tract of trigeminal nerve
Uv.	Uvula
Ventr. IV	Fourth ventricle
x	Cell group lateral to the descending vestibular nucleus
y	Cell group dorsal to the restiform body
z	Cell group dorsal to the caudal part of the descending vestibular nucleus
III, IV, V, VI, VII, XII	Motor cranial nerve nuclei

References

Adrian, E.D.: Afferent areas in the cerebellum connected with the limbs. Brain **66**, 289–315 (1943).

Aitken, J.T., Bridger, J.E.: Neuron size and neuron population density in the lumbosacral region of the cats' spinal cord. J. Anat. (Lond.) **95**, 38–53 (1961).

Allen, W.F.: Origin and distribution of the tractus solitarius in the guinea pig. J. comp. Neurol. **35**, 171–204 (1923).

Allen, W.F.: Distribution of the fibers originating from the different basal cerebellar nuclei. J. comp. Neurol. **36**, 399–439 (1924).

Altman, J., Carpenter, M.B.: Fiber projections of the superior colliculus in the cat. J. comp. Neurol. **116**, 157–178 (1961).

Angaut, P., Brodal, A.: The projection of the "vestibulocerebellum" onto the vestibular nuclei in the cat. Arch. ital. Biol. **105**, 441–479 (1967).

Avanzino, G.L., Hösli, L., Wolstencroft, J.H.: Identification of cerebellar projecting neurones in nucleus reticularis gigantocellularis. Brain Res. **3**, 201–203 (1966).

Bienfang, D.C.: Location of the cell bodies of the superior rectus and inferior oblique motoneurons in the cat. Exp. Neurol. **21**, 455–466 (1968).

Bowsher, D.: The topographical projection of fibres from the anterolateral quadrant of the spinal cord to the subdiencephalic brain stem in man. Psychiat. Neurol. (Basel) **143**, 75–99 (1962).

Brodal, A.: Modification of Gudden method for study of cerebral localization. Arch. Neurol. Psychiat. (Chic.) **43**, 46–58 (1940a).

Brodal, A.: Experimentelle Untersuchungen über die olivocerebellare Lokalisation. Z. ges. Neurol. Psychiat. **169**, 1–153 (1940b).

Brodal, A.: The cerebellum of the rabbit. A topographical atlas of the folia as revealed in transverse sections. J. comp. Neurol. **72**, 63–81 (1940c).

Brodal, A.: Experimental demonstration of cerebellar connexions from the peri-hypoglossal nuclei (nucleus intercalatus, nucleus praepositus hypoglossi and nucleus of Roller) in the cat. J. Anat. (Lond.) **86**, 110–129 (1952).

Brodal, A.: The reticular formation of the brain stem. Anatomical aspects and functional correlations. Ramsay Henderson Trust Lecture. Edinburgh and London: Oliver & Boyd 1957.

Brodal, A.: Fiber connections of the vestibular nuclei. In: Neural mechanisms of the auditory and vestibular systems. G.L. Rasmussen and W. Windle, Eds. Springfield (Ill.): Ch. C. Thomas 1960.

Brodal, A.: Anatomical organization and fiber connections of the vestibular nuclei. In: Neurological aspects of auditory and vestibular disorders. W.S. Fields and B.R. Alford, Eds. Springfield (Ill.): Ch. C. Thomas 1964a.

Brodal, A.: Anatomical observations on the vestibular nuclei, with special reference to their relations to the spinal cord and the cerebellum. Acta oto-laryng. (Stockh.) Suppl. **192**, 24–51 (1964b).

BRODAL, A.: Anatomical aspects and functional organization of the vestibular nuclei. In: NASA SP-115: Second symposium on the role of the vestibular organs in space exploration. Ames Research Center, Moffett Field, California 1966.

BRODAL, A.: Anatomical organization of cerebello-vestibulo-spinal pathways. In: Ciba Foundation Symposium: Myotatic, kinesthetic and vestibular mechanisms. A.V.S. DE REUCK and J. KNIGHT, Eds. London: Churchill Ltd. 1967a.

BRODAL, A.: Anatomical studies of cerebellar fibre connections with special reference to problems of functional localization. In: The cerebellum. Progress in Brain Research, vol. 25. J.P. SCHADÉ, Ed. Amsterdam: Elsevier Publ. Co. 1967b.

BRODAL, A., ANGAUT, P.: The termination of spinovestibular fibres in the cat. Brain Res. **5**, 494–500 (1967).

BRODAL, A., DRABLØS, P.A.: Two types of mossy fiber terminals in the cerebellum and their regional distribution. J. comp. Neurol. **121**, 173–187 (1963).

BRODAL, A., GOGSTAD, A.C.: Afferent connexions of the paramedian reticular nucleus of the medulla oblongata in the cat. An experimental study. Acta anat. (Basel) **30**, 133–151 (1957).

BRODAL, A., GRANT, G.: Morphology and temporal course of degeneration in cerebellar mossy fibers following transection of spinocerebellar tracts in the cat. An experimental study with silver methods. Exp. Neurol. **5**, 67–87 (1962).

BRODAL, A., HØIVIK, B.: Site and mode of termination of primary vestibulocerebellar fibres in the cat. An experimental study with silver impregnation methods. Arch. ital. Biol. **102**, 1–21 (1964).

BRODAL, A., POMPEIANO, O.: The vestibular nuclei in the cat. J. Anat. (Lond.) **91**, 438–454 (1957).

BRODAL, A., POMPEIANO, O.: The origin of ascending fibres of the medial longitudinal fasciculus from the vestibular nuclei. An experimental study in the cat. Acta morph. neerl.-scand. **1**, 306–328 (1958).

BRODAL, A., POMPEIANO, O., WALBERG, F.: The vestibular nuclei and their connections. Ramsay Henderson Trust Lectures. Edinburgh and London: Oliver & Boyd 1962.

BRODAL, A., ROSSI, G.F.: Ascending fibers in brain stem reticular formation of cat. Arch. Neurol. Psychiat. (Chic.) **74**, 68–87 (1955).

BRODAL, A., TORVIK, A.: Über den Ursprung der sekundären vestibulo-cerebellaren Fasern bei der Katze. Eine experimentell-anatomische Studie. Arch. Psychiat. Nervenkr. **195**, 550–567 (1957).

BRODAL, P., MARŠALA, J., BRODAL, A.: The cerebral cortical projection to the lateral reticular nucleus in the cat, with special reference to the sensorimotor cortical areas. Brain Res. **6**, 252–274 (1967).

BUCHANAN, A.R.: The course of the secondary vestibular fibers. J. comp. Neurol. **67**, 183–204 (1937).

CAJAL, S.R.Y.: Beitrag zum Studium der Medulla oblongata, des Kleinhirns und des Ursprungs der Gehirnnerven. Leipzig: J.A. Barth 1896.

CAJAL, S.R.Y.: Histologie du système nerveux de l'homme et des vertébrés. Paris: Maloine 1909–1911.

CAMMERMEYER, J.: The post-mortem origin and mechanism of neuronal hyperchromatosis and nuclear pyknosis. Exp. Neurol. **2**, 379–405 (1960).

CARPENTER, M.B.: Fiber projections from the descending and lateral vestibular nuclei in the cat. Amer. J. Anat. **107**, 1–22 1960a.

CARPENTER, M.B.: Experimental anatomical-physiological studies of the vestibular nerve and cerebellar connections. In: Neural mechanisms of the auditory and cerebellar connections. G.L. RASMUSSEN and W. WINDLE, Eds. Springfield (Ill.): Ch. C. Thomas 1960b.

CARPENTER, M.B., ALLING, F.A., BARD, D.S.: Lesions of the descending vestibular nucleus in the cat. J. comp. Neurol. **114**, 39–50 (1960).

CARPENTER, M.B., BARD, D.S., ALLING, F.A.: Anatomical connections between the fastigial nuclei, the labyrinth and the vestibular nuclei in the cat. J. comp. Neurol. **111**, 1–25 (1959).

CARPENTER, M.B., BRITTIN, G.M., PINES, J.: Isolated lesions of the fastigial nuclei in the cat. J. comp. Neurol. **109**, 65–89 (1958).

Carpenter, M.B., Hanna, G.R.: Lesions of the medial longitudinal fasciculus in the cat. Amer. J. Anat. **110**, 307–332 (1962).

Carpenter, M.B., McMasters, R.E.: Disturbances of conjugate horizontal movements in the monkey. II. Physiological effects and anatomical degeneration resulting from lesions in the medial longitudinal fasciculus. Arch. Neurol. (Chic.) **8**, 347–368 (1963).

Carpenter, M.B., Strominger, N.L.: The medial longitudinal fasciculus and disturbances of conjugate horizontal eye movements in the monkey. J. comp. Neurol. **125**, 41–66 (1965).

Clark, W.E. le Gros, Powell, T.P.S.: On the thalamo-cortical connexions of the general sensory cortex of Macaca. Proc. roy. Soc. B **141**, 467–487 (1953).

Cohen, B., Susuki, J.-I., Bender, M.B.: Eye movements from semicircular canal nerve stimulation in the cat. Ann. Otol. (St. Louis) **73**, 153–169 (1964).

Cohen, D., Chambers, W.W., Sprague, J.M.: Experimental study of the efferent projections from the cerebellar nuclei to the brainstem of the cat. J. comp. Neurol. **109**, 233–259 (1958).

Collier, J., Buzzard, E.F.: The degeneration resulting from lesions of posterior nerve roots and from transverse lesions of the spinal cord in man. Brain **26**, 559–591 (1903).

Corbin, K.B., Hinsey, J.C.: Intramedullary course of the dorsal root fibers of each of the first four cervical nerves. J. comp. Neurol. **63**, 119–126 (1935).

Courville, J., Brodal, A.: Rubrocerebellar connections in the cat. An experimental study with silver impregnation methods. J. comp. Neurol. **126**, 471–485 (1966).

Devito, R.V., Brusa, A., Arduini, A.: Cerebellar and vestibular influences on Deitersian units. J. Neurophysiol. **19**, 241–253 (1956).

Dohlman, G., Farkashidy, J., Salonna, F.: Centrifugal nerve-fibers to the sensory epithelium of the vestibular labyrinth. J. Laryng. **72**, 984–991 (1958).

Dow, R.S.: The fiber connections of the posterior parts of the cerebellum in the rat and cat. J. comp. Neurol. **63**, 527–548 (1936).

Dow, R.S.: Efferent connections of the flocculo-nodular lobe in Macaca mulatta. J. comp. Neurol. **68**, 297–305 (1938a).

Dow, R.S.: Effects of lesions in the vestibular part of the cerebellum in primates. Arch. Neurol Psychiat. (Chic.) **40**, 500–520 (1938b).

Duensing, F., Schaefer, K.P.: Die Aktivität einzelner Neurone der Formatio reticularis des nicht gefesselten Kaninchens bei Kopfwendungen und vestibulären Reizen. Arch. Psychiat. Nervenkr. **201**, 97–122 (1960).

Eager, R.P.: Efferent cortico-nuclear pathways in the cerebellum of the cat. J. comp. Neurol. **120**, 81–103 (1963).

Eager, R.P.: Patterns and mode of termination of cerebellar cortico-nuclear pathways in the monkey (Macaca mulatta). J. comp. Neurol. **126**, 551–565 (1966).

Eccles, J.C., Eccles, R.M., Iggo, A., Lundberg, A.: Electrophysiological studies on gamma motoneurons. Acta physiol. scand. **50**, 32–40 (1960).

Eckel, W.: Elektrophysiologische und histologische Untersuchungen im Vestibulariskerngebiet bei Drehreizen. Arch. Ohr.-, Nas.-, u. Kehlk.-Heilk. **164**, 487–513 (1954).

Engström, H., Rexed, B.: Über die Kaliberverhältnisse der Nervenfasern im N. stato-acusticus des Menschen. Z. mikr.-anat. Forsch. **47**, 448–455 (1940).

Erulkar, S.D., Sprague, J.M., Whistel, B.L., Dogan, S., Jannetta, P.J.: Organization of the vestibular projection to the spinal cord of the cat. J. Neurophysiol. **29**, 626–664 (1966).

Escolar, J.: The afferent connections of the 1st, 2nd and 3rd cervical nerves in the cat. An analysis by Marchi and Rasdolsky methods. J. comp. Neurol. **89**, 79–92 (1948).

Fernández, C., Fredrickson, J.M.: Experimental cerebellar lesions and their effect on vestibular function. Acta oto-laryng. (Stockh.) Suppl. **192**, 52–62 (1964).

Ferraro, A., Pacella, B.L., Barrera, S.E.: Effects of lesions of the medial vestibular nucleus. An anatomical and physiological study in Macacus rhesus monkeys. J. comp. Neurol. **73**, 7–37 (1940).

Flood, S., Jansen, J.: On the cerebellar nuclei in the cat. Acta anat. (Basel) **46**, 52–72 (1961)

Flood, S., Jansen, J.: The efferent fibres of the cerebellar nuclei and their distribution on the cerebellar peduncles in the cat. Acta anat. (Basel) **63**, 137–166 (1966).

FOERSTER, O., GAGEL, O.: Die Vorderseitenstrangdurchschneidung beim Menschen. Eine klinisch-patho-physiologisch-anatomische Studie. Z. ges. Neurol. Psychiat. **138**, 1–92 (1932).

FREDRICKSON, J.M., FIGGE, U., SCHEID, P., KORNHUBER, H.H.: Vestibular nerve projection to the cerebral cortex of the rhesus monkey. Exp. Brain Res. **2**, 318–327 (1966).

FREDRICKSON, J.M., SCHWARZ, D., KORNHUBER, H.H.: Convergence and interaction of vestibular and deep somatic afferents upon neurons in the vestibular nuclei of the cat. Acta oto-laryng. (Stockh.) **61**, 168–186 (1965).

FUSE, G.: Die innere Abteilung des Kleinhirnstiels (Meynert, IAK) und der Deiterssche Kern. Arb. Hirnanat. Inst. Zürich **6**, 29–267 (1912).

GACEK, R.R.: Efferent component of the vestibular nerve. In: Neural mechanisms of the auditory and vestibular systems. G.L. RASMUSSEN and W. WINDLE, Eds. Springfield (Ill.): Ch. C. Thomas 1960.

GACEK, R.R.: The course and central termination of first order neurons supplying vestibular endorgans in the cat. Acta oto-laryng. (Stockh.) Suppl. **254**, 1–66 (1969).

GACEK, R.R., RASMUSSEN, G.L.: Fiber analysis of the statoacoustic nerve of guinea pig, cat, and monkey. Anat. Rec. **139**, 455–463 (1961).

GEREBTZOFF, M.A.: Notes anatomiques. J. belge Neurol. Psychiat. No. **8**, 401–406 (1940).

GEREBTZOFF, M.A.: Les bases anatomiques de la physiologie du cervelet. Cellule **49**, 71–166 (1941).

GEREBTZOFF, M.A.: Cholinesterases. A histochemical contribution to the solution of some functional problems. London, New York, Paris and Los Angeles: Pergamon Press 1959.

GERNANDT, B.E., IRANYI, M., LIVINGSTON, R.B.: Vestibular influences on spinal mechanisms. Exp. Neurol. **1**, 248–273 (1959).

GLEES, P.: Terminal degeneration within the central nervous system as studied by a new silver method. J. Neuropath. exp. Neurol. **5**, 54–59 (1946).

GOODMAN, D.C., HALLETT, R.E., WELCH, R.B.: Patterns of localization in the cerebellar corticonuclear projections of the albino rat. J. comp. Neurol. **121**, 51–67 (1963).

GRANT, G., ASCHAN, G., EKVALL, L.: Nystagmus produced by localized cerebellar lesions. Acta oto-laryng. (Stockh.) Suppl. **192**, 78–84 (1964)

GRAY, L.P.: Some experimental evidence on the connections of the vestibular mechanism in the cat. J. comp. Neurol. **41**, 319–364 (1926).

HASHIMOTO, T.: Experimentelle Untersuchungen über die spinale Bahn des N. vestibularis, mit besonderer Berücksichtigung auf dem Gebiete des Deiters descendens et ascendens Winklers. Folia anat. jap. **6**, 537–598 (1928).

HASSLER, R.: Forels Haubenfaszikel als vestibuläre Empfindungsbahn mit Bemerkungen über einige andere sekundäre Bahnen des Vestibularis und Trigeminus. Arch. Psychiat. Nervenkr. **180**, 23–53 (1948).

HASSLER, R.: Die zentralen Apparate der Wendebewegungen. II. Die neuronalen Apparate der vestibulären Korrekturwendungen und der Adversivbewegungen. Arch. Psychiat. Nervenkr. **194**, 481–516 (1956).

HAUGLIE-HANSSEN, E.: Intrinsic neuronal organization of the vestibular nuclear complex in the cat. A Golgi study. Ergebn. Anat. Entwickl.-Gesch. **40**, 5, 1–105 (1968).

HELD, H.: Über eine directe acustische Rindenbahn und den Ursprung des Vorderseitenstranges beim Menschen. Arch. Anat. Physiol.-anat. Abth. 257–264 (1892).

HELD, H.: Die anatomische Grundlage der Vestibularisfunktionen. Beitr. Anat. etc., Ohr. **19**, 305–312 (1923).

HOHMAN, L.B.: The efferent connections of the cerebellar cortex; investigations based upon experimental extirpations in the cat. Res. Publ. Ass. nerv. ment. Dis. **6**, 445–460 (1929).

HYDÉN, H.: The neuron. In: The cell. S. BRACHET and A.E. MIRSKY, Eds. New York: Academic Press 1960.

INGVAR, S.: Zur Phylo- und Ontogenese des Kleinhirns nebst einem Versuche zu einheitlicher Erklärung der zerebellaren Funktion und Lokalisation. Folia neuro-biol. (Lpz.) **11**, 205–495 (1918).

ITO, M., HONGO, T., YOSHIDA, M., OKADA, Y., OBATA, K.: Antidromic and trans-synaptic activation of Deiters' neurones induced from the spinal cord. Jap. J. Physiol. **14**, 638–658 (1964).

Ito, M., Obata, K., Ochi, R.: The origin of cerebellar-induced inhibition of Deiter's neurones. II. Temporal correlation between the trans-synaptic activation of Purkinje cells and the inhibition of Deiters' neurones. Exp. Brain Res. **2**, 350–364 (1966).

Ito, M., Yoshida, M.: The origin of cerebellar-induced inhibition of Deiter's neurones. I. Monosynaptic initiation of the inhibitory postsynaptic potentials. Exp. Brain Res. **2**, 330–349 (1966).

Ito, M., Yoshida, M., Obata, K.: Monosynaptic inhibition of the intracerebellar nuclei induced from the cerebellar cortex. Experientia (Basel) **20**, 575 (1964).

Jacobsohn, L.: Über die Kerne des menschlichen Hirnstamms. Abh. Kön. Preuss. Akad. Wiss. Physik.-math. Kl. 1–70 (1909).

Jansen, J.: On the efferent connections of the cerebellum. In: Progr. Neurobiol. Amsterdam: Elsevier Publ. Co. 1956.

Jansen, J., Brodal, A.: Experimental studies on the intrinsic fibers of the cerebellum. II. The cortico-nuclear projection. J. comp. Neurol. **73**, 267–321 (1940).

Jansen, J., Brodal, A.: Experimental studies on the intrinsic fibers of the cerebellum. III. The cortico-nuclear projection in the rabbit and the monkey. Norske Vid.-Akad. Avh. I. Math.-Nat. Kl. No. **3**, 1–50 (1942).

Jansen, J., Brodal, A.: Das Kleinhirn. In: v. Möllendorff's Handbuch der mikroskopischen Anatomie des Menschen IV/8. Berlin-Göttingen-Heidelberg: Springer 1958.

Jansen, J., Jansen, J., Jr.: On the efferent fibers of the cerebellar nuclei in the cat. J. comp. Neurol. **102**, 607–632 (1955).

Johnson, T.N., Clemente, C.D.: An experimental study of the fiber connections between the putamen, globus pallidus, ventral thalamus, and midbrain tegmentum in cat. J. comp. Neurol. **113**, 83–101 (1959).

Kappers, C.U Ariëns, Huber, G.C., Crosby, E.C.: The comparative anatomy of the nervous system of vertebrates, including man. New York: Macmillan Co. 1936.

Kerr, F.W.L.: Facial, vagal and glossopharyngeal nerves in the cat. Afferent connections. Arch. Neurol. (Chic.) **6**, 264–281 (1962).

Koelliker, A.: Der feinere Bau des verlängerten Markes. Anat. Anz. **6**, 427–431 (1891).

Kohnstamm, O.: Ueber Ursprungskerne spinaler Bahnen im Hirnstamm, speciell über das Athemcentrum. Arch. Psychiat. Nervenkr. **32**, 681–684 (1899).

Kohnstamm ,O., Wolfstein, J.: Versuch einer physiologischen Anatomie der Vagusursprünge und des Kopfsympathicus. J. Psychol. Neurol. (Lpz.) **8**, 177–203 (1907).

Korneliussen, H.K.: Cerebellar corticogenesis in Cetacea, with special reference to regional variations. J. Hirnforsch. **9**, 151–185 (1967).

Kornhuber, H.: Physiologie und Klinik des zentralvestibularen Systems (Blick- und Stützmotorik). In: Hals-Nasen-Ohren-Heilkunde III/3. J. Berendes, R. Link and F. Zöllner, Eds. Stuttgart: Georg Thieme 1966.

Ladpli, R., Brodal, A.: Experimental studies of commissural and reticular formation projections from the vestibular nuclei in the cat. Brain Res. **8**, 65–96 (1968).

Landgren, S., Silfvenius, H., Wolsk, D.: Vestibular, cochlear and trigeminal projections to the cortex in the anterior suprasylvian sulcus of the cat. J. Physiol. (Lond.) **191**, 561–573 (1967).

Larsell, O.: The development and morphology of the cerebellum in the opossum. II. Later development and adult. J. comp. Neurol. **63**, 251–291 (1936a).

Larsell, O.: Cerebellum and corpus pontobulbare of the bat (Myotis). J. comp. Neurol. **64**, 275–302 (1936b).

Leidler, R.: Experimentelle Untersuchungen über das Endigungsgebiet des Nervus vestibularis. 2. Mitteilung. Arb. neurol. Inst. Univ. Wien **21**, 151–212 (1914).

Lewandowsky, M.: Untersuchungen über die Leitungsbahnen des Truncus cerebri und ihren Zusammenhang mit denen der Medulla spinalis und des Cortex cerebri. Neurobiol. Arb., Zweite Serie I, 63–147 (1904).

Lloyd, R.E.: On chromatolysis in Deiters' nucleus after hemisection of the cord. J. Physiol. (Lond.) **25**, 191–195 (1899).

Lorente de Nó, R.: Etudes sur le cerveau postérieur. III. Sur les connexions extra-cérébelleuses des fascicules afférents au cerveau, et sur la fonction de cet organe. Trav. Lab. Rech. Biol. Univ. Madr. **22**, 51–65 (1924).

Lorente de Nó, R.: Untersuchungen über die Anatomie und die Physiologie des Ohrlabyrinthes und des Nervus octavus. Kap. 9: Einige Experimente über den Nervenmechanismus der vestibulären Augenreflexe. Mschr. Ohrenheilk. **61**, 1066–1135 (1927).

Lorente de Nó, R.: Ausgewählte Kapitel aus der vergleichenden Physiologie des Labyrinthes. Die Augenmuskelreflexe beim Kaninchen und ihre Grundlagen. Ergebn. Physiol. **32**, 73–242 (1931).

Lorente de Nó, R.: Vestibulo-ocular reflex arc. Arch. Neurol. Psychiat. (Chic.) **30**, 245–291 (1933a).

Lorente de Nó, R.: Anatomy of the eighth nerve. The central projection of the nerve endings of the internal ear. Laryngoscope (St. Louis) **43**, 1–38 (1933b).

Lund, S., Pompeiano, O.: Descending pathways with monosynaptic action on motoneurones. Experientia (Basel) **21**, 602–603 (1965).

Løken, Aa. C., Brodal, A.: A somatotopical pattern in the lateral vestibular nucleus in man. Arch. Neurol. (Chic.) **23**, 350–357 (1970).

McMasters, R. E., Weiss, A. H., Carpenter, M. B.: Vestibular projections to the nuclei of the extraocular muscles. Degeneration resulting from discrete partial lesions of the vestibular nuclei in the monkey. Amer. J. Anat. **118**, 163–194 (1966).

MacNalty, A. S., Horsley, V.: On the cervical spino-bulbar and spino-cerebellar tracts and on the question of topographical representation in the cerebellum. Brain **32**, 237–255 (1909).

Mannen, H.: Arborisations dendritiques. Étude topographique et quantitative dans le noyau vestibulaire du chat. Arch. ital. Biol. **103**, 197–219 (1965).

Mano, N., Oshima, T., Shimazu, H.: Inhibitory commissural fibers interconnecting the bilateral vestibular nuclei. Brain Res. **8**, 378–382 (1968).

Marburg, O.: Mikroskopisch-topographischer Atlas des menschlichen Zentralnervensystems. Leipzig and Wien: F. Deuticke 1910.

Markham, C. H.: Midbrain and contralateral influences on brainstem vestibular neurons in the cat. Brain Res. **9**, 312–333 (1968).

Markham, C. H., Precht, W., Shimazu, H.: Effect of stimulation of interstitial nucleus of Cajal on vestibular unit activity in the cat. J. Neurophysiol. **29**, 493–507 (1966).

Matanao, S., Ôki, T., Zyo, K., Ban, T.: Experimental studies on the medial longitudinal fasciculus in the rabbit. III. Descending tectofugal tracts and the FLM. Med. J. Osaka Univ. **15**, 293–310 (1965).

Matano, S., Zyo, K., Ban, T.: Experimental studies on the medial longitudinal fasciculus in the rabbit. I. Fibers originating in the vestibular nuclei. Med. J. Osaka Univ. **14**, 339–370 (1964a).

Matano, S., Zyo, K., Ban, T.: Experimental studies on the medial longitudinal fasciculus in the rabbit. II. The mesencephalic component of FLM and the central tegmental, medial tegmental and rubrospinal tracts. Med. J. Osaka Univ. **15**, 169–191 (1964b).

Meessen, H., Olszewski, J.: A cytoarchitectonic atlas of the rhombencephalon of the rabbit. Basel and New York: S. Karger 1949.

Mehler, W. R., Feferman, M. E., Nauta, W. J. H.: Ascending axon degeneration following anterolateral cordotomy. An experimental study in the monkey. Brain **83**, 718–750 (1960).

Mettler, F. A.: Corticifugal fiber connections of the cortex of Macaca mulatta. The occipital region. J. comp. Neurol. **61**, 221–256 (1935).

Monakow, C. von: Experimenteller Beitrag zur Kenntnis des Corpus restiforme, des „äusseren Acusticuskerns" und deren Beziehungen zum Rückenmark. Arch. Psychiat. Nervenkr. **14**, 1–16 (1883).

Mugnaini, E., Walberg, F.: An experimental electron microscopical study on the mode of termination of cerebellar corticovestibular fibres in the cat lateral vestibular nucleus (Deiters' nucleus). Exp. Brain Res. **4**, 212–236 (1967).

Mugnaini, E., Walberg, F., Brodal, A.: Mode of termination of primary vestibular fibres in the lateral vestibular nucleus. An experimental electron microscopical study in the cat. Exp. Brain Res. **4**, 187–211 (1967).

Mugnaini, E., Walberg, F., Hauglie-Hanssen, E.: Observations on the fine structure of the lateral vestibular nucleus (Deiters' nucleus) in the cat. Exp. Brain Res. **4**, 146–186 (1967).

Muskens, L.J.J.: Experimentelle und klinische Untersuchungen über die Verbindungen der unteren Olive und ihre Bedeutung für die Fallrichtung. Arch. Psychiat. Nervenkr. **102**, 558–613 (1934).

Nauta, W.J.H.: Silver impregnation of degenerating axons. In: New research techniques of neuroanatomy. W.F. Windle, Ed. Springfield (Ill.): Ch. C. Thomas 1960.

Nauta, W.J.H., Kuypers, H.G.J.M.: Some ascending pathways in the brain stem reticular formation. In: Reticular formation of the brain. Henry Ford Hospital Symposium. H.H. Jasper, L.D. Proctor et al., Eds. Boston: Little, Brown & Co. 1958.

Nyberg-Hansen, R.: Origin and termination of fibers from the vestibular nuclei descending in the medial longitudinal fasciculus. An experimental study with silver impregnation methods in the cat. J. comp. Neurol. **122**, 355–367 (1964).

Nyberg-Hansen, R.: Anatomical demonstration of gamma motoneurons in the cat's spinal cord. Exp. Neurol. **13**, 71–81 (1965).

Nyberg-Hansen, R.: Sites of termination of interstitiospinal fibers in the cat. An experimental study with silver impregnation methods. Arch. ital. Biol. **104**, 98–111 (1966).

Nyberg-Hansen, R., Mascitti, T.: Sites and mode of termination of fibers of the vestibulospinal tract in the cat. An experimental study with silver impregnation methods. J. comp. Neurol. **122**, 369–387 (1964).

Olszewski, J., Baxter, D.: Cytoarchitecture of the human brain stem. New York and Basel: S. Karger 1954.

Osen, K.K.: Course and termination of the primary afferents in the cochlear nuclei of the cat. An experimental anatomical study. Arch. ital. Biol. **108**, 21–51 (1970).

Peterson, B.W.: Effect of tilting on the activity of neurons in the vestibular nuclei of the cat. Brain Res. **6**, 606–609 (1967).

Petras, J.M.: Cortical, tectal and tegmental fiber connections in the spinal cord of the cat. Brain Res. **6**, 275–324 (1967).

Pompeiano, O.: Organizzazione somatotopica delle risposte posturali alla stimolazione elettrica del nucleo di Deiters nel Gatto decerebrato. Arch. Sci. biol. (Bologna) **44**, 497–511 (1960).

Pompeiano, O.: Functional organization of the cerebellar projections to the spinal cord. In: The cerebellum. Progress in Brain Research, Vol. 25. J.P. Schadé, Ed. Amsterdam, London and New York: Elsevier Publ. Co. 1967.

Pompeiano, O., Brodal, A.: The origin of vestibulospinal fibres in the cat. An experimental-anatomical study, with comments on the descending medial longitudinal fasciculus. Arch. ital. Biol. **95**, 166–195 (1957a).

Pompeiano, O., Brodal, A.: Spino-vestibular fibers in the cat. An experimental study. J. comp. Neurol. **108**, 353–382 (1957b).

Pompeiano, O., Cotti, E.: Analisi microelettrodica delle proiezioni cerebello-deitersiane. Arch. Sci. biol. (Bologna) **43**, 57–101 (1959).

Pompeiano, O., Walberg, F.: Descending connections to the vestibular nuclei. An experimental study in the cat. J. comp. Neurol. **108**, 465–504 (1957).

Precht, W., Grippo, J., Wagner, A.: Contribution of different types of central vestibular neurons to the vestibulospinal system. Brain. Res. **4**, 119–123 (1967).

Precht, W., Shimazu, H.: Functional connections of tonic and kinetic vestibular neurons with primary vestibular afferents. J. Neurophysiol. **28**, 1014–1028 (1965).

Ranson, S.W., Davenport, H.K., Doles, E.A.: Intramedullary course of the dorsal root fibers of the first three cervical nerves. J. comp. Neurol. **54**, 1–12 (1932).

Rasmussen, A.T.: Secondary vestibular tracts in the cat. J. comp. Neurol. **54**, 143–171 (1932).

Rasmussen, A.T.: Origin and course of the fasciculus uncinatus (Russel) in the cat with observations on the other fibre tracts arising from the cerebellar nuclei. J. comp. Neurol. **57**, 165–197 (1933).

Rasmussen, G.L., Gacek, R.: Concerning the question of an efferent fiber component of the vestibular nerve of the cat. (Abstract). Anat. Rec. **130**, 361–362 (1958).

Rexed, B.: The cytoarchitectonic organization of the spinal cord in the cat. J. comp. Neurol. **96**, 415–495 (1952).

Rexed, B.: A cytoarchitectonic atlas of the spinal cord in the cat. J. comp. Neurol. **100**, 297–379 (1954).

Rossi, G., Cortesina, G.: The efferent innervation of the inner ear. Panminerva med. **4**, 478–500 (1962).

Rossi, G., Cortesina, G.: The "efferent cochlear and vestibular system" in Lepus cuniculus L. Acta anat. (Basel) **60**, 362–381 (1965).

Rossum, J. van: Corticonuclear and corticovestibular projections of the cerebellum. An experimental investigation of the anterior lobe, the simple lobule and the caudal vermis in the rabbit. Thesis. Assen: Van Gorcum 1969.

Sabin, F.R.: On the anatomical relations of the nuclei of reception of the cochlear and vestibular nerves. Johns Hopk. Hosp. Bull. **8**, 253–259 (1897).

Sadjadpour, K., Brodal, A.: The vestibular nuclei in man. A morphological study in the light of experimental findings in the cat. J. Hirnforsch. **10**, 299–323 (1968).

Scheibel, M.E., Scheibel, A.B.: Structural substrates for integrative patterns in the brain stem reticular core. In: Reticular formation of the brain. Henry Ford Hospital Symposium. H.H. Jasper and L.D. Proctor et al., Eds. Boston: Little, Brown & Co. 1958.

Scheibel, M.E., Scheibel, A.B.: Spinal motorneurons, interneurons and Renshaw cells. A Golgi study. Arch. ital. Biol. **104**, 328–353 (1966).

Schimert, J.S.: Die Endigungsweise des Tractus vestibulospinalis. Z. Anat. Entwickl.-Gesch. **108**, 761–767 (1938).

Shimazu, H., Precht, W.: Tonic and kinetic responses of cat's vestibular neurons to horizontal angular acceleration. J. Neurophysiol. **28**, 991–1013 (1965).

Shimazu, H., Precht, W.: Inhibition of central vestibular neurons from the contralateral labyrinth and its mediating pathway. J. Neurophysiol. **29**, 467–492 (1966).

Smith, C.A.: Microscopic structure of the utricle. Ann. oto-rhino-laryng. **65**, 450–470 (1956).

Smith, C.A., Rasmussen, G.L.: Nerve endings in the maculae and cristae of the chinchilla vestibule, with a special reference to the efferents. In: NASA SP-152: Third symposium on the role of the vestibular organs in space exploration. Pensacola, Florida. National Aeronautics and Space Administration, Washington, D.C. 1968.

Snider, R.S.: Alterations which occur in mossy terminals of the cerebellum following transection of the brachium pontis. J. comp. Neurol. **65**, 417–435 (1936).

Sotelo, C., Paley, S.L.: The fine structure of the lateral vestibular nucleus in the rat. I. Neurons and neuroglial cells. J. Cell Biol. **36**, 151–179 (1968).

Sprague, J.M., Ha, H.: The terminal fields of dorsal root fibers in the lumbosacral cord of the cat, and the dendritic organization of the motor nuclei. In: Organization of the spinal cord. J.C. Eccles and J.P. Schadé, Eds. Amsterdam, London and New York: Elsevier Publ. Co. 1964.

Stein, B.M., Carpenter, M.B.: Central projections of portions of the vestibular ganglia innervating specific parts of the labyrinth in the rhesus monkey. Amer. J. Anat. **120**, 281–318 (1967).

Sterling, P., Kuypers, H.G.J.M.: Anatomical organization of the brachial spinal cord of the cat. II. The motoneuron plexus. Brain Res. **4**, 16–32 (1967).

Szentágothai, J.: Die zentrale Innervation der Augenbewegungen. Arch. Psychiat. Nervenkr. **116**, 721–760 (1943).

Szentágothai, J.: The elementary vestibulo-ocular reflex arc. J. Neurophysiol. **13**, 395–407 (1950).

Szentágothai, J.: Die Rolle der einzelnen Labyrinthrezeptoren bei der Orientation von Augen und Kopf im Raume. Budapest: Akadémiai Kiado 1952.

Szentágothai, J.: Pathways and synaptic articulation patterns connecting vestibular receptors and oculomotor nuclei. In: The oculomotor system. Bender, M.B. Ed. New York: Hoeber Medical Division, Harper & Row 1964.

Szentágothai, J., Rajkovits, K.: Der Hirnnervenanteil der Pyramidenbahn und der prämotorische Apparat motorischer Hirnnervenkerne. Arch. Psychiat. Nervenkr. **197**, 335–354 (1958).

Tarlov, E.: The rostral projections of the primate vestibular nuclei. An experimental study in macaque, baboon and chimpanzee. J. comp. Neurol. **135**, 27–56 (1969).

Tarlov, E.: Organization of vestibulo-oculomotor projections in the cat. Brain Res. **20**, 159–179 (1970).

Thiele, F.H., Horsley, V.: A study of the degenerations observed in the central nervous system in a case of fracture dislocation of the spine. Brain **24**, 519–531 (1901).

Thomas, D.M., Kaufman, R.P., Sprague, J.M., Chambers, W.W.: Experimental studies of the vermal cerebellar projections in the brain stem of cat (fastigiobulbar tract). J. Anat. (Lond.) **90**, 371–385 (1956).

Tokumasu, K., Goto, K., Cohen, B.: Eye movements produced by the superior oblique muscle. Arch. Ophthal. **73**, 851–862 (1965).

Torvik, A.: Afferent connections to the sensory trigeminal nuclei, the nucleus of the solitary tract and adjacent structures. An experimental study in the cat. J. comp. Neurol. **106**, 51–142 (1956).

Torvik, A., Brodal, A.: The origin of reticulospinal fibers in the cat. An experimental study. Anat. Rec. **128**, 113–137 (1957).

Vachananda, B.: The major spinal afferent systems to the cerebellum and the cerebellar corticonuclear connections in Macaca mulatta. J. comp. Neurol. **112**, 303–351 (1959).

Valverde, F.: Reticular formation of the pons and medulla oblongata. A Golgi study. J. comp. Neurol. **116**, 71–100 (1961a).

Valverde, F.: A new type of cell in the lateral reticular formation of the brain stem. J. comp. Neurol. **117**, 189–195 (1961b).

Voogd, J.: The cerebellum of the cat. Structure and fibre connexions. Thesis. Assen: Van Gorcum 1964.

Vraa-Jensen, G.: On the correlation between the function and structure of nerve cells. Acta psychiat. scand. Suppl. **109**, 1–88 (1956).

Walberg, F.: Descending connections to the inferior olive. An experimental study in the cat. J. comp. Neurol. **104**, 77–173 (1956).

Walberg, F., Bowsher, D., Brodal, A.: The termination of primary vestibular fibers in the vestibular nuclei in the cat. An experimental study with silver methods. J. comp. Neurol. **110**, 391–419 (1958).

Walberg, F., Jansen, J.: Cerebellar corticovestibular fibers in the cat. Exp. Neurol. **3**, 32–52 (1961).

Walberg, F., Jansen, J.: Cerebellar corticonuclear projection studied experimentally with silver impregnation methods. J. Hirnforsch. **6**, 338–354 (1964).

Walberg, F., Mugnaini, E.: Distinction of degenerating fibres and boutons of cerebellar and peripheral origin in the Deiters' nucleus of the same animal. Brain Res. **14**, 67–75 (1969).

Walberg, F., Pompeiano, O.: Fastigiofugal fibers to the lateral reticular nucleus: an experimental study in the cat. Exp. Neurol. **2**, 40–53 (1960).

Walberg, F., Pompeiano, O., Brodal, A., Jansen, J.: The fastigiovestibular projection in the cat. An experimental study with silver impregnation methods. J. comp. Neurol. **118**, 49–76 (1962).

Walberg, F., Pompeiano, O., Westrum, L.E., Hauglie-Hanssen, E.: Fastigioreticular fibers in cat. An experimental study with silver methods. J. comp. Neurol. **119**, 187–199 (1962).

Warwick, R.: Representation of the extra-ocular muscles in the oculomotor nuclei of the monkey. J. comp. Neurol. **98**, 449–503 (1953).

Weiss, A.H., McMasters, R.E., Carpenter, M.B.: Secondary vestibular projections in the brain stem of the rhesus monkey. (Abstract). Anat. Rec. **148**, 349 (1964).

Wersäll, J.: Studies on the structure and innervation of the sensory epithelium of the cristae ampullares in the guinea pig. A light and electron microscopic investigation. Acta oto-laryng. (Stockh.) Suppl. **126**, 1–85 (1956).

Wilson, V.J., Kato, M., Peterson, B.W., Wylie, R.M.: A single-unit analysis of the organization of Deiters' nucleus. J. Neurophysiol. **30**, 603–619 (1967).

Wilson, V.J., Kato, M., Thomas, R.C.: Excitation of lateral vestibular neurones. Nature (Lond.) **206**, 96–97 (1965).

Wilson, V.J., Kato, M., Thomas, R.C., Peterson, B.W.: Excitation of lateral vestibular neurons by peripheral afferent fibers. J. Neurophysiol. **29**, 508–529 (1966).

Wilson, V.J., Wylie, R.M., Marco, L.A.: Projection to the spinal cord from the medial and descending vestibular nuclei of the cat. Nature (Lond.) **215**, 429–430 (1967).

WILSON, V.J., WYLIE, R.M., MARCO, L.A.: Organization of the medial vestibular nucleus. J. Neurophysiol. **31**, 166–175 (1968a).

WILSON, V.J., WYLIE, R.M., MARCO, L.A.: Synaptic inputs to cells in the medial vestibular nucleus. J. Neurophysiol. **31**, 176–185 (1968b).

WILSON, V.J., YOSHIDA, M.: Comparison of effects of stimulation of Deiters' nucleus and medial longitudinal fasciculus on neck, forelimb, and hindlimb motoneurons. J. Neurophysiol. **32**, 743–758 (1969a).

WILSON, V.J., YOSHIDA, M.: Monosynaptic inhibition of neck motoneurons by the medial vestibular nucleus. Exp. Brain Res. **9**, 365–380 (1969b).

WINKLER, C., POTTER, A.: An anatomical guide to experimental researches on the cat's brain. A series of 35 frontal sections. Amsterdam: W. Versluys 1914.

WOODBURNE, R.T., CROSBY, E.C., MCCOTTER, R.E.: The mammalian midbrain and isthmus regions. Part II. The fiber connections. A. The relations of the tegmentum of the midbrain with the basal ganglia in Macaca mulatta. J. comp. Neurol. **85**, 67–92 (1946).

YEE, J., CORBIN, K.B.: The intramedullary course of the upper five, cervical, dorsal root fibers in the rabbit. J. comp. Neurol. **70**, 297–314 (1939).

Addendum

Since this manuscript was submitted in 1969 relatively few studies dealing with anatomical aspects of the vestibular nuclei have appeared. On the whole they bring data which are in accord with and supplement previously published findings considered in this chapter. Below some relevant papers are listed. The titles will show the subjects treated.

In addition to these papers attention is directed to the monograph: "Basic Aspects of Central Vestibular Mechanisms", Progress in Brain Research, Vol. 37, 656 pp. Ed. by A. BRODAL and O. POMPEIANO, Elsevier Publ. Comp., Amsterdam, London, New York 1972. Apart from reviews this monograph contains some presentations of some new original findings on the organisation of the vestibular nuclei.

ALVAREZ, J., PÜSCHEL, M.: Transfer of material from efferent axons to sensory epithelium in the goldfish vestibular system. Brain Res. **37**, 265–278 (1972).

BERGSTRÖM, B.: Numerical analysis of the vestibular nerve in man. A preliminary report. Uppsala J. medical Sci. **77**, 205–207 (1972).

CARPENTER, M.B., STEIN, B.M., PETER, P.: Primary vestibulocerebellar fibers in the monkey. Distribution of fibers arising from distinctive cell groups of the vestibular ganglia. Amer. J. Anat. **135**, 221–250 (1972).

CORVAJA, N., GROFOVÁ, I., POMPEIANO, O.: The origin, course and termination of vestibulospinal fibers in the toad. Brain Behav. Evol. **7**, 401–423 (1973).

FUENTES, C., RAYMOND, J.: Chromatolyse irreversible et dégénérescence rétrograde dans le ganglion vestibulaire. Etude expérimentale. J. neurol. Sci. **17**, 69–80 (1972).

GACEK, R.R.: Anatomical demonstration of the vestibulo-ocular projections in the cat. Acta oto-Laryng. (Stockh.) Suppl. **293**, 63 (1971).

GRANT, G., BOIVIE, J., SILFVENIUS, H.: Course and termination of fibres from the nucleus z of the medulla oblongata. An experimental light microscopical study in the cat. Brain Res. **55**, 55–70 (1973).

GREGORY, K.M.: Central projections of the eighth nerve in frogs. Brain Behav. Evol. **5**, 70–88 (1972).

HILLMAN, D.E.: Light and electron microscopical study of the relationships between the cerebellum and the vestibular organ of the frog. Exp. Brain Res. **9**, 1–15 (1969).

Iurato, S., Luciano, L., Pannese, E., Reale, E.: Histochemical localization of acetylcholinesterase (AChE) activity in the inner ear. Acta oto-laryng. (Stockh.) Suppl. **279**, 1–50 (1971).

Korn, H., Sotelo, C., Crepel, F.: Electrotonic coupling between neurones in the rat lateral vestibular nucleus. Exp. Brain Res. **16**, 255–275 (1973).

Landholt, J. P., Topliff, E. D. L., Silverberg, I. D.: Size distribution analysis of myelinated fibers in the vestibular nerve of the pigeon. Brain Res. **54**, 31–42 (1973).

Mabuchi, M., Kusawa, T.: Mesodiencephalic projections to the inferior olive and the vestibular and perihypoglossal nuclei. Brain Res. **17**, 133–136 (1970).

Sotelo, C., Palay, S. L.: Altered axons and axon terminals in the lateral vestibular nucleus of the rat. Possible example of axonal remodeling. Lab. Invest. **25**, 653–671 (1971).

Sotelo, C., Palay, S. L.: The fine structure of the lateral vestibular nucleus in the rat. II. Synaptic organization. Brain Res. **18**, 93–115 (1970).

Tarlov, E., Roffler-Tarlov, S.: The representation of extraocular muscles in the oculomotor nuclei: experimental studies in the cat. Brain Res. **34**, 37–52 (1971).

Chapter II.

The Physiology of the Vestibular Nuclei*

By

W. PRECHT, Frankfurt a. M.

With 15 Figures

Contents

I. Introduction

The experiments of GOLTZ (1870), MACH (1873), BREUER (1891), EWALD (1892), BÁRÁNY (1907) and STEINHAUSEN (1931, 1933) can be considered as a very important first step in the development of the physiology of the vestibular system. They established a theory of the mechanics of the peripheral vestibular sensory mechanisms which is still basically valid today. The various sensory cells in the

* The author wishes to dedicate this article to Professor ROLF HASSLER on the occasion of his 60th birthday.

peripheral vestibular sensory organ serve as receptors for *linear* and *angular* accelerations about different axes, thus providing a three dimensionally organized sensory system for *orientation in space*. Various other sensory systems such as the visual, somatosensory and acoustic apparatus combine with the vestibular organs in assuring a high sensitivity for the adjustment of the body in space. Part of this regulation is achieved by means of *interaction in the vestibular nuclei* which integrate the activity of the various vestibular receptors as well as the activity of other sensory structures which converge directly or indirectly on the vestibular neurones. As the vertebrates developed from lower to higher forms other sensory systems such as the somatosensory and visual systems became more and more important in the regulation of posture; however, the vestibular nuclei still remain an important *integrative* structure that deserves the interest of anatomists as well as physiologists.

Most investigators have subdivided the rather extensive vestibular nuclear complex into four nuclei: the *lateral (Deiters')*, *medial*, *superior* and *descending* vestibular nuclei. Further subdivisions have been made on the basis of more sophisticated histological studies. For details of the topography, cytoarchitecture and fiber connections of the vestibular nuclei, the reader is referred to the monograph by BRODAL et al. (1962) and to Chapter D.I. of this volume. There is no doubt that recent anatomical studies have greatly advanced our knowledge of the *intrinsic*, *afferent* and *efferent* connections of the vestibular nuclei and have thus provided a sound basis for the interpretation of physiological data. As far as the afferent connections are concerned, the distribution of the *primary vestibular fibres* within the nuclear complex is of great importance. It has been shown by WALBERG et al. (1958) that none of the four vestibular nuclei receive an equally distributed number of fibres in all of their territory. Certain regions of the subdivisions are completely free of primary vestibular fibres. The lateral vestibular nucleus, for instance, is free of vestibular terminals in its dorsal part and the same holds true for the medial parts of the medial nucleus. Other *afferent systems*, such as fibres from (1) the cerebellar cortex and the cerebellar nuclei, (2) the spinal cord, (3) the reticular formation at various levels, and (4) the contralateral vestibular nuclei also send strong fibre contingents to the vestibular nuclei and partly supply those areas that are free of primary fibres as well as other territories. *Interneurones* in the vestibular nuclei may serve as morphological substrates for the interaction of neurones located in different subdivisions of the nuclear complex. By means of its *efferent* fibres the vestibular nuclei establish contacts with various parts of the central nervous system, in particular with the oculomotor nuclei, the spinal cord, the reticular formation and the cerebellum.

In the past most investigators dealing with physiological aspects of the vestibular nuclei have studied the behavioral effects of electrical stimulation or operative lesions. Analysis of disturbances of posture and ocular movements caused in these experiments has provided a good deal of important data concerning some functional aspects of the vestibular nuclei. More recently a new approach to vestibular physiology has been started by the application of *microphysiological techniques* which allow one to record electrical activities from single neurones both extra- and intracellularly. This technique has already proven to be most powerful in the investigation of the synaptology of the vestibular nuclei and a great deal of new data has been obtained concerning the functional organization of the various vestibular nuclei. In the account given in this Chapter, emphasis will be placed on the recent microphysiological studies and an attempt will be made to correlate our present-day knowledge of the anatomical and physiological features of the vestibular nuclei.

II. Labyrinthine Input to the Vestibular Nuclei

Numerous anatomical studies have contributed to the present knowledge of the histological organization of the vestibular nuclei and the distribution of *primary* vestibular fibres in various subdivisions of this voluminous *nuclear complex* in the *brain-stem* (for details, see BRODAL and POMPEIANO, 1957a; BRODAL et al., 1962; Chapter D.I. of this volume). Golgi studies by LORENTE DE NÓ (1933a) indicated that fibres from the various labyrinthine receptor organs have, in part, a different central representation. Recent degenerative investigations by STEIN and CARPENTER (1967) in the monkey and GACEK (1969) in the cat strongly support the idea of a *distinctive* as well as a partially *common* distribution of primary vestibular fibres arising from different receptors. It seems that the fibres innervating the cristae of the semicircular canals terminate mainly in the *interstitial* nucleus, the *superior*, oral parts of the *medial* and descending vestibular nuclei, whereas fibres coming from otolithic organs end mainly in the *descending* nucleus, *medial* vestibular nucleus, ventral parts of the *lateral* vestibular nucleus and group "Y" (STEIN and CARPENTER, 1967; GACEK, 1969).

Similarly, physiological studies of the vestibular input to the brain-stem during the last 20 years have greatly advanced our knowledge of the functional aspects of the vestibular nuclei. The analysis of *field potentials* generated by stimulation of the vestibular nerve and recorded in various parts of the central vestibular system, and the recording of *single unit activity* have combined in providing a better understanding of the functional connections within the vestibular system.

The development of the technique of recording with microelectrodes from single neurones in the central nervous system has provided us with a powerful tool for studying the characteristics of any neurone in the nervous system. As far as vestibular nuclei are concerned, this technique has also greatly advanced our knowledge of the response characteristics of vestibular neurones to stimulation of various inputs.

A. Stimulation of the Labyrinthine Organs

A great variety of stimulation techniques can be used in order to excite vestibular receptors and they will be briefly summarized in this section. It is generally accepted that *angular* as well as *linear* accelerations are the physiological or adequate stimuli for the vestibular receptors. However, the receptors also respond to *anodal* and *cathodal* polarizing currents applied to the inner ear. No movements of the cupula will occur during this form of stimulation (STEINHAUSEN, 1931, 1933). In the primary and most of the secondary vestibular neurones, cathodal stimulation generally increases the discharge frequencies and anodal stimulation has the opposite effect. This technique is known as *galvanic stimulation* and is frequently used in physiological studies (DOHLMAN, 1929; LOWENSTEIN, 1955; DE VITO et al., 1956; TRINCKER, 1964, 1965; KORNHUBER and DA FONSECA, 1964; WEBER and STEINER, 1965; FREDRICKSON et al., 1966). For studying central vestibular neurones, this technique is not favourable since all receptors are stimulated simultaneously owing to current spread, thus allowing no correlation between unitary response and a particular receptor.

Caloric stimulation of the labyrinth, by means of irrigation of the ear with hot or cold water, also succeeds in increasing or decreasing the discharge rate in primary and secondary vestibular neurones, thus leading to the well known caloric ocular nystagmus (BREUER, 1889; BÁRÁNY, 1907; DOHLMAN, 1925; GERNANDT, 1949; LOWENSTEIN, 1955; WEBER and STEINER, 1965). By using this form of stimulation, convection currents are provoked in the endolymph of the semicircular canals, causing the cupula to bend in one or the other direction, depending on the relative temperature of the water used with respect to body temperature. The caloric stimulation has the advantage over rotatory stimulation in that it allows *unilateral* stimulation of a particular canal.

Direct mechanical stimulation of the semicircular canals by means of compression and decompression deserves mention since this procedure has given us much information concerning the direction-specific mechanisms of the cupula endolymph system and the effects provoked thereby in related systems (EWALD, 1892; STEINHAUSEN, 1931, 1933; SZENTÁGOTHAI, 1943, 1952; TRINCKER, 1957, 1965).

Finally, stimulation with *short electric pulses* has proven to be a powerful method for studying the synaptic organization between peripheral afferents and central nervous structures.

B. Field Potentials in the Vestibular Nuclei Produced by VIIIth Nerve Stimulation

When a microelectrode is inserted into the vestibular nuclei, a characteristic field potential is evoked by a single electric shock of the *ipsilateral* vestibular nerve (MICKLE and ADES, 1954; GERNANDT, 1960; KUMOI et al., 1963; SHIMAZU and PRECHT, 1965; PRECHT and SHIMAZU, 1965). Figure 1 shows the field potentials correlated with the location of the microelectrode tip. As also shown in Fig. 2A, this potential complex consisted of an initial positive-negative deflection (P) followed by a large sharp negative (N_1) wave and a delayed small negative (N_2) potential (PRECHT and SHIMAZU, 1965). When the electrode tip moved through the border of the vestibular nucleus, N_1 potential amplitude decreased with fairly sharp gradients, especially at the ventral border of the nucleus (Fig. 1). It was found that the electrode tip was located within the vestibular nuclei when the amplitude of N_1 potential was more than one-third or one-fourth of the maximal N_1 amplitude. N_1 and N_2 potentials were evoked at approximately the same threshold intensity of VIIIth nerve stimulation. For obtaining field potentials *restricted* to the vestibular nuclei, the intensity of vestibular nerve stimulation has to be no more than two times the threshold intensity for the N_1 response, because with stronger stimulation, responses of complex shape are evoked in the adjacent *reticular formation* of the brain-stem (Fig. 2B). The field potential

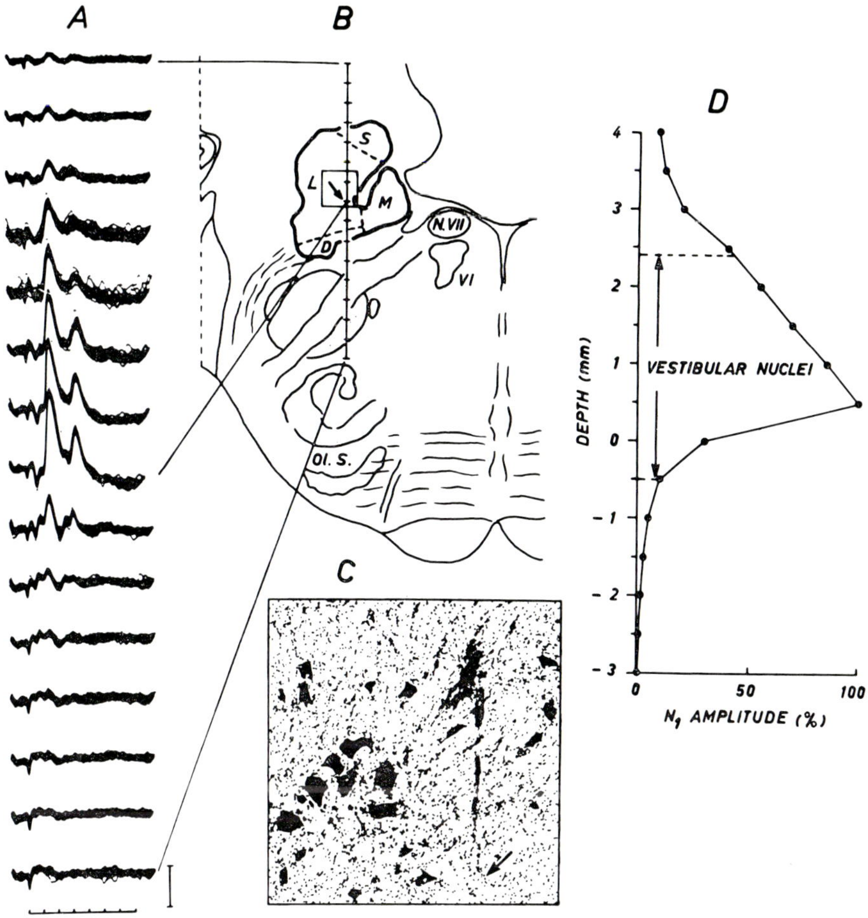

Fig. 1. Field potentials generated by stimulation of the vestibular nerve and recorded by a microelectrode in the ipsilateral vestibular nuclei of unanesthetized, decerebrate cat. A: potential fields evoked by single shocks of the vestibular nerve (the first downward deflection indicates stimulation artifact). Upward deflection indicates negativity of the microelectrode. Each record is composed of about 20 superimposed traces and was obtained from the site indicated by the scale in B. Time: 1 msec; voltage calibration: 0.5 mV. B: line drawing of histological section of the brain stem. The vertical line shows the insertion of the recording electrode. Scales on this line indicate 500 μ. Arrow indicates the site where coagulation was made with the microelectrode. S = superior nucleus; *L* — lateral nucleus; *M* — medial nucleus; *D* = descending nucleus; *Ol.S.* = superior olive; *N.VII* = seventh cranial nerve; *VI* = sixth cranial motor nucleus. C: microphotograph of the part surrounded by a square in B. Arrow indicates the position of the tip of the electrode. D: diagram showing relative amplitude of N_1 potential in A, correlated with the location of the electrode. Zero millimeters in the depth scale corresponds to the level of the surface in the midline of the fourth ventricle. Upper and lower borders of the vestibular nuclei are indicated by the two vertical arrows. Note the sharp decrease in amplitude of N_1 as the electrode approaches the ventral border of the vestibular nuclei (SHIMAZU and PRECHT, 1965)

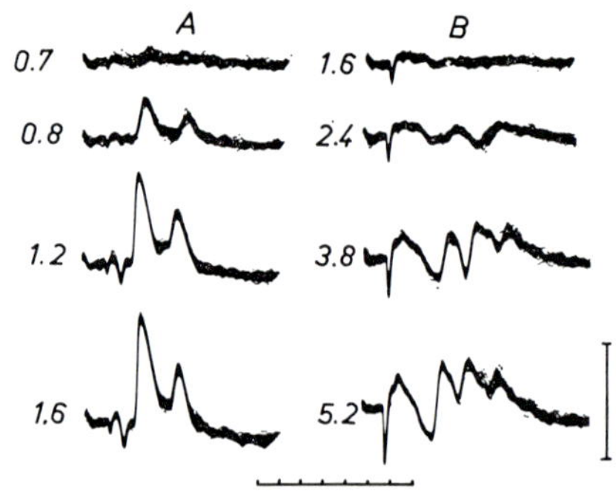

Fig. 2. Field potentials generated by single shock stimulation of the vestibular nerve and recorded by a microelectrode in the ipsilateral vestibular nuclei (A) and in the ipsilateral brain stem reticular formation of unanesthetized decerebrate cat (B). Upward deflection indicates negativity at the microelectrode and the first downward deflection indicates stimulation artifact. Each record is composed of about 20 superimposed traces. The numbers at the left side of each record represent stimulation voltages. The microelectrode was located in the lateral part of the medial vestibular nucleus (A) and in the reticular formation 3 mm beneath the ventral border of the medial vestibular nucleus. Note the higher threshold necessary to evoke field potentials in the reticular formation (B). Time 1 msec; voltage calibration: 1 mV (PRECHT and SHIMAZU, 1965)

complex is of similar configuration in all vestibular nuclei, although differences in the size of the amplitudes of the various components can be seen in different recording positions. Thus, the amplitude of the P-wave is larger the more *lateral* the electrode is placed, due to the proximity of the primary vestibular fibres (PRECHT and SHIMAZU, 1965). Both P and N_1 potentials dominate in the ventral portion of the Deiters' nucleus (ITO et al., 1968) as one would expect from the distribution of primary vestibular fibres in this nucleus (WALBERG et al., 1958; GACEK, 1969). Following stimulation of the lateral ampullary nerve, the N_2 wave appears to be relatively larger in the ventromedial part of the *medial* vestibular nucleus, whereas N_1 potential is larger in amplitude in the ventrolateral part of the same nucleus. The latter part is known to receive primary afferent fibres (WALBERG et al., 1958). Similarly, the N_1 potentials following stimulation of the anterior and posterior ampullary nerves and the utricular branch are found in slightly different positions, suggesting different central projection of peripheral organs (KUMOI et al., 1965). Further physiological evidence for a differential distribution of primary fibres will be given below.

The P potential has a latency of 0.66 ± 0.14 msec after a single pulse stimulation of the VIIIth nerve near its entry into the end organ (PRECHT and SHIMAZU, 1965). The summit of the positive wave may indicate the arrival of afferent impulses at the terminals (BROOKS and ECCLES, 1947). This potential follows repetitive stimulation up to frequencies of about 200/sec without change of its amplitude and proves to be very resistant to pentobarbital anaesthesia. These features suggest that the P-wave is generated by the compound action currents evoked conjointly in the primary vestibular fibres and in the efferent fibres which were found to exist also in mammals (GACEK, 1960).

The N_1 potential is the most conspicuous component of the field complex. It occurs about 0.4 msec after the arrival of the afferent impulses at the terminals with a latency of 1.06 ± 0.22 msec. The amplitude is decreased with high frequency stimulation, and the whole recovery period tested by double shocks is about 10 msec. N_1 potential was more sensitive to pentobarbital administration compared with the P-wave but less sensitive compared with N_2. It is assumed that N_1 potential consists of the synaptic and action currents generated mainly *monosynaptically* by primary vestibular fibres in secondary vestibular neurones (PRECHT and SHIMAZU, 1965). As a peculiar feature of vestibular nerve fibres repetitive action potentials are triggered by single shock stimulation. The action currents of these repetitively firing axons would also contribute to the N_1 and N_2 potentials (ITO et al., 1969b).

The latency of *N_2 potential* is 2.46 ± 0.26 msec. This potential is the one whose amplitude is most reduced during high frequency stimulation or under the influence of pentobarbital anaesthesia. The total recovery period tested by double shocks was usually more than 20 msec. These features suggest that N_2 potential is composed of synaptic and action currents generated by *multisynaptic* pathways in the vestibular nuclei (PRECHT and SHIMAZU, 1965). Possible *anatomical substrates for multisynaptic excitation* of vestibular neurones may be either *internuncial* neurones in the vestibular nuclei or *collaterals* of the axons leaving the nuclei (LORENTE DE NÓ, 1938; BRODAL et al., 1962). Since the stimulus intensity used for obtaining these field potentials is subthreshold for potentials in the reticular formation, a feedback from reticular neurones on vestibular units can be exluded for the generation of N_2. Likewise, generation of the field potential via a cerebellar loop was excluded by using cerebellectomized cats.

In summarizing the *field potential* analysis, it may be emphasized that characteristic potential sequences can be recorded in the vestibular nuclei following ipsilateral vestibular nerve stimulation. They are restricted to the vestibular nuclei if the stimulus intensity does not exceed two times of N_1 threshold. Recording of these field potentials thus allows a very fast *physiological identification* of the vestibular nuclei. A correlation of single spike activation with the various waves of the field potential will be given below.

C. Input from the Semicircular Canals

It is well known that all vertebrates have a structurally similar peripheral vestibular apparatus. Beginning from the true fishes, three semicircular canals (2 verticals and 1 horizontal) are found in all species, the horizontal or lateral canal being the last one appearing in phylogeny. They are approximately oriented according to the three dimensions of space. In the semicircular canals, the sensory *hair cells* are located in the *cristae ampullares* with the hairs facing the lumen. A normally transparent gelatinous structure, the so-called *cupula,* is superimposed on the cristae and hermetically separates the endolymph surrounding its utricular side from the one on the side of the canal. Thus the cupula is *mechanically coupled* with the endolymph, and any movement of the fluid will cause a deviation of the cupula to either the canal side or utricular side, leading to a deflection of the hairs embedded in the cupula (STEINHAUSEN, 1931, 1933). STEINHAUSEN's experiments directly proved and elucidated MACH's (1873) and BREUER's (1874, 1889, 1897) *theory* on the *mechanics* of the *semicircular canal mechanisms*, which now seems to be accepted by most scientists. Any *change in speed* of rotation will lead to a deflection of the cupula and the hairs of the sensory cells, owing to an *inertia movement* of the endolymph which is directed opposite to the direction of the progressing wall of the canal. Physically speaking, the semicircular canals are therefore *accelerometers* monitoring angular acceleration. More specifically, the cupula endolymph system has been considered as a *damped torsion pendulum* (STEINHAUSEN, 1931, 1933). Following Steinhausen's work, several investigators have dealt with the mathematical description of the cupula pendulum system, but a detailed description is beyond the scope of this Chapter (VAN EGMOND et al., 1949; GROEN et al., 1952; NIVEN and HIXSON, 1961; VALENTINUZZI, 1967).

Years before the centrally located vestibular nuclei were encroached upon by microelectrodes, several investigators had obtained oscillographic records from action potentials in the various branches of the vestibular nerve occuring spontaneously as well as in response to different kinds of stimuli given to the sensory vestibular organs of different animals (ASHCROFT and HALLPIKE, 1934; MOWRER, 1935; ROSS, 1936; LOWENSTEIN, and SAND 1936, 1940a, b; GERNANDT, 1949; LEDOUX, 1949; LOWENSTEIN, 1955; RUPERT et al., 1962; TRINCKER, 1964, 1965; GUALTIEROTTI and ALLTUCKER, 1967; LLINÁS et al., 1968; GOLDBERG and FERNÁNDEZ, 1971; PRECHT et al., 1971). All these studies combine in demonstrating that many *primary* vestibular neurones exhibit a *resting discharge*, even in the absence of any stimulus. The spontaneous activity is either *increased* or *decreased* in its rate, depending on the direction of the cupula deviation, thus showing a distinct *bi-directional* response pattern.

1. Input from the Horizontal Canals: Qualitative Aspects

LOWENSTEIN and SAND (1940a, b) have shown that the frequency of unit discharge recorded from the nerve branch of the horizontal canal *increases* when the cupula is deflected in an *utriculopetal* (ampullopetal) direction, and that spontaneous *firing ceases* when inertia movement of the endolymph causes the cupula to be bent in an *utriculofugal* (ampullofugal) direction. The maximum increase or decrease is related to the stimulus strength. Further, with increasing strengths, a recruitment of previously silent sensory units is observed. Using rotatory stimulation with the horizontal canal being in the plane of rotation, utriculopetal endolymph flow occurs on accelerated rotation towards the side of recording, and utriculofugal flow is generated when rotation is applied to the side contralateral to the recording side. For details of the peripheral mechanisms, see Chapter B.II. in this Handbook.

ADRIAN (1943) was the first to record from individual neurones in the vestibular nuclei (cat), i.e., from *secondary* vestibular units. The majority of the neurones responding to rotation give persistent low frequency discharges when the head is at rest. When the animal is rotated in the horizontal plane towards the recording side, the discharge frequency of a single unit increases, and it decreases on rotation opposite to the recording side. Thus, the second order neurones respond qualitatively in the same way as has been described for the primary neurones connected to the horizontal canals (LOWENSTEIN and SAND, 1940a, b) and will be called type-I units as designated by GERNANDT (1949) and DUENSING and SCHAEFER (1958). GERNANDT (1949) was recording from vestibular neurones of the cat and was able to confirm Adrian's finding that most units responding to stimulation of the horizontal semicircular canal increased their frequency of discharge during ipsilateral acceleration and showed the opposite reaction on contralateral rotation. In addition to type I responses, GERNANDT found units showing increase of their firing rate with acceleration in both directions and those whose frequency decreased with rotation in both directions. The former are classified by GERNANDT as type II and the latter as type III neurones. Although he was recording from the vestibular nerve, he assumed that he was recording from second order neurones also found in the vestibular nerve (interstitial nucleus of the VIIIth nerve). However, this assumption was not tested histologically or physiologically. ECKEL (1954) confirmed the three types of responses found by GERNANDT by recording from individual vestibular neurones in the vestibular nuclei of the rabbit. He was the first to localize histologically the recording points in the vestibular nuclei. In 1958, DUENSING and SCHAEFER reported their studies on horizontal canal activities recorded from neurones in the vestibular nuclei of the rabbit. They not only confirmed the neuronal types found by the earlier investigators, but were able to describe a new type of response which is characterized by a decrease of discharge frequency with ipsilateral acceleration and an increase with contralateral rotation, thus responding just opposite to the type-I neurones. They changed Gernandt's nomenclature by calling this new type of response type-II; and the former type-III and type-II were designated as type III and type-IV, respectively type-I remaining unchanged. In the following text, this nomenclature will be used. Recently, these four distinct types of responses of second order vestibular neurones, that can be recorded during horizontal angular acceleration, have also been described in the vestibular nuclei of the cat and some of their quantitative characteristics have been studied (SHIMAZU and PRECHT, 1965; PRECHT and SHIMAZU, 1965; SHIMAZU and PRECHT, 1966; PRECHT et al., 1966a).

2. Spontaneous Discharge of Vestibular Neurones

Before going into details of the response pattern of vestibular neurones to stimulation of the end organs, we would like to comment on the fact that both peripheral and central vestibular neurones show a *resting discharge* in the absence of any stimulation. This basic activity is so common among the labyrinthine receptors that it can be considered as an essential functional aspect of the system. Its cause, however, is still not known. On the other hand, some units in the nerve as well as in the vestibular nuclei are silent at rest and therefore show only a unidirectional response to rotation (LOWENSTEIN and SAND, 1940a, b; DUENSING and SCHAEFER, 1958; SHIMAZU and PRECHT, 1965; PRECHT et al., 1971a). The average frequency of spontaneous firing of the primary neurones in fishes, for example, was found to be around 20/sec, the individual neurones showing less than 4% deviation from the average firing rate (LOWENSTEIN and SAND, 1940a; GROEN et al., 1952). Similar regular resting discharge is seen in primary vestibular neurones of cats and monkeys, the rate of firing being not significantly influenced by anaesthetics (RUPERT et al., 1962; GOLDBERG and FERNÁNDEZ, 1971).

In decerebrate, as well as in encéphale isolé preparations, most of the *second order* vestibular neurones show a fairly regular resting activity ranging from 2–30/sec, and only occasionally, the basic rate amounts to 80–90/sec (ADRIAN, 1943; DUENSING and SCHAEFER, 1958; SHIMAZU and PRECHT, 1965). It seems that under pentobarbital anaesthesia, the number of spontaneously firing *central* units is significantly decreased in addition to the appearance of a general decrease of the excitability of most of the neurones when tested with electrical or adequate stimulation (GERNANDT, 1949; PRECHT and SHIMAZU, 1965). Under the influence of a light ether anaesthesia, the resting discharge appears to be in the range found in decerebrate animals (DUENSING and SCHAEFER, 1958).

Extracellular recording from single units in the various vestibular nuclei was performed in freely moving cats, and their activity was correlated to the states of *wakefulness* and *sleep* (BIZZI et al., 1964). Units recorded from *Deiters' nucleus* fire quite irregularly during wakefulness with an average frequency of 39/sec. The mean rate tends to decrease during *synchronized sleep*, and at the transition to the *desynchronized sleep* either no change or a slight increase of spontaneous firing occurs. Units located in the *superior nucleus* show a regular firing at an average frequency of 41/sec during quiet wakefulness. The mean rate of firing does not significantly change during the different stages of sleep. Units obtained from the *medial* and *descending vestibular nuclei* show a mean rate of spontaneous firing of 50/sec during relaxed wakefulness. During phases of desynchronized sleep, high *frequency bursts* (80–160 spikes/sec) occur which are strictly associated with the phenomenon of *rapid eye movements* characteristic for this state of sleep. Interestingly enough, no change in resting discharge is observed during *spontaneous eye movements* while the animals are awake. It was also shown that the discharge frequencies of most of the neurones tend to increase during *arousing stimuli* such as acoustic click stimulation. All these studies leave no doubt that resting discharge is a characteristic feature of many neurones in the *peripheral* and *central* vestibular system. This confirms EWALD's (1892) hypothesis of a *vestibular tone* which was based on the observation of loss of tone in the neck, limb and eye musculature, following bilateral labyrinthectomy, and on the presence of tonic asymmetries resulting from unilateral removal of the labyrinths.

While the origin of the "spontaneous" discharge found in the *primary neurones* still remains a matter of conjecture as far as the physiological mechanism is concerned, the "spontaneous" discharge of *second order neurones* is most likely not autochthonous in nature. It was shown that acute neurotomy of the VIIIth nerve nearly abolishes the resting discharge of many second order neurones, suggesting its reflex origin due to the tonic inflow of impulses from the labyrinths (GERNANDT and THULIN, 1952; SHIMAZU and PRECHT, 1966). Some time after the acute surgery, units regain to some degree their resting discharge, suggesting an additional excitatory impingement from sources other than the VIIIth nerve (PRECHT et al., 1966a). The reappearance of spontaneous activity in hemilabyrinthectomized animals parallels with the recovery of the symmetric ocular responses following bidirectional labyrinthine stimuli, pointing to the functional importance of a bilaterally balanced resting discharge activity (see Chapter F.X. of this Volume).

3. Quantitative Analysis of Type I Neurones

Modern, electronically controlled turntables allow the application of accurate values of angular acceleration for a protracted period of time which enables us to measure directly the constants of the equation for frequency response of single vestibular neurones to rotation. In the past, attempts have been made only to correlate sensation of rotation or ocular nystagmus directly with the activity of first order neurones of the semicircular canals (VAN EGMOND et al., 1949; HALLPIKE and HOOD, 1953a). These studies have not dealt adequately with the response characteristics of the second order vestibular neurones, which are intercalated between receptors and other central systems. Since type I vestibular neurones of the horizontal canals are the only neurones which are particularly well studied, their characteristics will be described in detail. Second order neurones of other canals may have similar characteristics. As mentioned above, type I second order vestibular neurones are characterized by an increase of their discharge rate during *ipsilaterally* directed angular acceleration in the horizontal plane and a decrease of firing during *contralateral* rotation. The horizontal canals of the cat are in plane of rotation when the stereotaxic frame holding the head is inclined 30° upward from the horizontal plane.

4. Mode of Increase and Decrease in Discharge Frequency

In Fig. 3 are plotted the serial changes of impulse frequencies of a tonic (A to D) and kinetic (E to H) type I vestibular neurone caused by ipsilateral rotations at different magnitudes of accelerations (SHIMAZU and PRECHT, 1965). As shown in each diagram of this figure, when the table was rotated in the ipsilateral direction with longlasting *constant* angular acceleration, the discharge frequency initially increased along an approximately *exponential* time course and then maintained a fairly *constant* value during the remainder of the acceleration. After the achievement of constant speed of rotation, the frequency decreased gradually to the level of the resting discharge characteristic for this neurone. Figure 4, shows examples of discharges of a tonic type I neurone at its maximum frequencies during different accelerations. It can be seen that the spike-to-spike interval of the tonically active neurones are fairly constant. Of all 122 type I units tested, 102 showed spontaneous activity (2–30/sec) at rest and had a similar response pattern during rotation. Nystagmic modulation of the type I frequency during the acceleration was rarely observed in decerebrate animals, but it is present in intact animals anaesthetized with ether (DUENSING and SCHAEFER, 1958).

Besides the tonically active type I neurones, there is another group of type I units which shows no spontaneous discharge or, in a few cases, only sporadic irregular discharges (less than 0.5/sec) in the resting condition. They will be called *kinetic* type I neurones as designated by SHIMAZU and PRECHT (1965). As shown in Fig. 3E to H, this type of neurone responds to ipsilateral rotation along an exponential time course after a remarkably long latency and *rapidly* reaches its maximum frequency. The decay in frequency was equally steep. Spike-to-spike intervals are more irregular than those of the tonic neurones. Figure 5A shows the replotting of the *increasing* phase of frequency response of a tonic and kinetic type I neurone. The relationship in each case corresponds closely to a straight line. Such an *exponential* increase was confirmed in two-thirds of the responses

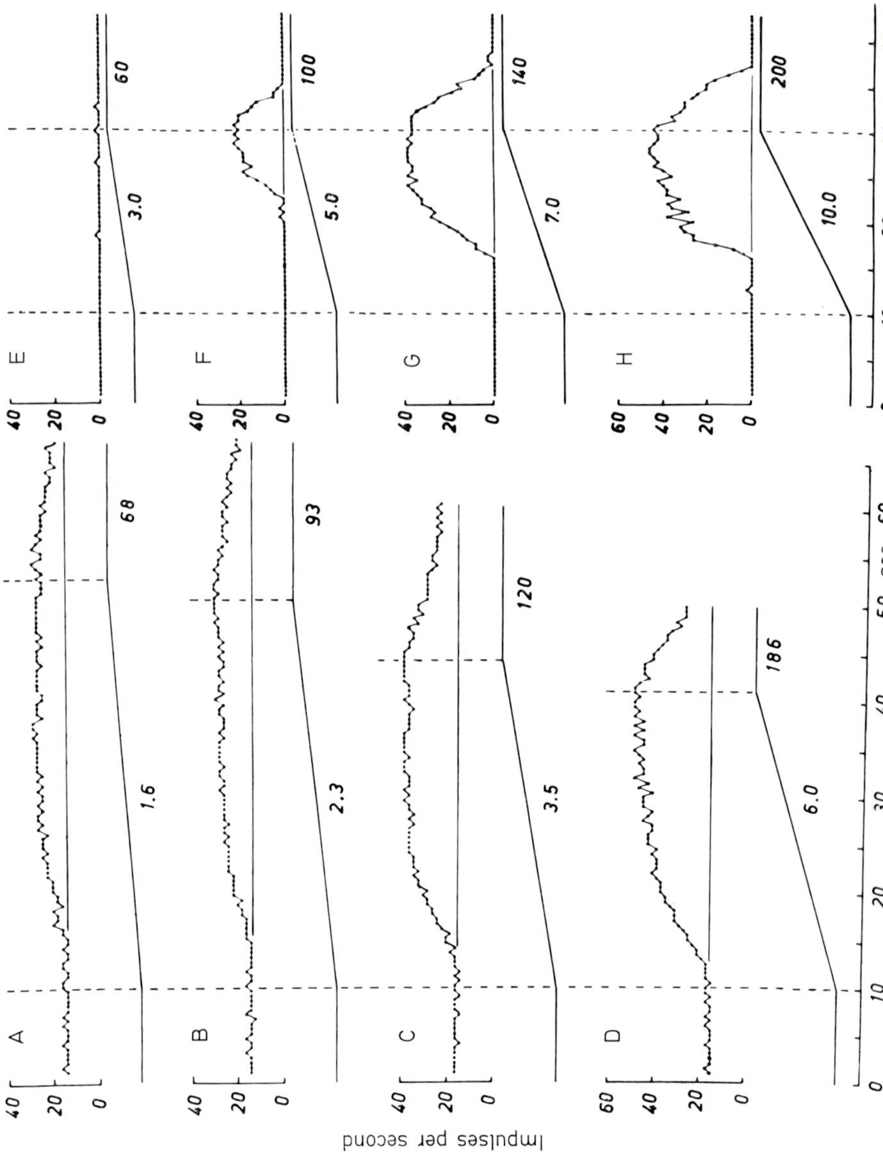

Fig. 3. Frequency diagrams of discharges of a tonic (A to D) and a kinetic (E to H) type I vestibular neurone in response to ipsilateral, horizontal, constant angular accelerations. The plane of the stereotaxic frame was inclined 30° upward from the horizontal position, such that the horizontal semicircular canals are approximately in a horizontal position. In each diagram (A to H), the ordinate represents spike per second of single unit discharges measured in each half-second. The horizontal line in each diagram (A to D) represents the average frequency over 10 sec before rotation. Onset of rotation is indicated by the left vertical broken line in each diagram, and cessation of acceleration (or beginning of constant speed rotation) by the right vertical broken line. Curve below each frequency diagram indicates the speed of rotation, though the transition at the beginning and the end of acceleration is not accurately shown in each schematic curve. The left-hand number in each diagram indicates the acceleration (degree/sec^2) and the right-hand number indicates the velocity (degree/sec) of constant rotation (SHIMAZU and PRECHT, 1965)

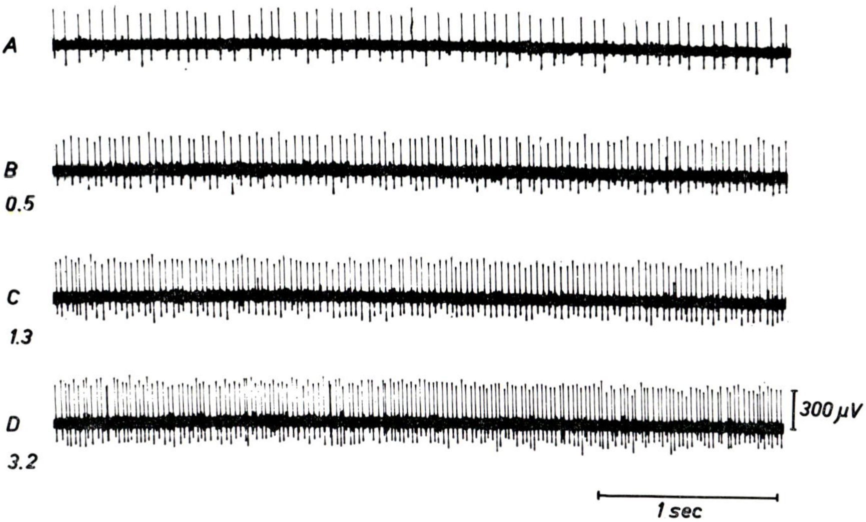

Fig. 4. Extracellularly recorded unit discharges of a tonic type I vestibular neurone in response to ipsilateral constant angular accelerations. Recording was done in a decerebrate and unanesthetized cat. A: record at resting condition. B, C, and D: records about 40 sec after the beginning of constant acceleration. The semicircular canals are in the plane of rotation. The constant acceleration (degree/sec²) applied is indicated on the left of each trace (SHIMAZU and PRECHT, 1965)

tested. This indicates that the following *equation* is applicable for the frequency response of vestibular neurones to ipsilateral constant angular acceleration (SHIMAZU and PRECHT, 1965):

$$f = f_{max} \, (1 - e^{\frac{-t}{p}}) \tag{1}$$

where f = frequency increase per second caused by angular acceleration; f_{max} = frequency increase at its maximum level; p = time constant of frequency response.

Figure 5B shows the values of p of type I neurones correlated to their basic frequencies of *spontaneous discharges*. It is statistically highly significant that the spontaneously nonactive or *kinetic* neurones (open circles) had *smaller* p values or steeper slopes (3.7 ± 0.8 sec) than the spontaneously active or *tonic* ones (8.1 ± 1.6 sec). The values of p, measured during the decrease in frequency after reaching constant speed of rotation, were approximately the same as those obtained during periods of increasing frequency.

VAN EGMOND et al. (1949) have calculated the coefficients of the equation for cupula deviation produced by rotation, using human sensation of rotation or nystagmus and an average of 8 sec or 10 sec was obtained for $\frac{F}{R}$ in equation 4 (see below). Recently GOLDBERG and FERNÁNDEZ (1971) have found that primary vestibular fibres in monkeys have time constants in the order of 6 sec. No separation between tonic and kinetic responses has been observed in the first order neurones of the monkey. These values are similar to the value of p for tonic vestibular neurones.

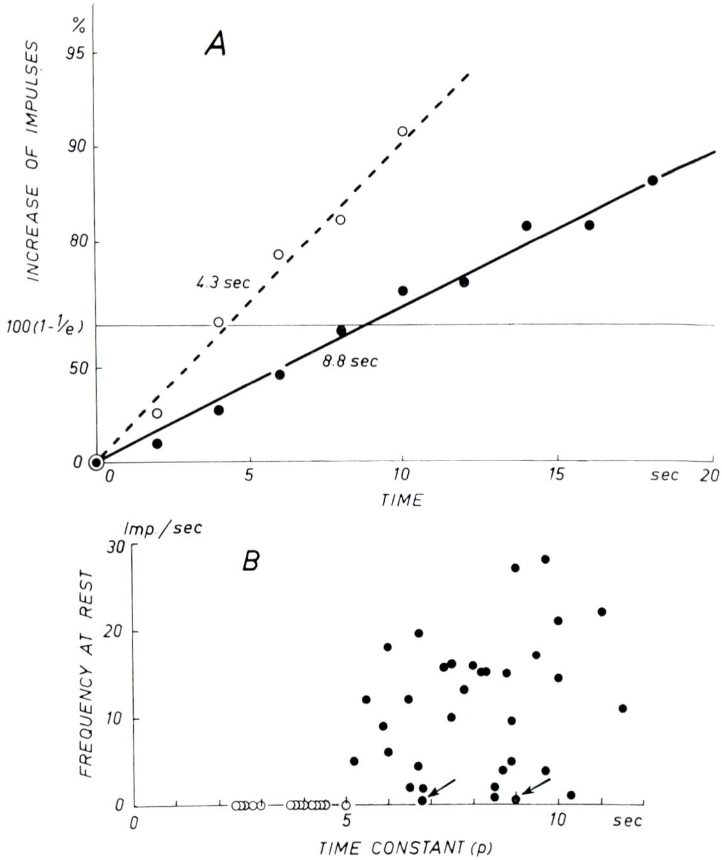

Fig. 5. Time constants of frequency responses to ipsilateral angular acceleration in tonic and kinetic type I vestibular neurones shown in Fig. 3. A: frequency diagram showing the responses of tonic (solid line) and kinetic (broken line) vestibular neurones to ipsilateral angular accelerations. The ordinate (logarithmic scale) represents the frequency increase (%) measured every 2 sec. Filled circles are taken from a tonic neurone during an acceleration of 6.0°/sec^2, and open circles represent the response of a kinetic neurone to an acceleration of 10°/sec^2. The points where both lines cross the horizontal line at 100 (1–1/e) indicate time constants of frequency responses of tonic and kinetic neurones, being 8.8 and 4.3 sec, respectively. B: diagram showing the discharge frequencies at rest and time constants of frequency responses to ipsilateral acceleration in tonic (filled circles) and kinetic (open circles) vestibular neurones (SHIMAZU and PRECHT, 1965)

5. Relation between Frequency Increase and Acceleration

It can be seen from Figs. 3 and 4 that the maximum frequency during acceleration is related to the magnitude of acceleration used. If one subtracts the average resting frequency of a particular neurone from the peak value of moving averages during different magnitudes of acceleration, one obtains a measure of the increase during rotation. In Fig. 6A, these values are plotted against the logarithmic scale of acceleration. Each series of points, calculated from records of a given type I neurone during various magnitudes of angular acceleration, appears to be distributed along a straight line within a range of 0.5–10°/sec² of acceleration. Assuming a linear relation, the following was obtained as the regression *equation* representing the relation between frequency increase and acceleration:

$$f_{max} = a + b \log A \tag{2}$$

where A is acceleration rate (degree/sec²). The points where the regression lines cross the abscissa in Fig. 6A indicate the threshold of each unit for frequency increase. Then *equation* 2 becomes:

$$f_{max} = b \log \frac{A}{T} \tag{3}$$

where T is the threshold for frequency increase by angular acceleration and b represents the gradient of the regression line (SHIMAZU and PRECHT, 1965).

Direct observation of the cupula movement led to the conclusion that the *cupula-endolymph system* is identical with a kind of *torsion pendulum*, and that the frictional coefficient of this system is much *higher* than the restoring force of the cupula. Under this condition, the movement of the pendulum shows an *overcritical damping* (STEINHAUSEN, 1931, 1933). VAN EGMOND et al. (1949) have theoretically deduced the equation for cupula deviations produced by a constant angular acceleration as follows:

$$X = A \frac{I}{R} \left(1 - e \frac{-Rt}{F}\right) \text{ approximation} \tag{4}$$

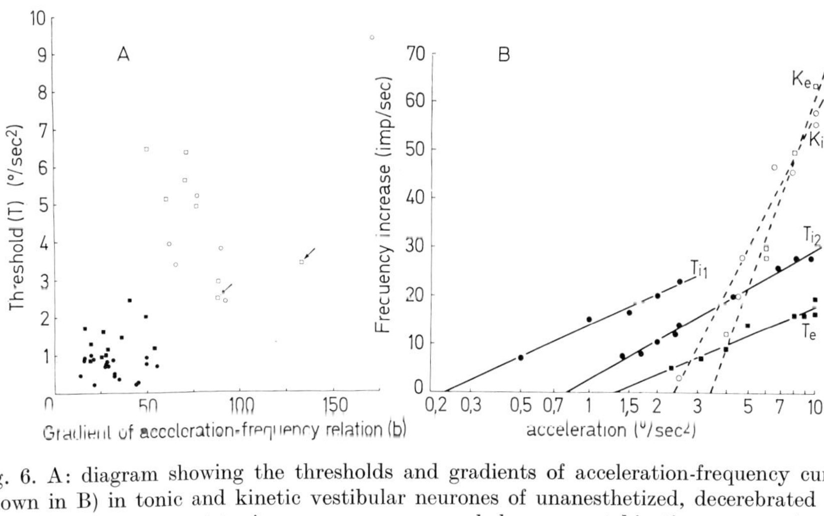

Fig. 6. A: diagram showing the thresholds and gradients of acceleration-frequency curves (shown in B) in tonic and kinetic vestibular neurones of unanesthetized, decerebrated cat. Filled symbols represent tonic neurones; open symbols represent kinetic neurones (except those indicated by arrows). Abscissa indicates *b* in equation 3. B: relation between acceleration rate and frequency increase at its maximum level in tonic (T) and kinetic (K) type I vestibular neurones. Ti_1, Ti_2 and Ki were obtained from animals in which the tympanic bulla was not opened. Te and Ke are from animals in which a stimulating electrode was placed on the ipsilateral vestibular nerve. Each solid or broken line indicates the regression line of points obtained from a single neurone tested with different accelerations. Abscissa is in logarithmic scale (SHIMAZU and PRECHT, 1965)

where X = the angular deviation of the endolymph in relation to the skull; A = the constant angular acceleration of rotation table; I = moment of inertia of the endolymph; F = moment of friction for unit angular velocity; and R = restoring force for unit angular deviation of the cupula. It appears that the *mode of increase* in impulse frequency of *vestibular neurones* shown in *equation 1* is quite similar in its form to the *mode of cupula deviation* with time. The frequency response of the primary vestibular neurones is also in agreement with the theoretical deduction from the torsion pendulum hypothesis (GROEN et al., 1952). Recent studies, have shown that even the simplest linear models which will approximate the response dynamics of the peripheral vestibular system, are more elaborate than a torsion pendulum (FERNÁNDEZ and GOLDBERG, 1971). Furthermore, distinct non-linearities of the system have been demonstrated and they will have to be considered more thoroughly in the future (SHIMAZU and PRECHT, 1965; FERNÁNDEZ and GOLDBERG, 1971; PRECHT et al., 1971a).

After infinite time, the deflection of the cupula is deduced from *equation 4* as follows:

$$X_{max} = A \frac{I}{R} \tag{5}$$

By comparing *equation 5* with *equation 3*, it can be deduced that the *maximal frequency increases* of *vestibular neurones* during long-lasting, constant angular acceleration are *proportional* to the *logarithm* of the *maximal angular deviations* of the cupula. A similar logarithmic stimulus-response relationship was found by analyzing ocular nystagmus induced by semicircular canal stimulation (VAN EGMOND et al., 1949; KOELLA, 1951; KOELLA et al., 1951; PRECHT et al., 1966a). In primary vestibular fibres it was found that for brief stimulation the response was a linear function of acceleration. As acceleration was prolonged, the response also became progressively nonlinear (GOLDBERG and FERNÁNDEZ, 1971).

It can be seen from Fig. 6B that the *gradients* of regression lines (b) are significantly *steeper* for *kinetic* type I neurones (85±30.5) as compared to the *tonic* type I (31.6±11.8). In Fig. 6B, the gradients of regression lines (b) of different type I neurones are plotted against their thresholds for frequency increase (T). Two distinct groups are apparent: the black symbols represent *tonic* neurones having a low threshold and a flat gradient whereas the open symbols show *kinetic* neurones being characterized by steep gradients and high thresholds. Some neurones show a mixed character and may form an intermediate type, though the number of these neurones seems to be quite small. It appears therefore, that under decerebrate and probably also encéphale isolé conditions, the type I vestibular neurones are divided into *two distinct groups* when tested with adequate stimulation of the horizontal semicircular canals. The *kinetic neurones* are characterized by lack of resting discharges, a high threshold for frequency increase, a rapid time course of frequency changes, and a steep gradient of the acceleration-frequency relationship, the *tonic neurones* showing the opposite of these characteristics (SHIMAZU and PRECHT, 1965). In using sinusoidal rotation of the head while recording from second order vestibular neurones MELVILL JONES and MILSUM (1970) found no significant differences in mean phase or gain between spontaneously active and inactive neurones. In both cases the action potential frequency was approximately in phase with stimulus angular velocity.

The precise response of the vestibular system to head deviation in space seems to be secured with the help of a *double safety mechanism*, at least as far as the horizontal canal system is concerned. The *low* threshold of *tonic* neurones assures the sensitivity of the responses, and their resting activity provides the vestibular tonus. The *high* threshold *kinetic* neurones respond with high frequency discharges and rapid changes in impulse frequency at higher acceleration magnitudes and may be a second factor essential for the assurance of high fidelity in vestibular responses. These characteristics may complement those of tonic neurones such as slow responsiveness and frequency saturation at higher acceleration rates.

As far as the *functional importance* of such a dual system is concerned, little can be said at the present time. Interestingly, HULK and JONGKEES (1948) found that the threshold of sensation of continued rotation after sudden stopping of the turntable is lower than that of afternystagmus, and with high stopping velocities durations of afternystagmus are larger than those of aftersensation. The *afternystagmus* cupulogram therefore, has a *steeper* slope than the *aftersensation* cupulogram, and they are crossed with each other similarly to the crossing of acceleration-frequency curves of tonic and kinetic neurones in Fig. 6A. This may imply that the oculomotor system receives a strong influence from the kinetic neurones in addition to the input from the tonic type I units.

6. Threshold of Vestibular Neurones

Threshold measurements of the vestibular organ have been reported by a great many authors. The values for the *perception* of angular acceleration in *man* found in different studies range between 0.035 and 8.2°/sec² (for summary, see CLARK, 1967). These discrepancies are probably due to the many differences in the methods and in the definitions of the threshold. Under optimal laboratory conditions, the *lowest thresholds* found for both *perception* of angular acceleration and *nystagmus* appears to be in the order of 0.1–0.2°/sec² (TUMARKIN, 1937; GROEN and JONGKEES, 1948; DE VRIES, 1949; HALLPIKE et al., 1952; HILDING, 1953; MONTANDON and RUSSBACH, 1956; PFALTZ and RICHTER, 1956; EK et al., 1959; DECHER, 1963).

The meaning of a "threshold" in the tonically active vestibular system has been extensively discussed by LOWENSTEIN (1956) and EK et al. (1959). LOWENSTEIN (1956) has suggested that theoretically a threshold hardly exists at all in *spontaneously* active peripheral vestibular units. By recording head movements during sinusoidal rotatory stimulation, it was found that stimuli as low as 0.04°/sec² were able to produce a measurable change, though the number of experiments had to be greater in studying the influence of such small stimuli (EK et al., 1959). With spontaneously active central neurones, precise determination of threshold acceleration is equally difficult, because even a slight fluctuation of the resting rate interferes with the identification of a small response. If so, the regression lines in Fig. 6A might not be straight in the region close to the abscissa, but could extend even to the point of 0°/sec² in an extreme case. However, with acceleration magnitudes lower than the thresholds determined by the procedure shown in Fig. 6A, no statistically significant changes in impulse frequency are observed in most of the neurones. Therefore, this method for determining the threshold of tonic neurones to constant angular acceleration appears to be a satisfactory one at present. The *mean threshold* of *tonic* vestibular neurones appears to be around $0.65 \pm 0.25°/sec^2$, lowest values being $0.2°/sec^2$ (SHIMAZU and PRECHT, 1965), thus showing perfect agreement with the threshold values for sensation of rotation or ocular nystagmus mentioned above. Similar values for thresholds of vestibular neurones have been reported by DUENSING and SCHAEFER (1958).

Determination of *thresholds* in *kinetic* neurones is more precise because of lack of resting discharge. A mean threshold of $4.65 \pm 1.84°/sec^2$ was found for this type of neurone (SHIMAZU and PRECHT, 1965). This value is significantly *higher* as compared to the threshold of tonic neurones. It appears that the *low threshold* of *tonic* vestibular neurones best reflects the high *sensitivity* of the vestibular system to angular acceleration.

7. Adaptation of Central Vestibular Neurones

Frequency decrease of sensory impulses, following a transient maximal response during application of a long-lasting constant stimulation, may be called an adaptation phenomenon. Using a protracted period of constant horizontal

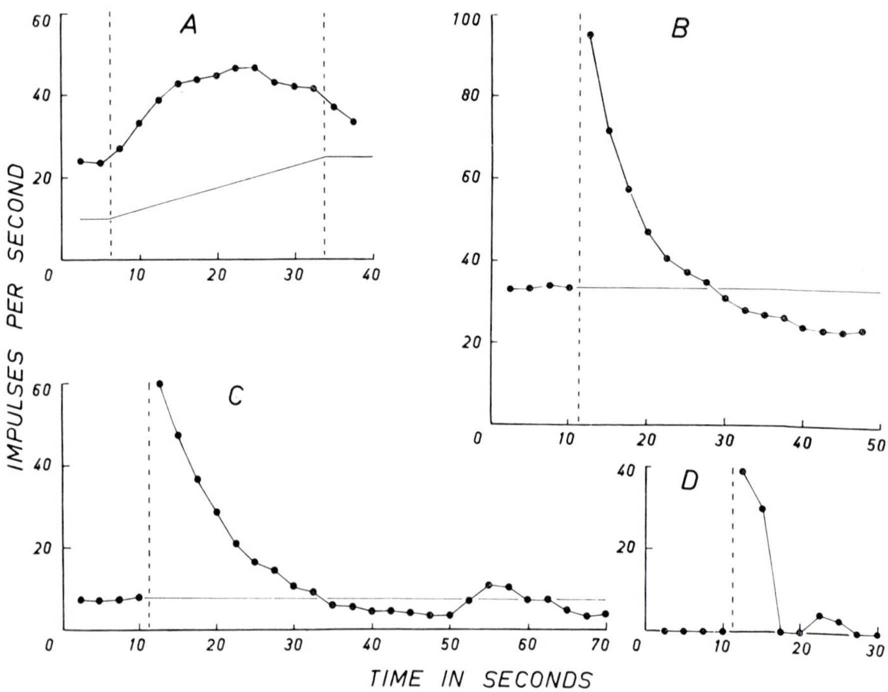

Fig. 7. Various response patterns of discharge frequencies of single vestibular neurones to horizontal rotation. A, B and C represent tonic neurones, and D, a kinetic neurone. A: response to ipsilateral constant angular acceleration ($7°/sec^2$). The left- and right-hand vertical lines indicate the onset and cessation of acceleration, respectively. The constant speed of rotation after acceleration was 195°/sec. B, C and D: responses to sudden arrest after constant speed (100°/sec in B, 65°/sec in C, and 150°/sec in D) of contralateral rotation. Horizontal lines in B and C indicate average frequencies during constant rotation. Vertical broken lines in B, C and D indicate the time when the turntable was stopped. A and B were obtained from an animal in which the contralateral labyrinth was destroyed. All records were obtained from unanesthetized, decerebrate cats (SHIMAZU and PRECHT, 1965)

angular acceleration, most of the second order vestibular neurones of the horizontal canals show *no significant* frequency *adaptation* as may be seen from Fig. 3 (SHIMAZU and PRECHT, 1965). Similar suggestions were made by ADRIAN (1943) and ROSS (1936).

As shown in Fig. 7 a small number of type I vestibular neurones are characterized by a slight *decrease* in frequency after attaining their peak value. All these neurones showed also a clear *undershoot* of discharge frequency when the turntable was stopped after constant speed of rotation. In some cases the frequency returned from this undershoot and still increased beyond the basic rate, i.e., *damped oscillatory* changes were observed (Fig. 7, C, D). None of the neurones which maintained their constant impulse rate during acceleration showed these oscillatory changes in frequency. This may indicate that the drop in frequency of some neurones is *not* a true *adaptation* but only an initial part of the frequency *oscillation*. At present, it is impossible to decide whether the oscillation is produced by *peripheral* or *central* mechanisms. Undershoots of impulse frequency have also been observed in the *peripheral* neurone (GROEN et al., 1952; LEDOUX, 1961) which may suggest that the cupula system does not always behave as an overcritical damped system, and part of the oscillatory phenomenon observed in central neurones may be caused by corresponding changes of primary vestibular afferent activity.

In an attempt to simulate the slow exponential change of cupula deflection occuring during angular acceleration by using slowly increasing polarizing currents, LOWENSTEIN (1955) found that the discharge rate of primary neurones connected to the semicircular canal shows only very slight adaptation. In the intact frog only 35% of the primary fibres showed no signs of adaptation in response to prolonged acceleration steps (PRECHT et al., 1971a). This finding is somewhat different from LOWENSTEIN's (1955) data on the isolated labyrinth and it may imply that in the intact preparation the efferent vestibular system may contribute to the frequency decline in response to constant acceleration (see ChapterC.IV.).

Even if there is a slight tendency for adaptation in some neurones, it is not significant enough to explain the considerable "adaptation" observed by HALLPIKE and HOOD (1953b) in human subjects under the condition of sustained cupula deflection. Single neurone studies would suggest that such an "adaptation" is not only produced by inherent mechanisms in the end organs or in the vestibular nuclei but rather may involve more complicated nervous activities such as a *habituation* phenomenon (ALBERT, 1965).

8. Other Horizontal Canal Responses

When an animal is subjected to horizontal angular acceleration, not only type I responses are found in the vestibular nuclei, but also other response patterns can be recorded which have been classified above as type II, III and IV neurones.

Type II vestibular neurones have been first described by DUENSING and SCHAEFER (1958). It seems that their absolute number is smaller as compared to type I neurones (DUENSING and SCHAEFER, 1958; SHIMAZU and PRECHT, 1965). As shown in Fig. 8, they increase their discharge frequency during *contralateral* rotation with an approximately *exponential* pattern and decrease it with *ipsilateral* acceleration, thus reacting just *opposite* to the main second-order sensory

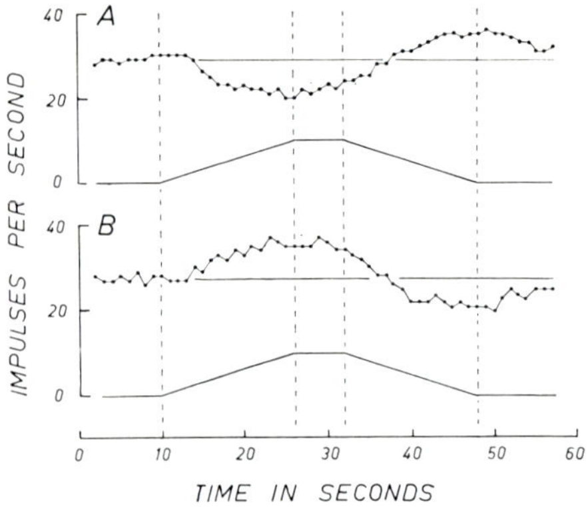

Fig. 8. Frequency diagrams of discharges of a type II vestibular neurone in response to constant angular acceleration and deceleration in unanesthetized, decerebrate cat. A: ipsilateral rotation. B: contralateral rotation. Ordinate represents spikes per second. The horizontal line in each diagram respresents the average frequency before rotation. Broken vertical lines indicate, from left to right, the onset and cessation of acceleration and those of deceleration. Acceleration and deceleration rates were 4.5°/sec² and constant speed of rotation after acceleration was 72°/sec (SHIMAZU and PRECHT, 1966)

neurone (type I) of the horizontal canals (Fig. 8). The *logarithmic* relation between acceleration rates and maximum frequency increase during constant angular accelerations are found in many type II neurones, this being very similar to type I units (SHIMAZU and PRECHT, 1965; SHIMAZU and PRECHT, 1966). The *thresholds* of type II neurones for frequency increase during contralateral accelerations range from 1.5–10°/sec² or more and are significantly *higher* than the thresholds of type I neurones (0.23–1.0°/sec²). Like type I neurones, type II resting discharges range between 1–30 impulses per second. The synaptic organization leading to type II responses has long been a matter of conjecture since this type of response has not been found by LOWENSTEIN in his extensive analysis of the *primary* afferent system in the *isolated* labyrinth. It should be briefly mentioned here that type II responses can be recorded in the vestibular nerve of the frog, whose vestibular nerve is not separated from the central nervous system. This type II response is still present after sectioning the VIIIth nerve distally to the recording point, which proves that the action potentials are not recorded from a primary afferent fibre but rather from *efferent* fibres. (For details see Chapter C.IV. of this Volume.) SHIMAZU and PRECHT (1966) have shown that at least *two different* type II neurones can be recorded in the vestibular nuclei of the cat. After removal of one labyrinth, type II neurones can be recorded both on the *intact* side as well as on the *deafferented* side. The latter type II was shown to be exclusively activated from the *contralateral* horizontal canal via *commissural fibres* crossing the midline. Type II responses recorded on the non-deafferented side and the functional importance of the crossed activation of the other group of type II neurones will be discussed below.

At the present stage, very little is known concerning the mechanisms producing type III and type IV responses found in a relatively small number in the vestibular nuclei. Both bilateral rotatory stimulation as well as hot and cold water irrigation of the ipsilateral ear succeed in producing these two types of response patterns (GERNANDT, 1949). It seems that type III is strongly influenced by extralabyrinthine sensory stimulation such as auditory or tactile stimuli (DUENSING and SCHAEFER, 1958); (SHIMAZU and PRECHT, 1965). Future work is needed to reveal more about their functional meaning.

9. Synaptology and Localization of Type I Neurones

A combination of single pulse stimulation of the vestibular nerve and rotatory stimulation allows us to study the *functional connections* of vestibular neurones. Once a unit is identified by adequate stimulation as a second order neurone of the horizontal canal or any other receptor, a single pulse stimulation of the vestibular nerve provides the means to study exactly the latency of the evoked response. Moreover, the response of a neurone to paired stimuli given at a short interval or high frequency of stimulation allows its classification as primary or secondary vestibular neurone (PRECHT and SHIMAZU, 1965; SHIMAZU and PRECHT, 1965).

As described above, there are two kinds of type I vestibular neurones, the *kinetic* and *tonic*, which are differentiated by characteristic frequency responses to horizontal angular accelerations. All of the type I neurones are excited by stimulation of the ipsilateral primary vestibular fibres, and none of them are inhibited (PRECHT and SHIMAZU, 1965). Most of the *kinetic* vestibular neurones are excited by vestibular nerve stimulation with fairly fixed latencies, and the spikes are superimposed on the N_1 peak of the field potential (Figs. 9A, 15Ea). Even with minimal intensity of stimulation, latencies cover only a small range, 1.2–2.0 msec, corresponding to about 0.6–1.4 msec after arrival of nerve impulses at the terminals of the afferent fibres. With stronger stimulation, the units are evoked with delays of 0.4–0.8 msec after arrival of presynaptic activity. The short latencies, their small fluctuations and their capability to follow faithfully at stimulation frequencies in excess of 100/sec, suggest that the *kinetic* neurones are mainly *monosynaptically* activated by primary afferent fibres.

Tonic type I vestibular neurones responded in a completely different manner (Fig. 9B). Stimulation of the VIIIth nerve near threshold in decerebrate and in unanaesthetized preparations excites the neurones with long and widely fluctuating latencies (6.7–9.3 msec). Though latencies of evoked spikes are gradually shortened with stronger stimuli (Fig. 9B), they are still within the range of the N_2 potential. The responses are effectively blocked by pentobarbital administration. In half of the type I neurones tested, these clear differences in latencies were obscured when the stimulation was very strong. Under this condition, kinetic neurones show *double* activation, the second spike falling on N_2, and tonic neurones are also repetitively activated with the first spike riding on N_1 potential. Even in these neurones, clear *differences* are found between *tonic* and *kinetic* neurones when tested with stimuli being near the threshold. Figure 9C summarizes the latency distribution for a larger sample of neurones in relation to N_1 and N_2 field potentials.

Multisynaptic pathways in the vestibular nuclei best explain the long-latency activation of tonic neurones with weak stimulation. Internuncial neurones in the vestibular nuclei or collaterals of the axons leaving them, might serve as an

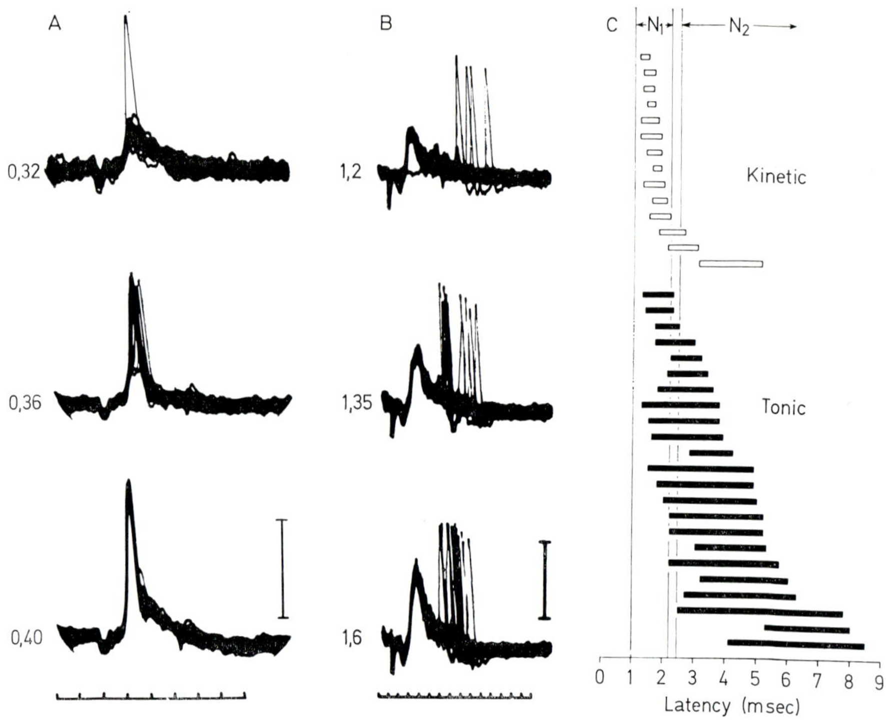

Fig. 9. Responses of kinetic (A) and tonic (B) type I vestibular neurones to electrical stimulation of the ipsilateral VIIIth nerve. All records were obtained from unanesthetized, decerebrate cat. A and B: 3/sec stimulation. Each record is composed of about 20 superimposed traces. The numerals on the left of each record indicate stimulation voltage. The first downward deflection indicates the stimulus artifact. N_1 field potential is seen in all records except the one at the bottom of A. Time: 1 msec; amplitude calibration: 1 mV. C: latency distribution of kinetic and tonic neurones. The horizontal extent of open oblongs (kinetic neurones) and filled oblongs (tonic neurones) indicates that latencies of the earliest spikes of each neurone evoked by weak stimulation of the ipsilateral vestibular nerve were distributed within these ranges. These results were obtained from 30 to 40 serial trials at 2–3/sec. N_1 and N_2, indicated by vertical lines, represent the ranges of N_1 and N_2 field potentials (PRECHT and SHIMAZU, 1965)

anatomical basis for multisynaptic excitation of vestibular neurones (LORENTE DE Nó, 1933b, 1938; BRODAL et al., 1962). *Lack of monosynaptic excitation* of about half of the tonic neurones may be explained by the histological findings that certain areas in the vestibular nuclei are *free* of *vestibular afferents* (WALBERG et al., 1958). It appears from several physiological studies, that type I neurones are most frequently found in the *medial* and *superior vestibular nuclei* (ADRIAN, 1943; DUENSING and SCHAEFER, 1958; SHIMAZU and PRECHT, 1965). This finding is in good agreement with anatomical data obtained by LORENTE DE Nó (1933a), STEIN and CARPENTER (1967) and GACEK (1969), suggesting that fibres from the cristae of the canals terminate mainly in the medial and superior vestibular nuclei. The existence of monosynaptic (mean latency 0.72 msec), disynaptic (1.0–1.6 msec) and polysynaptic excitatory postsynaptic potentials (EPSPs) has recently been shown in neurones located in the various subdivisions of the vestibular nuclear complex (Ito et al., 1969; Kawai et al., 1969). These studies further support the interpretation of the extracellular field and unitary potentials given above. In comparing the unitary components of the EPSPs recorded in non-Deiters' neurones with those in Deiters' neurones, Kawai et al., 1969, found that the former are characterized by significantly larger unitary EPSPs (up to 2 mV). Similarly, the mean least EPSPs in non-Deiters' neurones are 1.7 times as large as those in the Deiters' neurones. These findings would suggest that primary vestibular impulses activate non-Deiters' neurones more effectively. It is also indicated that non-Deiters' neurones may receive a smaller number of vestibular nerve fibres each of which having a higher efficacy of synaptic transmission.

10. Input from the Vertical Canals

Ewald's (1892) classical experiments on direct stimulation of the various semicircular canals, first pointed out the differences in reflex responses following stimulation of the horizontal canals with respect to those obtained by stimulation of the vertical canals. By recording DC potential changes during cupula movements in the vertical canals, Trincker (1957) found that utriculopetal cupula deflection is accompanied by a positive potential shift (decrease of afferent discharge) whereas utriculofugal movements lead to a negative potential shift (increase of afferent discharge). Thus, the *vertical canals* show just the opposite *polarity*, as compared to the horizontal canals.

Unlike the horizontal canal influences, the effects of *vertical canal* stimulation on neurones in the vestibular nuclei have not been studied in great detail. Frequency changes of neurones following stimulation of the vertical canals have been observed by Adrian (1943), Duensing and Schaefer (1959), Duensing (1968a, b). Markham (1968) has studied the effect of angular acceleration on *central* vestibular neurones when the vertical canals were in the plane of rotation. Since the anterior canal on one side is approximately in the same plane as the posterior canal on the other side, any attempt to bring one of them in the plane of a horizontally rotating table will result in placing both of them in this plane. By recording from the side where the anterior canal was in plane of rotation, Markham (1968) found that most units *increased* their resting discharge during *utriculofugal* endolymph flow in this canal and *decreased* by *utriculopetal* flow. These neurones may represent the *second order* neurones of the anterior canal. They seem to have *higher thresholds* for frequency increase during angular acceleration, as compared to the horizontal canal units, a finding which is in agreement with the higher threshold of vertical nystagmus reported by Decher (1963).

Histological checking of the recording points showed that the second order neurones of the anterior vertical canal are found in the same areas as type I neurones from the horizontal canal, i.e., mainly in the *medial* and *superior* vestibular nucleus (Shimazu and Precht, 1965; Markham, 1968). It appears that the *number* of units responding to vertical canal stimulation is smaller than the one for horizontal type I neurones (Markham, 1968). This may be related to the finding of Suzuki and Cohen (1966), that the muscle tension developed by stimulation of the anterior canal nerve is smaller, as compared to the stimulation of the horizontal canal nerve. Differences in *time course* of the primary vertical neurone have been shown by LEDOUX (1958). Similar to the horizontal canal system, adequate stimulation of the anterior canal reveals a *group of neurones* responding in an *inverse* manner as the one just described. It is very likely that these neurones receive their main excitatory input from the *contralateral posterior* canal being also in plane of rotation (MARKHAM, 1968). They are thus similar to the type II neurones of the horizontal canals which receive input from the opposite side (SHIMAZU and PRECHT, 1966). Neurones increasing their discharge rate to rotation in *both* directions have also been recorded (MARKHAM, 1968).

D. Input from the Otolith Organs

The function of the otolith organs appears to be the maintenance of a normal *position in space* which is characteristic for each animal. This is achieved with the aid of sensory cells located in the maculae of *utriculus* and *sacculus*, which are sensitive to both the *magnitude* and *direction* of *linear acceleration*, including that produced by gravity. It was BREUER (1891) who recognized that the only *adequate* stimulus for the otolith sensory hair cells is the *tangential* component of the forces acting on the maculae ("Scherungstheorie"). Later, STEINHAUSEN (1935), ULRICH (1935), VON HOLST (1950), VON HOLST et al. (1950), COHEN (1955), TRINCKER (1959) experimentally proved BREUER's theory and found no evidence for MAGNUS' idea of a "push-pull" mechanism (MAGNUS, 1924).

More detailed knowledge about the function of the otolith organs was obtained by recording the activities from *single neuronal elements* in this system and by *operative* interference on single receptor organs (MCNALLY and TAIT, 1934). It was first shown by ASHCROFT and HALLPIKE (1934), ROSS (1936) and LEDOUX (1949) that in the *frog*, the *utriculus* is especially concerned with *static* functions, whereas the *sacculus* proved to be mainly sensitive to *vibration*. In *fish* (Raja clavata), LOWENSTEIN and ROBERTS (1949, 1951) demonstrated that *both utriculus* and *sacculus* respond to changes in position of the animal. The same holds true for higher vertebrates.

Like other labyrinthine receptors the otolith organs display a moderate *resting discharge* (LOWENSTEIN and ROBERTS, 1949; RUPERT et al., 1962) which is either increased or decreased depending on the *direction* of the position change. Some neurones, *out-of-position receptors* and *into-level type*, always respond in the same way no matter to which side the animal is tilted and they adapt rapidly in contrast to the lack of significant adaptation of the main type of fibre (LOWENSTEIN and ROBERTS, 1949). Primary afferent discharge from utricular fibres has been recorded in the frog during different *states of gravity*, in the range of 1 G to 0 G, occuring during parabolic flights. It appears that the resting discharge increases during the first seconds of *weightlessness* and may be followed later by depression of discharge frequency (GUALTIEROTTI and ALLTUCKER, 1967). For further details on peripheral mechanisms, see Lowenstein's chapter in this Handbook.

ADRIAN (1943) was the first to record from *second order* neurones in the vestibular nuclei (cat) during altered positions of the head. All the neurones he found showed an *increase* in the discharge rate following lateral tilting of the head towards the side of recording and a *decrease* on tilt towards the other side. Linear accelerations in the horizontal plane away from the recording side also excited these neurones. In some cases, the same neurones were influenced by both *lateral tilt* and *for-and-aft* tilt, a finding which is in agreement with the data obtained by DUENSING and SCHAEFER (1959), HIEBERT and FERNÁNDEZ (1965). It was demonstrated by FUJITA et al. (1968) that the majority of second-order neurones are sensitive to displacements about *only one* of the axes, thus showing *"orthogonality"*, which seems to enable the nervous system to analyze head positions into different perpendicular components. Further investigations of second-order vestibular neurones in fishes (SCHOEN, 1957) and higher vertebrates (HIEBERT and FERNÁNDEZ, 1965; PETERSON, 1967, 1970; FUJITA et al., 1968) clearly demonstrated the existence of another less common type of neurone that behaved opposite to the pattern found by ADRIAN (1943) and neurones which responded with an increase or decrease on tilting in either direction. The latter responses were mainly found in neurones which showed polysynaptic activation following stimulation of the ipsilateral VIIIth nerve. The investigations on vertebrates thus showed utricular responses which were qualitatively similar to those recorded from utricular fibres in fish (LOWENSTEIN and ROBERTS, 1949). Some neurones appear to have *"phasic"* characteristics, in that they only show a transient increase of frequency during tilt, despite the maintenance of the new position (FUJITA et al., 1968). They may correspond to the "out-of-position" fibres mentioned above or their frequency change may be caused by afferents from semicircular canals. *Inhibition* as well as *excitation* of neurones during tilt in *either direction* has also been found by DUENSING and SCHAEFER (1959). It is not clear at present if in higher vertebrates inhibition of spontaneous frequency on ipsilateral tilt towards the side of recording, or on tilt towards either side of recording, is caused by the direct action of primary otolith neurones on second order neurones, or if inhibitory interneurones are involved. The presence of disynaptic IPSPs in some Deiters' neurones following stimulation of the ipsilateral VIIIth nerve could support the latter hypothesis (ITO et al., 1969b).

The *localization* of the vestibular neurones responding to tilt fits approximately with the distribution of utricular fibres described by LORENTE DE NÓ (1933a), STEIN and CARPENTER (1967) and GACEK (1969), which means that they are mainly found in the *Deiters' nucleus*, the *descending* nucleus and in the more caudal parts of the *medial* vestibular nucleus (PETERSON, 1967, 1970; FUJITA et al., 1968). Moreover, it was shown by PETERSON (1967, 1970) that within the Deiters' nucleus, the most sensitive neurones are located in the *ventral* part, a high percentage of them being activated *monosynaptically* after electric pulse stimulation of the ipsilateral VIIIth nerve. This finding is in good agreement with the distribution of primary fibres in the Deiters' nucleus as shown by WALBERG et al. (1958). Intracellular recordings from Deiters' neurones in response to ipsilateral VIIIth nerve stimulation (ITO et al., 1969b) show that monosynaptic EPSPs (latencies ranging from 0.6 to 1.0 msec) are only found in neurones located in the ventral portion of Deiters' nucleus, whereas neurones located in the dorsal portion show only di- or polysynaptic EPSPs in response to VIIIth nerve stimulation (latencies ranging from 1.0 to 1.8 and 1.9 to 2.2 msec, respectively). Recently, SHIMAZU and SMITH (1971) have demonstrated that in non-anesthetized decerebrate cats many neurones in the dorsal and middle part of the Deiters' nucleus were spontaneously active and were found to be highly sensitive to lateral tilting of the head. Apparently, monosynaptic linkage of vestibular neurones is not an essential prerequisite for sensitivity of response to natural stimulation in non-anesthetized animals (see also section on horizontal type I neurones). In anesthetized animals (PETERSON, 1970) the polysynaptic input to the dorsal Deiters' may have been partially blocked thus leading to a higher number of sensitive neurones located in the ventral Deiters' which is monosynaptically supplied by vestibular afferents. Different *firing patterns* have also been reported for neurones located in the ventral and dorsal half of Deiters' nucleus (HIEBERT and FERNÁNDEZ, 1965).

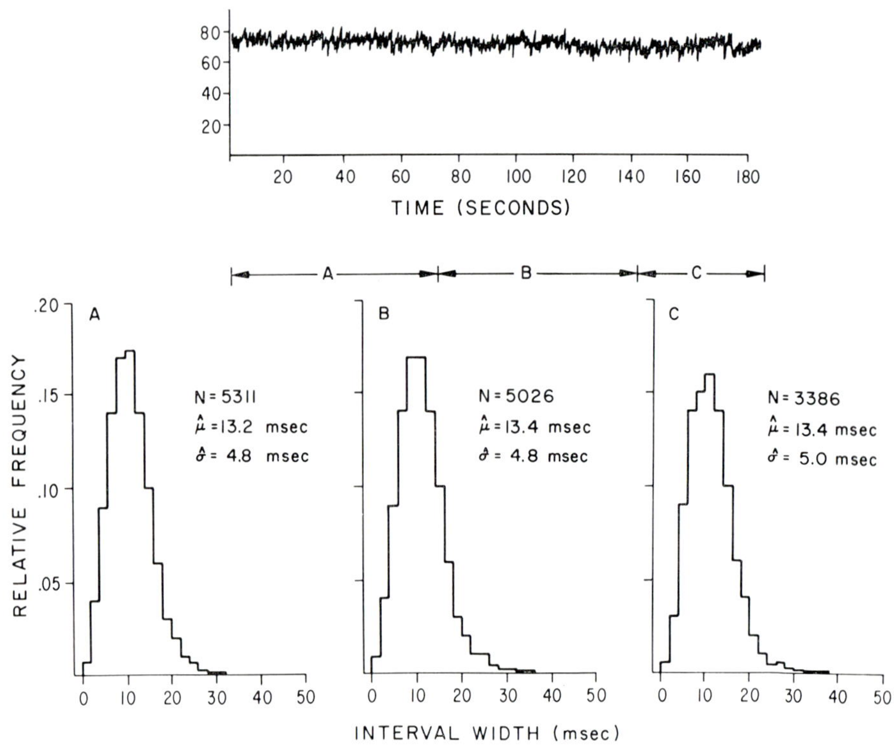

Fig. 10. Tonic response of Deiters' neurones over a protracted period of tilt. Upper record: integrated record of spike activity over a three minute period with the cat tilted 10° (ipsilateral side down) along a longitudinal axis. The ordinate (impulses/sec) was calibrated using trains of equally spaced pulses. A, B, and C: the similarity between the corresponding statistics from the consecutive sections, A, B and C, in the upper record is shown in the histograms for each section. Note the stationary or nonadapting characteristics of vestibular neurones during prolonged constant otolith stimulation (FUJITA, ROSENBERG and SEGUNDO, 1968)

Attempts have been made to study more precisely the *time course* of central vestibular neurones during *adequate* otolith stimulation. Closer inspection of the records shows that the frequencies of the neurones show a "*phasic-tonic*" pattern, characterized by an initial increase, followed by a tonic or steady level of discharge which is different from that found at horizontal plane and is *stationary or non-adapting* as long as the animal is held at a particular position (ADRIAN, 1943; SCHOEN, 1957; CRAMER, 1962; HIEBERT and FERNÁNDEZ, 1965; PETERSON, 1967; FUJITA et al., 1968). Figure 10 shows the nonadapting features of a *second order* neurone during a lateral tilt of 10°.

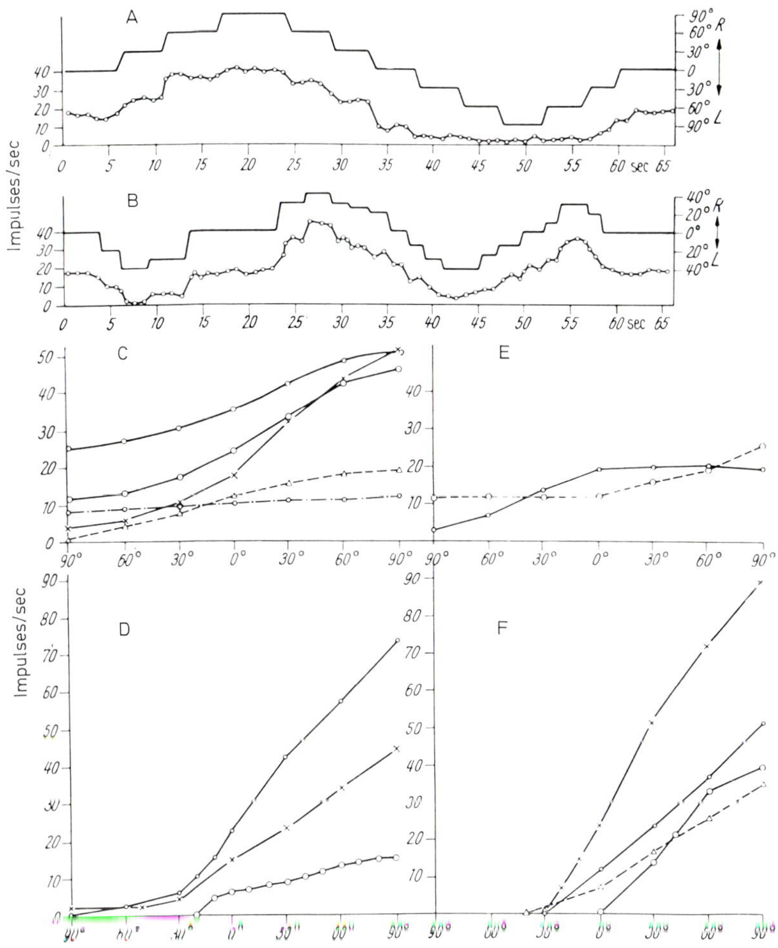

Fig. 11. Frequency diagrams of discharges of fish's (Tinca vulgaris) vestibular neurones in response to lateral tilt. A and B: continuous plot of frequency responses of two central vestibular neurones to stepwise tilt over the range shown in the diagrams. Ordinates on the right side represent the degrees of tilt toward the right and left side (zero degree indicates the normal position of the animal). The upper line in each diagram indicates the position of the head (in angular degrees) at a given time, and the lower line composed of open circles represents spikes per second of single unit discharge. C to F: each line in these diagrams indicates the average impulse frequency of single central vestibular neurone that has been repetitively subjected to the same lateral positions shown on the abscissa. Note the variety of responses of vestibular neurones to otolith stimulation (SCHOEN, 1957)

In 1950 VON HOLST demonstrated in free moving fishes, that the *tangential* or *shearing* force acting on the hair cells of the macula is a sinusoidal function of the *angular displacement* of the head. A similar relation has been found psychophysically by comparing the actual angular displacement of the head with the perception of position in space (SCHÖNE, 1962). Most of the primary utricular neurones tested by LOWENSTEIN and ROBERTS (1949) showed the same sinusoidal curves. By recording from second order utricular neurones in the brain stem of the fish, SCHOEN (1957) found that about one-third of the neurones show an approxi-

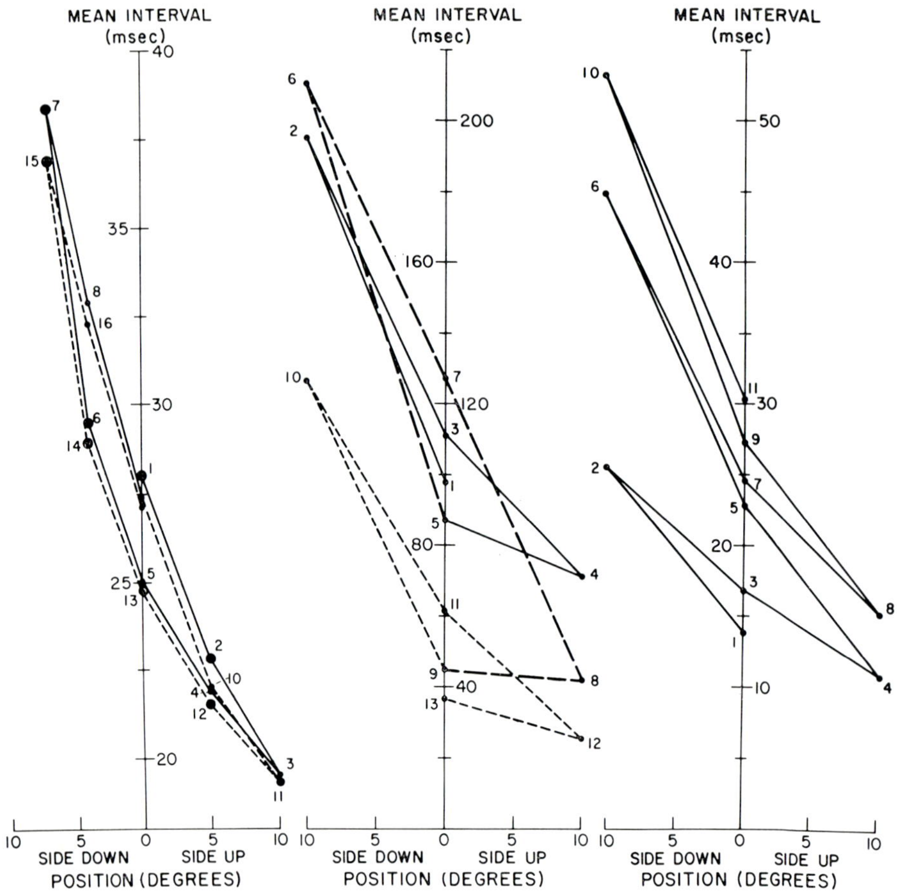

Fig. 12. Forms of the relation between mean interspike interval of Deiters' neurones and position of the head. Each point in the three diagrams derived from three different cells corresponds to a different station of angular displacement of the head whose order in the cycle is indicated by a number. For a given station the abscissa of the point is the position of the head with respect to gravity measured in degrees (recording side down or recording side up) by the angle between the basal stereotaxic reference plane and the horizontal. The ordinates are the mean interval in msec calculated over the stationary part of the spike train. The three curves represent recordings from three single cells responding in three different ways to the same kind of stimulation procedure. Their mode of response has been designated as (from the left to the right): "stable loop", "loop and creep" and "creep". For further details, see text (FUJITA, ROSENBERG and SEGUNDO, 1968)

mately sinusoidal time course when subjected to lateral angular displacement ranging from 0–90° in both directions (Fig. 11A, B). Other types of responses found are shown in Fig. 11C–F which is self explanatory.

Fujita et al. (1968) measured the interspike *interval histograms* of gravity-sensitive Deiters' neurones at 0-level and classified the histograms obtained in "*asymmetric*", "*symmetric*" and "*multimodal*". When the head of the cat is tilted laterally into different positions, the histograms are usually shifted along the interval axis, leaving its general shape and also that of the autocorrelograms unchanged. Figure 12 displays examples of second-order neurones whose stationary mean interval has been measured at different angles, showing that one particular position occurred more than one time during the test. Connecting the points in the order in which they were reached during the experiment resulted in three different forms (Fujita et al., 1968). They were classified as "*stable loops*", "*creep*" *forms*, and "*loop-creep*" forms (Fig. 12), the latter being the one most commonly found. It is concluded that "*multivaluedness*", i.e., to each position corresponded several values of mean intervals, is a characteristic feature of *gravity* sensitive *second-order* neurones, the basis of which is unknown. Multivaluedness, obviously, implies that on the basis of just one statistic of a particular cell, only a probabilistic statement about angular displacement of the head can be made. It is the combination of several statistics in a larger number of cells which eventually will provide the means to determine more exactly the position in space.

E. Receptor Convergence on Central Neurones

It was not until the studies by Duensing and Schaefer (1959), that a sound experimental basis was provided for the problem of *convergence of different labyrinthine receptors* onto *an individual cell* in the vestibular nuclei. Second-order neurones responding to horizontal canal stimulation were also subjected to rotations about *bitemporal* and *naso-occipital* axes. It was found that many of the horizontal semicircular canal units did also react to stimulation of the maculae and vertical canals, suggesting convergence of more than one receptor organ on a particular cell. In most of the cases, the responses evoked by stimulation of the otolith organs and those provoked by vertical canal stimulation had the same sign, i.e., they showed a *homonymous coupling*. Such type of coupling of otolith and semicircular canal system can be very useful for the proper adjustment of the eyes, when the head is moved in space. A few examples of convergence deserve mention. Most of the type I neurones of the *horizontal canal* also receive excitatory input from the *ipsilateral otolith* system and some of them in addition to that from the *ipsilateral posterior* canal. Type II and type III neurones of the horizontal canal also receive influences from the otolith organs and anterior and posterior canals. As mentioned above, *type II* seems to be divided into two distinct types of neurones. It has been shown by Shimazu and Precht (1966) that one of these two types is *monosynaptically* connected with the *ipsilateral* vestibular nerve and is still found following removal of the contralateral labyrinth. This monosynaptic excitation of type II neurones seems to be produced by impulses in primary afferents from some other end organs than the horizontal canal, because if the horizontal canal nerve had such strong excitatory connections with the vestibular neurones, this excitatory influence should produce type I response of these neurones during horizontal rotation (PRECHT and SHIMAZU, 1965). These data, therefore, suggest the *inhibitory interaction* within the vestibular nuclei between different labyrinthine sensory systems on the same side. Convergence in this case could function to *sharpen* incoming vestibular impulses related to head movement in space. *Disynaptically* evoked IPSPs have been occasionally recorded in those Deiters' neurones that were monosynaptically excited after stimulating the *ipsilateral* vestibular nerve (ITO et al., 1969b). Recently, in addition to mono- and polysynaptic EPSPs, polysynaptic IPSPs have also been recorded in vestibular neurones located in the non-Deiters' nuclei in response to weak ipsilateral vestibular nerve stimulation (KAWAI et al., 1969). Inhibitory neurones located *in* the vestibular nuclei are most likely responsible for the postsynaptic inhibitory potentials recorded in other vestibular neurones. Similarly, the horizontal canals may cause inhibition of certain central neurones by means of intercalated inhibitory interneurones, thus provoking this particular type II response.

It appears from the single unit analyses that many vestibular neurones are characterized by a high degree of *convergence* from different receptor organs, but that there are also neurones whose input derives from *only one type of receptor* organ (DUENSING and SCHAEFER, 1959; MARKHAM and CURTHOYS, 1972). Both of the *two groups* probably project to the various effector systems. At present we are far from knowing the exact synaptic organization and the functional implications of neurones that show convergence and those which are more or less concerned with one labyrinthine input. Earlier observations by LORENTE DE NÓ (1931) and KOELLA (1950) have shown that each semicircular canal may be able to provoke nystagmus in *all* of the eye muscles, and that position of the head can also affect nystagmic eye movements. Further studies have corroborated the concept of *mutual interaction* between *otolith* and *semicircular canal* organs. VON HOLST and GRISEBACH (1951) showed that the activity arising from the canal system can influence the recognition of the *subjective vertical* in man. In an attempt to study more quantitatively the influence of the otolith organs on caloric nystagmus, BERGSTEDT (1961a, b) found that the maximum intensity and duration of nystagmus increases in *direct proportion* with higher values of the *gravitational force* which, of course, is acting on the otolith organs. Otolith effects on nystagmus were also obtained by OWADA and OKUBO (1963); CRAMPTON (1966); and MILOJEVIC and VOOTS (1966). These data combine in showing that the otolith system can influence quite strongly the effects produced by stimulation of the semicircular canals. However, their influence is not essential since nystagmus occurs also during *weightlessness* (JACKSON and SEARS, 1966). It is almost a certainty that such interactions are not caused by the cupula system being sensitive to linear accelerations (GERNANDT, 1950a; BENSON et al., 1970) but rather by means of *central convergence* of otolith and canal activities, occurring either at the level of the vestibular nuclei or in the various effector systems. It is important to note that convergence described above is for the most part polysynaptic in nature and may well involve systems other than the vestibular nuclei which in turn feed back onto vestibular neurones. This statement is based on the findings that separate stimulation of individual canal nerves on one side with single electric shocks generally does *not* reveal short latency convergence of different canals on one single vestibular neurone (KASAHARA and UCHINO, 1971, WILSON, FELPEL (1972). It is not known whether otolith organs show short latency convergence on identified canal units.

F. Labyrinthine Influences on the Contralateral Vestibular Nuclei

It has been shown histologically that the bilateral vestibular nuclei are interconnected by *commissural fibres* crossing the midline beneath the fourth ventricle (GRAY, 1926; RASMUSSEN, 1932; FERRARO, 1940; LADPLI and BRODAL, 1968). Indirect pathways by way of the reticular formation may also serve as morphological substrates for the transmission of crossed influences (RAMÓN Y CAJAL, 1911; LORENTE DE NÓ, 1933b; LADPLI and BRODAL, 1968). DE VITO et al. (1956) have demonstrated physiologically that neurones located in the Deiters' nucleus can be influenced by polarizing currents applied to the *contralateral* labyrinth, a finding that has been confirmed by WEBER and STEINER (1965) and FREDRICKSON et al. (1966). Other investigators, however, did not succeed in finding any evidence for crossed activities using both adequate and electrical stimulation (GERNANDT and THULIN, 1952; MICKLE and ADES, 1954; GERNANDT et al., 1959). More recently, positive physiological evidence for crossing activity and its mediating pathways has been obtained by SHIMAZU and PRECHT (1966); PRECHT et al. (1966a); MARKHAM (1968); KASAHARA et al. (1968); MANO et al. (1968); and KASAHARA and UCHINO (1971).

1. Field Potentials in the Contralateral Vestibular Nuclei

As shown in Fig. 13, the *field potentials* recorded in the vestibular nuclei and generated by stimulation of the *contralateral* vestibular nerve (intensity of stimulation less than $2 \times N_1$) consist of an initial *positive*, or positive-negative deflection (latency 2.4 msec) and a later *slow negative* wave (latency 3.2 msec) mainly found in the *ventral* part of the *medial nucleus* and ventromedial part of the *superior* and *lateral* nuclei (SHIMAZU and PRECHT, 1966). The latency of the positive peak of this potential is about 0.4 msec longer than the latency of the compound action potential recorded superficially at the midline of the dorsal brainstem (Fig. 14B). This time differential corresponds to the latency of *antidromic* firing of type I neurones after single shock of the midline (Fig. 14E). From the analysis of the potentials in Fig. 14, recorded at different points along the pathway, it seems that the summit of the initial positive wave approximately corresponds in time to the arrival of the earliest impulses in the *contralateral* nuclei along the *commissural* fibre system. The presence of a *negative contralateral potential* following the positivity, with a delay of about 0.8 msec, may indicate that some vestibular neurones are *excited* by impulses conducted along the commissural fibres (Fig. 14D). Reduction of the amplitudes of the potential at the midline, following a second shock given at a short interval, indicates that the commissural fibres originate in the *vestibular nuclei* and do *not* represent primary vestibular fibres crossing the midline. This is in good agreement with anatomical studies (RASMUSSEN, 1932; and LADPLI and BRODAL, 1968). After *sagittal incision* of the dorsal brainstem (about 2 mm deep), the above mentioned potentials in the contralateral nuclei disappeared (Fig. 13C), suggesting that they are solely generated by the action of the *commissural* fibres and are *not* caused by vestibulo-reticular loops. However, when the intensity of vestibular nerve stimulation is raised to more than 2 times of N_1 threshold, complex potentials are observed throughout the contralateral vestibular nuclei and particularly in the *reticular formation* which are *not* changed by cutting the commissural fibres and thus may be caused by *vestibulo-reticular pathways* crossing *deeper* than the commissural fibres.

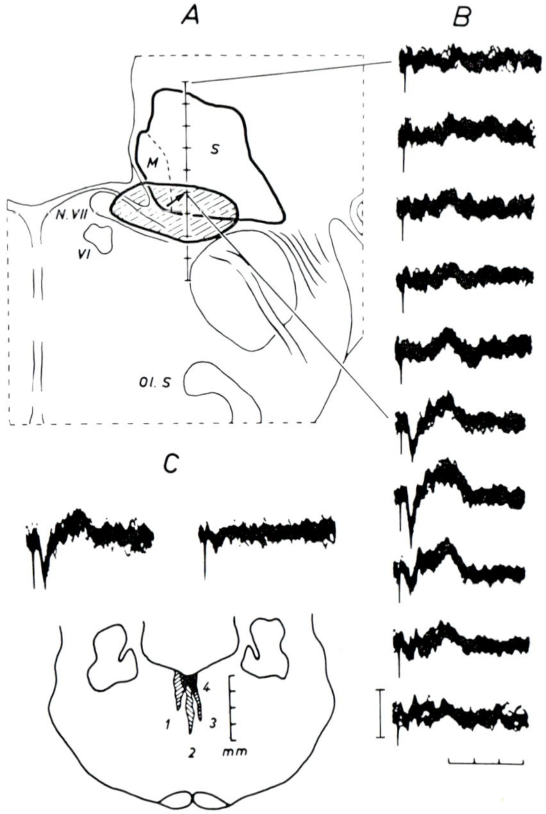

Fig. 13. Field potentials generated by stimulation of the vestibular nerve and recorded in the contralateral vestibular nuclei of unanesthetized and decerebrate cat. A: line drawing of a histological section of the brain stem. Vertical line shows the insertion of the electrode. Scales on this line indicate each 0.5 mm. Arrow indicates the site where coagulation was made with the microelectrode. Hatched area shows the region which produced field potentials of more than 30% of the maximum amplitude of positive potential. *S* = superior nucleus; *M* = medial nucleus; *Ol.S.* = superior olive; *N.VII* = VIIth cranial nerve; *VI* = VIth cranial motor nucleus. B: field potentials evoked by single shocks of the contralateral vestibular nerve and correlated with locations of electrode tip shown in A. Stimulation intensity was 1.2 V (2 times threshold for N_1 potential) in B and C. Time in B and C: 5 msec; amplitude calibration: 0.1 mV. C: field potential recorded in the contralateral vestibular nuclei following vestibular nerve stimulation (control on the left). Right-hand record: Effect of incision of the dorsal brain stem along the midline on the contralaterally evoked field potentials in the vestibular nuclei. Lower diagram: line drawing of histological section of the brain stem showing depth of incision. Contralateral vestibular field potentials were almost completely abolished by the incision, 1 to 3, and only slightly decreased by incision 4 (SHIMAZU and PRECHT, 1966)

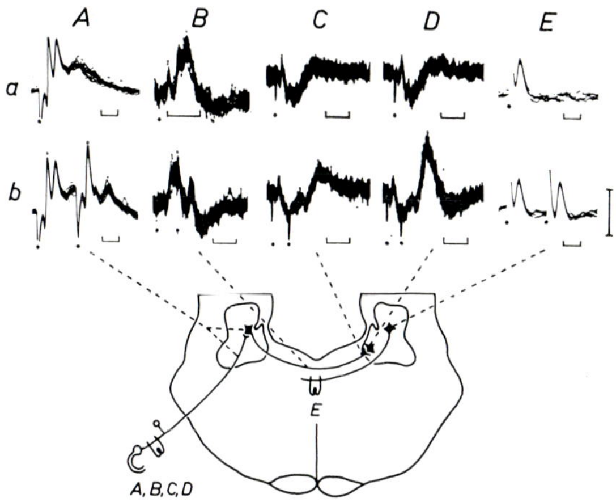

Fig. 14. Field potentials traced along the pathway from the ipsilateral to the contralateral vestibular nuclei after single shock of the vestibular nerve (A to D). All records were obtained from unanesthetized, decerebrate cats. Recording microelectrode was located in, A: ventrolateral part of the ipsilateral vestibular nuclei (note large P potential at this lateral recording point); B: midline about 0.5 mm deep beneath the IV ventricle; C and D: ventromedial part of the contralateral vestibular nuclei. In E: antidromically evoked action potentials of type I vestibular neurone in response to stimulation of the midline of the dorsal brain stem. In A to E, upper trace (a) shows the responses to single shock and lower trace (b) to double shocks. Each stimulus artifact is indicated by a dot below the record. Stimulation intensity was less than 2 times threshold for N_1 potential in A–D, and 0.4 V in E. Time: 1 msec for A and E, and 5 msec for B, C, and D. Amplitude calibration 0.6 mV for A and E, and 0.1 mV for B, C, and D. Inserted diagram below the records indicates the stimulated sites (A–E) and the structures to which the origin of recorded potentials were ascribed (broken lines) (Shimazu and Precht, 1966)

2. Excitation of Neurones from the Contralateral Labyrinth

Shimazu and Precht (1966) have demonstrated that some of the neurones which increase their discharge frequency during contralateral horizontal angular acceleration and decrease it with ipsilateral rotation (*type II neurones*) are mainly influenced by the *contralateral* horizontal canal. They can be recorded even if the *ipsilateral* labyrinth has been *removed*, but they are *not* found after cutting the commissural fibres. In line with these results, most of the *type II* neurones are *excited* by electrical stimulation of the *contralateral vestibular nerve*, the shortest latency being 3.2 msec which is consistent with the latency of the contralateral negative field potential described above. When this latency is compared with the values mentioned in the previous section, it can be deduced that some type II neurones may be *monosynaptically* activated by commissural fibres. Most of the type II neurones excited by weak stimulation of the contralateral VIIIth nerve are located in the region where contralaterally evoked potentials are predominantly found (Fig. 13A). According to Walberg et al. (1958), parts of this region are free from primary vestibular afferents. On the other hand, *degenerating synaptic terminals of commissural fibres* were described to show approximately the same distribution as the contralateral field potentials and the localization of type II neurones (Gray, 1926; Rasmussen, 1932; Ferraro et al., 1940; Ladpli and Brodal, 1968).

Neurones which respond to adequate stimulation of the *contralateral posterior* vertical canal are also found to be excited by electrical stimulation of the contralateral VIIIth nerve and are distributed approximately in the same territory as the type II neurones (MARKHAM, 1968). It is not clear at the present state, if these neurones are different ones or if different contralateral receptor organs converge on one and the same neurone. Some neurones located in Deiters' nucleus, particularly the ones which responded to tilt (SHIMAZU, 1967; SHIMAZU and SMITH, 1971), are also activated by contralateral vestibular nerve stimulation (DE VITO et al., 1956; PRECHT et al., 1967a).

3. Inhibition of Neurones from the Contralateral Labyrinth

Contralateral inhibition of some vestibular neurones located in the *lateral nucleus* was first described by DE VITO et al. (1956). MORUZZI and POMPEIANO (1957) and BATINI et al. (1957) suggested that the vestibular nuclei are subjected to inhibition arising from the contralateral labyrinth by studying *postural* changes following interruption of the vestibular nerve. A detailed study of the contralateral influences, provoked by stimulation of the semicircular canals, further elucidated the synaptology and some functional aspects of the *mutual interaction* between *bilateral* vestibular nuclei (SHIMAZU and PRECHT, 1966; PRECHT et al., 1966a; KASAHARA et al., 1968; MANO et al., 1968; MARKHAM, 1968).

Inhibition of Tonic Type I Neurones. Most of the *tonic* type I neurones identified by their responses to horizontal rotation have their *spontaneous discharges* distinctly *inhibited* by *weak* stimulation of the *contralateral* vestibular nerve (Fig. 15A–D), the intensity of which is subthreshold for reticular potentials (SHIMAZU and PRECHT, 1966). On all type I neurones tested after *interrupting the commissural* fibres by midline incision, the crossed *inhibitory influences* are completely *abolished* (like the excitation of type II neurones) and replaced by excitatory responses which are produced only with stimulation strong enough to produce *reticular evoked potentials.* Even with intact commissural fibres, excitation is also seen in some neurones following stimulation four to five times stronger than the threshold for N_1. Apparently, strong activation of reticulo-vestibular connections sometimes can overcome the inhibitory influences mediated through commissural fibres. As shown in Fig. 15D, in tonic type I neurones, the inhibition of the resting discharge occurs with a *latency* of about 4.0 msec on the average (SHIMAZU and PRECHT, 1966; KASAHARA et al., 1968; MARKHAM, 1968) and lasts for about 20–40 msec after single shock stimulation, which is in agreement with the time course of the IPSPs generated by contralateral vestibular nerve stimulation and recorded in vestibular neurones (SHIMAZU, 1967). High frequency stimulation is always more effective in producing inhibition because of *summation* of the IPSPs (SHIMAZU, 1967). When the value of the latency of inhibition (4.0 msec) is compared with the results described above, it can be deduced that tonic type I neurones are inhibited about 0.8 msec after the excitation of type II neurones. From these data, it may be assumed that *some of the type II neurones are intercalated inhibitory neurones* in the sense that they are *activated by contralateral horizontal canal stimulation* via *commissural* fibres and *exert inhibitory* influences on *homolateral type I neurones.* Like the type I neurones connected with the horizontal canals, the main second order sensory neurones from the *anterior vertical canals*

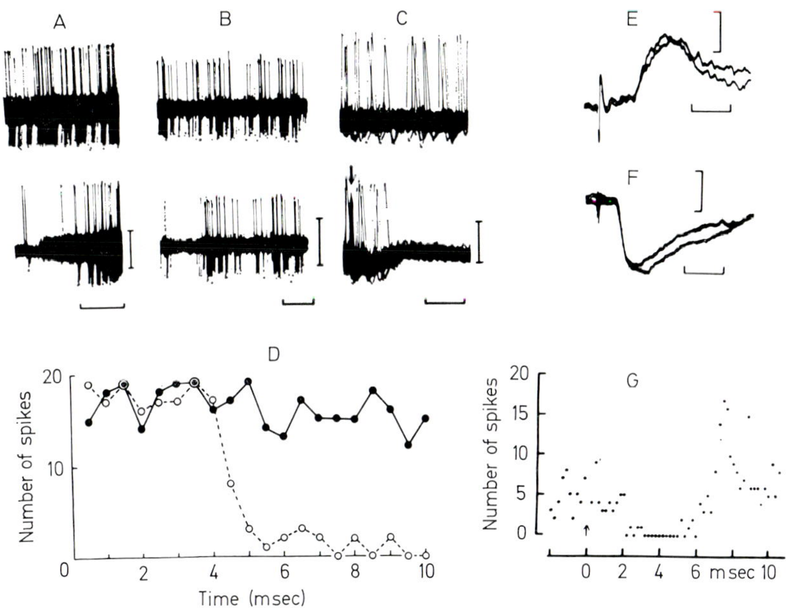

Fig. 15. Inhibition of the tonic and kinetic type I neurones induced by single shock of the contralateral vestibular nerve. Each record is composed of 50 (A, B) and 100 (C) superimposed traces at 2/sec. A to C, upper records show spontaneous discharges of extracellularly recorded tonic type I neurones. In lower records, a single shock was applied to the contralateral vestibular nerve at the onset of each sweep in A and B, and at the time indicated by the arrow in C. Stimulation intensity was 2 times threshold for N_1 potential. Amplitude: 0.5 mV. Time: 20 msec in A and B; 5 msec in C. D: distribution curves of the intervals between the shock artifact and all spikes in each trace (open circles), and of the intervals between the onset of the sweep and all spikes in each trace without stimulation (filled circles). Both curves were constructed using about 2,500 traces derived from 5 tonic type I units (Shimazu and Precht, 1966). E: intracellular recording from a medial vestibular nucleus neurone showing an excitatory postsynaptic potential (EPSP) generated by stimulation of the ipsilateral vestibular nerve. Time: 1 msec; Calibration: 2 mV. F: shows short latency inhibitory postsynaptic potential (IPSP) generated by contralateral vestibular nerve stimulation in the same neurone as shown in E. Time: 4 msec; Calibration: 5 mV. Upward deflection indicates positivity (Mano et al., 1968). G: spike distribution constructed with 10,000 sweeps for a kinetic type I neurone (repetitive background discharges were induced by ipsilateral cathodal polarization). Ordinate is the number of spikes counted at each interval of 0.2 msec and the abscissa is the time after the stimulation (arrow). Note earlier onset of inhibition in the kinetic neurone as compared to tonic neurones (D) (Kasahara et al., 1968)

have their resting discharge *inhibited* by stimulation of the contralateral vestibular nerve (Markham, 1968). It seems the latencies for inhibition of these neurones are somewhat *longer*, the inhibition appears to be *less* powerful and only about 60% of the neurones show significant reduction of their spontaneous discharge. Neurones being activated from the contralateral side show a reciprocal response during rotation with respect to the anterior canal units. They seem to be connected to the contralateral *posterior* canal. These *neurones* could also be considered as *inhibitory interneurones* mediating the *contralateral inhibition* found in neurones responding to *anterior canal stimulation*. Separate stimulation of each of the three canal nerves in each labyrinth has demonstrated a clear spatial distribution of the commissural inhibition (Kasahara and Uchino, 1971). Vestibular neurones were identified as horizontal or vertical canal units by stimulation of the ipsilateral vestibular nerve branches. On each of these identified neurones the contralateral inhibitory influence was investigated. It was confirmed that horizontal canal units were inhibited by contralateral horizontal canal stimulation. Furthermore, it was shown that anterior and posterior canal units were inhibited by stimulation of the contralateral posterior and anterior canals, respectively. The latencies of the IPSPs evoked in vertical canal neurones were similar to the ones described for type I neurones. Given the geometrical arrangement of the six semicircular canals, the specific mode of the inhibition observed in most of the neurones should be helpful for enhancing the sensitivity of the secondary vestibular neurones to angular accelerations of the head.

Inhibition of Kinetic Type I Neurones. In the study by Shimazu and Precht (1966), contralateral inhibition of *kinetic* type I neurones was already noted. Recent studies by Shimazu (1967); Kasahara et al. (1968); and Mano et al. (1968) show that the *latencies* of contralateral inhibition of *kinetic* neurones are significantly *shorter* than those in tonic cells. The spontaneously silent kinetic neurones were activated by means of *cathodal polarization* of the ipsilateral labyrinth in order to allow determination of the latency of inhibition of "spontaneous" discharge (Fig. 15G). A mean latency of 2.2 msec was found. With cells being recorded from intracellularly, IPSPs are found with a latency of about 2.0 msec following *contralateral vestibular nerve* stimulation. Direct stimulation of the contralateral *medial vestibular nucleus* produces IPSPs with latencies ranging from 1.0–1.3 msec. The conduction time of impulses along the commissural fibres was found to be about 0.55 msec. This suggests that *stimulation of the nucleus* produces IPSPs *monosynaptically* through *commissural fibres*. Hence, some of these fibres can also be *inhibitory* in nature besides the *excitatory* ones responsible for type II activation. Further, it appears from the studies by Mano et al. (1968) that the inhibitory commissural neurone itself is monosynaptically excited by primary vestibular afferents from the *ipsilateral* nerve. Kinetic type I neurones can thus be *inhibited* from the contralateral labyrinth by means of a *disynaptically* produced IPSP (Fig. 15F). *Monosynaptic excitation* of kinetic neurones after *ipsilateral* vestibular nerve stimulation has already been described above (Figs. 9A; 15E).

Finally it should be mentioned that commissural inhibition is blocked in one group of neurones by GABA antagonists (picrotoxin or bicuculline) and in another by the glycine antagonist strychnine (Precht et al., 1973a).

4. Functional Meaning of Crossed Inhibition

After removal of the contralateral labyrinth, the average *resting discharge* frequencies of tonic type I neurones seem to be *slightly higher*, suggesting *release* from the *tonically* acting commissural *inhibition*. Moreover, the *thresholds* for frequency increase of type I neurones on the *non-deafferented* side to horizontal angular acceleration are significantly *higher* as compared to animals with bilaterally *intact* labyrinths (Shimazu and Precht, 1966). Type I neurones located on the *acutely* deafferented side are very scarce but quite usual in *chronic* preparations where they are found to be inhibited by rotatory and electrical stimulation of the remaining contralateral horizontal canal (PRECHT et al., 1966a). It can be concluded from these results that during ipsilateral angular acceleration, discharge frequencies of type I neurones are enhanced not only by the *increased* activity of the ipsilateral horizontal canal but *also* by *decrease* of *crossed tonic inhibition*, resulting from decreased activity of the contralateral horizontal canal. In other words, withdrawal of inhibitory influence or *disinhibition* from the contralateral side elevates the *excitability* of type I neurones. During contralateral angular acceleration, the crossed inhibition acts on type I neurones *in addition* to decrease of excitation from the ipsilateral horizontal canal. These additive influences from the ipsi- and *contralateral labyrinths* will assure the highly *sensitive* responses of vestibular neurones and provide a basis for precisely organized efferent effects, such as those on the oculomotor apparatus under both normal and pathological conditions (see Chapter E.X.). It is important to emphasize that the commissural inhibition seems to be restricted to the canal systems. Second order vestibular neurones that respond to stimulation of the otolith system are not inhibited but rather excited by contralateral VIIIth nerve stimulation (see above).

III. Vestibular Nuclei in Relation to Other Systems

In the preceding sections of this Chapter, the labyrinthine input to the vestibular nuclei has been described. Numerous studies, however, have shown that the vestibular neurones are not only subjected to synaptic bombardment arising in the sensory organs of the vestibulum but receive also numerous fibres coming from central systems such as the *reticular formation*, the *cerebellum* and the *spinal cord*. Thus the vestibular nuclei are by no means a simple relay station carrying vestibular sensory information to various effector organs, but rather a very complicated structure *integrating* a variety of different inputs before the output reaches the stages of the final effector systems, such as the *oculomotor* apparatus, the *motoneurones* and interneurones of the spinal cord, the *reticular formation*, the *cerebellum* and other systems.

Other Chapters of this Handbook will provide a detailed description of the non-vestibular input as well as of the various outputs. Therefore, in this Chapter, only a short summary will be given trying to correlate the data described in the first part with those obtained for the various inputs and outputs.

A. Vestibulo-Cerebellar Interaction

Studies of the phylogenetic development of the cerebellum have shown that this organ originates from the rhomboidal lip of the fourth ventricle by an expansion of both octavolateral areas (LARSELL, 1923, 1929; HERRIK, 1924). The cerebellum can, for this reason, be considered as very closely related anatomically and functionally to the vestibular system. In all vertebrates, this close relation is represented by the presence of *primary* and *secondary vestibular fibres* projecting mainly to the *flocculonodular* region of the cerebellar cortex and to some of the deep cerebellar nuclei (for details see JANSEN and BRODAL, 1954; BRODAL et al., 1962).

Recent physiological studies have shown that in *frogs*, *primary vestibular fibres* end *monosynaptically* both as *climbing* fibres on Purkinje cells and as *mossy* fibres on granule cells in the flocculus of the cerebellar cortex. *Secondary vestibulo-cerebellar fibres* seem to end exclusively as *mossy* fibres in the flocculus of the frog (LLINÁS et al., 1967; PRECHT et al., 1970). In the *cat*, however, both *primary* and *secondary* vestibulo-cerebellar fibres end exclusively as *mossy* fibres in the "vestibulocerebellum" (PRECHT and LLINÁS, 1968a, 1969a, b; PRECHT et al., (1970); a finding which is in agreement with the anatomical studies by SNIDER (1936) and BRODAL and HOIVIK (1964). At present, we do, not know what kind of vestibular receptors are connected to the primary and secondary vestibulocerebellar fibres in the cat. Given the fact that secondary vestibulo-cerebellar fibres partly originate in the *descending* vestibular nucleus (BRODAL and TORVIK, 1957), which is known to receive afferents from the *utriculus* (STEIN and CARPENTER, 1967; PETERSON, 1967, 1970; GACEK, 1969), one may assume that otolithic influences are carried to the cerebellum. This does not exclude the possibility that in the cat also semicircular canal activity reaches the cerebellar cortex. In the frog it has indeed been shown that Purkinje cells respond very well to natural stimulation of the horizontal semicircular canals (PRECHT and LLINÁS, 1969b; LLINÁS et al., 1971). As described above four types of responses were recorded in the vestibular nuclei of mammals on horizontal rotation. Interestingly, these four types have also been found in recording from cerebellar Purkinje cells of the frog. Similar results have recently been obtained in mammals (unpublished observation) Further, some of the areas giving raise to vestibulo-cerebellar fibres (particularly group x) also receive *spinal* afferents (POMPEIANO and BRODAL, 1957a). This may provide a means by which *vestibular* and *somatic* afferent impulses could be integrated before they reach the cerebellum.

Besides the primary and secondary vestibulo-cerebellar fibres, indirect pathways via *vestibulo-reticulo-cerebellar* relays may provide even a greater basis for any kind of multisensory convergence. ANDERSON and GERNANDT (1954) described potentials recorded in the *lobulus simplex* and *culmen*, following vestibular nerve stimulation, as having *longer* latencies than those recorded in the vestibulo-cerebellum (PRECHT et al., 1970; PRECHT, LLINÁS, 1969a). These potentials may well be mediated through vestibulo-reticular-cerebellar pathways since no vestibular fibres have been found to terminate in this area of the cerebellum. As described above, the *fastigial nucleus* and parts of the *dentate nucleus* also receive *primary* and *secondary vestibular fibres*, a finding that has been confirmed physiologically by ARDUINI and POMPEIANO (1957) and PRECHT and LLINÁS (1968b).

It is well known that the cerebellum not only receives vestibular information, but it also *controls the vestibular nuclei* by means of *direct* corticofugal fibres (axons of Purkinje cells) and by fibres arising in the *nuclei fastigii* which in turn are under the inhibitory control of the cerebellar cortex (for detailed information on the anatomy, see JANSEN and BRODAL, 1954, 1958). In 1964, ITO and YOSHIDA discovered the *monosynaptic inhibitory* action of *Purkinje axons* on Deiters' neurones by recording from inside of these cells during stimulation of the *anterior lobe*. Similarly, the Purkinje axons were shown to have an inhibitory action onto the neurones in the *deep cerebellar nuclei* (ITO et al., 1964b). This direct demonstration of the *inhibitory nature of the Purkinje cells* explains the well known inhibitory action of cerebellar stimulation upon the *postural centers* of the brainstem (MORUZZI, 1950; BROOKHART, 1960), which is so clearly seen by the *disappearance* of *decerebrate rigidity* during stimulation of the *anterior lobe* (SHERRINGTON, 1898). Inhibition of *vestibular nystagmus* during stimulation of the "vestibulocerebellum" may also be explained by the inhibitory action of Purkinje cells on neurones located in the brainstem (FERNÁNDEZ and FREDRICKSON, 1963). Correspondingly, following lesions in the "vestibulocerebellum," *enhancement* of vestibular induced nystagmus, appearance of *spontaneous* nystagmus and *lack of habituation* of nystagmus are observed (HALSTEAD, 1935; SPIEGEL and SCALA, 1942; GRANT et al., 1964; ASCHAN et al., 1964). Recently it has been directly demonstrated that stimulation of the flocculus inhibits monosynaptically some vestibular neurones which project to the ocular motoneurones (FUKUDA et al., 1972; PRECHT et al., 1971b; BAKER et al., 1972; ITO et al., 1973). Discrete unilateral lesions in the nodulus seem to impair particularly otolithic influences on the oculomotor system (MANNI, 1950). For further information on these behavioral disturbances, see DOW and MORRUZZI (1958).

Following cerebellar stimulation, the Deiters' neurones not only show a postsynaptic inhibition caused by the Purkinje cell axons, but also distinct *disinhibitory* phenomena due to depression of tonic discharge from Purkinje cells by the action of the interneurones in the cerebellar cortex (ECCLES et al., 1967; ITO et al., 1968). *Disinhibition* partly explains the *excitatory* effects that have also been observed in Deiters' neurones following *anterior lobe* stimulation (DE VITO et al., 1956; POMPEIANO and COTTI, 1959). It also means that Purkinje cells can modulate their target neurones both in the excitatory as well as in the inhibitory direction. On the other hand, monosynaptic, postsynaptic excitatory potentials (EPSPs) also recorded in Deiters' neurones following cerebellar stimulation are most likely caused by axon reflexes through the *collaterals* of cerebellar afferents (ITO et al., 1965, 1969a). It is worthy to note that neurones located in the ventral part of the Deiters' nucleus do not receive Purkinje axons from the *anterior lobe* (WALBERG and JANSEN, 1961) and in these neurones only EPSPs are seen during cerebellar stimulation (ITO et al., 1969a). The smaller *ventral cells* in the Deiters' nucleus, however, receive fibres from the fastigial nuclei (BRODAL et al., 1962), flocculus (ANGAUT and BRODAL, 1967) and the vestibular nerve (WALBERG et al., 1958), while the dendrites and somata of the large and small *dorsal cells* are supplied by Purkinje axons from the anterior lobe and lack vestibular afferents (BRODAL et al., 1962; MUGNAINI and WALBERG, 1967). There is experimental evidence that Deiters' neurones responding to tilt (utricular stimulation) are inhibited by stimulation of the anterior vermis (SHIMAZU and SMITH, 1971).

In an attempt to study the effects of both *contralateral vestibular nerve* stimulation and stimulation of the *cerebellar vermis* on single neurones in the vestibular nuclei, SHIMAZU (1967) and SHIMAZU and SMITH (1971) found that Deiters' neurones inhibited during *cerebellar* stimulation (utricular units) are *not* inhibited but rather excited by stimulation of the *contralateral vestibular nerve*. On the other hand, *type I neurones* in the *medial* vestibular nuclei which are powerfully *inhibited* by stimulation of the *contralateral vestibular nerve* are *not* influenced by anterior lobe stimulation, thus showing *no convergence* between *cerebellar* and *commissural inhibition*. Stimulation of the vestibulo-cerebellum, however, inhibits the second order vestibular neurones of the horizontal canals (type I) which are also inhibited by the commissural path. Similar findings have been obtained for second order neurones receiving input from vertical canals (BAKER et al., 1972). Utricular units which are under inhibitory control of the anterior vermis are not influenced by stimulation of the vestibulo-cerebellum. Thus, it has been clearly demonstrated that various parts of the cerebellar cortex have differential connections with functional groups of vestibular neurones. Moreover, these physiological findings are for the most part in excellent agreement with the anatomical data showing that the projection of canal afferents and floccular afferents overlap in the vestibular nuclei (ANGAUT and BRODAL, 1967; GACEK, 1969).

The *type I neurones* in the medial and superior vestibular nuclei are *inhibited disynaptically*, during stimulation of the *contralateral fastigial nucleus* and monosynaptically excited by ipsilateral fastigial stimulation. Type II neurones are excited monosynaptically by contralateral fastigial stimulation (SHIMAZU, 1967). It is very likely that in this case type II neurones – as in the case of the inhibition initiated from the contralateral vestibular nerve – play the role of *inhibitory interneurones* acting on type I neurones. The purely *excitatory nature* of the tonic output of the cerebellar nuclei has been shown to hold true for various target neurones (for summary, see ECCLES et al., 1967). Since the fastigial nuclei, like the other cerebellar nuclei, are also under the *inhibitory* influence of the Purkinje cells of the cerebellar cortex, the latter may indirectly influence *vestibular neurones* by a mechanism known as *disfacilitation,* in addition to its direct corticofugal inhibitory action on some vestibular neurones. There is suggestive evidence for gamma-amino butyric acid (GABA) being the inhibitory transmitter substance released from Purkinje cell terminals (OBATA et al., 1967, 1970). For further details on the vestibulo-cerebellar interaction, Chapter D.III. of this volume may be consulted.

B. Vestibulo-Reticular Interrelationship

Neurones in the reticular formation have long been known for being influenced by a great variety of sense modalities converging upon them, which are integrated in this system before they reach the final motor output (MORUZZI, 1954; ROSSI and ZANCHETTI, 1957). The importance of the *vestibular* contribution to the reticular system appears to be particularly related to the coordination of postural and ocular movements. It is known from anatomical studies (CAJAL, 1911; PAPEZ, 1926; LORENTE DE NÓ, 1928, 1931, 1933b; FERRARO et al., 1940; SCHEIBEL and SCHEIBEL, 1958; BRODAL et al., 1962; LADPLI and BRODAL, 1968) that there are numerous connections between the *vestibular nuclei* and the *rhombencephalic reticular formation* in both directions. This has been confirmed by several physiological studies.

GERNANDT and THULIN (1952) and HENRIKSSON et al. (1962) found that single neurones in the bulbopontine reticular formation on both sides are influenced by adequate stimulation of the semicircular canals. The occurrence of *acoustic, somato-sensory* and *visual convergence* has been shown in reticular neurones being activated by labyrinthine stimulation (POTTHOFF et al., 1967). Using electrical stimulation of the *vestibular* nerve, *field potentials* have been recorded in the reticular formation (Fig. 2B), having a *higher* threshold than those recorded in the vestibular nuclei (PRECHT and SHIMAZU, 1965). Further, it has been shown that reticular neurones may be involved in the activation of vestibular neurones following stimulation of the contralateral vestibular nerve (SHIMAZU and PRECHT, 1966). Arousal reactions and convergence of non-vestibular sense modalities on vestibular neurones may be caused by similar reticulo-vestibular pathways (DUENSING and SCHAEFER, 1957a, b, 1958; BIZZI et al., 1964).

The behaviour of *vestibular neurones* and neurones located in a *dorsomedial region* of the rhombencephalic reticular formation (LORENTE DE NÓ'S, 1933b, vestibular part of the reticular formation) has been studied during *vestibular nystagmus* evoked by horizontal rotation (DUENSING and SCHAEFER, 1957a, b, 1958). It was found that the frequency of discharge of different types of *vestibular neurones* during the quick phase of nystagmus is influenced in five different ways. It deserves particular mention that the majority of the *type I neurones*, which presumably are the most important ones for *horizontal eye movements*, shows a *decrease* in frequency when the quick phase of the nystagmus is directed towards the recording side. Some of them also show a reciprocal pattern, others increase or decrease their frequency regardless of the direction the quick phase is beating. When recording was done from neurones located in the *reticular formation*, two groups of neurones were found. *One group* of cells highly *increases* their frequencies during the quick phase of nystagmus and *decreases* their discharge frequencies during the slow phase and *another group* shows the *opposite* reaction (DUENSING and SCHAEFER, 1957a). The authors point to the possibility that the *nystagmic rhythm* could be "*generated*" by this *dual system* of neurones located in the *dorsomedial* rhombencephalic *reticular formation*. This would mean that the nystagmic modulation seen in vestibular neurones may be caused by this system, an idea which is supported by the fact that LORENTE DE NÓ (1933a, b) found numerous fibres originating in this particular area of the reticular formation and ending in the *medial* vestibular nucleus. Further, he was able to show that the *quick phase* of the vestibular nystagmus disappears following destruction of this part of the *reticular formation*. Moreover, lesions in the *vestibular nuclei* do *not* abolish the quick component. It should be mentioned, however, that this hypothesis is not confirmed by SPIEGEL and PRICE'S (1939) finding showing that the *quick component* is *not* abolished following *reticular lesions*. These authors emphasize the importance of the *vestibular nuclei* in the generation of both slow and quick nystagmic components and consider the reticular pathways as dispensable (see also final section of this Chapter). Besides those reticular neurones which are very closely related to the components of the nystagmic rhythm, DUENSING and SCHAEFER (1957b) found other reticular neurones which showed only a rather *loose coupling* with the nystagmus. These reticular neurones are also influenced by *somatosensory*, *acoustic* stimuli and the state of *wakefullness* and seem to be dependent on the ascending reticular system of the brainstem. It is reasonable to assume that similar mechanisms of convergence may represent the neurophysiological basis of the arousal effects observed on vestibular nystagmus (COLLINS and GUEDRY, 1962).

It appears that the *reticular formation* of the *midbrain* has a similar *mutual* relationship with the vestibular nuclei. Pathways ascending from the *vestibular* nuclei to the *interstitial nucleus of Cajal* and adjacent structures have been described by GRAY (1926); BUCHANAN (1937); HASSLER (1948). The *descending* division from the *interstitial nucleus* to the *vestibular nuclei* has been described by POMPEIANO and WALBERG (1957) and is found to be a purely ipsilateral projection. Single neurones in the interstitial nucleus and adjacent areas have been shown to be influenced by *adequate* vestibular stimulation (DUENSING et al., 1963; GERNANDT, 1950b). This effect may be caused by certain second order vestibular neurones which could be *antidromically* excited on stimulation of the interstitial nucleus (MARKHAM et al., 1966; MARKHAM, 1968). Several investigators have studied the *stimulation effects* that one obtains during stimulation of the region of the *interstitial nucleus* (SZENTÁGOTHAI, 1943; HASSLER and HESS, 1954; FELDMAN et al., 1961) or *nucleus of Darkschewitsch* (SZENTÁGOTHAI and SCHAB, 1956; SCHEIBEL et al., 1961). It appears that the *interstitial nucleus* is involved in the coordination of *vertical* and *rotatory eye movements* in a facilitatory way, and the *nucleus of Darkschewitsch* is considered as an *inhibitory center* which exerts its effect on the oculomotor system. MARKHAM et al. (1966) showed that *type I vestibular neurones* of the horizontal canal are distinctly *inhibited* during stimulation of the ipsilateral interstitial nucleus, while *type II neurones* are *excited* with a lower threshold and a shorter latency, some probably monosynaptically. It is reasonable to assume that as in the case of the commissural or fastigial inhibition of type I, the type II neurones may again serve as *inhibitory interneurones*, particularly since *convergence* of excitation from the *contralateral* vestibular nerve and the *interstitial nucleus* on single type II neurones has been demonstrated to occur (MARKHAM, 1968). A similar but less intense inhibition was found for the vestibular neurones connected to the *anterior vertical canal* (MARKHAM, 1968). Stimulation of the *contralateral* interstitial nucleus, or strong stimulation of the *ipsilateral* one, and stimuli given to the more laterally located reticular formation, invariably caused *excitation* of type I neurones.

Since the *interstitial nucleus* projects directly to all ocular motoneurones except for those which innervate the medial and lateral recti muscles, it may be assumed that the powerful inhibitory action, particularly on the neuronal substrate for horizontal eye movement in the vestibular nuclei, may aid in the performance of vertical eye movements. Inhibition of *nystagmus* following stimulation of the mesencephalic reticular formation found by YULES et al. (1966b) may be caused by similar mechanisms. The midbrain reticular nuclei may, in addition, provide a means by which *other sensory systems* and *higher centers*, such as the basal ganglia or cerebral cortex, could override or modulate the vestibulo-ocular system. *Convergence* of *labyrinthine* and *cerebral* activity on neurones located in the *ponto-mesencephalic reticular formation* has been described by AZZENA et al. (1967). Experiments by SPIEGEL (1933) demonstrated that eye movements elicited by stimulation of the *cerebral cortex* change their direction following destruction of the vestibular nuclei, indicating the important role the vestibular nuclei play in the cortical control of the eye muscles for lateral eye movements. Since no direct cortico-vestibular fibres have been described, it is likely that cortical induced eye movements are mediated by intercalated systems, such as the midbrain areas just described. Stimulation of a circumscribed area, including the reticular formation medial to the *nucleus reticularis thalami* and the *geniculate bodies*, causes *central nystagmus*, its neurophysiological mechanism being not clear at the present stage (LACHMANN et al., 1958a, b). It becomes apparent that further physiological studies are needed in order to elucidate more detailed functional mechanisms of the vestibulo-reticular interaction.

C. Vestibulo-Spinal Interactions

Since separate Chapters of this volume provide a full description of problems related to vestibulospinal mechanisms, only a few data will be discussed here. A relatively small number of spinal afferents ascending mainly with the dorsal spinocerebellar tract have been described to end in the caudalmost region of the *descending* and *medial vestibular nucleus*, the dorsocaudal part of the *Deiters' nucleus* (hind-limb region) and in the cell groups x and z (POMPEIANO and BRODAL, 1957a; BOWSHER, 1962; BRODAL and ANGAUT, 1967). These parts of the vestibular nuclei do not seem to receive *primary* vestibular afferent fibres (WALBERG et al., 1958). In addition to this direct spinovestibular pathway, one has to keep in mind that *spino-reticulo-vestibular* connections allow ample possibilities for spinal activity to reach the vestibular nuclei (see BRODAL et al., 1962). Further, axon collaterals of fibres of the olivocerebellar tract ending in the vestibular nuclei may convey spinal impulses (LORENTE DE NÓ, 1924; ITO et al., 1964a; ALLEN et al., 1971). Since some of the areas receiving *direct* spinal afferents also project to the vestibulocerebellum (see above), the cerebellum seems to be also indirectly involved in the operation of the vestibulospinal system. According to the anatomical connection briefly outlined above, it is not surprising that many neurones in the vestibular nuclei were shown to be influenced by *stimulation* of the *spinal cord* or *afferent nerves*. POMPEIANO and COTTI (1959), FELDMANN et al. (1961), ITO et al. (1964a), WILSON et al. (1965, 1966a, b, 1967b) and PRECHT et al. (1966b, 1967a) convincingly demonstrated that in the cat the early direct *spinal input* to the vestibular nuclei is mainly *excitatory*, although some late inhibitory effects were also seen. Recently ALLEN et al. (1971) have demonstrated that Deiters' neurones receive a combination of an early EPSP (through olivo-vestibular fibres) and later IPSP through olivo-cerebello-vestibular paths from the peripheral nerves of the dominant limb, while only EPSPs were produced from the nerves of the nondominant limb. This indicates that there are two types of excitatory convergence onto Deiters' neurones from the inferior olivary nucleus; one is activated from the nerves of the dominant limb and always associated with the convergence of inhibition from Purkinje cells, and the other is activated from the nondominant limb and free from the inhibitory convergence of Purkinje cells. In animals anesthetized with Chloralose TEN BRUGGENCATE et al. (1971) found in addition to the sharp IPSP (mediated through climbing fibre activation of Purkinje cells) prolonged IPSP disinhibition sequences which they ascribed to activation of the mossy fibre-granule cell path. Both hindlimb and forelimb areas of *Deiters' nuclei* receive excitatory influences, a finding which also suggests that not only direct spino-vestibular fibres are responsible for the transmission of spinal impulses. Further, in about half of the Deiters' neurones studied, strong stimulation of the spinal cord at C_3 not only caused antidromic activation of the cells but also produced EPSPs (probably monosynaptic) and to a lesser degree polysynaptic and monosynaptic IPSPs (ITO et al., 1964b). These short latency spinal-evoked IPSPs may partly explain the inhibitory effects caused by conditioning sciatic nerve stimulation on utricular evoked test responses in decerebellate animals (Gernandt, 1970). No evidence was found for axon collaterals of Deiters' neurones producing recurrent inhibition as it is seen in spinal motoneurones (Eccles et al., 1954). Many cells located in the *medial* and *superior vestibular nuclei* were also excited by spinal stimulation and amongst those which responded to horizontal rotation particularly type II and type III neurones (Precht et al., 1967a). The generalized facilitation of many vestibular neurones by impulses arising in the periphery of the body may contribute to the *tonic resting discharge* of these neurones, which in turn can be modified by labyrinthine and other extralabyrinthine sources, such as the cerebellum or higher centers. *Summative convergence* of adequate *somatic* (joint movements) and *vestibular stimulation* on single vestibular neurones has been demonstrated and discussed by Fredrickson et al. (1966). *Proprioceptive* influences arising in the joints of the neck can produce eye movements (Magnus, 1924) and seem to alter vestibular induced eye movements (Koella, 1947; Koella et al., 1956) and finally lesions in the cervical cord may cause nystagmus (Booth, 1952). In short, it may be assumed that the data briefly outlined above provide a neurophysiological basis for the long known interaction of the vestibular and the proprioceptive systems. Both systems are of great importance in the regulation of posture (Sherrington, 1906).

By means of the *vestibulospinal* tracts and *vestibulo-reticulo-spinal* pathways, the vestibular nuclei are enabled to exert influences onto spinal *motoneurones* and interneurones. Deiters' nucleus gives origin to the uncrossed vestibulospinal tract so that the rostroventral part projects to cervico-thoracic levels and the dorsocaudal part to the lumbar segments of the cord, thus indicating a clear somatotopical arrangement (Pompeiano and Brodal, 1957b). The *medial vestibular nucleus* sends fibres mainly to the *cervical* cord via the descending branch of the medial longitudinal fasciculus (Nyberg-Hansen, 1964).

The somatotopical arrangement within the Deiters' nucleus has been basically confirmed by a number of *physiological studies*, showing that cells in the dorsocaudal half of the nucleus and those in the rostroventral part are projecting to different levels of the spinal cord, although most authors found a considerable overlapping between the two areas (Ito et al. 1964b; Wilson et al., 1965, 1967b; Precht et al., 1966b, 1967a). The percentage of cells being driven monosynaptically by stimulation of the vestibular nerve is much higher in the *rostroventral* area of the Deiters' nucleus (Wilson et al., 1966a, 1967b; Precht et al., 1966b, 1967a), a finding which is also in good agreement with the anatomy (Walberg et al., 1958). Further evidence for the functional differentiation of the two parts in the Deiters' nucleus is added by the fact that neurones located dorsocaudally are more frequently found to be spontaneously active (Wilson et al., 1966a), although they have much less monosynaptic input from the labyrinth. Parenthetically, this finding parallels to the presence of spontaneous discharge of tonic type I neurones in the medial vestibular nucleus, the majority of which have been shown to be innervated through polysynaptic pathways (Precht and Shimazu, 1965). As described above, only neurones in the dorsocaudal part of Deiters' nucleus are the target of the monosynaptic *inhibitory* pathway arising from Purkinje cells in the *anterior lobe* of the cerebellum (Ito and Yoshida, 1964). It may be recalled that only a modest number of Deiters' neurones respond to adequate stimulation of the *semicircular canals*, but many cells react to stimulation of the *otolith system* (see above). These findings may suggest that Deiters' nucleus is functionally more involved in the regulation of *tonic labyrinthine reflexes* on the head, the body and on the oculomotor system (see below). Interestingly, Deiters' neurones projecting to the cervico-thoracic region of the spinal cord appear to be frequently activated in response to ipsilateral tilting and inhibited to tilting in the opposite direction, whereas most neurones projecting to the lumbosacral segments are activated in response to tilting in either direction (PETERSON, personal communication). This differential projection could give rise to differences in postural responses between fore- and hindlimb motoneurones.

In good agreement with the anatomical data, physiological studies have shown that neurones having a particularly marked monosynaptic labyrinthine input, and being located in the *medial* and *descending vestibular nucleus*, also participate to some extent in the output to the spinal cord via the *descending longitudinal* fasciculus (PRECHT et al., 1966b, 1967a; WILSON et al., 1967a, 1968a, b). However, a higher percentage of these cells is found to be antidromically excited by stimulation of the *ascending longitudinal fasciculus*. It appears that antidromic activation of the main *second order* vestibular neurones of the *horizontal canals* (type I) from the spinal cord occurs extremely rarely, whereas, particularly type III neurones are more frequently activated by stimulation of their axons at the cervical cord. Otolithic influences on those neurones in the *descending* nucleus, which are antidromically activated from the spinal cord, have also been shown (PETERSON, 1970). At present, it seems difficult to compare the degree of functional importance of each type of vestibular neurone with respect to changes of spinal activities during stimulation of the semicircular canals described by GERNANDT and THULIN (1953); WAGNER et al., 1967; EHRHARDT and WAGNER, 1970).

Since both the neurones in the *rostroventral Deiters' nucleus* and in the *medial* and *descending vestibular nucleus* receive strong *monosynaptic* input from the labyrinth, and both of these groups project to higher levels of the spinal cord and probably do not send their axons beyond thoracic levels, it may be emphasized that the *cervico-thoracic* cord is more directly influenced by the vestibular impulses than the lumbosacral motor systems. As mentioned above, *vestibulo-reticulo-spinal* pathways provide another means by which the vestibular nuclei can indirectly exert crossed and uncrossed influences onto the spinal cord.

Only a few comments on the nature and mode of action of the vestibulospinal tracts will be given. Numerous investigators have shown that the *vestibular nuclei* exert a *facilitatory influence* on the *postural tonus* (antigravity muscles), as well as on the reflex activities of the spinal cord (SHERRINGTON, 1898; MAGNUS, 1924; FULTON et al., 1930; BACH and MAGOUN, 1947; THULIN, 1953; ANDERSON and GERNANDT, 1956; POMPEIANO, 1958; BRODAL et al., 1962). It has been directly demonstrated by LUND and POMPEIANO (1965) and GRILLNER et al. (1966, 1970) that the axons of Deiters' neurones provoke monosynaptic EPSPs in *alpha extensor motoneurones*, particularly in those innervating neck muscles (WILSON and YOSHIDA, 1968, 1969a), as well as in inhibitory interneurones for flexor motoneurones. Interestingly, some fibres originating in the medial vestibular nuclei are able to exert a *monosynaptic inhibitory* action on many *neck* extensor motoneurones (WILSON and YOSHIDA, 1969b). Electrical stimulation of the ipsilateral labyrinth often produced disynaptic IPSPs in neck motoneurones, very probably by means of a relay in the medial nucleus. Thus, the vestibular nuclei are also inhibitory to certain spinal motoneurones. Direct vestibulospinal influences on spinal *interneurones* for extensor motoneurones should also be considered. Similarly, the *gamma motoneurones* of the extensor muscles receive an excitatory influence from the Deiters' nucleus (CARLI et al., 1966, 1967; DIETE-SPIFF et al., 1967). Interestingly, a fast pathway from Deiters' nucleus to extensor muscle spindles has been found, and it appears that some fusimotor effects may be mediated by fibres larger than gamma efferents (GRANIT et al., 1959; CARLI et al., 1966). In using natural stimulation it has been shown that extensor alpha motoneurones of the hindlimbs reacted to movements of the head mostly with brief discharge increase regardless of the direction of the head movement (EHRHARDT and WAGNER, 1970). After the neck afferents were eliminated the facilitation of extensor alpha motoneurones previously observed *during* the movement was now abolished, and marked facilitation for the period of *maintained head position* appeared. In flexor neurones frequency decrease was the rule. The neck afferents therefore, have an inhibitory influence upon labyrinthine reflexes arising in the otoliths during maintained head positions, which, of course, is important for proper co-operation of neck- and labyrinthine reflexes in the control of posture. Direct evidence for convergence of *cortical, proprioceptive* and *vestibular impulses* on *spinal interneurones* has been given by ERULKAR et al. (1966). These findings further support the importance of the interaction of *proprioceptive* and *vestibular* impulses for the maintenance of the postural reflexes at different levels of the central nervous system.

D. Vestibulo-Ocular Relationship

It has long been recognized that the various vestibular receptors are capable of influencing the extraocular muscles in a very distinct way. Particularly well studied are the effects of stimulation and ablation of individual *semicircular canals* on various eye muscles (BREUER, 1889; EWALD, 1892; BÁRÁNY, 1907; LORENTE DE NÓ, 1928, 1931, 1933b; SZENTÁGOTHAI, 1943, 1950, 1952; FLUUR, 1959, 1960; MONEY and SCOTT, 1962; COHEN et al., 1964; SUZUKI and COHEN, 1966; CLARK and BURNS, 1967). It appears that a rather precise projection exists between the *horizontal* semicircular canal and the ipsilateral medial and contralateral lateral rectus muscle; the *anterior canal* and the ipsilateral superior rectus and contralateral inferior oblique; the *posterior canal* and the ipsilateral superior oblique and contralateral inferior rectus muscle (SZENTÁGOTHAI, 1950; FLUUR, 1959; COHEN et al., 1964; ITO et al., 1973). The shortest reflex connections between these labyrinthine organs and the ocular muscles consist of *three* neurones, i.e., (1) the *primary* vestibular neurone connecting the sensory cells in the crista ampullaris with the neurones in the vestibular nuclei; (2) the *secondary* vestibular neurones sending their axons to the oculomotor nuclei via the ascending branch of the medial longitudinal fasciculus; and (3) the *motoneurones* innervating the various extraocular muscles. Similarly, the otolith organs are able to influence the position of the eyes, a phenomenon which is known as the *tonic labyrinthine reflex* on the eyes (VAN DER HOEVE and KLEYN, 1917; KLEYN and MAGNUS, 1920; KLEYN, 1921; LORENTE DE No, 1932; SCHOENE, 1962; SUZUKI et al., 1969). Recent studies have shown that ocular motoneurons also receive disynaptic EPSPs from the utriculus, i.e. a three neuronal arc characterizes both the canal and otolith inputs to motoneurones (Schwindt et al. 1973; BAKER et al., 1973). It should also be emphasized that not all vestibular neurones projecting into the medial longitudinal fasciculus are part of a bisynaptic pathway since many vestibular neurones do not receive primary vestibular fibres but are rather influenced by means of multisynaptic intranuclear circuits (WALBERG et al., 1958; PRECHT and SHIMAZU, 1965).

In addition to these well-known elementary and selective three neuronal pathways, any semicircular canal can establish functional contact with any one of the extraocular muscles by means of a far more complex system of connections involving partly the *reticular formation*. Further, even fibres ascending in the medial longitudinal fasciculus, may exert *indirect* influences on the eye muscles by means of pathways involving the *interstitial nucleus of Cajal* and other midbrain nuclei (LORENTE DE NÓ, 1931, 1933b; SZENTÁGOTHAI, 1943; HASSLER and HESS, 1954; SZENTÁGOTHAI and SCHAB, 1956; SCHEIBEL et al., 1961; HYDE and TOCZEK, 1962; MARKHAM et al., 1966). It is beyond the scope of this Chapter to go into details of this rather complex problem. Some of the aspects have already been discussed in connection with problems on the vestibulo-reticular interaction. For further details the reader is referred to Chapter D.IV. of this Volume. Since we are primarily concerned with the vestibular nuclei, their role in the vestibulo-ocular relationship will be evaluated. There is no doubt that the *vestibular nuclear complex* is of great importance for the maintenance of *symmetric* control of eye movements. As far as vestibular induced eye movements are concerned, both the direct bisynaptic pathway and the more complex pathways through the reticular formation involve the vestibular nuclei. This seems to hold true also for some cortical induced eye movements (SPIEGEL, 1933).

Anatomical connections: Several attempts have been made in the past to evaluate the anatomical basis of the well-known ocular movements following labyrinthine stimulation, by studying the distribution of secondary vestibular fibres among the various motor nuclei of the eye muscles (BUCHANAN, 1937; SZENTÁGOTHAI, 1943; BRODAL and POMPEIANO, 1957b; CARPENTER and MCMASTERS, 1963; CARPENTER et al., 1963; MCMASTERS et al., 1966; TARLOV, 1970: GACEK, 1971). The *somatotopical* distribution of the motoneurones of the different ocular nerves in the oculomotor complex has also been studied and is, of course, of great importance for an evaluation of the data obtained by the first kind of approach (SZENTÁGOTHAI, 1942; BENDER and WEINSTEIN, 1943; WARWICK, 1953). It appears from the anatomical studies in *monkeys* by MCMASTERS et al. (1966) that fibres arising in the *superior vestibular nucleus* ascend exclusively and project mainly to the ipsilateral nuclei of the extraocular muscles (particularly strong projections are found in the trochlear nucleus and the dorsal nucleus of the IIIrd nucleus). The rostral part of the *descending vestibular nucleus* has bilateral projections to the abducens nucleus, oculomotor nuclei and to the contralateral trochlear nucleus. Ascending fibres arising in the *medial vestibular nucleus* project bilaterally and asymmetrically to all motor nuclei. Only the ventral part of the *Deiters' nucleus* takes part in the projection to the contralateral abducens the trochlear nuclei and to specific parts of the oculomotor complex bilaterally. A comparison between the patterned eye movements obtained by stimulation of individual semicircular ducts and the anatomical data, seems to indicate that most of the short latency effects on the eye muscles could be mediated by fibres arising in the medial and lateral vestibular nuclei, though the other nuclei are, of course, also involved. Further, the number of fibres coming from the medial and lateral nuclei is most abundant to those nuclei being concerned with *horizontal* eye movement and less powerful to nuclei innervating muscles whose function is concerned with vertical eye movements. This may also suggest that the *vestibular nuclei* are particularly important for *conjugate horizontal* eye movements (SPIEGEL, 1933; BENDER and WEINSTEIN, 1944; McMASTERS et al., 1966). A recent study of the vestibulo-ocular projection in the *cat* (TARLOV, 1970; GACEK, 1971) has shown that there are differences from the findings obtained with monkeys (McMASTERS et al., 1966). In the cat vestibular projections to the extraocular motor nuclei arise only in the superior vestibular nucleus (SV) and in rostral portions of the medial vestibular nucleus (MV), the regions which receive the central projections of the semicircular canal ganglia. The majority of SV fibres pass rostromedially into the *ipsilateral* MLF from which they enter the ipsilateral IVth and IIIrd nuclei. Some fibres cross the midline at the level of the IIIrd nuclei. From the MV, fibres pass into the ipsilateral and a few in the contralateral VIth nucleus. Ascending fibres pass in the contralateral MLF to the motor nuclei bilaterally.

Closer inspection of the synaptic knobs in the oculomotor nuclei has shown that they are of extraordinary size both in fish (HORSTMANN, 1954) and mammals (SZENTÁGOTHAI, 1964). Two types of synaptic boutons have been differentiated by SZENTÁGOTHAI (1964) in the oculomotor nuclei of cats. The large *A-type terminal* belonging to secondary vestibular neurones seems to assure a powerful and localized connection between the vestibular nuclei and the ocular motoneurones. *Type B terminals*, on the other hand, are of small caliber and the branches are distributed over a wide area. A great deal of convergence seems to be required in order to excite motoneurones along this type of synapse. Degeneration studies indicate that type-B synapses belong to axons of reticular cells and arise partly from the medial vestibular nucleus. At the present stage we have no idea as to whether both of these terminals are only excitatory in nature as will be described below. *Inhibitory synapses* have to be postulated since *reciprocal inhibition* (see below) has been found to exist in the oculomotor system (SZENTÁGOTHAI and SCHAB, 1956; FLUUR, 1959; PRECHT et al., 1967b; RICHTER and PRECHT, 1968).

Physiological aspects: As described above, stimulation of the peripheral vestibular organs has resulted in the concept of short latency *crista reflexes*, mediated over MLF which may be superceded by a complex reticular path. Numerous attempts have been made in the past trying to interrupt these pathways by means of localized lesions or to stimulate the vestibular nuclei and adjacent structures in order to elicit patterned eye movements. *Large unilateral lesions* in the *vestibular nuclei* lead to disequilibrium symptoms and spontaneous nystagmus directed toward the intact side (SHANZER and BENDER, 1959). *Smaller unilateral lesions of the vestibular nuclei* may provoke horizontal, vertical and rotatory nystagmus towards the intact side, as well as towards the side of the lesion (LEIDLER, 1916; FERRARO et al., 1940; CRANMER, 1951; CARPENTER et al., 1960; BENDER and SHANZER, 1964). It seems that *rotatory* nystagmus is caused by lesions, particularly of the caudal part of the vestibular nuclei, whereas rostral lesions provoke preferably *vertical* nystagmus (LEIDLER, 1916). Small, properly placed lesions can also successfully abolish the eye movements produced by one particular canal (SHANZER, 1965). Operative interference with the MLF, of course, will interrupt most of the short reflex pathways connecting the labyrinth with the eye muscles, and hence the short latency crista reflexes can no longer be evoked (SZENTÁGOTHAI, 1950, 1952). *Bilateral lesions* of the vestibular nuclei did completely *abolish* the *rapid eye movements* typical for desynchronized sleep. This drastic effect is due to the destruction of second-order vestibular neurones (POMPEIANO and MORRISON, 1965).

In short, it may be stated that *unilateral lesions* in the vestibular nuclei lead to *asymmetric disturbances* of the *tonic* innervation of the motor nuclei of the eye muscles, thus producing a variety of symptoms most of which, however, are transient in nature. Since a lesions does not only destroy the cell bodies in a particular area but also fibres only passing through the nucleus, the data obtained from these studies should be very critically evaluated. The same holds true for any kind of effects evoked by electric stimulation in the vestibular nuclei.

Conjugate ocular deviations can be evoked by stimulating various sites in the brainstem including the vestibular nuclei (SZENTÁGOTHAI, 1943; HASSLER, 1948, 1956; CRANMER, 1951; HYDE and ELIASSON, 1957; LACHMAN et al., 1958; HYDE and EASON, 1959; HYDE and TOCZEK, 1962; BENDER and SHANZER, 1964). Stimulation of the *medial vestibular nucleus* (CRANMER, 1951) produces *horizontal* nystagmus to the same side, a finding that fits well with the somatotopical distribution of the second order neurones of horizontal canals in the vestibular nuclei (see preceding sections). Stimulation of the *lateral vestibular nucleus* evokes nystagmus towards the side of the stimulation, and spontaneous nystagmus can be potentiated or inhibited depending on the side of stimulation (YULES and GAULT, 1966; YULES et al., 1966a).

More recently, attempts have been made to study the activities of *single neurones* in the *ocular motor* nuclei at rest, as well as during vestibular stimulation (SASAKI, 1963; SCHAEFER, 1965; MANNI et al., 1965; MANNI and DESOLE, 1966; GERNANDT et al., 1966; PRECHT et al., 1967b, 1969; YAMANAKA and BACH Y RITA, 1968; HORCHOLLE and TYC-DUMONT, 1968; RICHTER and PRECHT, 1968; BAKER et al., 1969; PRECHT and BAKER, 1972; HIGHSTEIN et al., 1971). Ocular motoneurones are in many aspects similar to spinal motoneurones. There are, however, some differences, such as a shorter time constant, shorter duration of afterhyperpolarization and lack of recurrent inhibition (SASAKI, 1963; BAKER and PRECHT, 1972). The rates of discharges during stimulation or during saccadic eye movements are usually much higher (maximal frequencies of more than 500/sec were observed) in ocular motoneurones as compared to spinal motoneurones (SASAKI, 1963;

SCHAEFER, 1965; PRECHT et al., 1967b, 1969; FUCHS and LUSCHEI, 1970; ROBINSON, 1970). Given the high *tetanus frequency* for *extraocular muscles* (COOPER and ECCLES, 1930), the high frequency of discharge of ocular motoneurones seems to be very useful for the performance of precise saccadic eye movements. When the discharge of an ocular motoneurone is recorded during vestibular nystagmus, its frequency of discharge is modulated in close relation with the different phases of nystagmus (SCHAEFER, 1965; PRECHT et al., 1967b, 1969; YAMANAKA and BACH Y RITA, 1968; HORCHOLLE and TYC-DUMONT, 1968; SHIMAZU, 1972; MAEDA et al., 1971a, b; BAKER and BERTHOZ, 1971, 1974). Neurones showing no discharge at rest, as well as tonically active motoneurones, seem to be involved in the performance of *both* phases of nystagmus (SCHAEFER, 1965; PRECHT et al., 1967b, 1969). The effect of different magnitudes of horizontal angular acceleration on *abducens motoneurones* were studied by PRECHT et al. (1967b, 1969) in decerebrate and decerebellate cat and it was found that these neurones increase their frequencies during contralateral angular acceleration very much in the same way as has been described for type I *vestibular* neurones by SHIMAZU and PRECHT (1965). *Tonic* as well as *silent* motoneurones have similar low thresholds (0.5 ± 0.27 and $0.63 \pm 0.4°/\text{sec}^2$ respectively) and are also not significantly different in their *gradients* of the *logarithmic* acceleration-frequency relationship. Hence, it may be concluded that the motoneurones are not clearly separated in tonic and kinetic types of neurones, a feature that has been found to be quiet characteristic for type I vestibular neurones (SHIMAZU and PRECHT, 1965).

Synaptology of the excitatory and inhibitory vestibulo-ocular reflex: As already mentioned above anatomical studies strongly suggested a disynaptic linkage between the vestibular nerve and the ocular motoneurones. Furthermore, these studies led to the assumption that the vestibular nuclei are the link between the VIIIth nerve and the motoneurones. Recent physiological studies have fully confirmed the anatomical work and the functional organization described above. It has been shown that stimulation of the contralateral *VIIIth nerve* causes *disynaptic* excitation of abducens and trochlear motoneurones and that stimulation of the *medial vestibular nucleus* generates in the same motoneurones *monosynaptic* EPSPs (BAKER et al., 1969; RICHTER and PRECHT, 1968; PRECHT and BAKER, 1972). When recordings were obtained from vestibular axons terminating in these nuclei monosynaptic activation was obtained following VIIIth nerve stimulation. Similar studies have been performed with neurones located in the IIIrd nucleus (HIGHSTEIN et al., 1971). In short it can be stated that the excitatory reflex from the horizontal and posterior canals is mediated through the medial vestibular nucleus and the one from the anterior canal appears to run through the y-group (for summary see ITO et al., 1973). It should be added that single shock stimulation of the VIIIth nerve generally produces double activation of vestibular axons terminating in the ocular motor nuclei. This double firing corresponds well with the double activation of vestibular neurones described above and indicates that both N_1 and N_2 components of the vestibular field potential are also represented in the output to the oculomotor system. Reticular paths are thus dispensable for the early di- and polysynaptic activations. Interestingly, in fish a monosynaptic vestibulo-ocular reflex has been demonstrated (KIDOKORO, 1969).

It has long been known that during conjugate eye movements the antagonistic muscles show a reduction in muscle tone. This effect is in part caused by a decrease of the excitatory input to the motor nuclei occurring as the result of a combined action of peripheral receptor mechanisms *and* commissural inhibition both of which decrease the firing rate of vestibular neurones innervating the antagonistic muscles (for details see PRECHT et al., 1966a; PRECHT et al., 1969; PRECHT (1972). However, disfacilitation is not the only mechanism by which antagonistic inhibition is achieved. This has been demonstrated by the finding that inhibition of the antagonist is not abolished by midsagittal section of the brain stem (RICHTER and PRECHT, 1968). Hence, the vestibular nuclei can also actively inhibit ocular motoneurones. This statement is fully supported by the demonstration of *disynaptic* and *monosynaptic* IPSPs in motoneurones of the IIIrd, IVth and VIth nuclei following stimulation of the ipsilateral *VIIIth nerve* and *nucleus* respectively (HIGHSTEIN et al., 1971; PRECHT and BAKER, 1972. BAKER et al., 1969). In the case of the IIIrd and IVth nuclei stimulation of the *superior* vestibular nucleus produces monosynaptic IPSPs in motoneurones, whereas in the VIth nucleus stimulation of the *medial* vestibular nucleus causes this effect. The functional organization of canal-induced inhibition is such that (I) the horizontal canal inhibits the ipsilateral lateral rectus and contralateral medial rectus muscle (2) the anterior canal the contralateral superior oblique and ipsilateral inferior rectus muscle, and (3) the posterior canal inhibits the ipsilateral inferior oblique and contralateral superior rectus muscle (RICHTER, PRECHT, 1968; BAKER et al., 1969; 1973; PRECHT, BAKER, 1972; ITO et al., 1973). All these pathways are mediated through the superior vestibular nucleus with the exception of the one to the ipsilateral lateral rectus (medial vestibular nucleus). There is evidence for GABA as the synaptic transmitter of the inhibitory vestibulo-ocular pathway (PRECHT et al. 1973b).

Thus it has clearly been demonstrated that the *vestibular nuclei* are the link in the *excitatory* as well as in the *inhibitory disynaptic vestibulo-ocular reflexes*. On the basis of intracellular recordings obtained from abducens motoneurones and vestibular axons during nystagmus it has been suggested that rhythmic membrane potential changes in the motoneurones originate from the vestibular nuclei (SHIMAZU, 1972). The excitatory and inhibitory vestibulo-ocular pathways being influenced at the level of the vestibular nuclei by the commissural inhibitory system may serve as the "basic circuit" for vestibular induced nystagmus. The reticular formation may be essential for subserving the maintenance of background activities for rhythmic function of the bilateral vestibular nuclei. At present, however, the role and synaptology of vestibulo-reticulo-oculomotor paths is not clear yet. It has been assumed that they are important for both excitation and inhibition (LORENTE DE NÓ, 1933b; SZENTÁGOTHAI and SCHAB, 1956) of ocular motoneurones. On the other hand, it has recently been shown that even long latency inhibitory and excitatory events recorded in motoneurones following VIIIth nerve stimulation appear to be more closely related to vestibulo-cerebello-vestibular interactions than to reticular activity (PRECHT et al., 1971b; BAKER et al., 1972). Further microphysiological and anatomical studies are needed for a better understanding of the role of vestibulo-reticular interactions in vestibular induced eye movements.

References

Adrian, E.D.: Discharges from vestibular receptors in the cat. J. Physiol. (Lond.) **101**, 389–407 (1943).

Albert, H.H. von: Untersuchungen zur Habituation des postrotatorischen Nystagmus. Dtsch. Z. Nervenheilk. **187**, 503–506 (1965).

Allen, G.I., Sabah, N.H., Toyama, K.: Effect of fore- and hindlimb nerve stimulation on Deiters' neurones. Brain Res. **25**, 645–650 (1971).

Anderson, S., Gernandt, B.E.: Cortical projection of vestibular nerve in cat. Acta oto-laryng. (Stockh.) **116**, 10–18 (1954).

Anderson, S., Gernandt, B.E.: Ventral root discharge in response to vestibular and proprioceptive stimulation. J. Neurophysiol. **19**, 524–543 (1956).

Angaut, P., Brodal, A.: The projection of the "vestibulocerebellum" onto the vestibular nuclei in the cat. Arch. ital. Biol. **105**, 441–479 (1967).

Arduini, A., Pompeiano, O.: Microelectrode analysis of units of the rostral portion of the nucleus fastigius. Arch. ital. Biol. **95**, 56–70 (1957).

Ashcroft, D.W., Hallpike, C.S.: On the function of the saccule. J. Laryng. **49**, 450–460 (1934).

Aschan, G., Ekvall, L., Grant, G.: Nystagmus following stimulation in the central vestibular pathways using permanently implanted electrodes. Acta oto-laryng. (Stockh.) **58**, Suppl. 192, 63–77 (1964).

Azzena, G.B., Giretti, M.L., Derin, P.L.: Convergence of labyrinthine and cerebral nystagmogenic impulses on brain stem units. Exp. Neurol. **19**, 401–411 (1967).

Bach, L.M.N., Magoun, H.W.: The vestibular nuclei as an excitatory mechanism for the cord. J. Neurophysiol. **10**, 331–337 (1947).

Baker, R., Berthoz, A.: Organization of vestibular nystagmus in oblique oculomotor system. J. Neurophysiol. **37**, 195—217 (1974).

Baker, R., Berthoz, A.: Spontaneous nystagmus recorded in trochlear motoneurones following labyrinthine lesion. Brain Res. **32**, 239–245 (1971).

Baker, R.G., Mano, N., Shimazu, H.: Postsynaptic potentials in abducens motoneurons induced by vestibular stimulation. Brain Res. **15**, 577–580 (1969).

Baker, R., Precht, W.: Electrophysiological properties of trochlear motoneurons as revealed by IVth nerve stimulation. Exp. Brain Res. **14**, 127—157 (1972).

Baker, R., Precht, W., Berthoz, A.: Synaptic connections to trochlear motoneurons determined by individual vestibular nerve branch stimulation in the cat. Brain Res. **64**, 402—406 (1973).

Baker, R., Precht, W., Llinás, R.: Cerebellar modulatory action on the vestibulo-trochlear pathway in the cat. Exp. Brain Res. **15**, 364—385 (1972).

Bárány, R.: Physiologie and Pathologie des Bogengangsapparates beim Menschen. Wien: Franz Deutick 1907.

Batini, C., Moruzzi, G., Pompeiano, O.: Cerebellar release phenomena. Arch. ital. Biol. **95**, 71–95 (1957).

Bender, M.B., Shanzer, S.: Oculomotor pathways defined by electric stimulation and lesions in the brainstem of monkey. In: The Oculomotor System. New York: Hoeber 1964.

Bender, M.B., Weinstein, E.A.: Functional representation in the oculomotor and trochlear nuclei. Arch. Neurol. Psychiat. **49**, 98—106 (1943).

Bender, M.B., Weinstein, E.A.: Effects of stimulation and lesion of the medial longitudinal fasciculus in the monkey. Arch. Neurol. Psychiat. (Chic.) **52**, 106–113 (1944).

Benson, A.J., Guedry, F.E., Melvill Jones, G.: Response of semicircular canal dependent units in vestibular nuclei to rotation of a linear acceleration vector without angular acceleration. J. Physiol. (Lond.) **210**, 475–494 (1970).

Bergstedt, M.: The effect of gravitational force on the vestibular caloric test. Acta oto-laryng. (Stockh.) **53**, 551–562 (1961a).

Bergstedt, M.: Studies of positional nystagmus in the human centrifuge. Acta oto-laryng. (Stockh.) Suppl. **165**, 1–144 (1961b).

Bizzi, E., Pompeiano, O., Somogyi, J.: Spontaneous activity of single vestibular neurons of unrestrained cats during sleep and wakefulness. Arch. ital. Biol. **102**, 308–330 (1964).

Booth, C. B.: Does nystagmus occur in lesions of the cervical cord? Arch. Neurol. Psychiat. (Chic.) **67**, 69–71 (1952).

Bowsher, D.: The topographical projection of fibres from the anterolateral quadrant of the spinal cord to the subdiencephalic brain stem in man. Psychiat. et Neurol. (Basel) **143**, 75–99 (1962).

Breuer, J.: Über die Funktion der Bogengänge des Ohrlabyrinthes. Wien. med. Jahrb. **4**, 72–124 (1874).

Breuer, J.: Neue Versuche an den Ohrbogengängen. Pflügers Arch. ges. Physiol. **44**, 135–152 (1889).

Breuer, J.: Über die Funktion der Otolithen-Apparate. Pflügers Arch. ges. Physiol. **48**, 195–306 (1891).

Breuer, J.: Über Bogengänge und Raumsinn. Pflügers Arch. ges. Physiol. **68**, 596–648 (1897).

Brodal, A., Angaut, P.: The termination of spino-vestibular fibres in the cat. Brain Res. **5**, 494–500 (1967).

Brodal, A., Høivik, B.: Site and mode of termination of primary vestibulocerebellar fibres in the cat. Arch. ital. Biol. **102**, 1–21 (1964).

Brodal, A., Pompeiano, O.: The vestibular nuclei in the cat. J. Anat. (Lond.) **91**, 438–454 (1957a).

Brodal, A., Pompeiano, O.: The origin of ascending fibres of the medial longitudinal fasciculus from the vestibular nuclei. Acta morph. neerl.-scand. **1**, 306–328 (1957b).

Brodal, A. Pompeiano, O., Walberg, F.: The Vestibular Nuclei and Their Connections: Anatomy and Functional Correlations. London: Oliver and Boyd 1962.

Brodal, A., Torvik, A.: Über den Ursprung der sekundären vestibulocerebellaren Fasern bei der Katze. Eine experimentell anatomische Studie. Arch. Psychiat. Neurol. **195**, 550–567 (1957).

Brookhart, J. M.: The Cerebellum. Handbook of Physiology, Sect. I, Neurophysiology, II, Washington, D. C., American Physiological Society, 1960.

Brooks, C. M., Eccles, J. C.: Electrical investigation of the monosynaptic pathway through the spinal cord. J. Neurophysiol. **10**, 251–273 (1947).

Bruggencate, ten G., Sonnhof, U., Teichmann, R., Weller, E.: A study of the synaptic input to Deiters' neurones evoked by stimulation of peripheral nerves and spinal cord. Brain Res. **25**, 207–211 (1971).

Buchanan, A. R.: The course of the secondary vestibular fibres in the cat. J. comp. Neurol. **67**, 183–204 (1937).

Carli, G., Diete-Spiff, K., Pompeiano, O.: Skeletomotor and fusimotor control of gastrocnemius muscle from Deiters' nucleus. Experientia (Basel) **22**, 583 (1966).

Carli, G., Diete-Spiff, K., Pompeiano, O.: Responses of the muscle spindles and of the extrafusal fibres in an extensor muscle to stimulation of the lateral vestibular nucleus in the cat. Arch. ital. Biol. **105**, 209–242 (1967).

Carpenter, M. B., Alling, F. A., Bard, D. S.: Lesions of the descending vestibular nucleus in the cat. J. comp. Neurol. **114**, 39–49 (1960).

Carpenter, M. B., McMasters, R. E.: Disturbances of conjugate horizontal eye movements in the monkey. II. Physiological effects and anatomical degeneration resulting from lesions of the medial longitudinal fasciculus. Arch. Neurol. (Chic.) **8**, 347–368 (1963).

Carpenter, M. B., McMasters, R. E., Hanna, G. R.: Disturbances of conjugate horizontal eye movements in the monkey. I. Physiological effects and anatomical degeneration resulting from lesions of the abducens nucleus and nerve. Arch. Neurol. (Chic.) **8**, 231–247 (1963).

Clark, D. L., Burns, R. D.: Specific subtotal labyrinthectomy of the superior semicircular canals of the kangaroo rat. J. comp. Neurol. **129**, 285–292 (1967).

Clark, B.: Thresholds for the perception of angular acceleration in man. Aerospace Med. **38**, 443–450 (1967).

Cohen, B., Suzuki, J. I., Shanzer, S.: Semicircular canal control of eye movements. In: The Oculomotor System. Ed. by M. B. Bender. New York: Hoeber 1964. pp. 163.

Cohen, M. J.: The function of receptors in the statocyst of the lobster Homarus americanus. J. Physiol. (Lond.) **130**, 9–34 (1955).

COLLINS, W.E., GUEDRY, F.E.: Arousal effects and nystagmus during prolonged constant angular acceleration. Acta oto-laryng. (Stockh.) **54**, 349–362 (1962).

COOPER, S., ECCLES, J.C.: The isometric responses of mammalian muscles. J. Physiol. (Lond.) **69**, 377–385 (1930).

CRAMER, R.L.: Response of mammalian gravity receptors to sustained tilt. Aerospace Med. **33**, 663–666 (1962).

CRAMPTON, G.H.: Does linear acceleration modify cupular deflection? In: Second Symposium on The Role of the Vestibular Organs in Space Exploration. Washington: NASA 1966.

CRANMER, R.: Nystagmus related to lesions of the central vestibular apparatus and the cerebellum. Ann. Otol. (St. Louis) **60**, 186–196 (1951).

DECHER, D.: Neues zur Labyrinthphysiologie. Die Drehreiz-Schwellen der verticalen Bogengänge. Arch. Ohr.-, Nas.-, u. Kehlk.-Heilk. **181**, 395–407 (1963).

DIETE-SPIFF, K., CARLI, G., POMPEIANO, O.: Comparison of the effects of stimulation of the VIIIth cranial nerve, the vestibular nuclei or the reticular formation on the gastrocnemius muscle and its spindles. Arch. ital. Biol. **105**, 243–272 (1967).

DOHLMAN, G.: Physikalische und physiologische Studien zur Theorie des kalorischen Nystagmus. Acta oto-laryng. (Stockh.) Suppl.**5**, (1925).

DOHLMAN, G.: Experimentelle Untersuchungen über die galvanische Vestibularisreaktion. Acta oto-laryng. (Stockh.) Suppl. **8**, 1–48 (1929).

DOW, R.S., MORUZZI, G.: The Physiology and Pathology of the Cerebellum. Minneapolis: The University of Minnesota Press 1958.

DUENSING, F., SCHAEFER, K.P.: Die Neuronenaktivität in der formatio reticularis des Rhombencephalons beim vestibulären Nystagmus. Arch. Psychiat. Nervenkr. **196**, 265–290 (1957a).

DUENSING, F., SCHAEFER, K.P.: Die "locker-gekoppelten" Neurone der Formatio reticularis des Rhombencephalons beim vestibulären Nystagmus. Arch. Psychiat. Nervenkr. **196**, 402–420 (1957b).

DUENSING, F., SCHAEFER, K.P.: Die Aktivität einzelner Neurone im Bereich der Vestibulariskerne bei Horizontalbeschleunigungen unter besonderer Berücksichtigung des vestibulären Nystagmus. Arch. Psychiat. Nervenkr. **198**, 225–252 (1958).

DUENSING, F., SCHAEFER, K.P.: Über die Konvergenz verschiedener labyrinthärer Afferenzen auf einzelne Neurone des Vestibulariskerngebietes. Arch. Psychiat. **199**, 345–371 (1959).

DUENSING, F., SCHAEFER, K.P., TREVISAN, C.: Die Raddrehung vermittelnde Neurone in der zentralen Funktionsstruktur der Labyrinthstellreflexe auf Kopf und Augen. Arch. Psychiat. Nervenkr. **204**, 113–132 (1963).

DUENSING, F.: Die Aktivität der von den vertikalen Bogengängen abhängigen Neurone im Hirnstamm des Kaninchens. I. Mitteilung. Drehbeschleunigungen in Seitenlage. Arch. klin. exp. Ohr.- Nas.-, u. Kehlk.-Heilk. **192**, 32–50 (1968a).

DUENSING, F.: Die Aktivität der von den vertikalen Bogengängen abhängigen Neurone im Hirnstamm des Kaninchens. II. Mitteilung. Drehbeschleunigungen in verschiedenen Positionen. Arch. klin. exp. Ohr.-, Nas.-, u. Kehlk.-Heilk. **192**, 51–62 (1968b).

ECCLES, J.C., FATT, P., KOKETSU, K.: Cholinergic and inhibitory synapses in a pathway from motor axon collaterals to motoneurones. J. Physiol. (Lond.) **126**, 524–562 (1954).

ECCLES, J.C., ITO, M., SZENTÁGOTHAI, J.: The Cerebellum as a Neuronal Machine. Berlin-Heidelberg-New York: Springer 1967.

ECKEL, W.: Elektrophysiologische und histologische Untersuchungen im Vestibulariskerngebiet bei Drehreizen. Arch. Ohr.-, Nas.-, u. Kehlkopf. Heilk. **164**, 487–513 (1954).

EHRHARDT, K.J., WAGNER, A.: Labyrinthine and neck reflexes recorded from spinal single motoneurones in the cat. Brain Res. **19**, 87–104 (1970).

EK, J., JONGKEES, L.B.W., KLIJN, A.J.: The threshold of the vestibular organ. Acta oto-laryng. (Stockh.) **50**, 292–300 (1959).

ERULKAR, S.D., SPRAGUE, D.M., WHITSEL, B.L., DOGAN, S., JANNETTA, P.J.: Organization of the vestibular projection to the spinal cord of the cat. J. Neurophysiol. **29**, 626–664 (1966).

EWALD, J.R.: Physiologische Untersuchungen über das Endorgan des N. Oktavus. Wiesbaden: Bergmann 1892.

FELDMAN, S., WAGMAN, J.H., BENDER, M.B.: Anterior brainstem and sciatic nerve connections to vestibular nuclei in cat. J. Neurophysiol. **24**, 350–362 (1961).

FERNÁNDEZ, C., FREDRICKSON, J.M.: Experimental cerebellar lesions and their effect on vestibular function. Acta oto-laryng. (Stockh.) Suppl. **192**, 52–62 (1963).

FERNÁNDEZ, C., GOLDBERG, J.M.: Physiology of peripheral neurons innervating semicircular canals of the squirrel monkey. II. Response to sinusoidal stimulation and dynamics of peripheral vestibular system. J. Neurophysiol. **34**, 661–675 (1971).

FERRARO, A., PACELLA, B.L., BARRERA, S.E.: Effects of the lesions of the medial vestibular nucleus. An anatomical and physiological study in macacus rhesus monkeys. J. comp. Neurol. **73**, 7–36 (1940).

FLUUR, E.: Influences of semicircular ducts on extraocular muscles. Acta oto-laryng. (Stockh.) Suppl. **149**, 1–46 (1959).

FLUUR, E.: Vestibular compensation after labyrinthine destruction. Acta oto-laryng. (Stockh.) **52**, 367–375 (1960).

FREDRICKSON, J.M., SCHWARZ, D., KORNHUBER, H.H.: Convergence and interaction of vestibular and deep somatic afferents upon neurons in the vestibular nuclei of the cat. Acta oto-laryng. (Stockh.) **61**, 168–188 (1966).

FUCHS, A.F., LUSCHEI, E.S.: Firing patterns of abducens neurons of alert monkeys in relationship to horizontal eye movement. J. Neurophysiol. **33**, 382–392 (1970).

FUJITA, Y., ROSENBERG, J., SEGUNDO, J.P.: Activity of cells in the lateral vestibular nucleus as a function of head position. J. Physiol. (Lond.) **196**, 1—18 (1968).

FUKUDA, J., HIGHSTEIN, S.M., ITO, M.: Cerebellar inhibitory control of the vestibulo-ocular reflex in rabbit IIIrd nucleus. Exp. Brain Res. **14**, 511—526 (1972).

FULTON, J.F., LIDDEL, E.G.T., RIOCH, D.McK.: The influence of unilateral destruction of vestibular nuclei upon posture and the knee-jerk. J. Physiol. (Lond.) **70**, XXII (1930).

GACEK, R.R.: Efferent component of the vestibular nerve. In: Neural Mechanism of the Auditory and Vestibular Systems. Springfield, Ill.: C. C. Thomas 1960.

GACEK, R.R.: The course and central termination of first order neurons supplying vestibular endorgans in the cat. Acta oto-laryng. (Stockh.) **254**, 1–66 (1969).

GACEK, R.R.: Anatomical demonstration of the vestibulo-ocular projections in the cat. Acta otolaryng. (Stockh.) Suppl. **293**, 1—63 (1971).

GERNANDT, B.E.: Response of mammalian vestibular neurons to horizontal rotation and caloric stimulation. J. Neurophysiol. **12**, 173–184 (1949).

GERNANDT, B.E.: The effect of the centrifugal force upon the nerve discharge from the horizontal canal. Acta physiol. scand. **21**, 61–72 (1950a).

GERNANDT, B.E.: Midbrain activity in response to vestibular stimulation. Acta physiol. scand. **21**, 73–81 (1950b).

GERNANDT, B.E.: Generation of labyrinthine impulses, descending vestibular pathway, and modulation of vestibular activity by proprioceptive, cerebellar, and reticular influences. In: Neural Mechanisms of the Auditory and Vestibular Systems. Springfield, Ill.: Thomas 1960.

GERNANDT, B.E.: Discharges from utricular receptors in the cat. Exp. Neurol. **26**, 203–219 (1970).

GERNANDT, B.E., IGARASHI, M., ADES, H.W.: Effects of prolonged caloric stimulation upon oculomotor, vestibulo-spinal and segmental spinal activity. Exp. Neurol. **14**, 249–263 (1966).

GERNANDT, B.E., IRANYI, M., LIVINGSTON, R.B.: Vestibular influences on spinal mechanisms. Exp. Neurol. **1**, 248–273 (1959).

GERNANDT, B.E., THULIN, C.A.: Vestibular connections of the brainstem. Amer. J. Physiol. **171**, 121–127 (1952).

GERNANDT, B.E., THULIN, C.A.: Vestibular mechanisms of facilitation and inhibition of cord reflexes. Amer. J. Physiol. **172**, 653–660 (1953).

GOLDBERG, J.M., FERNÁNDEZ, C.: Physiology of peripheral neurons innervating semicircular canals of the squirrel monkey. Resting discharge and response to constant angular accelerations. J. Neurophysiol. **34**, 635–660 (1971).

GOLTZ, F.: Über die physiologische Bedeutung der Bogengänge des Ohrlabyrinthes. Pflügers Arch. ges. Physiol. **3**, 172–192 (1870).

GRANIT, R., POMPEIANO, O., WALTMAN, B.: Fast supraspinal control of mammalian muscle spindles: extra- and intrafusal coactivation. J. Physiol. (Lond.) **147**, 385–398 (1959).

GRANT, G., ASCHAN, G., EKVALL, L.: Nystagmus produced by localized cerebellar lesions. Acta oto-laryng. (Stockh.) **58**, Suppl. 192, 78–84 (1964).

GRAY, L.P.: Some experimental evidence on the connections of the vestibular mechanism in the cat. J. comp. Neurol. **41**, 319–364 (1926).

GRILLNER, S., HONGO, T., LUND, S.: Descending pathways with monosynaptic action on motoneurones. Acta physiol. scand. **68**, Suppl. 277, 60 (1966).

GRILLNER, S., HONGO, T., LUND, S.: The vestibulospinal tract. Effects on alpha-motoneurons in the lumbosacral spinal cord in the cat. Exp. Brain Res. **10**, 94–120 (1970).

GROEN, J.J., JONGKEES, L.B.W.: The threshold of angular acceleration perception. J. Physiol. (Lond.) **107**, 1–7 (1948).

GROEN, J.J., LOWENSTEIN, O., VENDRIK, A.J.H.: The mechanical analysis of the responses from the end organs of the horizontal semicircular canal in the isolated elasmobranch labyrinth. J. Physiol. (Lond.) **117**, 329–346 (1952).

GUALTIEROTTI, T., ALLTUCKER, D.S.: Prolonged recording from single vestibular units in the frog during plane and space flight, its significance and techniques. Aerospace Med. **38**, 513–517 (1967).

HALLPIKE, C.S., HOOD, J.D.: The speed of the slow component of ocular nystagmus induced by angular acceleration of the head: its experimental determination and application to the physical theory of the cupular mechanism. Proc. roy. Soc. B **141**, 216–230 (1953a).

HALLPIKE, C.S., HOOD, J.D.: Fatigue and adaptation of the cupular mechanism of the human horizontal semicircular canal: an experimental investigation. Proc. roy. Soc. B **141**, 542–567 (1953b).

HALLPIKE, C.S., HOOD, J.D., BYFORD, G.H.: The design, construction and performance of a new type revolving chair. Acta oto-laryng. (Stockh.) **42**, 511–538 (1952).

HALSTEAD, W.: The effects of cerebellar lesions upon the habituation of postrotational nystagmus. Comp. Psychol. Monogr. **12**, 1 (1935).

HASSLER, R.: Forels Haubenfaszikel als vestibuläre Empfindungsbahn mit Bemerkungen über einige andere sekundäre Bahnen des Vestibularis and Trigeminus. Arch. Psychiat. Nervenkr. **180**, 23–53 (1948).

HASSLER, R., HESS, W.R.: Experimentelle und anatomische Befunde über die Drehbewegungen und ihre nervösen Apparate. Arch. Psychiat. Nervenkr. **192**, 488–526 (1954).

HENRIKSSON, N.G., SCHMIDT, R.S., FERNÁNDEZ, C.: Crossed vestibular connections in the frog. Acta oto-laryng. (Stockh.) **54**, 292–302 (1962).

HERRICK, C.J.: Origin and evolution of the cerebellum. Arch. Neurol. Psychiat. (Chic.) **11**, 621–652 (1924).

HIEBERT, T.G., FERNÁNDEZ, C.: Deitersian response to tilt. Acta oto-laryng. (Stockh.) **60**, 180–190 (1965).

HIGHSTEIN, S.M., ITO, M., TSUCHIYA, T.: Synaptic linkage in the vestibulo-ocular reflex pathway of rabbit. Exp. Brain Res. **13**, 306–326 (1971).

HILDING, A.C.: Studies on otic labyrinth. III. On the threshold of minimal perceptible angular acceleration. Ann. Otol. (St. Louis) **62**, 5–14 (1953).

HOEVE, J. VAN DER, DE KLEYN, A.: Tonische Labyrinthreflexe auf die Augen. Pflügers Arch. ges. Physiol. **169**, 241–262 (1917).

HOLST, E. VON: Die Tätigkeit des Statolithenapparates im Wirbeltierlabyrinth. Naturwissenschaften **37**, 265–272 (1950).

HOLST, E. VON, GRISEBACH, E.: Einfluß des Bogengangsystems auf die „subjektive Lotrechte" beim Menschen. Naturwissenschaften **38**, 67–68 (1951).

HOLST, E. VON, KAISER, H., SCHOEN, L., ROEBIG, G., GÖLDNER, G.: Die Arbeitsweise des Statolithenapparates bei Fischen. Z. vergl. Physiol. **32**, 60–120 (1950).

HORCHOLLE, G., TYČ-DUMONT, S.: Activités unitaires des neurones vestibulaires et oculomoteurs au cours du nystagmus. Exp. Brain Res. **5**, 16–31 (1968).

HORSTMANN, E.: Über kernspezifische Synapsenformen im Mittelhirn von Knochenfischen. Z. Zellforsch. **40**, 139–150 (1954).

HULK, J., JONGKEES, L. B. W.: The turning test with small regulable stimuli. II. The normal cupulogram. J. Laryng. **62**, 70–75 (1948).

HYDE, J. E., EASON, R. G.: Characteristics of ocular movements evoked by stimulation of brain-stem of cat. J. Neurophysiol. **22**, 666–678 (1959).

HYDE, J. E., ELIASSON, S. G.: Brainstem induced eye movements in cats. J. comp. Neurol. **108**, 139–172 (1957).

HYDE, J. E., TOCZEK, S.: Functional relation of interstitial nucleus to rotatory movements evoked from zona incerta stimulation. J. Neurophysiol. **25**, 455–466 (1962).

ITO, M., KAWAI, N., UDO, M.: The origin of cerebellar induced inhibition and facilitation in the neurones of Deiters' and intracerebellar nuclei. XXIII Intern. Congr. Physiol. Sci. Abstr. 997. Tokyo 1965.

ITO, M., NISIMARU, N., YAMAMOTO, M.: Specific neural connections for the cerebellar control of vestibulo-ocular reflexes. Brain Res. **60**, 238—243 (1973).

ITO, M., KAWAI, N., UDO, M., MANO, N.: Axon reflex activation of Deiters neurones from the cerebellar cortex through collaterals of the cerebellar afferents. Exp. Brain Res. **8**, 249–268 (1969a).

ITO, M., HONGO, T., OKADA, Y.: Vestibular-evoked postsynaptic potentials in Deiters' neurones. Exp. Brain Res. **7**, 214—230 (1969b).

ITO, M., HONGO, T., OKADA, Y., SATO, N.: Cerebellar-evoked disinhibition in dorsal Deiters' neurones. Exp. Brain Res. **6**, 247–264 (1968).

ITO, M., HONGO, T., YOSHIDA, M., OKADA, Y., OBATA, K.: Antidromic and trans-synaptic activation of Deiters' neurones induced from the spinal cord. Jap. J. Physiol. **14**, 638–658 (1964a).

ITO, M., YOSHIDA, M.: The cerebellar-evoked monosynaptic inhibition of Deiters' neurones. Experientia (Basel) **20**, 515–516 (1964).

ITO, M., YOSHIDA, M., OBATA, K.: Monosynaptic inhibition of the intra-cerebellar nuclei induced from the cerebellar cortex. Experientia (Basel) **20**, 575–576 (1964b).

JACKSON, M. M., SEARS, C. W.: Effect of weightlessness upon the normal nystagmic reaction. Aerospace Med. **37**, 719–721 (1966).

JANSEN, J., BRODAL, A.: Aspects of Cerebellar Anatomy. Oslo: Johan Grundt Tanum 1954.

JANSEN, J., BRODAL, A.: Das Kleinhirn. In: v. Möllendorffs Handbuch der mikroskopischen Anatomie des Menschen IV/8. Berlin-Göttingen-Heidelberg: Springer 1958.

KASAHARA, M., UCHINO, Y.: Selective mode of commissural inhibition induced by semicircular canal afferents on secondary vestibular neurons in the cat. Brain Res. **34**, 366—369 (1971).

KASAHARA, M., MANO, M., OSHIMA, T., OZAWA, S., SHIMAZU, H.: Contralateral short latency inhibition of central vestibular neurones in the horizontal canal system. Brain Res. **8**, 376–378 (1968).

KAWAI, N., ITO, M., NOZUE, M.: Postsynaptic influences on the vestibular non-Deiters' nuclei from primary vestibular nerve. Exp. Brain Res. **8**, 190–200 (1969).

KIDOKORO, Y.: Cerebellar and vestibular control of fish oculomotor neurones. In: Neurobiology of Cerebellar Evolution and Development. Ed. by R. LLINÁS, Chicago: Amer Med. Assn. Educ. and Res. Fdn. 1969.

KLEYN, A. DE: Tonische Labyrinth- und Halsreflexe auf die Augen. Pflügers Arch. ges. Physiol. **186**, 82–97 (1921).

KLEYN, A. DE, MAGNUS, R.: Tonische Labyrinthreflexe auf die Augenmuskeln. Pflügers Arch. ges. Physiol. **178**, 179–192 (1920).

KOELLA, W.: Die Beeinflussbarkeit des postrotatorischen Augennystagmus durch propriozeptive Halsreflexe beim Kaninchen. Helv. physiol. Acta **5**, 430–440 (1947).

KOELLA, W.: Gleichgewichtsorgan und Augenmuskelsystem im Lichte der Koordinationslehre. Vjschr. naturforsch. Ges. Beiheft, **95**, (1950).

KOELLA, W.: Bogengangsfunktion und Weber-Fechnersches Gesetz. Z. Biol. **104**, 285–288 (1951).

Koella, W., Kesselring, R., Kälin, R.: Quantitative Beziehungen zwischen Vestibularisreiz und Augennystagmus beim Kaninchen. Helv. physiol. pharmacol. Acta **9**, 389–405 (1951).

Koella, W.P., Nakao, H., Evans, R.L., Wada, J.: Interaction of vestibular and proprioceptive reflexes in the decerebrate cat. Amer. J. Physiol. **185**, 607–613 (1956).

Kornhuber, H.H., DaFonseca, J.S.: Optovestibular integration in the cat's cortex: A study of sensory convergence on cortical neurons. In: The Oculomotor System. Ed. by M.B. Bender. New York: Hoeber 1964.

Kumoi, T., Hosomi, H., Matsumura, H.: An analysis of the vestibular evoked potentials in response to stimulation of the ampullar nerve. Kobe J. med. Sci. **9**, 79–88 (1963).

Kumoi, T., Hosomi, H., Matsumura, H., Amatsu, M., Asai, R.: An analysis of the vestibular evoked potentials in response to stimulation of the vestibular nerve branches. In: International Symposium on Vestibular and Oculomotor Problems. Tokyo: Auspices of University of Tokyo 1965.

Lachmann, J., Bergman, F., Monnier, M.: Central nystagmus elicited by stimulation of the meso-diencephalon in rabbit. Amer. J. Physiol. **193**, 328–334 (1958b).

Lachmann, J., Bergman, F., Weinmann, J., Welner, A.: Central nystagmus. II. Relationship between central and labyrinthine nystagmus. Amer. J. Physiol. **195**, 267–270 (1958a).

Ladpli, R., Brodal, A.: Experimental studies of commissural and reticular formation projections from the vestibular nuclei in the cat. Brain Res. **8**, 65–96 (1968).

Larsell, O.: The cerebellum of the frog. J. comp. Neurol. **36**, 89–112 (1923).

Larsell, O.: The comparative morphology of the membraneous labyrinth and the lateral line organs in their relation to the development of the cerebellum. In: The Cerebellum. Baltimore: William and Wilkins 1929.

Ledoux, A.: Activité électrique des nerfs des canaux semicirculaires du saccule et de l'utricle chez la grenouille. Acta oto-rhino-laryng. belg. **3**, 335–349 (1949).

Ledoux, A.: Les canaux semi-circulaires. Etude électro-physiologique. Contribution a l'effort d'uniformisation des épreuvés vestibulaires. Essai d'interprétation de la semiologie vestibulaire. Acta oto-rhino-laryng. belg. **12**, 109–348 (1958).

Ledoux, A.: L'adaptation du systéme vestibulaire périphérique. Acta oto-laryng. (Stockh.) **53**, 307–316 (1961).

Leidler, R.: Experimentelle Untersuchungen über das Endigungsgebiet des Nervus vestibularis. Z. Mitteilung. Arb. a. d. Neur. Inst. Wien Univ. **21**, 151–212 (1916).

Llinás, R., Precht, W., Bracchi, F., Huertas, J.: The inhibitory cerebello-vestibular system in the frog. Proc. Internat. Union Physiol. Sci. **7**, Abst. 806, 269, 1968.

Llinás, R., Precht, W., Clarke, M.: Cerebellar Purkinje cell responses to physiological stimulation of the vestibular system in the frog. Exp. Brain Res. **13**, 408–431 (1971).

Llinás, R., Precht, W., Kitai, S.T.: Climbing fibre activation of Purkinje cell following primary vestibular afferent stimulation in the frog. Brain Res. **6**, 371–375 (1967).

Lorente de Nó, R.: Etudes sur le cerveau postérieur. III. Sur les connexions extracérébelleuses des fascicules afférents au cerveau, et sur la fonction de cet organe. Trav. Lab. Rech. Biol. **22**, 51–65 (1924).

Lorente de Nó, R.: Die Labyrinthreflexe auf die Augenmuskeln nach einseitiger Labyrinthexstirpation nebst einer kurzen Angabe über den Nervenmechanismus der vestibulären Augenbewegungen. Berlin-Wien: Urban and Schwarzenberg 1928.

Lorente de Nó, R.: Ausgewählte Kapitel aus der vergleichenden Physiologie des Labyrinths. Die Augenmuskelreflexe beim Kaninchen und ihre Grundlagen. Ergebn. Physiol. **32**, 71–242 (1931).

Lorente de Nó, R.: The regulation of eye positions and movements induced by the labyrinth. Laryngoscope (St. Louis) **42**, 233–332 (1932).

Lorente de Nó, R.: Anatomy of the eighth nerve. The central projection of the nerve endings of the internal ear. Laryngoscope (St. Louis) **43**, 1–38 (1933a).

Lorente de Nó, R.: Vestibulo-ocular reflex arc. Arch. Neurol. Psychiat. (Chic.) **30**, 245–291 (1933b).

Lorente de Nó, R.: Analysis of the activity of the chains of internuncial neurons. J. Neurophysiol. **1**, 207–244 (1938).

LOWENSTEIN, O.: The effect of galvanic polarization on the impulse discharge from sense endings in the isolated labyrinth of the Thornback ray (Raja clavata). J. Physiol. (Lond.) **127**, 104–117 (1955).

LOWENSTEIN, O.: Peripheral mechanisms of equilibrium. Brit. med. Bull. **12**, 114–118 (1956).

LOWENSTEIN, O., ROBERTS, T.D.M.: The equilibrium function of the otolith organs of the Thornback ray. J. Physiol. (Lond.) **110**, 392–415 (1949).

LOWENSTEIN, O., ROBERTS, T.D.M.: The localization and analysis of the responses to vibration from the isolated elasmobranch labyrinth. A contribution to the problem of the evolution of hearing in vertebrates. J. Physiol. (Lond.) **114**, 471–489 (1951).

LOWENSTEIN, O., SAND, A.: The activity of the horizontal semicircular canals of the dog fish, Scyllium canicula. J. exp. Biol. **13**, 416–428 (1936).

LOWENSTEIN, O., SAND, A.: The individual and integrated activity of the semicircular canals of the elasmobranch labyrinth. J. Physiol. (Lond.) **99**, 89–101 (1940a).

LOWENSTEIN, O., SAND, A.: The mechanism of the semicircular canal. A study of the responses of single-fibre preparations to angular accelerations and rotation at constant speed. Proc. roy. Soc. Biol. **129**, 256–275 (1940b).

LUND, S., POMPEIANO, O.: Descending pathways with monosynaptic action on motoneurones. Experientia (Basel) **21**, 602–603 (1965).

MACH, E.: Physikalische Versuche über den Gleichgewichtssinn des Menschen. Wien. Akad. Sitzungsberichte III **68**, 124–143 (1873).

MAEDA, M., SHIMAZU, H., SHINODA, Y.: Inhibitory postsynaptic potentials in the abducens motoneurons associated with the quick relaxation phase of vestibular nystagmus. Brain Res. **26**, 420–424 (1971a).

MAEDA, M., SHIMAZU, H., SHINODA, Y.: Rhythmic activities of secondary vestibular efferent fibers recorded within the abducens nucleus during vestibular nystagmus. Brain Res. **34**, 361—365 (1971b).

MAGNUS, R.: Körperstellung. Berlin: Springer 1924.

MANNI, E.: Localisazzioni cerebellari corticali nella cavia. II. Effeti de lesioni delle parti vestibolari del cerveletto. Arch. Fisiol. **50**, 110–123 (1950).

MANNI, E., AZZENA, G.B., CASEY, H., DOW, R.S.: Influence of the labyrinth on unitary discharge of the oculomotor nucleus and some adjacent formations. Exp. Neurol. **12**, 9–24 (1965).

MANNI, E., DESOLE, C.: Responses of oculomotor units to stimulation of single semicircular canals. Exp. Neurol. **15**, 206–219 (1966).

MANO, M., OSHIMA, T., SHIMAZU, H.: Inhibitory commissural fibres interconnecting the bilateral vestibular nuclei. Brain Res. **8**, 378–382 (1968).

MARKHAM, C.H.: Midbrain and contralateral labyrinth influences on brainstem vestibular neurons in the cat. Brain Res. **9**, 312–333 (1968).

MARKHAM, C.H., CURTHOYS, I.S.: Labyrinthine convergence on cat brain stem vestibular neurons using natural and electrical stimulation. In: Progress in Brain Research, Vol. 37, Basic Aspects of Central Vestibular Mechanisms. Amsterdam: Elsevier 1972.

MARKHAM, C.H., PRECHT, W., SHIMAZU, H.: Effect of stimulation of interstitial nucleus of Cajal on vestibular unit activity in the cat. J. Neurophysiol. **29**, 493–507 (1966).

MELVILL JONES, G., MILSUM, J.H.: Characteristics of neural transmission from the semicircular canal to the vestibular nuclei of cats. J. Physiol. (Lond.) **209**, 295–316 (1970).

MICKLE, W.A., ADES, H.W.: Rostral projection pathway of the vestibular system. Amer. J. Physiol. **176**, 243–252 (1954).

MILOJEVIC, B., VOOTS, R.J.: Simultaneous stimulation of the otolithic organs and semicircular canals. Acta oto-laryng. (Stockh.) **61**, 92–100 (1966).

MONEY, K.E., SCOTT, J.W.: Functions of separate sensory receptors of non-auditory labyrinth of the cat. Amer. J. Physiol. **202/6**, 1211–1220 (1962).

MONTANDON, A., RUSSBACH, A.: Etude de quelques syndromes vestibulaires par l'épreuvé giratoire liminaire. Acta oto-laryng. (Stockh.) **46**, 264–275 (1956).

MORUZZI, G.: Problems in Cerebellar Physiology. Springfield, Ill.: Ch. C. Thomas 1950.

MORUZZI, G.: The physiological properties of the brainstem reticular system. In: Brain Mechanisms and Consciousness. Oxford: Blackwell 1954.

MORUZZI, G., POMPEIANO, O.: Inhibitory mechanisms underlying the collapse of decerebrate rigidity after unilateral fastigial lesions. J. comp. Neurol. **107**, 1–26 (1957).

MOWRER, O.H.: The electrical response of the vestibular nerve during adequate stimulation. Science **81**, 180–181 (1935).

MUGNAINI, E., WALBERG, F.: An experimental electron microscopical study on the mode of termination of cerebellar cortico-vestibular fibres in the cat lateral vestibular nucleus (Deiters' nucleus). Exp. Brain Res. **4**, 212–236 (1967).

MCMASTERS, R.E., WEISS, A.H., CARPENTER, M.B.: Vestibular projections to the nuclei of the extra-ocular muscles. Degeneration resulting from discrete partial lesions of the vestibular nuclei in the monkey. Amer. J. Anat. **118**, 163–194 (1966).

MCNALLY, W.J., TAIT, J.: The function of the utricular macula of the frog. Acta oto-laryng. (Stockh.) **20**, 73–76 (1934).

NIVEN, J.I., HIXON, W.C.: Frequency response of the human semicircular canals. I. Steady state ocular nystagmus response to high level, sinusoidal angular acceleration. USNSAM and NASA Joint Report No. 58, Pensacola, Florida, (1961).

NYBERG-HANSEN, R.: Origin and termination of fibers from the vestibular nuclei descending in the medial longitudinal fasciculus. An experimental study with silver impregnation methods in the cat. J. comp. Neurol. **122**, 355–367 (1964).

OBATA, K., ITO, M., OCHI, R., SATO, N.: Pharmacological properties of the postsynaptic inhibition by Purkinje cell axons and the action of γ-aminobutyric acid on Deiters' neurones. Exp. Brain Res. **4**, 43–57 (1967).

OBATA, K., TAKEDA, K., SHINOZAKI, H.: Further study on pharmacological properties of the cerebellar-induced inhibition of Deiters' neurones. Exp. Brain Res. **11**, 327–342 (1970).

OWADA, K., OKUBO, K.: The otolithic reaction on nystagmus by caloric stimulations. Acta oto-laryng. (Stockh.) Suppl. **179**, (1963).

PAPEZ, J.W.: Reticulospinal tracts in the cat. Marchi method. J. comp. Neurol. **41**, 365–399 (1926).

PETERSON, B.W.: Effect of tilting on the activity of neurons in the vestibular nuclei of the cat. Brain Res. **6**, 606–609 (1967).

PETERSON, B.W.: Distribution of neural responses to tilting within vestibular nuclei of the cat. J. Neurophysiol. **33**, 750–767 (1970).

PFALTZ, C.R., RICHTER, H.R.: Photoelektrische Nystagmusregistrierung. Pract. oto-rhino-laryng. (Basel) **18**, 263–271 (1956).

POMPEIANO, O.: Responses to electrical stimulation of the intermediate part of the cerebellar anterior lobe in the decerebrate cat. Arch. ital. Biol. **96**, 330–360 (1958).

POMPEIANO, O., BRODAL, A.: Spino-vestibular fibres in the cat. An experimental study. J. comp. Neurol. **108**, 353–382 (1957a).

POMPEIANO, O., BRODAL, A.: The origin of vestibulospinal fibres in the cat. Arch. ital. Biol. **95**, 166–195 (1957b).

POMPEIANO, O., COTTI, G.: Analisi microelettrodica delle proiezioni cerebello-deitersiane. Arch. Sci. biol. (Bologna) **43**, 57–101 (1959).

POMPEIANO, O., Morrison, A.R.: Vestibular influences during sleep. I. Abolition of the rapid eye movements of desynchronized sleep following vestibular lesions. Arch. ital. Biol. **103**, 569–595 (1965).

POMPEIANO, O., WALBERG, F.: Descending connections to the vestibular nuclei. An experimental study in the cat. J. comp. Neurol. **108**, 465–503 (1957).

POTTHOF, P.C., RICHTER, H.P., BURANDT, H.R.: Multisensorische Konvergenzen an Hirnstammneuronen der Katze. Arch. Psychiat. Nervenkr. **210**, 36–60 (1967).

PRECHT, W.: Vestibular and cerebellar control of oculomotor functions. Bibl. ophthal. (Basel), **82**, 71 88 (1972).

PRECHT, W., BAKER, R.: Synaptic organization of the vestibulo-trochlear pathway. Exp. Brain Res. **14**, 158—184 (1972).

PRECHT, W., BAKER, R., LLINÁS, R.: Cerebellar control of ipsilateral vestibular inhibition of trochlear motoneurons. Proc. Internat. Union Physiol. Sci., Vol. 9, 1971b.

PRECHT, W., BAKER, R., OKADA, Y.: Evidence for GABA as the synaptic transmitter of the inhibitory vestibulo-ocular pathway. Exp. Brain Res. **18**, 415—428 (1973b).

PRECHT, W., GRIPPO, J., RICHTER, A.: Effect of horizontal angular acceleration on neurons in the abducens nucleus. Brain Res. **5**, 527–531 (1967b).

PRECHT, W., GRIPPO, J., WAGNER, A.: Untersuchungen zur Organisation des vestibulospinalen Systems. Pflügers Arch. ges. Physiol. **291**, 6 (1966b).

PRECHT, W., GRIPPO, J., WAGNER, A.: Contribution of different types of central vestibular neurons to the vestibulospinal system. Brain Res. **4**, 119–123 (1967a).

PRECHT, W., KITAI, S.T., LLINÁS, R.: Vestibular input to the cerebellum. In: The Cerebellum in Health and Disease. W.H. GREEN, Inc., St. Louis (1970).

PRECHT, W., LLINÁS, R.: Functional organization of the direct vestibular nerve projection to the flocculus and nodulus in the cat cerebellum. Federation Proc., 1968a.

PRECHT, W., LLINÁS, R.: Direct vestibular afferents to cat cerebellar nuclei. Proc. Internat. Union Physiol. Sci., Vol. VII, Abst. 1063, p. 355 (1968b).

PRECHT, W., LLINÁS, R.: Functional organization of the vestibular afferents to the cerebellar cortex of frog and cat. Exp. Brain Res. **9**, 30–52 (1969a).

PRECHT, W., LLINÁS, R.: Comparative aspects of the vestibular input to the cerebellum. In: Neurobiology of Cerebellar Evolution and Development. Ed. by R. LLINÁS. Chicago: Amer. Med. Assn. Educ. and Res. Fdn., pp. 677–702, 1969b.

PRECHT, W., LLINÁS, R., CLARKE, M.: Physiological responses of frog vestibular fibers to horizontal angular rotation. Exp. Brain Res. **13**, 378–407 (1971a).

PRECHT, W., RICHTER, A., GRIPPO, J.: Responses of neurones in cat's abducens nuclei to horizontal angular acceleration. Pflügers Arch. **309**, 285–309 (1969).

PRECHT, W., SHIMAZU, H.: Functional connections of tonic and kinetic vestibular neurones with primary vestibular afferents. J. Neurophysiol. **28**, 1014–1028 (1965).

PRECHT, W., SHIMAZU, H., MARKHAM, CH.H.: A mechanism of central compensation of vestibular function following hemilabyrinthectomy. J. Neurophysiol. **29**, 996–1010 (1966a).

PRECHT, W., SCHWINDT, P.C., BAKER, R.: Removal of vestibular commissural inhibition by antagonists of GABA and glycine. Brain Res. **62**, 222–226 (1973a).

RAMÓN Y CAJAL, S.: Histologie du Système Nerveux de l'Homme et des vertébrés. Paris: Maloine 1911.

RASMUSSEN, A.T.: Secondary vestibular tracts in the cat. J. comp. Neurol. **54**, 143–172 (1932).

RICHTER, A., PRECHT, W.: Inhibition of abducens motoneurones by vestibular nerve stimulation. Brain Res. **11**, 701–705 (1968).

ROBINSON, D.A.: Oculomotor unit behavior in monkey. J. Neurophysiol. **33**, 393–404 (1970).

ROSS, J.A.: Electrical studies on the frog's labyrinth. J. Physiol. (Lond.) **86**, 117–146 (1936).

ROSSI, G.F., ZANCHETTI, A.: The brainstem reticular formation. Anatomy and physiology. Arch. ital. Biol. **95**, 199–438 (1957).

RUPERT, A., MOUSHEGIAN, G., GALAMBOS, R.: Microelectrode studies of primary vestibular neurons in cat. Exp. Neurol. **5**, 100–109 (1962).

SASAKI, K.: Electrophysiological studies on oculomotor neurons of the cat. Jap. J. Physiol. **13**, 287–302 (1963).

SCHAEFER, K.P.: Die Erregungsmuster einzelner Neurone des Abducens-Kernes beim Kaninchen. Pflügers Arch. ges. Physiol. **284**, 31–52 (1965).

SCHEIBEL, A., MARKHAM, C., KOEGLER, R.: Neural correlates of the vestibular ocular reflex. Neurology **11**, 1055–1065 (1961).

SCHEIBEL, M.E., SCHEIBEL, A.B.: Structural substrates for integrative patterns in the brain reticular core. In: Reticular Formation of the Brain. Boston: Little Brown and Co. 1958.

SCHOEN, L.: Mikroableitungen einzelner zentraler Vestibularisneurone von Knochenfischen bei Statolithenreizen. Z. vergl. Physiol. **39**, 399–417 (1957).

SCHÖNE, H.: Über den Einfluß der Schwerkraft auf die Augenrollung und auf die Wahrnehmung der Lage im Raum. Z. vergl. Physiol. **46**, 57–87 (1962).

SCHWINDT, P.C., RICHTER, A., PRECHT, W.: Short latency utricular and canal input to ipsilateral abducens motoneurons. Brain Res. **60**, 259–262 (1973).

SHANZER, S.: Effect of brainstem lesions on individual semicircular canal responses. XXIII Internat. Congr. Physiol. Sci., Tokyo, No. 984, 1965.

SHANZER, S., BENDER, M.B.: Oculomotor responses on vestibular stimulation of monkeys with lesions of the brainstem. Brain **82**, 669–682 (1959).

SHERRINGTON, C.S.: Decerebrate rigidity and reflex co-ordination of movements. J. Physiol. (Lond.) **22**, 319–332 (1898).

SHERRINGTON, C.S.: The Integrative Action of the Nervous System. New Haven: Yale University Press 1906.

SHIMAZU, H.: Mutual interactions between bilateral vestibular nuclei and their significance in motor regulation. In: Neurophysiological Basis of Normal and Abnormal Motor Activities. New York: Raven Press 1967.

SHIMAZU, H.: Vestibulo-oculomotor relations: dynamic oculomotor reactions. In: Progress in Brain Res. Vol. 37, Basic Aspects of Central Vestibular Mechanisms. Amsterdam: Elsevier 1972.

SHIMAZU, H., PRECHT, W.: Tonic and kinetic responses of cat's vestibular neurons to horizontal angular acceleration. J. Neurophysiol. **28**, 991–1013 (1965).

SHIMAZU, H., PRECHT, W.: Inhibition of central vestibular neurones from the contralateral labyrinth and its mediating pathway. J. Neurophysiol. **29**, 467–492 (1966).

SHIMAZU, H., SMITH, C.M.: Cerebellar and labyrinthine influences on single vestibular neurons identified by natural stimuli. J. Neurophysiol. **34**, 493–508 (1971).

SNIDER, R.S.: Alterations which occur in mossy terminals of the cerebellum following transection of the brachium pontis. J. comp. Neurol. **65**, 417–435 (1936).

SPIEGEL, E.A.: Role of vestibular nuclei in cortical innervation of the eye muscles. Arch. Neurol. Psychiat. (Chic.) **29**, 1084–1097 (1933).

SPIEGEL, E.A., PRICE, J.B.: Origin of the quick component of labyrinthine nystagmus. Arch. Otolaryng. **30**, 576–588 (1939).

SPIEGEL, E.A., SCALA, N.P.: Positional nystagmus in cerebellar lesions. J. Neurophysiol. **5**, 247–260 (1942).

STEINHAUSEN, W.: Über den Nachweis der Bewegung der Cupula in der intakten Bogengangsampulle des Labyrinthes bei der natürlichen rotatorischen und calorischen Reizung. Pflügers Arch. ges. Physiol. **228**, 322–328 (1931).

STEINHAUSEN, W.: Über die Beobachtung der Cupula in den Bogengangsampullen des lebenden Hechts. Pflügers Arch. ges. Physiol. **232**, 500–512 (1933).

STEINHAUSEN, W.: Über die durch die Otolithen ausgelösten Kräfte. Pflügers Arch. ges. Physiol. **235**, 538–544 (1935).

STEIN, B.M., CARPENTER, M.B.: Central projections of portions of the vestibular ganglia innervating specific parts of the labyrinth in the rhesus monkey. Amer. J. Anat. **120**, 281–318 (1967).

SUZUKI, J.I., COHEN, B.: Integration of semicircular canal activity. J. Neurophysiol. **29**, 981–995 (1966).

SUZUKI, J.I., TOKUMASU, K., GOTO, K.: Eye movements from single utricular nerve stimulation in the cat. Acta oto-laryng. (Stockh.) **68**, 350–392 (1969).

SZENTÁGOTHAI, J.: Die innere Gliederung des Oculomotorius-Kernes. Arch. Psychiat. **115**, 127–135 (1942).

SZENTÁGOTHAI, J.: Die zentrale Innervation der Augenbewegungen. Arch. Psychiat. **116**, 721–760 (1943).

SZENTÁGOTHAI, J.: The elementary vestibulo-ocular reflex arc. J. Neurophysiol. **13**, 395–407 (1950).

SZENTÁGOTHAI, J.: Die Rolle der einzelnen Labyrinthrezeptoren bei der Orientation von Augen und Kopf im Raume. Budapest: Akadémiai Kiado 1952.

SZENTÁGOTHAI, J.: Pathways and synaptic articulation patterns connecting vestibular receptors and oculomotor nuclei. In: The Oculomotor System. Ed. by M.B. BENDER. New York: Hoeber 1964.

SZENTÁGOTHAI, J., RAJKOVITS, K.: Über den Ursprung der Kletterfasern des Kleinhirns. Z. Anat. Entwickl.-Gesch. **121**, 130–141 (1959).

SZENTÁGOTHAI, J., SCHÁB, R.: A midbrain inhibitory mechanism of the oculomotor activity. Acta physiol. Acad. Sci. hung. **9**, 89–98 (1956).

TARLOV, E.: Organization of vestibulo-oculomotor projections in the cat. Brain Res. **20**, 159–179 (1970).

THULIN, C.A.: Motor effects from stimulation of the vestibular nuclei and the reticular formation. Acta physiol. scand. **28**, Suppl. 103 (1953).

TRINCKER, D.: Bestandspotentiale im Bogengangssystem des Meerschweinchens und ihre Änderung bei experimentellen Cupula Ablenkungen. Pflügers Arch. ges. Physiol. **264**, 351–382 (1957).

TRINCKER, D.: Neuere Untersuchungen zur Elektrophysiologie des Vestibular-Apparates. Naturwissenschaften **10**, 344–350 (1959).

TRINCKER, D.: Kennlinien der Receptoren und primären Neurone des nicht-akustischen Säuger Labyrinthes. Pflügers Arch. ges. Physiol. **281**, 87 (1964).

TRINCKER, D.: Physiologie des Gleichgewichtsorgans. In: Hals-Nasen-Ohren-Heilkunde, Band III, Teil 1. Stuttgart: Georg Thieme 1965.

TUMARKIN, I.A.: Some observations on the function of the labyrinth. Proc. roy. Soc. Med. **30**, 599–610 (1937).

ULRICH, H.: Die Funktion der Otolithen, geprüft durch direkte mechanische Beeinflussung des Utriculusotolithen am lebenden Hecht. Pflügers Arch. ges. Physiol. **235**, 545–553 (1935).

VALENTINUZZI, M.: An analysis of the mechanical forces in each semicircular canal of the cat under single and combined rotations. Bull. Mathem. Biophysics **29**, 267–289 (1967).

VAN EGMOND, A.A.J., GROEN, J.J., JONGKEES, L.B.W.: The mechanics of the semicircular canal. J. Physiol. (Lond.) **110**, 1–17 (1949).

VITO, R.V. DE, BRUSA, A., ARDUINI, A.: Cerebellar and vestibular influences on Deitersian units. J. Neurophysiol. **19**, 241–253 (1956).

VRIES, H.L., DE: The minimum perceptible angular acceleration under various conditions. Acta oto-laryng. (Stockh.) **37**, 218–229 (1949).

WAGNER, A., EHRHARDT, J., PRECHT, W.: Erregende und hemmende Einflüsse des vestibulo-spinalen Systems auf die Motorik. Pflügers Arch. ges. Physiol. **297**, S. R. 13 (1967).

WALBERG, F., BOWSHER, D., BRODAL, A.: The termination of primary vestibular fibres in the vestibular nuclei in the cat. An experimental study with silver methods. J. comp. Neurol. **110**, 391–419 (1958).

WALBERG, F., JANSEN, J.: Cerebellar cortico-vestibular fibres in the cat. Exp. Neurol. **3**, 32–52 (1961).

WARWICK, R.: Representation of the extraocular muscles in the oculo-motor nuclei of the monkey. J. comp. Neurol. **98**, 449–504 (1953).

WEBER, G., STEINER, F.A.: Labyrinthär erregbare Neurone im Hirnstamm und Kleinhirn der Katze. Helv. physiol. pharmacol. Acta **23**, 61–81 (1965).

WILSON, V.J., FELPEL, L.P.: Specificity of semicircular canal input to neurons in the pigeon vestibular nuclei. J. Neurophysiol. **35**, 253–264 (1972).

WILSON, V.J., KATO, M., PETERSON, B.W.: Convergence of inputs on Deiters neurones. Nature (Lond.) **211**, 1409–1411 (1966a).

WILSON, V.J., KATO, M., THOMAS, R.C., PETERSON, B.W.: Excitation of lateral vestibular neurones by peripheral afferent fibres. J. Neurophysiol. **29**, 508–529 (1966b).

WILSON, V.J., KATO, M., PETERSON, B.W., WYLIE, R.M.: A single-unit analysis of the organization of Deiters' nucleus. J. Neurophysiol. **30**, 603–619 (1967b).

WILSON, V.J., KATO, M., THOMAS, R.C.: Excitation of lateral vestibular neurones. Nature (Lond.) **206**/4979, 96–97 (1965).

WILSON, V.J., WYLIE, R.M., MARCO, L.A.: Projection to the spinal cord from the medial and descending vestibular nuclei of the cat. Nature (Lond.) **215**, 429–430 (1967a).

WILSON, V.J., WYLIE, R.M., MARCO, L.A.: Organization of the medial vestibular nucleus. J. Neurophysiol. **31**, 166–175 (1968b).

WILSON, V.J., WYLIE, R.M., MARCO, L.A.: Synaptic inputs to cells in the medial vestibular nucleus. J. Neurophysiol. **31**, 176–185 (1968a).

WILSON, V.J., YOSHIDA, M.: Vestibulospinal and reticulospinal effects on hindlimb, forelimb and neck alphamotoneurones. Proc. nat. Acad. Sci. (Wash.) **60**, 836–840 (1968).

WILSON, V.J., YOSHIDA, M.: Comparison of effects of stimulation of Deiters' nucleus and medial longitudinal fasciculus on neck, forelimb, and hindlimb motoneurons. J. Neurophysiol. **32**, 743–758 (1969a).

WILSON, V.J., YOSHIDA, M.: Monosynaptic inhibition of neck motoneurones by the medial vestibular nucleus. Exp. Brain Res. **9**, 365–380 (1969b).

YAMANAKA, Y., BACH-Y RITA, P.: Conduction velocities in the abducens nerve correlated with vestibular nystagmus in cats. Exp. Neurol. **20**, 143–155 (1968).

YULES, R. B., GAULT, F. P.: The relationship of nystagmus to lateral vestibular nucleus stimulation. Exp. Neurol. **15**, 475–483 (1966).

YULES, R. B., KREBS, C.Q., GAULT, F. P.: Physiology of the lateral vestibular nucleus. Exp. Neurol. **16**, 172–180 (1966a).

YULES, R. B., KREBS, C.Q., GAULT, F. P.: Reticular formation control of vestibular system. Exp. Neurol. **16**, 349–358 (1966b).

Chapter III.

Cerebello-Vestibular Interrelations*

By

O. POMPEIANO, Pisa (Italy)

With 15 Figures

Contents

I. Introduction

The basic investigations on cerebello-vestibular relations started with the experiments of MAGNUS (1914) and DE KLEIJN and MAGNUS (1920), who reported that labyrinthine reflexes were constantly present in cerebellectomized animals. The statement by DE KLEIJN and MAGNUS (1920) that the essential pathways mediating the labyrinthine reflexes do not course through the cerebellum was supported by later investigators (DUSSER DE BARENNE, 1923, 1937; RADEMAKER, 1931). This finding, however, did not disprove the hypothesis of a cerebellar control of the brainstem mechanisms underlying the labyrinthine reflexes.

The problem of the functional relations between the vestibular system and the cerebellum will be discussed from the following points of view: i) effects of the vestibular input on the cerebellum; ii) input-output relation of the vestibular volleys at cerebellar level, and finally iii) effects of the cerebellar output on the vestibular nuclei and their related functions.

* The manuscript of this article was sent to the Editor in June 1968. Further contributions to the subject have been summarized in the following book: A. Brodal and O. Pompeiano (Eds.): Progress in Brain Research. Vol. 37. Basic aspects of central vestibular mechanisms. XI, 656 pp. Amsterdam: Elsevier Publ. Co. 1972.

II. Vestibular Influence on the Cerebellum

It is generally assumed that the primary vestibulocerebellar fibers end in the flocculus, nodulus, ventral part of the uvula and the fastigial nucleus; a few probably end in the lingula (cf. Brodal et al., 1962). These primary afferents terminate not only in the ipsilateral (Dow, 1936) but also, to a lesser extent, in the contralateral half of the cortical areas mentioned above (Brodal and Høivik, 1964). This study showed that both the ventral and the dorsal paraflocculus also receive a certain number of primary vestibular fibers. Moreover, no evidence of terminations of primary vestibular fibers in the fastigial nucleus was found, while there were some in the ventral part of the dentate nucleus (Brodal and Høivik, 1964). These observations are of interest because they make it clear that the "vestibulocerebellum", defined on the basis of its vestibular influx, extends considerably beyond the confines of the classic "vestibulocerebellum" of comparative anatomy.

Secondary vestibulocerebellar fibers, *i.e.*, fibers from the vestibular nuclei to the cerebellum, have also been traced to the flocculus, nodulus, uvula and fastigial nucleus, chiefly ipsilaterally (Dow, 1936). The secondary vestibular fibers originate mainly in the ipsilateral descending and medial vestibular nuclei and in the group X of Brodal and Pompeiano (1957) (Brodal and Torvik, 1957; Carpenter et al., 1959a, 1960; Carpenter 1960a, b; Brodal et al., 1962).

The physiological observations on vestibular influences on the cerebellum, although still rather scanty, are on the whole in agreement with the anatomical organization of the relevant connections. The arrival of impulses from the labyrinth at the cerebellar cortex is indicated by changes in its electrical activity. Camis (1919, 1928) reported that in dogs rotation yielded potential changes in the cerebellar nuclei and not in the cerebellar cortex. Changes in the electrical activity of the cerebellum were actually observed when one electrode was placed in the fastigial nucleus and the other in the dentate nucleus after removal of the overlying cortex. Price and Spiegel (1937) recorded the electrocerebellogram by the unipolar method (active electrode above the caudal part of the vermis) and observed an increase in the amplitude and number of the fast oscillations after stimulation of the labyrinth. In unanesthetized decerebrate cats, Dow (1939) studied the cerebellar responses elicited by single shocks applied to the VIII nerve. Evoked potentials occurred only in the flocculonodular lobe, the lingula, the uvula and the fastigial nucleus. The latency in the midline cerebellar structures was of the order of 4.5 msec, but occasionally a response was led from the base of the nodulus after only 0.6 msec. This response can be ascribed to transmission along the myelinated primary vestibular fibers. Cerebellar action potential in the ipsilateral flocculus had a latency of 3 msec. A response was also found in the contralateral flocculus in one experiment, but the latency of this response was not given. The close correspondence between anatomical and physiological projections shows that these potentials were due to stimulation of the labyrinthine component of the VIII nerve. The arrival of labyrinthine volleys in the vestibulocerebellum has also been shown in birds (Gualtierotti and Passerini, 1958, 1959; Gualtierotti et al., 1959) and in amphibia (Chang and Kostyuk, 1960).

In none of these studies is any mention made of the possible projection of vestibular volleys to cerebellar cortical areas other than the flocculonodular lobe.

Following stimulation of the peripheral branches of the VIII nerve, responses were found by ANDERSSON and GERNANDT (1954) in the culmen of the anterior lobe and lobulus simplex. The potentials evoked had latencies of 6 to 8 msec, *i.e.*, slightly longer than those found by Dow (1939). Since no primary or secondary vestibular fibers end in the cerebellar cortex of the culmen and lobulus simplex, the responses recorded by ANDERSSON and GERNANDT (1954) are presumably not transmitted along these pathways. They must be assumed to follow some circuitous route, but more specific indications are not available. More recently, RIVA-SANSEVERINO and URBANO (1965a, b, c), working with "encéphale isolé," unanesthetized cats, found that natural stimulation of the labyrinth effected by rotating the animal around its longitudinal axis produced marked increases in the voltage of the electrical potentials not only of the uvula, nodulus and flocculus, but also of the folium-tuber vermis, lobulus paramedianus, crus II and the paraflocculus. In particular, the paraflocculus (dorsal and ventral) was the structure most responsive to labyrinthine stimulation. These effects were still present in the "encéphale isolé" preparation after transverse section of the brainstem at intercollicular level, but they were abolished after bilateral labyrinthectomy. Other indirect evidence suggests the arrival of labyrinthine volleys to the paraflocculus (INFANTELLINA et al., 1963). Because terminal degenerating endings of primary vestibular fibers have now been anatomically demonstrated in the ventral and dorsal paraflocculus (BRODAL and HØIVIK, 1964), the primary vestibulocerebellar projection might be considered the best candidate for mediator of the parafloccular activation following labyrinthine stimulation. However this corticocerebellar response disappeared after lesion of the pontobulbar reticular formation which did not affect the vestibular system. This finding, together with the observation that labyrinthine stimulation also affects cerebellar cortical areas (such as folium-tuber vermis, lobulus paramedianus and crus II) that do not receive primary or secondary vestibular fibers, lead these authors to conclude that the reticular formation is responsible for the transmission of vestibular volleys to the paraflocculus as well as to the other nonvestibular cerebellar cortical areas so far examined.

It is of interest that while few if any primary vestibular fibers pass into the reticular formation (WALBERG et al., 1958; CARPENTER, 1960b), the second-order vestibular neurons originating in all four main vestibular nuclei largely project to this brainstem structure (BRODAL et al., 1962; MATANO et al., 1964; CARPENTER, 1960a, b; McMASTERS et al., 1966; LADPLI and BRODAL, 1968). It appears, however, that most of these vestibuloreticular fibers reach the reticular nuclei which do not project to the cerebellum. Among the nuclei of the reticular formation projecting onto the cerebellum, the lateral reticular nucleus (nucleus of the lateral funiculus) receive vestibular afferents only from the ipsilateral nucleus of Deiters, while the nucleus reticularis tegmenti pontis receives fibers from the contralateral superior and lateral vestibular nuclei (LADPLI and BRODAL, 1968). Further physiological experiments are required to find out whether the evoked potentials recorded from the nonvestibular cerebellar cortical areas during labyrinthine stimulation are mediated by these precerebellar reticular nuclei or by some circuitous route.

The vestibular volleys affect not only the cerebellar cortex but also the cerebellar nuclei. So far, however, only the fastigial nucleus has been explored (Arduini and Pompeiano, 1956a, b, 1957a, b). In decerebrate cats the effects of stimulation of the labyrinth on the spike discharges of single units of the fastigial nucleus were recorded by means of microelectrodes. Only the rostral part of the fastigial nucleus, which was under the influence of the ipsilateral vermis of the

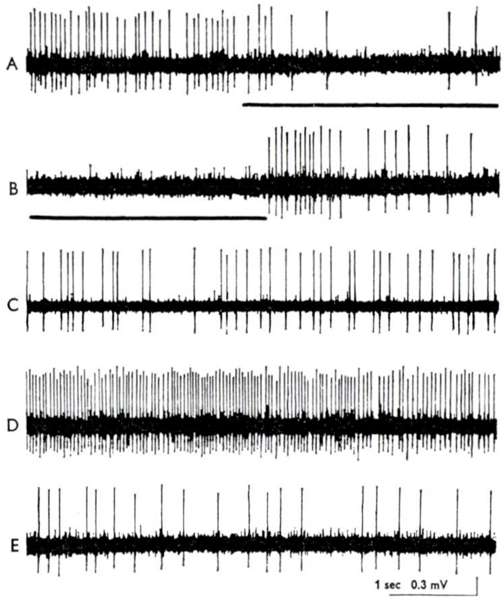

Fig. 1. Effects of stimulation of the cerebellar cortex and labyrinth upon spontaneous spike discharge of unit in the rostromedial portion of the fastigial nucleus. Decerebrate cat. A: the black line indicates d.c. stimulation (0.2 mA) of the ipsilateral hemivermis (lobuli IV and V) of anterior lobe; B: immediately after A. End of stimulation and recovery; C: control; D: cathodal polarization (0.4 mA) of the ipsilateral labyrinth; E: control (Arduini and Pompeiano, 1957b)

anterior lobe, was explored. It was possible to influence fastigial units affected by stimulation of this cortical region by galvanic cathodal stimulation of either labyrinth (Fig. 1). In particular, galvanic (cathodal) polarization of the ipsilateral labyrinth (0.1–0.8 mA) resulted in an increased rate of firing of practically all the units in the rostral part of the fastigial nucleus which were affected by cerebellar polarization. Stimulation of the contralateral labyrinth was ineffective in about one half of the units, while in the other elements there was an increase in the spike discharge. About half the rostrofastigial units unaffected by cerebellar polarization of the vermal cortex of the anterior lobe were driven by stimulation of the ipsilateral labyrinth. This observation suggests that probably not all the fastigial neurons, which are triggered by labyrinthine volleys, are under the control of the cerebellar cortex.

The vestibular impulses entering the rostral portion of the fastigial nucleus may reach this by way of primary and secondary vestibulofastigial fibers or by a route passing through the reticular formation. There is no physiological evidence in support of either of these alternatives, but the anatomical data are entirely compatible with the first one. It is true that the region of the vestibular complex which projects onto the cerebellum, namely the ventrolateral part of the descending nucleus (BRODAL and TORVIK, 1957), does not receive primary vestibular fibers, or only a modest number. This anatomical study, however, does not entirely exclude the possibility that cerebellar fibers arise in other parts of the nuclear complex as well, since negative results with the method of retrograde chromatolysis are not decisive.

It can be concluded from all these studies that vestibular volleys reach the vestibulocerebellum. There are, however, several gaps in our knowledge. In particular, it would be of interest to know: i) whether impulses originating from the vestibular end organs in the cristae and in the maculae contribute to these cerebellar evoked responses; ii) whether there is a selective distribution of afferents from the various receptor regions in the labyrinth to particular subdivisions of the flocculonodular lobe and the fastigial nucleus; iii) whether labyrinthine volleys impinge upon the dentate nucleus; iv) whether the amplitude of the cerebellar responses evoked by labyrinthine volleys coursing along primary and secondary vestibulocerebellar fibers is modified by activation of the vestibuloreticular interconnections, and finally v) where the neural circuits responsible for the arrival of labyrinthine volleys to corticocerebellar regions others than the vestibulocerebellum are located.

III. Input-Output Relation of the Vestibular Volleys at Cerebellar Level

After the demonstration that labyrinthine volleys impinge upon the cerebellum the problem is to find out how these volleys are integrated at corticocerebellar and nucleocerebellar level. The pioneer investigations of CAJAL (1909–1911) have led to refined developments concerning microstructure, geometrical arrangements, and numerical assessment of corticocerebellar neurons (ECCLES et al., 1967). There are only two kinds of afferent fibers conveying information to the cerebellum, the climbing fibers and the mossy fibers, and there is only one type of efferent fiber from the cerebellum, the axon of the Purkinje cells; these fibers terminate in the cerebellar nuclei and in the vestibular nuclei. The climbing fiber is uniquely distributed to a single Purkinje cell (CAJAL, 1909–1911; HÁMORI and SZENTÁGOTHAI, 1966; FOX et al., 1967; ECCLES et al., 1967) on which it has a potent excitatory action (cf. ECCLES et al., 1967). Impulses initiated in climbing fibers excite Purkinje cells very powerfully across single synapses.

On the other hand, the mossy fiber input is characterized by enormous divergence, and it has both excitatory and inhibitory actions on Purkinje cells. For our present purpose it is sufficient to outline the two major pathways. The excitatory pathway is by way of mossy fibers to granule cells which discharge impulses along their axons, the parallel fibers that give excitatory synapses to Purkinje cells (ECCLES et al., 1967).

The inhibitory pathway is by way of mossy fibers to granule cells, to parallel fibers to basket and stellate cells that give a dense array of inhibitory synapses on the Purkinje cells. Another inhibitory pathway is given by the parallel fibers to the Golgi cells, which are inhibitory on the dendrites of the granular cell. It is assumed that this pathway works as a negative feedback on the main afferent system to the cerebellar cortex, represented by the mossy fibers. It is of interest that the density of the Golgi cells within the granular layer of the cerebellar cortex of the vestibulocerebellum is higher than that in the other parts of the cerebellum (BRODAL and DRABLOS, 1963; BRODAL and HØIVIK, 1964).

The mossy fiber action is effected in the rectangular lattice determined principally by the parallel course of the parallel fibers for about 3 mm along a cerebellar folium and by the basket cell axons that extend for up to 1 mm perpendicular to this. A sharply focused mossy fiber input would give a "beam" of parallel fiber impulses that results in a 3 mm strip of excited Purkinje cells "on-beam", and the action of the basket cells results in a zone of inhibited Purkinje cells 1 mm "off-beam" on either side (ECCLES et al., 1967). As pointed out by ECCLES et al. (1967), this arrangement gives excellent opportunities for the integration of the inputs by the various mossy fibers that have overlapping excitatory and inhibitory actions, these arbitrary zones of potential interaction being limited to a few square millimeters.

It has been suggested that there is no significant transfer of information from each small zone to another in the cerebellar cortex because the only association pathways would be the Purkinje axon collaterals that are weakly inhibitory (ECCLES et al., 1967). The absence of excitatory association paths gives an areal restriction for any particular input, so that impulses passing to some focus in the cerebellar cortex via mossy or climbing fibers influence only a few square millimeters of cerebellar cortex at most.

These concepts, which have been developed on the basis of work performed on the cerebellar cortex of the anterior lobe, are likely also to be valid for the cortical areas of the vestibulocerebellum, since the neuronal constituents of the cerebellar cortex follow the same stereotyped and simple geometrical arrangement in all the cortical regions of this structure.

There is anatomical evidence indicating that the primary vestibular fibers (SNIDER, 1936; BRODAL and HØIVIK, 1964) and possibly also the secondary vestibular fibers end as mossy fibers (CARREA et al., 1947; SZENTÁGOTHAI and RAJKOVITS, 1959; GRANT, 1962). It is a moot point whether all the mossy fibers within the flocculonodular lobe originate in the vestibular afferent system and all the vestibulocerebellar afferents end as mossy fibers, at least in mammals.

In the frog, for instance, the VIII nerve primary fibers activate Purkinje cells via the mossy-parallel fiber as well as the climbing fiber system (MATTHEWS et al., 1958; LLINÁS and BLOEDEL, 1966/1967, 1967; LLINÁS et al., 1967). It has been suggested that these two afferent systems in the frog may relay different types of information to this cerebellum, the mossy fiber being a tonic operator while the climbing fiber operates as a phasic relay system. Anatomical and physiological research is required to find out whether these two systems are related to specific types of receptors in the vestibular organ.

The possibility that these projection characteristics are also present in mammals is weakened by the anatomical evidence so far produced, which indicates that vestibular fibers terminate only as mossy fiber afferents. It should be stated that negative results in this connection are not decisive, since it is extremely difficult to identify degenerating climbing fibers with silver impregnating methods. However, even assuming that all the vestibulocerebellar afferents terminate as mossy fibers, it is still not known whether the climbing fibers ending within the vestibulocerebellum originate in the inferior olive, as described for other cortical regions (Szentágothai and Rajkovits, 1959) or how volleys coursing along this climbing fiber system interact with labyrinthine impulses, which apparently reach the flocculonodular lobe through the mossy fiber system. It is of interest that the inferior olive receives spinal ascending fibers as well as descending projections from higher centers (cf. Jansen and Brodal, 1958; Eccles et al., 1967).

Much electrophysiological work is required to follow the signal transfer of labyrinthine volleys in the corticocerebellar efferent system. As far as the activity of the fastigial neurons are concerned, however, it is clear that labyrinthine stimulation excites the fastigial nuclei of both sides (Arduini and Pompeiano, 1957b), which are known to exert a tonic excitatory influence on the vestibular nuclei of both sides (pp. 431–436). This indicates that the labyrinthine volleys are one of the main excitatory inputs to the fastigial nuclei, which in their turn create a tonic excitatory background in the vestibular nuclei. The same neurons are also excited through collaterals from other mossy fiber and climbing fiber pathways (Eccles et al., 1967). The demonstration that the Purkinje cells are inhibitory in function (pp. 436–444) suggests that this tonic activity of the vestibular nuclei may be depressed by the efferent impulses of the Purkinje neurons, triggered not only by the peripheral labyrinthine volleys but also by extralabyrinthine volleys which may originate both from higher centers and from the periphery.

IV. Influence of the Lobus Flocculonodularis on Vestibular Functions

The same cortical area of the cerebellum which receives primary or secondary vestibular afferents, namely the flocculonodular lobe, projects back to the vestibular nuclei (Dow, 1936, 1938a; Brodal et al., 1962; Voogd, 1964). It appears therefore that most of the influence from this cerebellar lobe must be exerted through the vestibular nuclei. Direct cerebellofugal fibers from the flocculus to the oculomotor nuclei are postulated by some authors (Löwy, 1916; Marburg, 1924; Kuzume, 1926a, b; Gerebtzoff, 1941) but have not been confirmed (cf. Jansen and Brodal, 1958).

A comparison of the distribution of the floccular and the nodular-uvular projections with the areas of termination of other afferent fiber contingents to the vestibular nuclei by Angaut and Brodal (1967) indicates that the terminal areas of fibers from the flocculus in the superior, medial and descending vestibular nuclei coincide with the sites of termination of the primary vestibular fibers (Walberg et al., 1958). On the other hand there is a striking similarity between the afferents from the nodulus-uvula and those from the hook bundle of Russell (Walberg et al., 1962). It is known that neurons of the superior, descending and medial vestibular nuclei project rostrally via the ascending medial longitudinal fascicle to higher centers, particularly to the oculomotor nuclei (BRODAL and POMPEIANO, 1958), while cells from the medial and descending nucleus also project to the cerebellum (BRODAL and TORVIK, 1957) and to the spinal cord via the descending medial longitudinal fascicle (POMPEIANO and BRODAL, 1957a; CARPENTER, 1960a, b; NYBERG-HANSEN, 1964; WILSON et al., 1967b, 1968a).

An interesting point which emerges from anatomical studies (ANGAUT and BRODAL, 1967) is that even the lateral vestibular nucleus receives fibers from the vestibulocerebellum (cf. DOW, 1936, 1938a; GEREBTZOFF, 1941). While the floccular efferents reach all parts of Deiters' nucleus, the fibers originating from nodulus-uvula impinge only upon the dorsocaudal part of Deiters' nucleus, which projects to the lumbosacral segments of the spinal cord (POMPEIANO and BRODAL, 1957a).

Physiological studies clearly indicate that the projections from the vestibulocerebellum onto the vestibular nuclei are involved in the control of the equilibrium and of the motor activity of the extrinsic eye muscles.

Ablation experiments. Ablation of the nodulus and/or uvula has been performed in several animal species (DOW, 1938b; MANNI, 1950; FERNÁNDEZ, 1960; FERNÁNDEZ and FREDRICKSON, 1964; GRANT et al., 1964).

Ablation of the nodulus alone or of the nodulus and adjacent segments of the paleocerebellum in particular (DOW, 1938b; SPIEGEL and SCALA, 1941, 1942; CARREA and METTLER, 1947; MANNI, 1950; DI GIORGIO, 1950b; FERNÁNDEZ, 1960; FERNÁNDEZ et al., 1960a, b; FERNÁNDEZ and FREDRICKSON, 1964) revealed a syndrome of disequilibrium characterized by oscillations of the body from side to side during standing or moving. The gait is unsteady and broad-based. Falling frequently occurs. Unlike the deficit produced by lesions in other regions of the cerebellum, this syndrome does not generally involve any disturbance in posture or in the range, rate, force or direction of voluntary movements. However, extension of the ipsilateral foreleg has been reported by GRANT et al. (1964) after lesion of the nodulus and uvula in the rabbit. Since this cortical area projects to the hindlimb region of Deiters' nucleus, changes of postural tonus should be expected in the hindlimb rather than in the forelimb.

In addition to the signs of disequilibrium mentioned above, lesions in the nodulus elicit positional nystagmus in cat (SPIEGEL and SCALA, 1942; FERNÁNDEZ, 1960; FERNÁNDEZ et al., 1960a, b; ALLEN and FERNÁNDEZ, 1960; FERNÁNDEZ and FREDRICKSON, 1964) and rabbit (GRANT et al., 1964). This effect is consistently observed in supine and hanging-head positions and is frequently seen in the right lateral and/or left lateral positions. It is always direction-fixed, *i.e.*, it occurs in the same direction regardless of the position. In every case the direction is vertical toward the lower eyelid. Control experiments suggest that it is the lesion of the nodulus, and not that of the uvula, which produces disequilibrium and positional nystagmus.

Recent experiments by GRANT et al. (1964) show that unilateral lesion of the nodulus and the ventral part of the uvula also produces positional nystagmus in rabbit. This is mainly horizontal, beating to the side of the lesion. However, positional, horizontal nystagmus is also described after unilateral lesion of the uvula.

Another syndrome occurs after ablation of the nodulus and the ventral part of the uvula, characterized by prolonged vestibular reactions to rotatory and caloric tests (FERNÁNDEZ and FREDRICKSON, 1964). On unilateral lesion of both the nodulus and the uvula there is in particular asymmetry in the rotatory test, nystagmus beating to the side of the lesion being predominant. In animals intoxicated with alcohol positional nystagmus appears, beating to the right in the right lateral and to the left in the left lateral position of the body. Even this alcohol-induced positional nystagmus dominated towards the side of this lesion (GRANT et al., 1964). However, when the unilateral lesion is restricted to the uvula, both alcohol-induced positional nystagmus and nystagmus induced by rotation showed an asymmetrical beating which was more pronounced from the side of the lesion (GRANT et al., 1964). Comparison of these experiments with the previous group, where both uvula and nodulus were ablated, yields the impression of a crossed effect. It is known in fact that the uvula projects on the caudal part of the fastigial nucleus from which the hook bundle of Russell originates.

The experimental evidence so far presented suggests that the disturbances in equilibrium and eye movements following ablation of the nodulus are due to release of the vestibular nuclei from cerebellar inhibition. The effects of unilateral lesion of the nodulus would then be referred to asymmetrical disinhibition of the vestibular nuclei.

The symptoms of ablation of the flocculus (KUZUME, 1926a, b; LORENTE DE NÓ, 1931; CARREA and METTLER, 1947; FERNÁNDEZ and FREDRICKSON, 1964) and lingula (FULTON and CONNOR, 1939; CONNOR, 1941; CONNOR and GERMAN, 1941; MANNI, 1950) are generally considered similar to those elicited by lesions of the nodulus. According to some authors, however, unilateral ablation of the flocculus (always associated with some damage to the overlying paraflocculus) yielded contradictory results (FERNÁNDEZ and FREDRICKSON, 1964). Some animals presented disequilibrium and postural nystagmus, while others exhibited little or no vestibular disturbance. It is possible that the signs of the former group may have been due at least in part to vascular disturbances, edema or surgical trauma involving the cerebellopontine angle.

It should be pointed out that the occurrence of positional nystagmus produced by ablation of the flocculonodular lobe requires the presence of signals from vestibular receptors indicating positional changes of the head. The nystagmus is in fact abolished after bilateral labyrinthectomy (DOW, 1938b; SPIEGEL and SCALA, 1942) or bilateral cocainization of the middle ear (FERNÁNDEZ, 1960). On the other hand, the disequilibrium following unilateral lesion of the flocculus, nodulus and lingula is still present in the guinea pig subjected to bilateral labyrinthectomy followed by compensation (MANNI, 1950).

Stimulation experiments have been limited particularly to the nodulus and uvula (ASCHAN et al., 1964; FERNÁNDEZ and FREDRICKSON, 1964; COHEN et al., 1965).

Repetitive electrical stimulation of the nodulus in unrestrained, unanesthetized cats (FERNÁNDEZ and FREDRICKSON, 1964) did not produce eye movements. However, electrical stimulation of the nodulus during nystagmus elicited by both rotatory or caloric tests produced a consistent inhibitory effect. ASCHAN et al. (1964) found that in unrestrained, unanesthetized rabbits, stimulation of the lateral part of the nodulus provoked nystagmus that was influenced by the position of the body. Moreover, stimulation of the same cortical area inhibited alcohol-induced nystagmus in the ipsilateral position.

All these experiments support the opinion that in cat the nodulus has an inhibitory action upon the vestibular responses, at least on the vestibulo-ocular reflex arc. Experiments based on stimulation of the flocculus have apparently not been performed systematically, nor has the unit activity been recorded from vestibular or oculomotor nuclei during stimulation of the flocculonodular lobe.

The data available are too scanty to permit any conclusion as to whether the different projections of the nodulus-uvula and the flocculus to the vestibular nuclei are reflected functionally. It is of interest, however, that both ablation (DOW, 1938b; MANNI, 1950; GRANT et al., 1964) and stimulation experiments (ASCHAN et al., 1964; FERNÁNDEZ and FREDRICKSON, 1964; COHEN et al., 1965) lead to an asymmetrical reaction if performed unilaterally; this finding fits in with the observation that the projections of the nodulus to the vestibular nuclei are almost exclusively ipsilateral. Further and detailed studies are obviously needed before satisfactory correlation will be possible between physiological and anatomical observations on the efferent projections of the vestibulocerebellum.

V. Influence of the Corpus Cerebelli on Vestibular Functions

The cerebellar efferent connections to the vestibular nuclei do not originate exclusively in the vestibulocerebellum. There is in fact a heavy projection from the anterior and the posterior vermis of the cerebellum and the fastigial nucleus to all the vestibular nuclei, including the lateral vestibular nucleus of Deiters, which is an important link in the pathways mediating cerebellar influences to the cord.

There are two main routes by which the cerebellar vermis can influence the vestibular nuclei (BRODAL et al., 1962; VOOGD, 1964; POMPEIANO, 1966a, 1967; BRODAL, 1966, 1967a, b) and in particular the nucleus of Deiters. There is a direct pathway and an indirect one that involves a synapse in the fastigial nucleus. The direct cerebellovestibular pathway to Deiters' nucleus arises mainly in the vermis of the anterior lobe (WALBERG and JANSEN, 1961; EAGER, 1963; VOOGD, 1964) and to a lesser extent in the posterior vermis (DOW, 1936; WALBERG and JANSEN, 1961; EAGER, 1963), and its fibers end in the dorsal half of the ipsilateral nucleus. This projection originating from the vermal cortex of the anterior lobe is somatotopically organized (WALBERG and JANSEN, 1961; VOOGD, 1964). The other cerebellovestibular pathway passing via the fastigial nucleus is more complex (BRODAL et al., 1962; VOOGD, 1964; POMPEIANO, 1966a, 1967; BRODAL, 1966, 1967a, b). First of all there is an orderly arrangement in the projection from the anterior and posterior vermis onto the rostral and caudal part of the fastigial nucleus. This was inferred from findings made in Marchi studies (JANSEN and BRODAL, 1940, 1942) and even though later studies with silver-impregnation methods (VACHANANDA, 1959; EAGER, 1963; GOODMAN et al., 1963; WALBERG and JANSEN, 1964; VOOGD, 1964) have shown that the localization is not so sharp as originally supposed, the main principle appears to be valid. There are marked differences between the projections from the two parts of the fastigial nucleus onto the vestibular nuclei, however (WALBERG et al., 1962); those from the rostral part, receiving their cerebellar input from the anterior vermis, end in the dorsal part of the ipsilateral nucleus of Deiters, *i.e.*, in the same region as the direct fibers. The fibers from the caudal part of the fastigial nucleus, being influenced from the caudal vermis, cross in the hook bundle and enter the contralateral nucleus of Deiters, where they terminate in the ventral part of the nucleus. Both these fastigial projections to the ipsilateral and contralateral Deiters' nucleus show a pattern of somatotopical localization. It should be pointed out that other vestibular nuclei besides the Deiters' nucleus receive efferent projections from these cerebellocortical regions.

The cerebellovestibular fiber connections considered so far are all, whether direct or synaptically interrupted in the fastigial nucleus, derived ultimately from the anterior and posterior vermis, *i.e.*, from cerebellar regions referred to as the spinocerebellum, since they receive the bulk of afferent impulses from the cord. It may be more appropriate to distinguish three and not two functionally different zones within the cerebellar vermis. The most rostral part is the vermis of the anterior lobe (Larsell's lobuli I–V) which receives most of its afferent impulses from the spinal cord via various spinocerebellar systems (LUNDBERG, 1964; OSCARSSON, 1965). The most caudal part, the pyramis and uvula (Larsell's lobuli VIII and IX, the nodulus being lobulus X) is likewise largely impinged upon by spinal impulses. The middle part, Larsell's lobuli VI–VII, is activated chiefly by auditory and visual impulses according to physiological studies (SNIDER and STOWELL, 1944; FADIGA and PUPILLI, 1964). Recent experiments have given evidence for a projection of afferents from the eye muscle receptors to lobuli VI and VII and to the caudal part of lobulus V (FUCHS and KORNHUBER, 1969).

The first section of this chapter will be devoted to a study on the functional significance of the middle part of the cerebellar vermis which controls mainly the activity of the oculomotor neurons. The remaining sections will be devoted to functional considerations on the most rostral and most caudal zones of the cerebellar vermis, which control the activity of the spinal cord.

A. Cerebellar Control of Oculomotor Nuclei

Ablation experiments. — *Ocular deviations* and *spontaneous nystagmus* have been described by some authors after bilateral total or unilateral cerebellectomy (cf. DOW and MORUZZI, 1958; DOW and MANNI, 1964). Nystagmus following hemicerebellectomy is generally of the horizontal type with the rapid phase towards the normal side (SIMONELLI and DI GIORGIO, 1931; MANNI and DOW, 1963). This symptom is never long-lasting (DI GIORGIO, 1950c). It is of interest that nystagmus is also found after isolated unilateral lesions of the vermis and roof nuclei (BAUER and LEIDLER, 1912; LEIDLER, 1919; CRANMER, 1951).

Spontaneous nystagmus occurs far more easily after hemicerebellectomy or after unilateral lesion of the vermis and fastigial nuclei than after total or any symmetrical cerebellar ablation. It is difficult to believe that the vestibular nuclei are less easily injured when cerebellectomy is complete, or that they are usually encroached upon asymmetrically as a consequence of surgical accidents during this operation. A more likely explanation (DOW and MORUZZI, 1958) is that the nystagmus is related to an imbalance between the labyrinthine systems of the two sides of the body, which occurs particularly when the vestibular system is activated by small head movements (LEIDLER, 1919) or certain head positions (SPIEGEL and SCALA, 1941, 1942; CARREA and METTLER, 1947; DI GIORGIO, 1950b; FERNÁNDEZ et al., 1960a, b; ALLEN and FERNÁNDEZ, 1960).

FERRARO and BARRERA (1938) pointed out that nystagmus is not present after different cerebellar lesions in a resting position, but can appear in any direction of gaze following total cerebellectomy or wide cerebellar lesions. It is more pronounced after lesions of the lobuli VII to X and fastigial nuclei. Its intensity has been correlated with the degree of labyrinthine hyperexcitability, which can be determined by studying postrotatory nystagmus.

These observations suggest that whenever the vestibular nuclei are deprived of the cerebellar control, previously subliminal labyrinthine reflexes (static or kinetic) can produce so-called spontaneous nystagmus. The influence of the position of the head can be interpreted by assuming that the tonic barrage of otolithic impulses influences the ampullary reflexes. This conclusion is supported by the observation that neurons in the medial and descending vestibular nuclei, which are known to mediate ampullary reflexes, respond to macular stimulations (PETERSON, 1967). The interrelations between cervical, macular, and ampullary reflexes have been investigated by GROEBBELS (1927a, b), LORENTE DE NÓ (1931), KOELLA (1947a, b) and HAHN (1952).

Cerebellar ablations affect not only the spontaneous oculomotor activity but also the *labyrinthine induced nystagmus*. DE KLEIJN (1925) showed that postrotatory nystagmus was still present after cerebellectomy in the rabbit (DUSSER DE BARENNE, 1937; SPIEGEL and SCALA, 1942; DI GIORGIO, 1950b). This agrees with the findings of Magnus and his associates that vestibular reflexes are preserved after total cerebellectomy (MAGNUS, 1914; DE KLEIJN and MAGNUS, 1920). However, the threshold to galvanic labyrinthine stimulation decreased following total cerebellectomy (HAHN, 1951) or destruction of the posterior vermis (DI GIORGIO and HAHN, 1951) and increased after strychninization of this area (DI GIORGIO and HAHN, 1951). Asymmetrical cerebellar lesions may also modify vestibular reflexes (SIMONELLI and DI GIORGIO, 1926). Postrotatory nystagmus was decreased when the animal was rotated toward the intact side and increased after rotation toward the treated side, particularly after hemicerebellectomy (SIMONELLI and DI GIORGIO, 1931; DI GIORGIO, 1950a, c) and after unilateral ablation of the posterior vermis and fastigial nuclei (BAUER and LEIDLER, 1912). HOSHINO (1921) obtained modifications of postrotatory nystagmus following lesions of the "ophthalmotropogenic zone" of the cerebellum (p. 429) and removal of the posterior vermis. FERRARO and BARRERA (1938) reported that postrotatory responses in monkeys were prolonged following destruction of various cerebellar parts. A similar result was observed in cats with bilateral ablation of the anterior lobe and cranial parts of fastigial and interpositus nuclei (CHAMBERS and SPRAGUE, 1955b). There is apparently an optimal angular speed for detection of postrotatory changes induced by experimental cerebellar lesions (BILLIA, 1952), which may explain the negative results reported in the literature (RADEMAKER, 1931; BUCHANAN, 1938). It can be concluded therefore that the cerebellar efferent system originating in the posterior vermis exercises a clearcut effect on vestibular nystagmus.

Postrotatory nystagmus is subject to habituation if repeatedly produced. It appears now that the cerebellum can influence habituation to repeated rotations. In pigeons, in fact, habituation was less readily produced and more poorly retained after cerebellectomy. Moreover, it was reduced when cerebellar lesions were induced after habituation had already been established (HALSTEAD, 1935; HALSTEAD et al., 1937). These defects in habituation were also found in guinea pigs after removal of the vermal cortex limited to lobuli VII and VIII (DI GIORGIO and PESTELLINI, 1948). It is possible that habituation is a true conditioned reflex supported by the cerebellum (HALSTEAD et al., 1937).

It is also possible that habituation is simply another manifestation of the release of the vestibular nuclei (DI GIORGIO and PESTELLINI, 1948) on the excitability of the final common pathway. These theories remain to be proved (MENZIO, 1950).

BECHTEREW (1883) showed that nystagmus normally resulting from labyrinthectomy immediately stopped if the second labyrinth was destroyed soon after the first one was damaged. However, when the second labyrinthectomy was performed after compensation for the first was complete and nystagmus had gradually disappeared, it resulted in nystagmus in the opposite direction (cf. BECHTEREW, 1883; MAGNUS, 1924; CAMIS, 1928). The central mechanisms responsible for compensation of vestibular function following hemilabyrinthectomy have since been investigated (PRECHT et al., 1966). SPIEGEL and DEMETRIADES (1925) showed that Bechterew's compensatory nystagmus also occurred in cerebellectomized animals. If cerebellar lesions were effected during the compensatory period following unilateral labyrinthectomy, nystagmus reappeared in the opposite direction (DEMETRIADES and SPIEGEL, 1927). The same cerebellar lesions were incapable of producing nystagmus in the normal rabbit. Apparently the cerebellum is involved in the mechanisms responsible for compensation after unilateral labyrinthectomy (cf. CARPENTER et al., 1959 b). Its ablation allows the imbalance to become manifest but in the opposite direction.

Stimulation experiments. The earlier investigators frequently observed conjugate ocular movements after stimulation of the cerebellum (cf. DOW and MANNI, 1964), but often their reports gave no exact indication of the cerebellar area stimulated. It is very likely, however, that these early workers stimulated the folium and tuber vermis (lobule VII), and the folia immediately anterior and posterior, the declive (lobule VI) and the pyramis (lobule VIII). The area which elicited eye movements upon stimulation actually includes HOSHINO's (1921) "opththalmotropogenic zone". Experiments performed on intact unanesthetized rabbits (HOSHINO, 1921) showed that stimulation of an area near the rostral end of the sulcus paramedianus on the medial part of the lobulus simplex produced horizontal deviation of both eyes toward the side stimulated.

BREMER (1935) pointed out that the depth of the cerebellar folia is rather shallow in these cerebellar regions, and that it was possible that the underlying white matter was being stimulated.

Ocular effects have also been described following stimulation of the deeper structures of the cerebellum (cf. DOW and MORUZZI, 1958; DOW and MANNI, 1964;

Cohen et al., 1965; Azzena and Giretti, 1967). Unfortunately, because of the numerous pathways which can be indiscriminately activated by the deep stimulating electrodes, it is difficult to assess the functional significance of those data.

It should be mentioned that cerebellar stimulation influences not only the position of the eyes but also the nystagmus elicited by labyrinthine stimulation (Gratscher, 1919; Hoshino, 1921; Dow, 1935).

Electrophysiological experiments. The effects of stimulation of the cerebellar cortex on the unitary discharge of the oculomotor (III cranial nerve) nucleus was investigated in curarized guinea pigs (Manni et al., 1965b). High-frequency repetitive stimulation of the lateral half of Larsell's lobulus VI and VII and also of the ansoparamedian lobule of one side (Larsell's lobules H VII a, b) generally produced inhibition of the ipsilateral oculomotor units and activation of the contralateral ones. Similar but more evident patterns of activation or inhibition were shown by most of the units located in the vicinity of the oculomotor nuclei.[1]

Great caution must be exercised in the attribution of these responses to stimulation of the Purkinje cells. Because of the inhibitory influence of these neurons on the cerebellar nuclei (pp. 436–444), opposite effects would be expected when the cerebellar cortex and the underlying nuclei are stimulated. On the contrary, when the effects of deep cerebellar stimulation on the units of the oculomotor nuclei were investigated (Azzena and Giretti, 1967), it was found that ipsilateral inhibition and contralateral excitation of the oculomotor units generally occurred during stimulation of the dentate nucleus. The similarity between these responses and those elicited by stimulation of the corresponding corticocerebellar region suggests that the last effect is due at least in part to antidromic excitation of some cerebellar afferent fibers and to monosynaptic excitation, through collaterals, of neurons of the dentate nucleus.

In contrast to stimulation of the dentate nucleus, fastigial and interposite nucleus stimulation provoked facilitation of the oculomotor units regardless of which side was stimulated.

All the units recorded were also strikingly modified by labyrinthine stimulation (Manni et al., 1965a; Azzena and Giretti, 1967). Thus a convergence of labyrinthine and cerebellar impulses on the oculomotor units was shown (di Giorgio, 1955; Manni et al., 1965b; Azzena and Giretti, 1967). Since all these experiments (Manni et al., 1965b; Azzena and Giretti, 1967) were performed in curarized animals it is impossible to correlate these results with the movements evoked by cerebellar stimulation.

In some experiments Azzena and Giretti (1967) recorded evoked potentials from the region of the oculomotor nuclei following single-shock stimulation of each of the three cerebellar nuclei. Latencies as short as 0.2 msec were recorded following stimulation of the contralateral dentate or interposite nuclei. In the case of stimulation of the fastigial nucleus the latencies ranged from 1.0 to 1.2 msec. Because of the short latency of the evoked potential recorded from the oculomotor nuclei on single-shock stimulation of the contralateral interposite and dentate nuclei, the authors assume that the connection between dentate or interposite

1 The effects of corticocerebellar stimulation on the rhythmical responses of the oculomotor cells induced by the caloric labyrinthine stimulation were also studied (Manni et al., 1965b), but the results obtained were inconsistent.

nuclei and oculomotor nuclei is a direct one. The existence of a direct cerebello-oculomotor pathway is still debated. Fibers from the cerebellum to the oculomotor nucleus were traced by some authors (KLIMOFF, 1896; WALLENBERG, 1905; LÖWY, 1916; ALLEN, 1924; MARBURG, 1924; KUZUME, 1926a, b; SACHS and FINCHER, 1927; WINKLER, 1927; RASMUSSEN, 1933; LE GROSS CLARK, 1936; GEREBTZOFF, 1941; cf. JANSEN and BRODAL, 1958) but they were not confirmed by later workers (RANSON and INGRAM, 1932; JANSEN and BRODAL, 1958; CARPENTER et al., 1958; CARPENTER, 1959, 1960b). More recently CARPENTER and STROMINGER (1964) described a direct cerebello-oculomotor pathway in monkey, connecting the dentate nucleus with the contralateral oculomotor nucleus and neighboring structures. No information, however, is available on the efferent projection from the small-celled part of the dentate nucleus, which should be considered part of the vestibulocerebellum since it receives primary vestibular afferents (BRODAL and HØIVIK, 1964).

In the case of fastigial stimulation, the impulses directed towards the oculomotor nuclei are probably mediated by the vestibular nuclei and the medial longitudinal fascicle. Since the latencies of the evoked potentials recorded in this investigation from the oculomotor nuclei after fastigial stimulation range from 1.0 to 1.2 msec, it seems reasonable to suppose that a synapse is intercalated within the vestibular nuclei along the fastigio-oculomotor pathway.

In summary, the middle part of the vermis, corresponding to Larsell's lobuli VI–VII, exerts a control on both the spontaneous and the reflex ocular movements. The anatomical connections between this cortical cerebellar area and the middle third of the fastigial nucleus, which projects to the vestibular nuclei through both crossed and uncrossed pathways (WALBERG et al., 1962), supports the conclusion that cerebellar control of the oculomotor activity is mediated in part by the vestibular nuclei. However a control of both spontaneous and reflex oculomotor activity seems also to be exerted by more laterally placed corticocerebellar regions as well as by the interposite and dentate nuclei. Much more work is required to define the extent and the nature of this control. The physiological demonstration that this cortical area is activated chiefly by auditory and visual impulses (SNIDER and STOWELL, 1944; FADIGA and PUPILLI, 1964) has led to the suggestion that "lobules VI and VII might supervise, without being necessarily responsible for the coordination of ocular movements brought about by visual and auditory stimuli" (DOW and MORUZZI, 1958). Unfortunately there is no evidence so far that the vestibular neurons respond to optic or acoustic stimuli (FREDRICKSON et al., 1966). As pointed out above, this cerebellar cortical region also receives proprioceptive impulses from the extra-ocular muscles (FUCHS and KORNHUBER, 1969).

B. Cerebellar Control of Postural Tonus

Facilitation of the vestibular activity by the fastigial nuclei. SPRAGUE and CHAMBERS (1953) were the first to consider the fastigial nucleus as a tonogenic structure whose background activity is under the control of cerebellopetal impulses reaching the fastigial nucleus either directly or by way of collaterals of fibers reaching the cerebellar cortex. It will be shown that Deiters' nucleus plays an important role in transmitting the impulses originating from the fastigial nucleus to the extensor muscles. Experiments involving destruction or stimulation point to the lateral vestibular nucleus as an important structure which exerts a facilitatory influence on the myotatic reflexes of extensor muscles, which are essential for postural tonus (cf. BRODAL et al., 1962). Lesion experiments have shown that unilateral destruction of the fastigial nucleus, similarly to the unilateral lesion of Deiters' nucleus, abolishes the extensor rigidity in the ipsilateral limbs which on the other hand increases in the contralateral limbs (SPRAGUE and CHAMBERS, 1953).

The results of SPRAGUE and CHAMBERS (1953) were confirmed by MORUZZI and POMPEIANO (1955a, b, 1956b, c), BATINI and POMPEIANO (1955, 1956a, 1957) and STELLA et al. (1955), who also reported that extensor rigidity was sharply reduced when only the rostral part of the ipsilateral fastigial nucleus had been acutely or chronically destroyed. This syndrome was called "ipsilateral fastigial atonia" by MORUZZI and POMPEIANO (1955a, b, 1956b, c). The same effect was observed when the rostral lesion was made after bilateral and symmetrical destruction of the caudal parts of the fastigial nucleus, where the crossed fastigiobulbar fibers originate (BATINI and POMPEIANO, 1956b, c, 1958a, b).

The conclusion drawn from these experiments was that the direct fastigiobulbar pathway exerts a tonic facilitatory influence on the extensor mechanisms of the ipsilateral side of the body. The increase in the decerebrate rigidity contralateral to the rostrofastigial lesion is due at least in part to release of the decerebrate rigidity from crossed inhibitory influences, which are greatly reduced when the ipsilateral limbs are made atonic by the lesion (MORUZZI and POMPEIANO, 1955c, d, 1957b). This observation, incidentally, explains the reappearance of a bilateral rigidity following symmetrical lesion of the contralateral fastigial nucleus.

More detailed analysis of the postural effects produced by more localized lesions within the rostral part of the fastigial nucleus led to a more complex picture (BATINI and POMPEIANO, 1956b, c, 1958a, b). Symptoms similar to those characterizing ipsilateral fastigial atonia can also be produced by unilateral destruction limited to the large-celled rostromedial part of the fastigial nucleus (Fig. 2C, D). Destruction of the rostrolateral part yielded the exact reverse of this postural asymmetry, *i.e.*, a further release of the ipsilateral extensor tonus and a reduction in the spasticity of the contralateral limbs (Fig. 2A, B). The latter operation was followed by abolition of the typical inhibition of the decerebrate rigidity elicited by stimulation of the overlying anterior hemivermis (MORUZZI and POMPEIANO, 1954, 1956a, 1957a), an observation hinting that the inhibitory pathway from the vermal cortex had been selectively destroyed. It will be shown later that this lesion interrupts the long cerebellar corticovestibular projection which has an inhibitory function on Deiters' nucleus. While the increase in the ipsilateral rigidity is due to release of the postural tonus from tonic inhibition, the decrease in the decerebrate rigidity contralateral to the side of the rostrolateral fastigial lesion is due at least in part to crossed inhibitory influences originating from the stretch receptors of the ipsilateral limbs made spastic by the lesion (MORUZZI and POMPEIANO, 1955c, d, 1957b).

Turning now to the function of the crossed fastigiobulbar projection, it has been shown that an acute (MORUZZI and POMPEIANO, 1955a, b, 1956b, c) or chronic (BATINI and POMPEIANO, 1955, 1956a, 1957; COHEN et al., 1958) electrolytic lesion limited to the caudal part of one fastigial nucleus increases the extensor

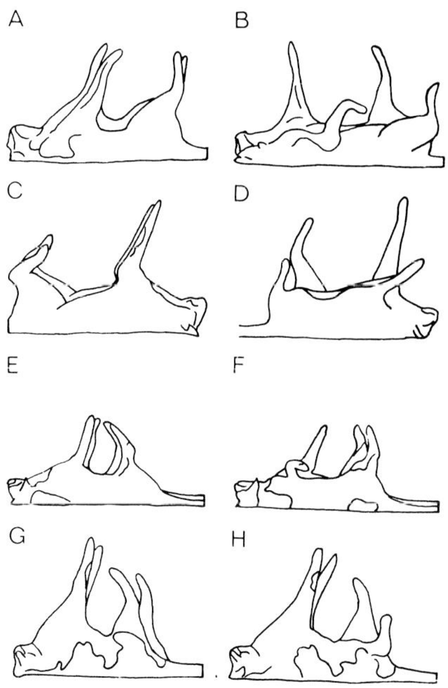

Fig. 2. Effects of localized fastigial lesions on the decerebrate rigidity. A: symmetrical distribution of extensor rigidity after chronic electrolytic destruction of the caudal half of both fastigial nuclei followed, 16 days later, by intercollicular decerebration. B: ipsilateral increase and contralateral decrease of extensor rigidity after electrolytic lesion of the rostrolateral part of the left fastigial nucleus made in the same decerebrate preparation. C: new experiment. Symmetrical distribution of extensor rigidity after chronic electrolytic destruction of the caudal half of both fastigial nuclei followed, 14 days later, by intercollicular decerebration. D: the same cat after electrolytic lesion of the rostromedial part of the left fastigial nucleus. Note marked decrease in extensor rigidity on the left side and increase of extensor rigidity on the right side (Batini and Pompeiano, 1958b). E: new experiment. Symmetrical distribution of extensor rigidity after precollicular decerebration. F: disappearance of extensor rigidity of the right foreleg after lesion of the rostral part of the caudal third of the left fastigial nucleus. G: another experiment showing symmetrical rigidity after precollicular decerebration. H: disappearance of extensor rigidity of the right hindleg following lesion of the caudal pole of the left fastigial nucleus (Pompeiano, 1962)

tonus in the ipsilateral limbs, while this disappears or is strikingly reduced in the contralateral limbs. This syndrome has been called "crossed fastigial atonia". The opposite posture, *i.e.*, ipsilateral inhibition and crossed facilitation of extensor tonus is observed when the caudal part of one fastigial nucleus is stimulated electrically. It was concluded therefore that the caudal pole of the fastigial nucleus exerts a tonic excitatory influence on the extensor motoneurons of the contralateral side. These motoneurons actually collapse under the impact of the crossed inhibitory barrage as soon as they are deprived of the support of the fastigiobulbar facilitation. On the other hand, the increased ipsilateral rigidity after caudofastigial lesion can be attributed to release of the decerebrate rigidity from crossed inhibitory influences which are greatly reduced when the contralateral limbs are made atonic by the fastigial lesion (Moruzzi and Pompeiano, 1955c, d, 1957b).

There is little doubt that the fastigial nucleus exerts a tonic facilitatory influence on the tonogenic structures of the brainstem. This effect is thought to be mediated via the direct and crossed fastigiobulbar pathways originating to a large extent in the rostral and caudal parts of the fastigial nucleus (Jansen and Jansen, 1955; Batini and Pompeiano, 1955, 1956a, 1957). This does not mean that the tonic facilitatory influences are mediated via Deiters' nucleus, even if this exerts a facilitatory influence on the extensor tonus. Several arguments support this conclusion, however.

First of all it has been shown that the same postural asymmetries as are produced by rostral or caudal fastigial lesions after conventional decerebration can still be observed superimposed on vestibular rigidity (Moruzzi and Pompeiano, 1955e, f, 1957b). This term refers to the rigidity which occurs in the flaccid deafferentated forelimb following acute postbrachial transection of the spinal cord, because it disappears after unilateral section of the vestibular nerve (Stella, 1944a; Batini et al., 1956a–e, 1957) or lesion of Deiters' nucleus (Batini et al., 1956a–c, 1957). Thus the vestibular component of extensor rigidity is influenced by the efferent projections from the fastigial nucleus in the same way as the rigidity in a decerebrate animal.

Secondly, it has been shown that the unilateral disappearance of the decerebrate rigidity brought about by the fastigial lesion is due not only to crossed inhibitory influences originating in the stretch receptors of the contralateral side, but also to a tonic inhibitory influence arising in the labyrinthine receptors of the opposite side of the body (Moruzzi and Pompeiano, 1955e, f, 1957b). It has already been reported that the decerebrate rigidity was abolished in the right forelimb when the caudal portion of the left fastigial nucleus had been destroyed. If the left VIII nerve was then severed intracranially, not only did the extensor rigidity disappear in the left foreleg, but the previously atonic forelimb of the right side became rigid. In other words, the postural mechanisms of the brainstem, particularly those localized in the vestibular nuclei, are overruled by inhibitory reflexes arising in the contralateral labyrinthine receptors when they are deprived of the support of the fastigial facilitation. The reciprocal response of the vestibular nuclei to the labyrinthine volleys arising on each side of the body is also substantiated by the electrophysiological experiments (de Vito et al., 1956; Pompeiano and Cotti, 1959g). Pathways mediating crossed vestibular effects have been investigated recently by both anatomical (Ladpli and Brodal, 1968) and physiological investigations (Shimazu and Precht, 1965, 1966; Precht and Shimazu, 1965; Shimazu, 1967; Kasahara et al., 1968; Wilson et al., 1968b; Mano et al., 1968).

A final piece of evidence in support of the view that Deiters' nucleus is involved in the fastigial influence on the postural tonus has been obtained by experiments showing that the effects of stimulation or destruction of the fastigial nucleus are somatotopically organized. Experiments of stimulation (Pompeiano, 1960a–c) or unit recording of Deiters' nucleus (Ito et al., 1964a, b; Wilson et al., 1965, 1966a, b, 1967a) indicate that the vestibulospinal tract is somatotopically organized according to a pattern similar to that described anatomically (Pompeiano and Brodal, 1957; Nyberg-Hansen and Mascitti, 1964). In view of the functional organization of the efferent projection originating in the fastigial nucleus, and particularly in the caudal part of this nucleus, when the lesion is limited to the rostral or the caudal part of the caudal region of the fastigial nucleus the ensuing atonia is restricted to the contralateral forelimb and hindlimb respectively (Fig. 2E–H).

The effects of localized stimulation of the same nuclear regions are discrete but opposite in character (POMPEIANO, 1961, 1962, 1966a, 1967). The somatotopical pattern in the postural responses to local stimulation or destruction of the caudal part of the fastigial nucleus is perfectly consistent with the pattern of localization shown by our anatomical findings (WALBERG et al., 1962) in the projection of the caudal part of the nucleus fastigii onto the contralateral nucleus of Deiters. These findings, therefore, strongly support the conclusion that the tonic facilitatory influence exerted by the caudal part of the fastigial nucleus on the extensor mechanisms of the contralateral side of the body is mediated via Deiters' nucleus. The same conclusion can be extended to the rostral part of the fastigial nucleus (particularly the rostromedial part of this nucleus), which also exerts an excitatory influence on the extensor mechanisms of the ipsilateral side of the body via the Deiters' nucleus.

The general conclusion of all these experiments, namely that the fastigial nucleus exerts an excitatory influence on the vestibular nuclei, is supported by

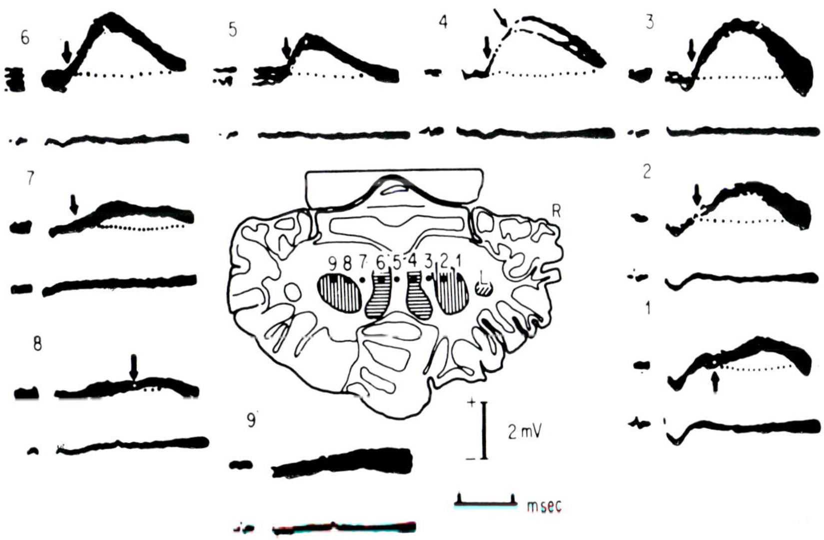

Fig. 3. Monosynaptic excitation of Deiters' neuron from fastigial nuclei region. Diagram in the center shows a horizontal section of the cerebellum. *L*, lateral nucleus. *R*, right side. Spots 1–9 represent electrolytic marks made by the stimulating electrodes. Records were taken from a Deiters' neuron with pulses of 0.08 msec duration and 10 V strength. Figure on each record indicates the site of cathode. Anode was formed by the left side partner except when the spot 9 was used as cathode against anode at 8. Lower traces, extracellular records. Dotted lines superposed on the upper traces indicate the time course of the lower traces. Vertical arrows point to the moment of onset of EPSPs. Oblique arrow in the record 4 indicates the diverging point of the two sets of the potential curves which were separated spontaneously during stimulation with constant pulses (ECCLES et al., 1967)

recent experiments showing that neurons in Deiters' nucleus receive an excitatory impingement during fastigial stimulation (cf. ECCLES et al., 1967). It is not surprising that the intracellular EPSP recorded by these authors is monosynaptic (Fig. 3) because of the histologically well-documented fastigiofugal projection to these vestibular nuclei (WALBERG et al., 1962; BRODAL et al., 1962). In the vestibular neurons the effect of fastigial stimulation is not restricted to the fastigial nuclei but also arises from a rather wide area surrounding these nuclei (Fig. 3). This may be due to contamination by axon reflexes through collaterals of the cerebellar afferents. Figure 3 (trace 4) also shows that the stimulation of the fastigial nucleus evoked a delayed EPSP superposed upon the monosynaptic EPSP. On account of the small difference (0.4 msec) in the onset times of these EPSPs, the delayed EPSPs can be ascribed to transsynaptic activation of some fastigial neurons.

Inhibition of the fastigiovestibular activity by the cerebellar cortex. The function of the anterior and posterior parts of the cerebellar vermis should now be considered. First the function of the vermis of the anterior lobe will be examined. It has been shown anatomically that the vermal cortex of the anterior lobe projects to the rostral third of the fastigial nucleus (JANSEN and BRODAL, 1940, 1942, 1958), which in turn projects to ipsilateral brainstem structures, particularly to the ipsilateral vestibular nuclei (WALBERG et al., 1962; BRODAL et al., 1962). There is also a direct projection from the vermal cortex of the anterior lobe to the ipsilateral vestibular nuclei, and particularly to Deiters' nucleus (WALBERG and JANSEN, 1961; BRODAL et al., 1962).

The most marked effect of high-frequency electrical stimulation of this cortical region in a decerebrate animal is the classic inhibition of the rigidity of the ipsilateral limbs followed by extensor rebound (LÖWENTHAL and HORSLEY, 1897; SHERRINGTON, 1897, 1898; BREMER, 1922; DENNY BROWN et al., 1929). This effect is somatotopically organized (HAMPSON et al., 1945, 1946, 1952). It is of interest that the inhibition of the decerebrate rigidity disappears after total destruction of the fastigial nucleus (SPRAGUE and CHAMBERS, 1953; MORUZZI and POMPEIANO, 1954, 1956a, 1957a; CHAMBERS and SPRAGUE, 1955a; STELLA et al., 1955; POMPEIANO, 1958) or lesions limited to the rostral part of the fastigial nucleus (MORUZZI and POMPEIANO, 1954, 1956a, 1957a; BATINI and POMPEIANO, 1955, 1956a, 1957; STELLA et al., 1955). A reversal of the inhibitory response can be obtained by lowering the repetition rate of the electrical pulses applied to the anterior vermis (MORUZZI, 1950a, b). After stereotaxically oriented and histologically controlled lesions of the rostrolateral part of the fastigial nucleus (Fig. 4A), MORUZZI and POMPEIANO (1954, 1956a, 1957a) found that high-frequency stimulation of the ipsilateral vermis of the anterior lobe yielded a clearcut increase of the extensor rigidity in the ipsilateral limbs with the same parameters of stimulation which usually produces the typical inhibition of the decerebrate rigidity. Under this experimental condition an augmentatory effect, otherwise concealed by an overwhelming inhibition, becomes apparent. On the other hand, clearcut inhibitory effects can be elicited by stimulating the vermis of the anterior lobe with the same parameters of stimulation if the rostromedial part of the fastigial nucleus is damaged and the rostrolateral part spared. Therefore both excitatory and inhibitory pathways are activated by vermal stimulation.

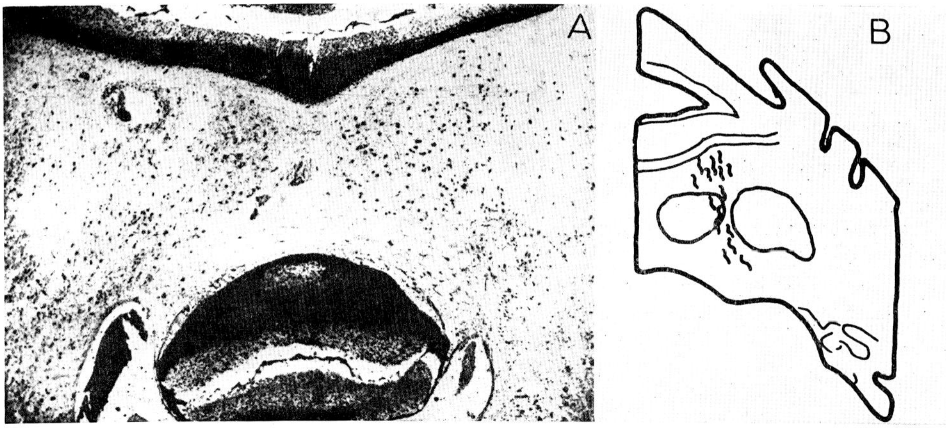

Fig. 4. Intrafastigial course of the cerebellar corticovestibular fibers. A: microphotograph showing a dorsolateral lesion of the rostral part of a fastigial nucleus yielding reversal of the inhibitory response of the vermal part of the anterior lobe. The lesion occupies the rostrolateral and dorsal, parvicellular part of the right fastigial nucleus, while the rostromedial, magnocellular part is intact. Stimulation of the right hemivermis of the anterior lobe increased the ipsilateral extensor rigidity, while the inhibitory response was still obtained from the left hemivermis (Moruzzi and Pompeiano, 1957a). B: diagrammatic representation of the cerebellar corticovestibular fibers mainly directed to Deiters' nucleus, on their way through the cerebellum (Walberg and Jansen, 1961). These corticofugal fibers penetrate the rostrolateral part of the fastigial nucleus, *i.e.*, that region whose destruction abolishes the inhibitory effects on decerebrate rigidity induced by vermal stimulation of the anterior lobe

It would be interesting to know whether the inhibitory and augmentative effects on the decerebrate rigidity elicited by stimulation of the vermis of the anterior lobe are due to influences exerted on Deiters' nucleus, which is known to facilitate the extensor mechanisms. Experiments by de Vito et al. (1956) and Pompeiano and Cotti (1959a–g, 1960) have shown that surface-positive polarization of the vermal cortex of the anterior lobe or single-shock stimulation of this cortical area produced a decrease in some cases and an increase in the frequency of discharge of units in the ipsilateral Deiters' nucleus in others. Some units were not influenced even with supramaximal stimulation.

It may well be assumed that the disappearance of decerebrate rigidity during repetitive stimulation of the vermis of the anterior lobe is due to inhibition of the discharge of Deiters' nucleus. On the other hand, the units of Deiters' nucleus which show an increase in their discharge following cerebellar polarization may facilitate the extensor mechanisms. As mentioned above, repetitive stimulation of the vermis of the anterior lobe can increase the extensor rigidity under certain experimental conditions.

The most impressive results of these investigations (Pompeiano and Cotti, 1959a–c, g) was the demonstration that functionally the projection of the vermis of the anterior lobe onto Deiters' nucleus was very localized. Among the 76 units recorded, 48 were influenced only by a threshold stimulation of a single lamella of the ipsilateral vermis of the anterior lobe (Fig. 5). Similar effects were also obtained when polarization of the cerebellar cortex was performed (Fig. 6). That

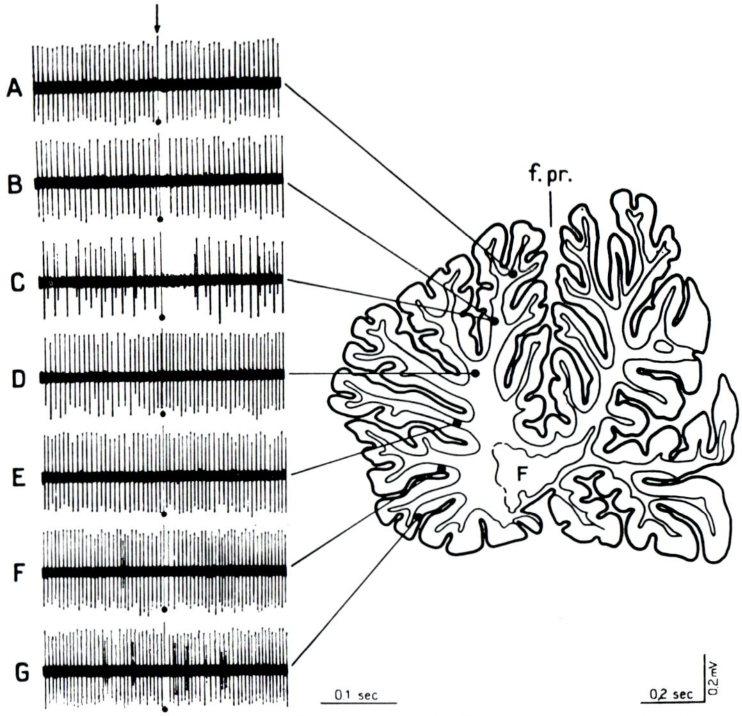

Fig. 5. Inhibition of the spontaneous discharge of a Deiters' neuron produced by stereotaxic stimulation of the cerebellar vermis. The ipsilateral hemivermis of the anterior lobe was stimulated with rectangular pulses (1.5 V, 1 msec) at the sites indicated in the schematic drawing. F: nucleus fastigii; f.pr.: fissura prima. The inhibitory response is present only in records A–C. Time calibration of 0.1 sec applies only to record C (POMPEIANO and COTTI, 1959g)

these localized responses are due to activity in the cerebellar cortex immediately underlying the electrode is apparent from the fact that local application of cocaine chlorhydrate or Nembutal to the active folium raised the threshold from 0.1–0.2 to 0.4–0.8 mA (Fig. 6). This demonstration of a functional localization within the projection of the vermis of the anterior lobe onto Deiters' nucleus fits in with our anatomical findings, demonstrating a localization in the projection of the anterior lobe onto Deiters' nucleus (BRODAL et al., 1962). They even indicate that the localization is sharper than it has been possible to show in the anatomical studies.

It would be interesting to know by what mechanisms stimulation of the vermal cortex of the anterior lobe can either inhibit or facilitate the discharge of ipsilateral vestibular neurons. Let us start with the inhibitory effects. MORUZZI and POMPEIANO (1957a) put forward the hypothesis that the abolition of the vermal inhibition of the anterior lobe following electrolytic lesion of the rostrolateral part of the fastigial nucleus is due to destruction of fastigial neurons or to interruption of long cerebellar corticofugal fibers passing through the rostrolateral part of the fastigial nucleus. Later anatomical studies (WALBERG and JANSEN, 1961; EAGER, 1963) showed that long corticofugal fibers to the vestibular nuclei from the vermal cortex of the anterior lobe pass through the rostrolateral part of the fastigial

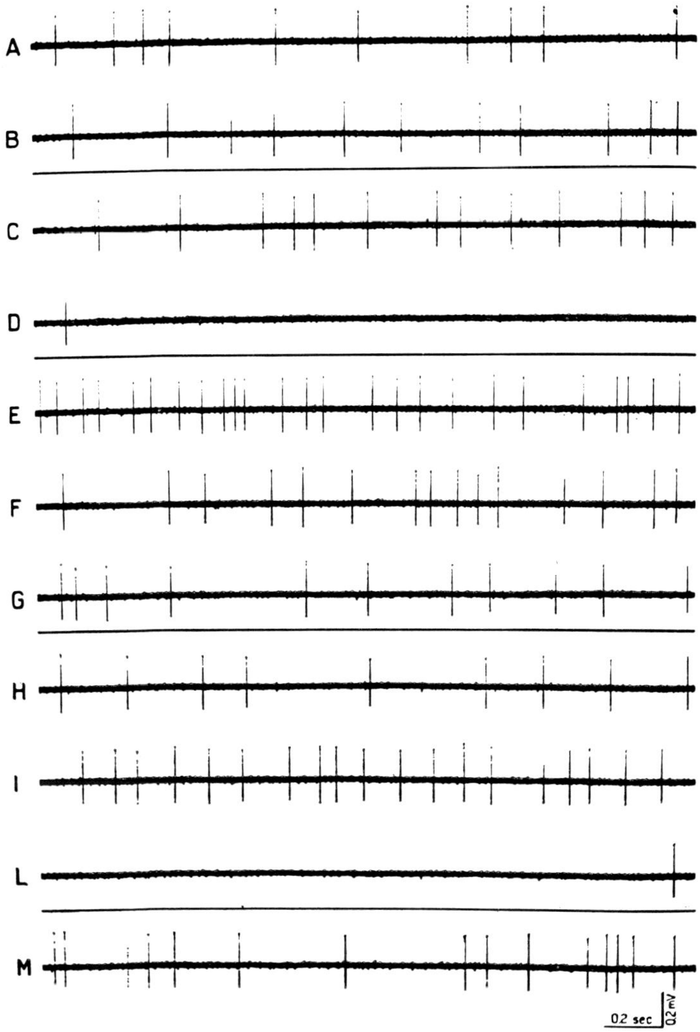

Fig. 6. Inhibition of a single unit in the right Deiters' nucleus to anodal polarization of a single folium in the cortex of the vermis of the anterior lobe. Decerebrate and curarized cat. A: spontaneous discharge. B: no response to polarization of the right side of folium Vb with 0.4 mA. C: control after stimulation. D: arrest of discharge on polarization with 0.3 mA of the right side of the most ventral folium of sublobulus V A. E: control after stimulation. F: spontaneous activity after local application on the active lamella of 6% Nembutal for 1 min. G: no effect on polarization with 0.3 mA of the right side of the most ventral folium of sublobulus V A (cf. record D). H: control after stimulation. I: spontaneous activity after washing the cortex with Ringer solution for 2 min. L: on polarization with 0.3 mA of the point stimulated in D and G the arrest of discharge reappears. M: control after stimulation (Pompeiano and Cotti, 1959g)

nucleus (Fig. 4B). It has been suggested therefore (Brodal et al., 1962) that the long cerebellar corticovestibular fibers are responsible not only for the vermal inhibition of the decerebrate rigidity but also for the inhibition of Deiters' neurons elicited by stimulation of the vermal cortex of the anterior lobe (DE VITO et al., 1956; POMPEIANO and COTTI, 1959a–c, g). According to BRODAL et al. (1962) "the pathway for the inhibitory action on these units is related to the rostrolateral part of the fastigial nucleus through which the long cerebellar corticovestibular fibres pass, making it likely that the stimulation of these fibres is involved in the effect".

Experiments involving intracellular recording from Deiters' neurons strongly support this hypothesis (cf. ECCLES et al., 1967). Stimulation of the vermal cortex

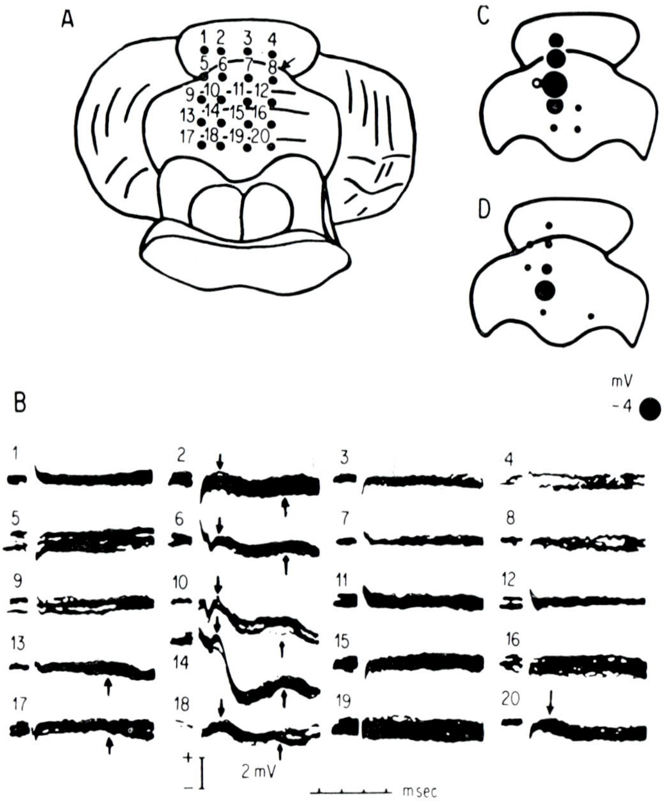

Fig. 7. Monosynaptic inhibitory zone in the cerebellum for Deiters' neurons. A, frontal view of the cerebellum. Black dots 1–20 indicate the sites of stimulation provided by four multipolar stimulating electrodes. Each of these electrodes was made of 5 pieces of enamel wire stuck on a shaft of steel needle. They were mounted on a micromanipulator and inserted into the culmen in the caudodorsal to rostroventral direction. B, intracellular records taken in a Deiters' neuron during stimulation at each spot of A. The figure attached to each record refers to the position of cathode, while the anode was served by the caudal partner except when spots 1–4 were used as cathode against anode at their rostral partners. Pulse duration was 0.2 msec and pulse amplitude was 10 V. Downward arrows indicate the onset time of the monosynaptic IPSPs. Upward arrows point to the delayed onset of IPSPs. C and D plot for two Deiters' neurons, respectively, sizes of the monosynaptic IPSPs at the sites of stimulation. In C an open circle indicates the size of the depolarization produced by monosynaptic EPSP (ITO et al., 1968)

of the anterior lobe in anesthetized cats did in fact produce IPSPs in Deiters' neurons (Ito and Yoshida, 1964, 1966), identified by their antidromic invasion from the vestibulospinal tract (Ito et al., 1964a, b). Latency measurements indicate that the inhibitory impulses travel directly through the cerebellum at a relatively slow conduction velocity of 15–20 m/sec and impinge on Deiters' neurons monosynaptically (Fig. 7). The demonstration of long inhibitory fibers between the cerebellar cortex and Deiters' neurons is of particular interest since the inhibitory neurons identified in the mammalian CNS so far are mostly short-axoned (cf. Eccles, 1964). Several groups of experiments suggest that this monosynaptic inhibitory pathway to Deiters' neurons originates from Purkinje cells. First, the cerebellar area which gives rise to the monosynaptic inhibition of Deiters' neurons is localized on the ipsilateral vermis and also the medial portion of the paravermis of both the anterior and the posterior lobes of the cerebellum (Ito and Kawai, 1964; Ito et al., 1965, 1968) from which long cerebellodeitersian fibers originate (Walberg and Jansen, 1961; Eager, 1963). Secondly, cerebellar monosynaptic inhibition is absent in neurons of the ventral portion of Deiters' nucleus, which is the portion not impinged upon by the Purkinje axons from the anterior and posterior lobes (cf. Brodal et al., 1962). Thirdly, there is an excellent temporal correlation between the activation of Purkinje cells in the anterior lobe of the cerebellum through the cerebellar afferent fibers, particularly through the climbing fibers (Eccles et al., 1964, 1966), and the inhibitory events in Deiters' neurons (Ito et al., 1964c, 1966).[2]

Much like IPSPs in spinal motoneurons and the other nerve cells (Eccles, 1964), the IPSPs in Deiters' neurons are reversed to a depolarizing potential by intracellular injection either of hyperpolarizing currents or of chloride ions. It is of interest, however, that while the ionic mechanisms generating the IPSPs in Deiters' neurons appear to be the same as those generating IPSPs in spinal motoneurons (cf. Eccles et al., 1967), there is a large discrepancy between Deiters' neurons and motoneurons in the pharmacology of their inhibition (Obata, 1965; Obata et al., 1967; cf. Eccles et al., 1967). Preliminary experiments seem to indicate that GABA may be responsible for the inhibitory action of these cells (cf. Curtis and Watkins, 1965; Kuriyama et al., 1966; Obata et al., 1967). However, more neurochemical and neuropharmacological investigations are required to determine the nature of the inhibitory transmitter of the Purkinje neurons.

Regarding the facilitatory responses of some Deiters' units obtainable by stimulation of the vermis of the anterior lobe (de Vito et al., 1956; Pompeiano and Cotti, 1959a–g) the possibility was put forward that these effects could be due to excitation of rostrofastigial neurons from which the ipsilateral fastigiovestibular projection originates.

---

2 It is of interest that the cerebellar corticovestibular fibers in cat are in synaptic contact with all parts of Deiters' neurons, *i.e.*, soma, proximal and distal dendritic trunks, and spine-like projections (Mugnaini and Walberg, 1967). Since these Purkinje cells are inhibitory, all the axonal endings of the Purkinje cells in Deiters' nucleus, *i.e.*, axodendritic as well as axosomatic synapses in this nucleus are inhibitory. There is a school of thought that inhibitory synapses are situated on somata and proximal dendrites (Eccles et al., 1967). The presence of endings of fibers from the cerebellar cortex on the distal dendrites of these cells, therefore, suggests that conditions are probably not so schematic as one might think.

The belief that the short-axon Purkinje neurons could excite this fastigio-vestibular projection was grounded on the observation that an increase in the decerebrate rigidity actually occurs after interruption of the inhibitory pathway represented by the long cerebellodeitersian projection. This hypothesis has been questioned by Ito and his group. They made intracellular recordings and found that Deiters' neurons sometimes receive monosynaptic (and polysynaptic) EPSP from the vermal cortex of the anterior lobe (ITO and YOSHIDA, 1964, 1966; ITO and KAWAI, 1964; ITO et al., 1965). This effect has been attributed to antidromic excitation of some cerebellar afferent fibers and to monosynaptic excitation through collaterals of neurons of Deiters' nucleus. Excitatory influences in Deiters' nucleus actually originate from various muscle and skin nerves (POMPEIANO and COTTI, 1959d, e, g; DUMONT, 1960; GIAQUINTO et al., 1963; TYC-DUMONT, 1964; FREDRICKSON et al., 1964, 1966; WILSON et al., 1965, 1966a, b, 1967a).

An alternative or complementary mechanism to explain the excitation of Deiters' neurons on vermal stimulation is that stimulation of the cerebellar cortex can induce inhibition of Purkinje cells through several pathways. Since an abundant inhibitory bombardment is spontaneously acting upon Deiters' neurons, the resulting depression of this tonic inhibitory bombardment of the subcortical neurons will cause disinhibition in the subcortical neurons and, correspondingly, late facilitation in the vestibular neurons. That this depolarization is due to removal of background IPSPs is shown by the fact that it is reversed by the intracellular injection of hyperpolarizing currents and/or chloride ions, the equilibrium potential being at the same level as for the IPSPs (cf. ECCLES et al., 1967). The disinhibition phenomenon following cerebellar stimulation has been ascribed to inhibition of Purkinje cells through the basket and stellate cells. Disinhibition would also be induced by the inhibition of the granular cells through Golgi cells, which would depress the excitatory bombardment of the Purkinje neurons by granular cells.

Much like Deiters' neurons, even the neurons of the fastigial nucleus can be either inhibited (Fig. 1A, B) or excited by stimulation of the ipsilateral vermal cortex (ARDUINI and POMPEIANO, 1956a, b, 1957a, b). One result of this is that units localized in the rostral half of the fastigial nucleus were frequently but not constantly affected by bipolar d.c. stimulation (0.1 to 0.8 mA) of the ipsilateral vermal cortex of the anterior lobe.

Recent experiments show that both monosynaptic IPSP and EPSP can be elicited from the vermal cortex (ITO et al., 1964d; cf. ECCLES et al., 1967). The monosynaptic inhibitory effects are attributed to stimulation of Purkinje neurons, while the monosynaptic excitatory effects are attributed to excitation through axo-axonic reflex of spinocerebellar afferents giving collaterals to the fastigial neurons.

The spontaneous discharge of the fastigial neurons (ARDUINI and POMPEIANO, 1956a, b, 1957a, b) is probably due not only to collaterals of cerebellar afferents, but also to reverberation between the fastigial nucleus and the descending vestibular nucleus (cf. BRODAL et al., 1962; ECCLES et al., 1967). Similar circuits may be formed between the fastigial nucleus and the precerebellar reticular nuclei (cf. ECCLES et al., 1967). The result of all these experiments is that the fastigial nucleus, similarly to Deiters' nucleus, can be considered as a reflex center which receives excitatory signals from extracerebellar sources and thereby generates out-going excitatory signals, while the cerebellar cortex controls them by inhibition (ITO et al., 1964a–c, 1966; ECCLES, 1965; ECCLES et al., 1967). It is not known, however, whether all the fastigial neurons are under the inhibitory control of the vermal cortex.[3]

The function of the posterior vermis of the cerebellum, which projects to the caudal part of the fastigial nucleus (JANSEN and BRODAL, 1940, 1942, 1958) must now be considered. It has already been shown that acute (MORUZZI and POMPEIANO, 1955a, b, 1956b, c) or chronic (BATINI and POMPEIANO, 1955, 1956a, 1957; COHEN et al., 1958) electrolytic lesions restricted to the caudal part of the fastigial nucleus increase the extensor tonus in the ipsilateral limbs but reduce it strikingly in the contralateral limbs. This syndrome, which has been called "crossed fastigial atonia" is also observed following unilateral ablation of the pyramis and uvula, which project onto the caudal part of the fastigial nucleus. The opposite effect, *i.e.*, ipsilateral inhibition and crossed facilitation of extensor rigidity is observed not only when the caudal part of the fastigial nucleus is stimulated electrically (MORUZZI and POMPEIANO, 1955a, b, 1956b, c), but also during stimulation of the pyramis and uvula (BREMER, 1922; HAMPSON et al., 1945, 1946, 1952; SPRAGUE and CHAMBERS, 1954; CHAMBERS and SPRAGUE, 1955a; MORUZZI and POMPEIANO, 1956c).

If we accept that the short-axon Purkinje neurons projecting to the cerebellar nuclei, like the long-axon Purkinje neurons projecting directly to Deiters' nucleus, are inhibitory in function, we should expect that unilateral stimulation or destruction of the posterior vermis give rise to effects opposite in sign with respect to those elicited by stimulation or destruction of the caudal part of the corresponding fastigial nucleus. On the contrary, the results obtained appear to be the same. Further experiments are required to explain this discrepancy.

An electrophysiological study of the responses of single units in Deiters' nucleus to stimulation of the posterior vermis and of the caudal part of the fastigial nucleus might shed some light on the problem of the functional organization of the efferent projections from the posterior vermis to Deiters' nucleus. Furthermore, a study of this kind might indicate whether the ipsilateral hemivermis of

3 Histological (PETROFF, 1955; WERSÄLL, 1956, 1960; ENGSTRÖM, 1958; RASMUSSEN and GACEK, 1958; ENGSTRÖM and WERSÄLL, 1958; CARPENTER et al., 1958, 1959a; GACEK, 1960; CARPENTER, 1960b; IURATO and TAIDELLI, 1964; WERSÄLL et al., 1967), histochemical (DOHLMAN, 1960; DOHLMAN et al., 1958; IRELAND and FARKASHIDY, 1961; ROSSI and CORTESINA, 1962, 1963, 1965; HILDING and WERSÄLL, 1962; ROSSI, 1964) and physiological investigations (SALA, 1962, 1963a–c, 1964, 1965; SCHMIDT, 1963; GLEISNER and HENRIKSSON, 1964) have shown the existence of centrifugal fibers in the vestibular nerve, which have been traced to all subdivisions of the labyrinth. The suggestion of RASMUSSEN and GACEK (1958) and GACEK (1960) that these efferent vestibular fibers are derived from the nucleus of Deiters is apparently shared by ROSSI and CORTESINA (1962, 1965), who in addition assert the origin of some such fibers in particular small cell groups. Stimulation of the area of Deiters' nucleus also gives rise to efferent vestibular activity (SALA, 1965). Since the vestibular complex is under the facilitatory and inhibitory control of the fastigial nuclei and the vermal cortex respectively, the result would be that these cerebellar structures control the background activity of the second-order vestibular neurons not only directly through the cerebello-vestibular projections but also indirectly by exciting or inhibiting the efferent control system. Experimental evidence seem to suggest a predominantly inhibitory function of this efferent vestibular system (GLEISNER and HENRIKSSON, 1964; SALA, 1965).

the anterior lobe and the contralateral hemivermis of the posterior lobe are able to influence the activity of the same or of separate units in Deiters' nucleus. Anatomical evidence suggests that the pathways from the two regions of the vermis have different terminal regions in this nucleus (Brodal et al., 1962).

C. Cerebellar Control of *α* Motoneurons

The *α* motoneurons may be played upon directly by cerebellofugal volleys impinging upon the vestibular nuclei, without involvement of the *γ* system.

It is known that decerebrate rigidity is abolished by acute (Sherrington, 1898) or chronic (Sherrington, 1898; Terzuolo and Terzian, 1951a, b; Terzian and Terzuolo, 1954) deafferentation. However, following postbrachial transection of the spinal cord, the flaccidity of the bilaterally deafferentated forelimbs is replaced by extensor rigidity (Liliestrand and Magnus, 1919; Stella, 1944b, c; Batini et al., 1956a–e, 1957). The same results occur after complete cerebellectomy (Stella, 1944b) or after anatomical or functional ablation of the vermal cortex of the anterior lobe (Pollock and Davis, 1931; Stella, 1944b, c; Terzuolo and Terzian, 1954; Batini et al., 1956a–e, 1957) or electrolytic destruction of the two fastigial nuclei (Batini et al., 1956a–e, 1957). It appears therefore that the flaccidity of the deafferentated legs is not exclusively due to sheer lack of reflex excitation, but results from active inhibition of the nonmyotatic component of the postural tonus arising in the lumbosacral segments of the spinal cord or in the cerebellum (Stella, 1944b, c, 1946). The membrane of the *α* motoneurons actually depolarizes 10–15 mV during "release" obtained by removal of tonic inhibition from the lower cord or from the cerebellum (Gidlof, 1966).

Stella (1944b, c) maintained that this *α* rigidity, which is released by complete cerebellectomy or by postbrachial transection of the spinal cord, is mainly labyrinthine in origin, since it disappeared ipsilaterally to the acute section of the VIII nerve.[4] Batini et al. (1956a–e, 1957) were able to confirm Stella's observations. However, if the opposite VIII nerve was also sectioned an extensor hypertonus appeared in the previously flaccid forelimb, and the rigidity became symmetrical in the forequarters. It has already been mentioned that the collapse of the nonmyotatic rigidity brought about by severing the ipsilateral VIII nerve is not only related to the abolition of the tonic inflow of labyrinthine impulses, but also to an inhibitory effect of afferent volleys arising from the vestibular receptors of the opposite side.

It is of interest, however, that bilateral destruction of the labyrinths (Pollock and Davis, 1927, 1930b, 1931) or bilateral section of the VIII nerve (Batini et al., 1956a–e, 1957) abolishes the opisthotonus which occurs in normal decerebrate animals after cerebellectomy (Bremer, 1922; Camis, 1922, 1923; Pollock and Davis, 1923, 1927, 1930a, b, 1931) or bilateral destruction of the fastigial nucleus (Sprague and Chambers, 1953; Batini and Pompeiano, 1955, 1956a, 1957; Batini et al., 1956a–e, 1957), as well as in animals where the cerebellar lesion was made on a background of *α* rigidity (Stella, 1944a, b; Batini et al., 1957).

---

4 It is of interest that unilateral section of the VIII nerve does not affect the decerebrate rigidity (Sherrington, 1898) but ipsilaterally to the section of the VIII nerve it strongly decreases the most intense rigidity in the decerebrate, cerebellectomized cat (Magnus, 1914).

The influence exerted by the labyrinths on the extensor reflexes of the neck muscles, as demonstrated in these experiments, is probably mediated by the vestibulospinal fibers arising in Deiters' nucleus. It has been shown that in the latter nucleus, primary vestibular fibers end chiefly in its rostroventral part (POMPEIANO and BRODAL, 1957b; WALBERG et al., 1958), *i.e.*, in the region which sends fibers mainly to the cervical segments of the spinal cord (POMPEIANO and BRODAL, 1957a). Anatomical (HAUGLIE-HANSSEN, 1968; MUGNAINI et al., 1967) and physiological (ITO et al., 1964a; ECCLES et al., 1967; WILSON et al., 1966b, 1967a) observations have basically confirmed this finding. Opisthotonus can be obtained selectively after bilateral lesion of the rostrolateral parts of the fastigial nucleus (BATINI and POMPEIANO, 1958b), *i.e.*, after interruption of the long corticofugal fibers which have an inhibitory action on Deiters' neurons. Hence opisthotonus appears to be a labyrinthine phenomenon (probably mediated by Deiters' nucleus) which is tonically inhibited by the cerebellum. Furthermore, it has been shown that even the rigidity of the deafferentated forequarters that occurs after postbrachial transection of the spinal cord is clearly inhibited by electrical stimulation of the vermal part of the anterior lobe (STELLA, 1944a; TERZUOLO and TERZIAN, 1953). Obviously these inhibitory effects are not mediated by the γ route.

All these experiments strongly suggest that the cerebellar influence on Deiters' nucleus can affect the α motoneurons directly, *i.e.*, after interruption of the γ loop.

Several experiments have shown that Deiters' nucleus can actually exert its influence directly on the α extensor motoneurons. In fact, α rigidity disappears after unilateral lesion of Deiters' nucleus (BATINI et al., 1957). The conclusion derived from this research, namely that the vestibulospinal tract exerts an excitatory influence on the α extensor motoneurons, is also supported by the observation that single shock stimulation of Deiters' nucleus exerts a monosynaptic excitatory influence on extensor motoneurons (Fig. 8A–D) (LUND and POMPEIANO, 1965, 1968; POMPEIANO, 1966b; SHAPOVALOV, 1966; SHAPOVALOV et al., 1967–1968). The maximal amplitude of this supraspinal monosynaptic EPSP recorded from motoneurons of lumbosacral segments of the spinal cord corresponded on average to 24% of the maximal amplitude of the homonymous monosynaptic Ia EPSP. This early EPSP was often followed by a late disynaptic EPSP of larger amplitude. In contrast, the vestibulospinal tract produced a disynaptic IPSP on flexor motoneurons (Fig. 8E–H) (LUND and POMPEIANO, 1965, 1968) due to facilitation of the reciprocal I a inhibitory pathway from extensor to flexor motoneurons (GRILLNER et al., 1966).

The demonstration that the vestibulospinal tract impinges monosynaptically on extensor motoneurons is apparently inconsistent with recent anatomical findings (NYBERG-HANSSEN and MASCITTI, 1964) showing that the vestibulospinal fibers terminate only in Rexed's laminae VII and VIII (1954) and not in layer IX, where the motoneurons are located. One should consider that the dendrites of the motoneurons, on which synaptic contacts are present, extend dorsally into laminae VIII and VII (CAJAL, 1909–1911; LORENTE DE NÓ, 1938; AITKEN and BRIDGER, 1961; SPRAGUE and HA, 1964). Scattered degenerated vestibulospinal fibers can also be observed in layer IX, where the motoneurons are situated (ERULKAR et al., 1966). On the other hand, the polysynaptic effects

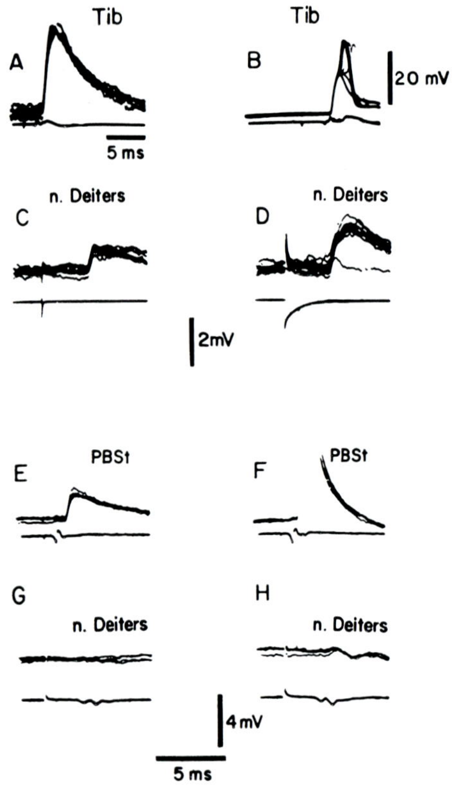

Fig. 8. Monosynaptic excitatory connections from the ipsilateral Deiters' nucleus to extensor motoneurons. A–D are from a tibial (Tib), E–H from a posterior biceps-semitendinosus (PBSt) motoneuron. Upper traces in each record are intracellular recordings with microelectrode. For voltage calibration see inset. Lower traces are records from L7 dorsal root entry zone. A and E show the maximal monosynaptic Ia EPSPs, B and F antidromic spikes obtained by slightly higher stimulus intensities applied to the homonymous nerves, C and G show effects of stimulation of Deiters' nucleus with low, and D and H with high stimulus intensities (Lund and Pompeiano, 1965)

on extensor or flexor motoneurons are likely to be due to the interneurons located in layers VIII and VII, where most of the vestibulospinal fibers terminate.

Since Deiters' nucleus is particularly involved in the phenomenon of the cerebellar inhibition of the decerebrate rigidity, we should know what type of change in membrane potential affects the a motoneurons during corticocerebellar stimulation.

It has already been shown that the long cerebellar corticovestibular fibers are responsible for the vermal inhibition of Deiters' neurons. The collapse of the extensor rigidity induced by high-frequency stimulation of the vermis of the anterior lobe is therefore due to inhibition of tonogenic centers (particularly the Deiters' nucleus), which are responsible for decerebrate rigidity.

This hypothesis is supported by the fact that the hyperpolarization of extensor motoneurons induced by stimulation of the vermis of the anterior lobe is not

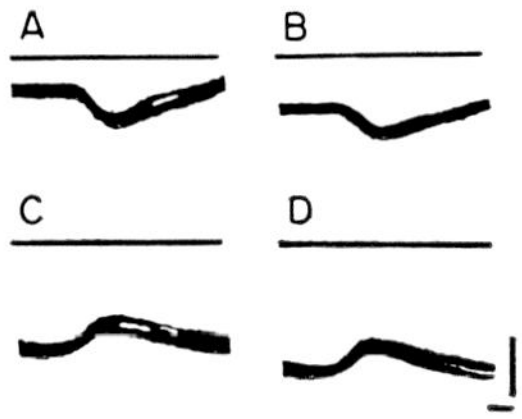

Fig. 9. Absence of reversal of the increase in membrane potential due to cerebellar inhibition during the flow of inward current. A: inhibitory postsynaptic potential recorded from a biceps-semitendinosus motoneuron following stimulation of the quadriceps nerve. Cerebellar inhibition increases the membrane potential (B). In C and D a steady inward current is applied so that a reversal of the inhibitory postsynaptic potential into a depolarizing one is obtained. Cerebellar inhibitory stimulation applied in this condition still increases the membrane potential. The top line is only a reference, and the major displacement in d.c. potential between the upper and the lower pairs of records is not a measure of the hyperpolarization of the membrane due to the flow of inward current. Time, 1 msec. Calibration, 5 mV (TERZUOLO, 1959)

reversed by passing hyperpolarizing current through the membrane (Fig. 9), nor it is associated with the conductance changes which determine the IPSP (TERZUOLO, 1959; LLINÁS, 1964). The conclusion drawn from these observations was that the cerebellar inhibition is due to suppression of tonic excitatory influences acting upon the motoneurons. The demonstration (LUND and POMPEIANO, 1965, 1968; POMPEIANO, 1966b; GRILLNER et al., 1966) that Deiters' nucleus exerts a direct monosynaptic excitatory influence on extensor motoneurons and on interneurons which inhibit flexor motoneurons leads to the conclusion that the inhibition of decerebrate rigidity induced by cerebellar stimulation is due to a striking disfacilitation of the extensor motoneurons as a consequence of an abrupt suppression of the vestibulospinal excitatory input to the extensor motoneurons.

This new interpretation of cerebellar inhibition differs from the old one, *i.e.*, that the inhibition of decerebrate rigidity elicited by stimulation of the vermis of the anterior lobe or of the fastigial nucleus is due to excitation (through cerebello-fastigio-reticular pathways) of the inhibitory region of the reticular formation (cf. MAGOUN and RHINES, 1947; SNIDER et al., 1949). If this were so, the hyperpolarization produced by cerebellar stimulation would present the same characteristics as the hyperpolarization produced by stimulation of the medial reticular formation. It is known, however, that the last effect is not due to a suppression of tonic excitatory influences acting on the motoneurons but is due to true IPSPs, because the IPSP can be reversed by passing hyperpolarizing current through the membrane, and is associated with conductance changes typical of the IPSP induced by peripheral afferent volleys (JANKOWSKA et al., 1964a, b, 1968; LLINÁS and TERZUOLO, 1964, 1965).

D. Cerebellar Control of γ Motoneurons

The cerebellar control of γ motoneurons is likely to be mediated at least in part by the vestibular nuclei. It has been shown that spindle discharge is increased by natural labyrinthine stimulation (ELDRED et al., 1953; GRANIT et al., 1955; VAN DER MEULEN and GILMAN, 1965; GILMAN and VAN DER MEULEN, 1966;

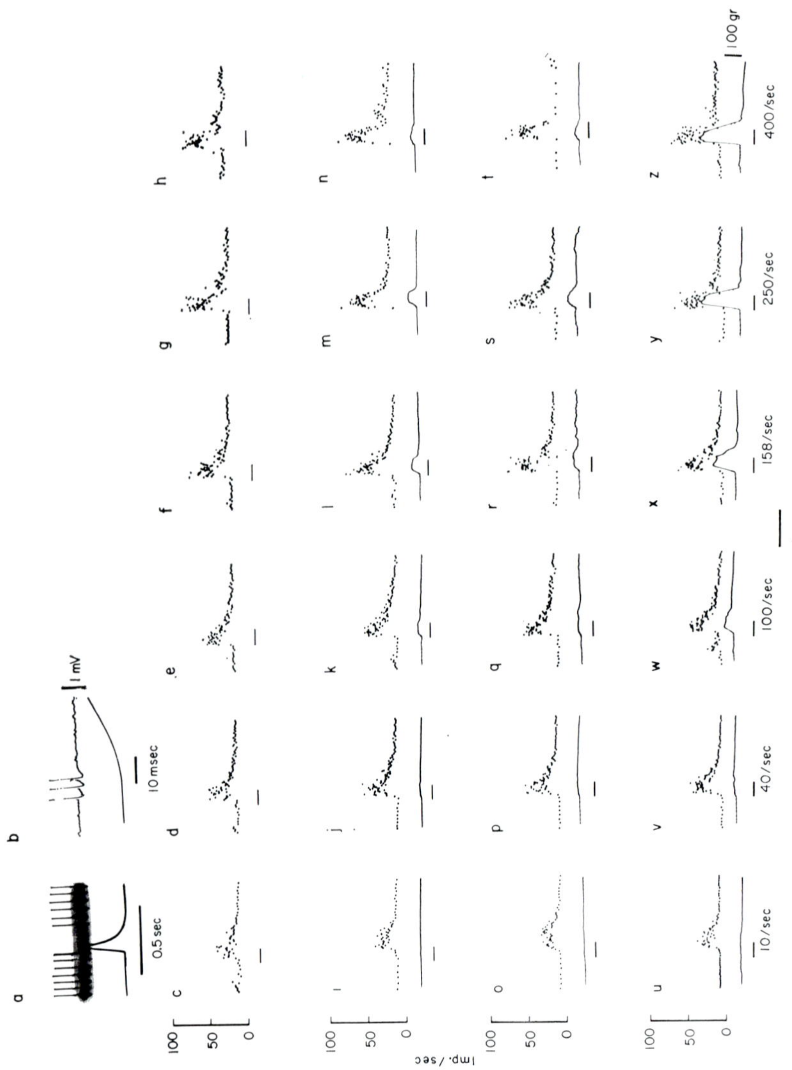

Fig. 10. Excitation of a muscle spindle receptor (conduction velocity of receptor fiber: 111 m/sec) in isotonic and isometric conditions, on stimulation of the fastigial nucleus. Left gastrocnemius-soleus muscle, dorsal roots intact. Precollicular decerebrate cat. *a*, *b*: classification of the receptor. 4 mm initial extension. *a*: the "pause" during a maximal twitch; *b*: the "evoked" spike and two "early discharge" spikes on an expanded sweep for determination of conduction time. *c–z*: the caudal part of the right fastigial nucleus was stimulated at the frequencies indicated at the bottom of the figure (10 V, 0.5 msec pulses). Records taken at 8 sec intervals. *c–h*: spindle excitation in slack muscle. *i–z*: spindle excitation in muscle at an initial extension of 0 (*i–n*), 2 mm (*o–t*) and 4 mm (*u–z*). Stimulus parameters similar to those used in investigating responses in slack muscle. The period of stimulation is indicated by a bar beneath each appropriate record. In these records, upper trace: spindle receptor discharge. Each dot represents an action potential, the instantaneous frequency of which is given by its height above zero on the calibration scale on the left hand side. Lower trace: tension record (Carli and Pompeiano, 1968)

POPPELE, 1967) or by electrical stimulation of the vestibular nerve (ANDERSSON and GERNANDT, 1956; DIETE-SPIFF et al., 1966, 1967a, b) and the vestibular nuclei (GRANIT et al., 1959; CARLI et al., 1966a–c, 1967a–d; POMPEIANO et al., 1967a, b).

These vestibular influences on the fusimotor neurons are likely to be under the excitatory and the inhibitory control originating from the fastigial nucleus and the vermal cortex respectively. Recent experiments have shown in fact that stimulation of the fastigial nucleus increases the activity in the ipsilateral extensor γ motoneurons (HENATSCH et al., 1964a, b; MANNI et al., 1964). Stimulation of a fastigial nucleus, however, produced generally ipsilateral inhibition of the stretch reflex. The fact that intracerebellar stimulation elicits opposite effects on the α and γ motoneurons has been considered an indication of the independent control of the cerebellum on the two spinal systems. It should be pointed out that stimulation of the fastigial nucleus, particularly at rostral level, may stimulate not only fastigial excitatory neurons but also cerebellar corticovestibular fibers as well as efferent cerebellofugal fibers originating from other regions of the cerebellar nuclei. There have been experiments (CARLI and POMPEIANO, 1968) to study the effects of stimulation of the caudal part of the fastigial nucleus on muscle spindle receptor discharge and on extrafusal contraction recorded from the extensor muscles of the contralateral hindlimb. In decerebrate cats, repetitive stimulation of the caudal part of the contralateral fastigial nucleus at an intensity just above the threshold for induction of an increase in the forelimb rigidity consistently produced extrafusal contraction of gastrocnemius-soleus muscle. Parallel with this event there was a consistent activation of muscle spindle receptors of the same muscles (Fig. 10). Both primary and secondary muscle spindle receptor endings were activated in this way during the concomitant evoked contraction. Spindle activation was generally obtained at a repetition frequency lower than that responsible for extrafusal contraction. However, when both spindle activation and extrafusal contraction occurred they increased parallel to an increase in the frequency of stimulation applied to the fastigial nucleus. Muscle spindle excitation occurred with the muscle contracting either isotonically (Fig. 10c–h) or isometrically (Fig. 10i–z). This activation persisted in spite of the development of tension in the contracting extrafusal muscle fibers. The excitation of spindle receptors from the fastigial nucleus was genuinely fusimotor, since this response could still be obtained after differential block of extrafusal end plates with gallamine triethiodide. On the other hand, the extrafusal contraction persisted even after deafferentation of the hindlimb. A comparison of these results and those obtained by stimulation of different vestibular structures indicates that the fusimotor neurons to the extensor muscles, like the skeletomotor neurons innervating the same muscles, are excited by the fastigiovestibular pathways.

While the fastigial nucleus exerts these excitatory influences, the afferent discharge arising from the muscle spindles of gastrocnemius muscle is substantially decreased or even blocked during stimulation of the vermal part of the anterior lobe (GRANIT and KAADA, 1952). It is very likely that the direct cerebellovestibular pathway, which has an inhibitory action on Deiters' neurons, is responsible for the effect. In other words, the depression of the fusimotor discharge like that of the α rigidity, is probably due not to IPSPs of the γ motoneurons but to disfacilitation caused by cerebellar inhibition of Deiters' neurons and probably also of the fastigial nucleus.

Recent experiments indicate that there are two different types of fusimotor neurons which influence the static and the dynamic properties of primary afferents to stretch respectively (Matthews, 1962, 1964). It is generally assumed that γ activity leading to intrafusal contraction is an important feature of the extensor rigidity (Hunt, 1951; Kobayashi et al., 1952; Granit and Kaada, 1952; Eldred et al., 1953; Granit, 1955). Experiments performed in cats anesthetized with mixtures of nitrous oxide and Fluothane or ether, however, indicate that primary spindle afferents from extensor muscles lose their responsiveness to some extent after intercollicular decerebration (Barrios et al., 1968). At least in this experimental condition it appears that decerebration does not enhance the activity of primary spindle afferents by release of fusimotor activity. It is of interest, however, that a reduction of fusimotor activity to extensor muscles is caused in the decerebrate preparation by a transverse section of the spinal cord (Kobayashi et al., 1952; Diete-Spiff et al., 1962; Voorhoeve and van Kanten, 1962; Barrios et al., 1968). It appears now that in the decerebrate cat there is a background activity in both static and dynamic fusimotor efferents to extensor muscle spindles (Jansen and Matthews, 1962; Jansen, 1966). Since spinalization results in a severe decrease in the activity of static fusimotor efferents without a corresponding loss of function of the dynamic fusimotor efferents (Alnaes et al., 1965; Jansen, 1966; cf. however Barrios et al., 1968), it was concluded that activity in the static fusimotor efferents depends mainly upon descending suprasegmental activation, whereas the dynamic fusimotor neurons are activated by dorsal root inflow (cf. Hunt, 1951).

It would be interesting to know the origin of this supraspinal control on static fusimotor efferents, and also the role exerted by the cerebellum in these mechanisms. The tonogenic structures of the brainstem, particularly Deiters' nucleus, which are responsible for the decerebrate rigidity are likely to contribute to these static effects. Experiments involving intracellular recording indicate that Deiters' nucleus exerts a monosynaptic effect on static γ motoneurons innervating extensor muscles (Bergmans and Grillner, 1968). This conclusion is supported by other experiments showing that acceleration of group II afferent extensors occurs on stimulation of Deiters' nucleus (Carli et al., 1967a). This means that static γ motoneurons are accelerated (Appelberg et al., 1966; Brown et al., 1967). The short latency of these responses and the comparatively slight susceptibility to anesthesia (Pompeiano et al., 1967a, b) support the conclusion that the vestibulospinal tract is monosynaptically connected with these γ motoneurons.

It would also be of interest to know whether the cerebellum can influence static fusimotor neurons through the vestibular system. In studying the cerebellar control of muscle spindle function, Granit et al. (1955) found that the α–γ linkage, *i.e.*, the initiation of the motoneuronal discharge due to the activity in the γ loop, can be experimentally destroyed by anatomical and functional inactivation of the anterior lobe. Cooling or ablation of the anterior lobe of the cerebellum in particular increased the extensor rigidity but silenced the spindle discharge, *i.e.*, the spindle behaves passively, pausing during contraction. Matthews (1958) also observed a decrease in the action of γ motoneurons in anemic decerebrate preparations. This severe decrease of muscle spindle afferent activity was also associated with a decline of spindle reactivity, which included both the response to maintained passive muscle stretch and the reflex reaction to a natural labyrinthine or cutaneous stimulus.

VAN DER MEULEN and GILMAN (1965) observed a similar decrease of spindle response to maintained stretch and to other natural stimuli (external reactivity) following acute ablation of the entire cerebellum. Some recovery of the γ mechanisms occurs in the chronically decerebellate animal, however (HIGGINS and GLASER, 1964; DENNY-BROWN and GILMAN, 1965; VAN DER MEULEN and GILMAN, 1965; DENNY-BROWN, 1966; VAN DER MEULEN et al., 1966; GLASER and HIGGINS, 1966; GILMAN and McDONALD, 1967a, b). A recording of spindle activity a few days after total cerebellectomy is enough to show a recovery of the spindle responses to external stimulus. In these preparations, however, the responses of primary spindle receptor afferents in the gastrocnemius muscle to static muscle stretch are still reduced (GILMAN and McDONALD, 1967a, b). This cerebellar facilitation of the responses to static stretch of primary afferent endings in gastrocnemius spindles is both crossed and uncrossed (GILMAN, 1968). These observations indicate that the cerebellum is a supraspinal structure responsible for support of activity of static fusimotor efferents. It is still not known whether this effect is mediated by the crossed and uncrossed fastigiovestibular projections.

The demonstration that supraspinal structures do not exert a striking tonic influence on γ dynamic fusimotor efferents (ALNAES et al., 1965; JANSEN, 1966) does not exclude the possibility that some influence is exerted by cerebellovestibular volleys on this type of fusimotor neurons. Recent experiments indicate that the dynamic response of a primary ending to slow stretches increases during labyrinthine polarization, while it is abolished by high-rate stimulation of the anterior lobe of the cerebellum (JANSEN and MATTHEWS, 1962).

It appears therefore that there are two supraspinal mechanisms that affect the activity of static and dynamic fusimotor neurons respectively. More experiments are required to assess the role of the vestibular nuclei in the transmission of the cerebellar influences to both static and dynamic fusimotor neurons.

E. Cerebellar Control of Primary Afferents

The vestibular nuclei exert a depolarizing influence not only on the motoneurons, but also on the central endings of primary afferents to the spinal cord. Presynaptic inhibition through primary afferent depolarization can thus be evoked by the vestibular nuclei, and it is therefore possible that the cerebellum affects transmission through primary afferents by influencing the activity of the vestibular nuclei. CARPENTER et al. (1962, 1966) demonstrated that electrical stimulation of localized points of the medulla and caudal pons, including the region of the medial longitudinal fasciculus (MLF) and the medial vestibular nucleus, evoked primary afferent depolarization in the decerebrate cat, as shown by the appearance of negative dorsal root potentials and by excitability tests made according to WALL's technique (1958). The enhancement of excitability was found in both Ia and Ib muscle afferents and cutaneous fibers. These effects were abolished by section of the ventral quadrants of the spinal cord. Before a conclusion to the effect that the descending projection originating from the vestibular nuclei is responsible for this presynaptic inhibitory effect is justified, three points should be discussed.

i) It is probable that when the MLF was electrically stimulated in the experiments of CARPENTER et al. (1962, 1966), even the reticulospinal fibers coursing along this tract were excited.

ii) Presynaptic inhibition involved the lumbar segments, while the MLF is known to terminate mainly at midthoracic level (cf. POMPEIANO and BRODAL, 1957a; BRODAL et al., 1962; NYBERG-HANSEN, 1964; WILSON et al., 1967b, 1968a).

iii) The effects obtained by stimulating the area of the medial vestibular nuclei were ipsilateral while anatomical evidence (cf. BRODAL et al., 1962; NYBERG-HANSEN, 1964) suggests that the effects should be both crossed and uncrossed.

It is not apparent from these experiments involving brainstem stimulation how reflex transmission is effected by the primary afferent depolarization elicited by these supraspinal volleys. Experiments performed on unanaesthetized, decerebrate cats (COOK et al., 1968a, b, c) indicate that repetitive stimulation of the VIII cranial nerve elicits negative dorsal root potentials from the lumbar segments of the cord not only ipsilaterally but also contralaterally (cf. also ERULKAR et al., 1966). Depolarization of group I muscle afferents from both extensor and flexor nerves as well as of group II cutaneous afferents contribute to these dorsal root potentials (COOK et al., 1968a, b, c). Experiments involving chronic hemisection of the spinal cord at T10–12 indicate that the supraspinal effects on the group I primary afferents are abolished if the hemicord ipsilateral to the side of the section is stimulated. This suggests that the effects are not due to excitation from the MLF of propriospinal pathways. This observation together with the fact that these effects can be obtained in normal decerebrate cats by stimulating not only the ventral funiculus, where the MLF is located, but also the lateral funiculus, indicate that primary afferent depolarization is due to supraspinal descending volleys originating from the brainstem reticular formation. The vestibular nuclei, however, are responsible for the transmission of labyrinthine volleys to the reticular formation, as is apparent from the abolition of these effects after electrolytic lesion of these nuclei. Moreover, primary afferent depolarization of the group Ia muscular as well as group II cutaneous fibers was elicited when the MLF was stimulated not only at medullary but also at mesencephalic level.

Experiments were also performed to find out whether the vestibular apparatus modulated spinal sensory input while descending vestibular volleys evoked a motor response. Repetitive stimulation of the VIII cranial nerve evoked extrafusal contraction of the gastrocnemius-soleus muscle as well as negative dorsal root potentials at threshold frequencies of 100–200/sec. The amplitude of both responses increased in parallel with further increases in the stimulus intensity or frequency. A parallelism also exists between the excitability changes of the group I extensor afferents and the extrafusal contraction.

To test whether the vestibulum-induced primary afferent depolarization and associated presynaptic inhibition would uncouple the motoneurons from their segmental afferent input, the effect of VIII nerve stimulation on the extensor monosynaptic reflex was studied at different time intervals. The extensor monosynaptic reflex was not depressed but actually enhanced during conditioning stimulation of the VIII nerve. A parallelism was found between enhancement of the monosynaptic reflex and increase in excitability of the intraspinal terminals of the group I fibers arising from the same extensor muscles.

It is known that presynaptic depolarization of the primary afferents to spinal motoneurons results in a reduced postsynaptic efficacy of the orthodromic volley (ECCLES, 1964). This would tend to decrease the size of the monosynaptic reflex. This decrease, however, has to be weighed against the facilitation that results from postsynaptic depolarization of the α motoneurons. During stimulation of the VIII nerve the depression in synaptic transmission of the group I muscle afferent volleys due to presynaptic inhibitory mechanisms is apparently overwhelmed by the large increase in motoneuronal discharge.

The extent to which the cerebellum is able to affect these vestibular mechanisms is also of interest. It has been shown that large negative dorsal root potentials can be evoked from the cerebellar cortex, which are due to primary afferent depolarization in group Ib and cutaneous afferents but not in Ia afferents (CARPENTER et al., 1966). These effects are produced on stimulation of the most lateral strip of the intermediate region on both sides and cannot be relayed through the vestibular nuclei, since this cortical area projects to the interpositus and not to the fastigial nucleus. Stimulation of this area actually causes increased extensor rigidity (POMPEIANO, 1958) which may be relayed at least partly in the reticular formation (MAFFEI and POMPEIANO, 1961, 1962). On the other hand, no depolarization of the primary afferents was evoked from the anterior vermis, whereas

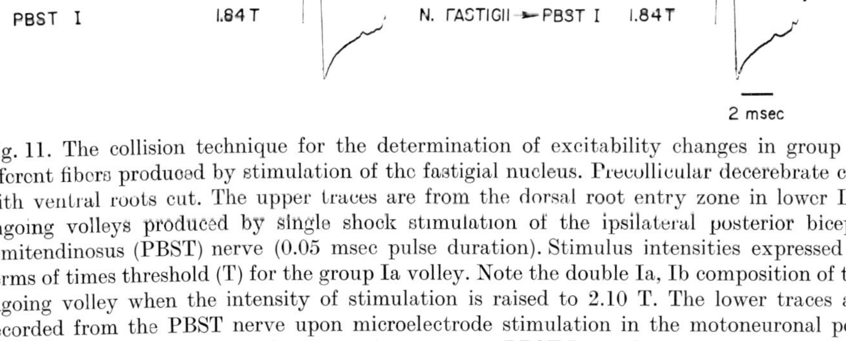

Fig. 11. The collision technique for the determination of excitability changes in group Ia afferent fibers produced by stimulation of the fastigial nucleus. Precollicular decerebrate cat, with ventral roots cut. The upper traces are from the dorsal root entry zone in lower L7. Ingoing volleys produced by single shock stimulation of the ipsilateral posterior biceps-semitendinosus (PBST) nerve (0.05 msec pulse duration). Stimulus intensities expressed in terms of times threshold (T) for the group Ia volley. Note the double Ia, Ib composition of the ingoing volley when the intensity of stimulation is raised to 2.10 T. The lower traces are recorded from the PBST nerve upon microelectrode stimulation in the motoneuronal pool with 0.1 msec pulses. The antidromic testing response (PBST I) is enhanced during conditioning stimulation of the contralateral caudal part of the fastigial nucleus at 500/sec, 0.3 msec pulse duration, 1.4 times the threshold for crossed forelimb extension (N. FASTIGII→PBST I). Both these centrally evoked group I volleys are collided with an orthodromic volley initiated in the Ia afferents of the PBST nerve (1.84 T). This indicates that fastigial stimulation increases the excitability of the central endings of the group Ia fibers (COOK et al., 1968d)

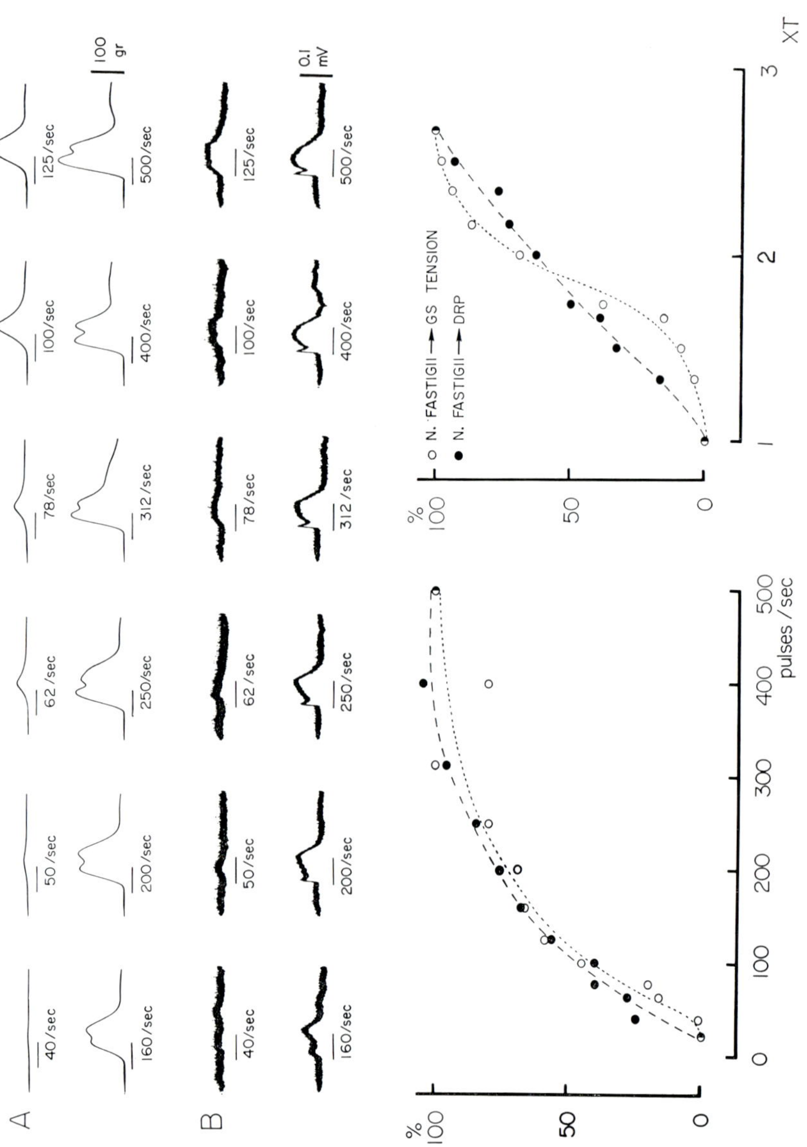

Fig. 12. Muscle contractions and dorsal root potentials evoked by stimulation of the fastigial nucleus. Precollicular, decerebrate cat. A: muscle contraction of the left gastrocnemius-soleus muscle (GS) recorded isometrically at an initial extension of 6 mm. Ipsilateral dorsal roots L7–S2 intact. B: dorsal root potentials (DRPs) recorded from lower L6 on the left side. The filament was cut 15 mm from the dorsal root entry zone and placed on two electrodes, one close to the entry zone and the other on the cut end. Upwards deflection denotes negativity of the central electrode. Effects of repetitive stimulation of the caudal part of contralateral fastigial nucleus with 0.5 msec rectangular pulses, and at the frequencies indicated below each record. The stimulus intensity used corresponded to 2.0 times the threshold (T) for crossed forelimb extension obtained at 500/sec. The amplitude of these responses has been plotted in the left graph. In the right graph both muscle tension and dorsal root potentials (elicited by stimulation of the fastigial nucleus at 500/sec) are plotted as a function of the stimulus intensities expressed in multiples of T (COOK et al., 1968d)

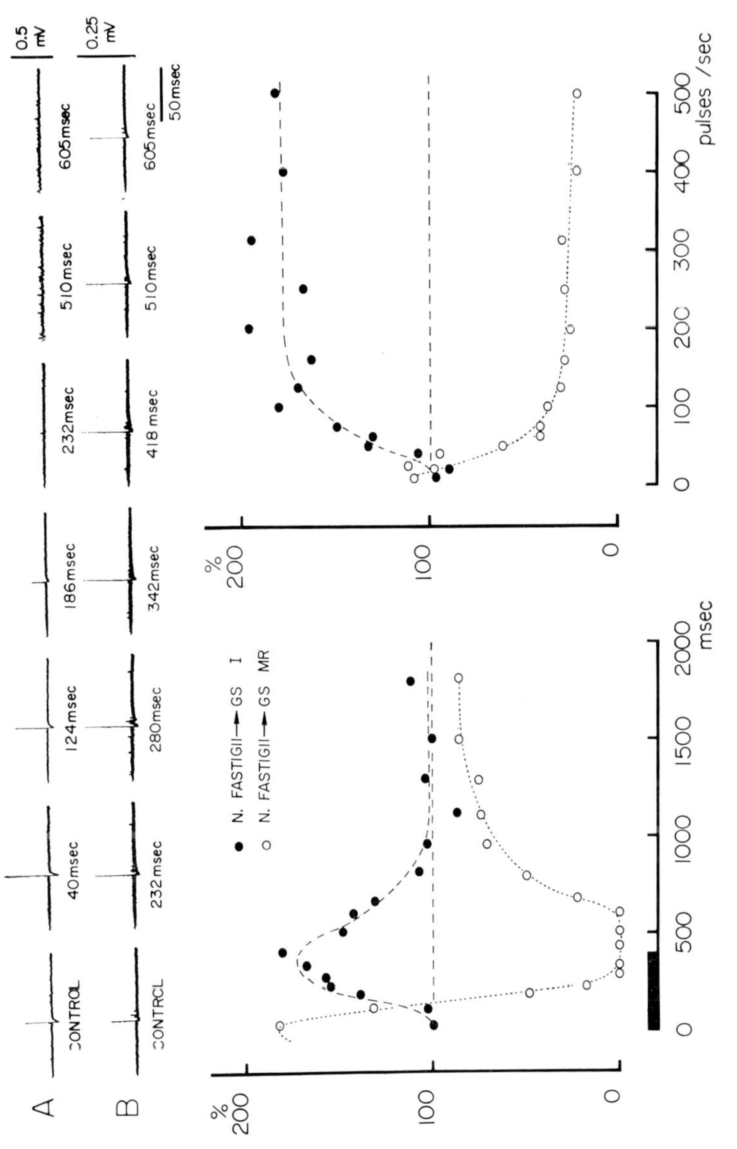

Fig. 13. Gastrocnemius-soleus (GS) monosynaptic reflexes (A) and group I antidromic volleys recorded from GS nerve (B) conditioned by stimulation of the caudal part of the contralateral fastigial nucleus. Precollicular decerebrate cat with ventral roots cut. The fastigial nucleus was stimulated at 500/sec, 0.2 msec pulse duration, 2.0 times the threshold for crossed forelimb extension. Intervals between onset of conditioning volleys and test volley indicated in msec. The amplitudes of the antidromic volleys (dots) and monosynaptic reflexes (circles) partially illustrated in A and B are plotted in the left graph. In the right graph the amplitudes of the extensor monosynaptic reflex and the group I antidromic volley from GS nerve are plotted as a function of the frequency of fastigial stimulation. The interval between beginning of the conditioning tetanus and the testing shock was 415 msec for the antidromic volley and 573 msec for the monosynaptic reflex (Cook et al., 1968d)

there was a profound inhibition of ipsilateral extensor motoneurons from this region. The conclusion drawn from these experiments was that the cerebellum does not affect presynaptic transmission through the group Ia fibers. Recent experiments, however, have shown that both fastigial nuclei and the cerebellar cortex are able to affect transmission through this pathway (Cook et al., 1968d).

Stereotaxic stimulation of the fastigial nucleus is particularly effective in the production of primary afferent depolarization (PAD) in group Ia fibers (Fig. 11) and also in group II cutaneous afferents (Cook et al., 1968d). Stimulation of the fastigial neurons without contamination of the long inhibitory corticofugal fibers directed to the vestibular nuclei can be obtained on stimulation of the caudal part of the fastigial nucleus. Since a crossed fastigiovestibular projection originates in this fastigial nucleus, the large PAD on both group Ia and cutaneous afferents can be recorded contralaterally to the stimulated side. It has been shown previously that the hook bundle of Russell exerts an excitatory influence on the extensor motoneurons. Figure 12 clearly shows a parallelism between tension recorded from the extensor muscle and PAD elicited by repetitive stimulation of this cerebellar efferent projection. The effect of fastigial stimulation on the extensor monosynaptic reflex and on the excitability changes of the central endings of the group Ia fibers was also studied at different time intervals (Fig. 13). In these experiments the extensor monosynaptic reflex generally showed an early facilitation followed by a late depression. This effect can be attributed to the large amount of presynaptic depolarization which greatly reduces the postsynaptic efficacy of the orthodromic volley. This fastigial influence on primary afferents is probably at least partly due to fastigiofugal excitation of the vestibular nuclei; however it is possible that direct impingement of the hook bundle of Russell on the same descending reticular system excited by the vestibular nuclei also plays some role.

A final group of experiments has been devoted to the effect of stimulation of the cerebellar cortex on the level of polarization of the intraspinal terminals of the primary afferents (Cook et al., 1968d). In contrast to previous negative results (Carpenter et al., 1966), stimulation of the vermal cortex of the anterior lobe produced an hyperpolarization of the central endings of primary afferents in some instances as shown by the occurrence of positive dorsal root potentials (Fig. 14). Moreover, the same vermal cortex stimulation can also depress the PAD in the group Ia and group II cutaneous afferents elicited by repetitive stimulation of the ipsilateral VIII nerve (Fig. 14), while ablation of the vermal cortex or of the whole cerebellum enhances these effects. The positive dorsal root potential elicited by vermal stimulation can thus be referred to removal of primary afferent depolarization produced by the vestibular activity.

In summary, the vestibulum-induced PAD in group Ia muscular and group II cutaneous afferents may serve as a negative feedback to transmission from these afferents to motoneurons. This effect is potentiated by the activity of the fastigial nuclei and is under the inhibitory control of the cerebellar cortex. The release of the vestibular activity following cerebellectomy is therefore responsible not only for an increase in motoneuronal discharge, but also for an increase in the presynaptic depolarization of the primary afferents induced by orthodromic VIII nerve volleys.

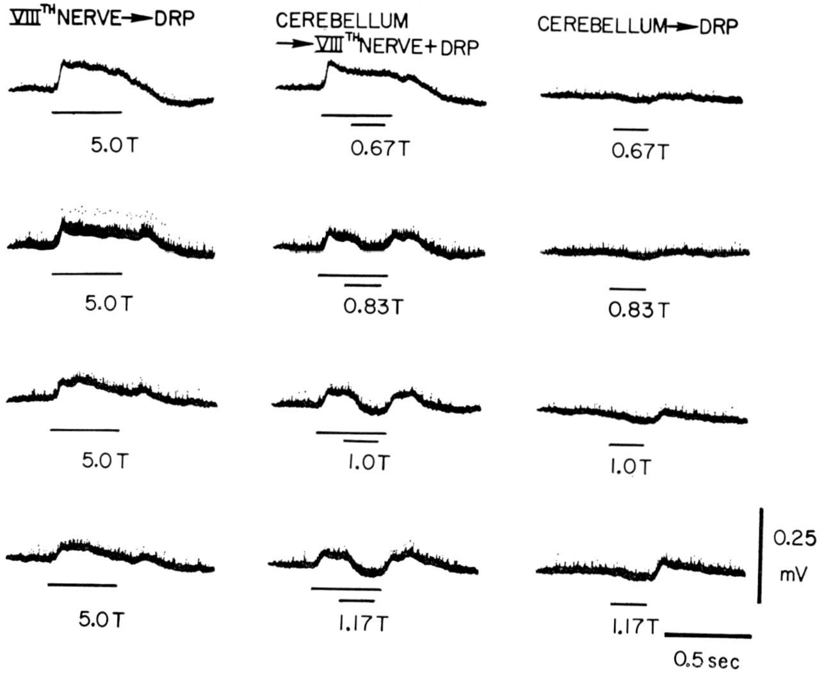

Fig. 14. Cerebellar inhibition of the dorsal root potentials evoked by VIII nerve stimulationl Precollicular decerebrate cat. Dorsal root potentials (DRPs) recorded from the most cauda. dorsal rootlet in L6 on the left side. The filament was cut 15 mm from the dorsal root entry zone and placed on two electrodes, one close to the entry zone and the other on the cut end. Upwards deflection denotes negativity of the central electrode. The DRPs in the left column are evoked by stimulating the VIII nerve with rectangular pulses at 500/sec, 0.2 msec pulse duration, 5.0 times the threshold (T) for the monosynaptic response of the second order vestibular neurons to VIII nerve stimulation as recorded from the ascending medial longitudinal fascicle. The right column shows the effects of stimulation of the ipsilateral vermal cortex of the cerebellar anterior lobe with trains at 500/sec, 0.2 msec pulse duration, and at different stimulus intensities (from 0.67 to 1.17) expressed in multiples of the threshold for the inhibition of the ipsilateral forelimb rigidity. Cerebellar stimulation produces a positive DRP followed by a negative DRP as rebound. The middle column illustrates the effects of combined stimulation of the VIII nerve and the cerebellum at strengths given in the corresponding records. Note the removal of the negative DRP evoked from the VIII nerve during cerebellar stimulations (Cook et al., 1968d)

F. Cerebellar Control of Transmission through Ascending Spinal Pathways

We should also consider whether descending impulses originating from the vestibular nuclei affect the transmission of somatic afferent volleys through ascending spinal pathways, and whether the cerebellum can influence these vestibular mechanisms.

There is no experimental evidence so far indicating that the vestibular volleys exert any influence on the transmission of somatic afferent volleys through both the dorsal and the ventral spinocerebellar tracts.

In the spinal cord there are ascending pathways that are distinct from the spinocerebellar tracts (cf. Lundberg, 1964), whose neurons are activated by group II and III muscle afferents, skin and high threshold joint afferents (the flexion reflex afferents: FRA), *i.e.*, by the same afferents as evoke the flexion reflex (Eccles and Lundberg, 1959). The neurons with axons projecting to the ventral quadrants, which contribute particularly to the spinoreticular pathway, have a bilateral receptive field. Recent experiments performed on unanesthetized decerebrate cats have shown the existence of a supraspinal control system which excites the above pathway ascending in the contralateral ventral quadrant of the spinal cord from the lumbar segments to the brainstem (Holmqvist et al., 1960b). It is not possible to decide from these experiments whether these neurons belong to a vestibulospinal or a reticulospinal pathway. Experimental evidence indicated that the axons of this pathway, which may reach a conduction velocity of 100 m/sec, descend in the ipsilateral ventral quadrant of the cord and reach the lower thoracic and lumbar segments to make monosynaptic connections with the ascending pathway. It is of interest that this brainstem response appeared at a low stimulus strength when the electrode was placed superficially in the region of the lateral recess of the fourth ventricle. Stereotaxic stimulation of the brainstem actually indicates that the lowest threshold values are found in the region of the brainstem where the axons of the vestibulospinal tract are located (Busch, 1964). It therefore seems reasonable to suggest that this supraspinal control system originates in Deiters' nucleus. It appears that this system can be influenced from the cortex of the cerebellar anterior lobe (Holmqvist et al., 1960b); the control system influencing the right ascending pathway is organized as follows. There are two excitatory cortical areas of the cerebellar anterior lobe; the right area consists of the whole of the intermediate cortex and the lateral strip of the vermal cortex, while the left area consists of a lateral strip of the intermediate cortex. Stimulation of both these cortical areas elicits discharges in the ascending pathway. These are due to volleys coursing in cerebellofugal fibers which make a monosynaptic connection in the brainstem with the neurons of the descending pathway. Double

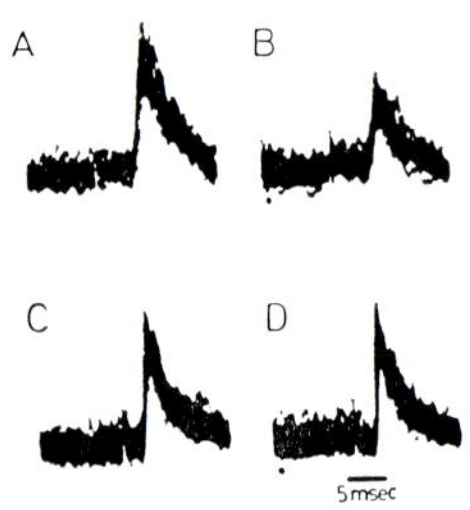

Fig. 15. Cerebellar inhibition of the discharge evoked in the ventral ascending spinal pathway. Ascending discharge recorded from the dissected right half (except dorsal column) of the spinal cord at Th 8. The test discharge in the upper records (shown alone in A) was evoked by a single stimulus applied at the left rostral corner of the intermediate cortex of the anterior lobe. The test discharge in the lower records (shown alone in C) was evoked by submaximal stimulation of the intact left spinal half (dorsal column removed) in the midthoracic region. In B and D a single conditioning stimulus was applied to the left anterior vermis. This conditioning stimulus inhibits the former (B) but not the latter (D) test response (Holmqvist et al., 1960b)

shock stimulation of the cerebellar cortex was usually needed to evoke this discharge. The shortest time necessary for the impulses originating in the cerebellar cortex to reach the brainstem was about 2 msec, thus suggesting a relay station in the cerebellar nuclei. Because of the inhibitory function recently attributed to the Purkinje cells, the question arises as to whether these effects are due to antidromic excitation of cerebellopetal pathways giving collaterals to the fastigial nuclei. This stimulation would lead to excitation of the fastigiovestibular projection through an axo-axonic reflex. If this hypothesis is correct, a bilateral lesion of the fastigial nuclei will abolish these responses. The interesting point is that the discharge evoked in the ascending spinal pathway on stimulation of the excitatory areas was completely inhibited by stimulation of the inhibitory area, which consisted of the cerebellar cortex between the two excitatory areas. The inhibition was exerted at the level of the brainstem nucleus and not of the spinal nucleus of the ascending tract (Fig. 15). The inhibition appeared in response to single stimuli and had a conduction time of about 1 msec from the cerebellar cortex to the brainstem. This short-latency inhibitory response is likely to be due to the activity of Purkinje cells which project from the anterior lobe cortex directly to Deiters' nucleus. The Deiters' neurons respond only to stimulation of cutaneous and high-threshold muscle afferents, and not to stimulation of the group I a muscle afferents (GIAQUINTO et al., 1963; WILSON et al., 1965, 1966a) and this effect is mediated at least in part by volleys coursing along the spinoreticular pathway. It seems likely that there is a positive feedback loop between Deiters' nucleus and the neurons of this ascending spinal hindlimb tract, and that this mechanism is under the inhibitory control of the cerebellar cortex.

It should be recalled that transmission from hindlimb nerves to this ascending pathway is controlled by another supraspinal system (HOLMQVIST et al., 1960a). This control is inhibitory and is tonically active in the decerebrate preparation to the degree that transmission from the nerves can be completely suppressed. The centers responsible are located in the brainstem and the tonic control is uninfluenced by stimulation of the cerebellum leading to complete collapse of decerebrate rigidity and also by ablation of cerebellum and the vestibular nuclei. Presumably the inhibitory effect is exerted on the interneurons mediating excitation from the nerves and would not interfere with the monosynaptic transmission originating in the vestibular nuclei.

VI. Conclusion

Electrophysiological experiments have clearly proved the existence of functional relationships between the vestibular system and the flocculonodular lobe and the corpus cerebelli. It is striking that while labyrinthine volleys impinge upon a restricted cerebellar cortical area (the flocculonodular lobe), the vestibular nuclei are under the cerebellofugal control not only of the vestibulocerebellum but also of a cortical area (namely the vermis) that does not receive primary or secondary vestibular afferent volleys. This cortical area actually integrates impulses from different sources, particularly from spinal, acoustic and visual inputs. Unfortunately there is no direct information on the input-output relation of the different types of labyrinthine and extralabyrinthine volleys at corticocerebellar level.

The experimental evidence so far presented indicates that the vestibular nuclei receive excitatory impulses through both the primary vestibular afferents and the fastigiovestibular pathways but are under the inhibitory control of Purkinje neurons. The long-axon Purkinje neurons, which contribute to the direct cerebello-vestibular projection, have a particularly inhibitory action on the vestibular neurons. The possibility that this function can also be applied to the short-axon Purkinje neurons projecting to the fastigial nucleus is supported by some electrophysiological experiments. There are, however, still some difficulties in the interpretation of the results obtained in some experiments based on cerebellar stimulation and ablation.

Most of the findings reviewed in this report relate to the cerebellar control of vestibular influences exerted on the oculomotor nuclei and on spinal motoneurons. More recent experiments, however, indicate that labyrinthine volleys can control not only the activity of the oculomotor and spinal motoneurons, but also the transmission of sensory volleys. The vestibular system may affect somatic afferent transmission at the same time as descending vestibular volleys elicit a motoneuronal discharge, particularly in the spinal cord. This mechanism of sensorimotor integration appears to be under the control of the cerebellum. It is thus possible for this structure to contribute to an appropriate integration of the somatic sensory input and the corresponding motor output.

References

Aitken, J.T., Bridger, J.E.: Neuron size and neuron population density in the lumbosacral region of the cat's spinal cord. J. Anat. (Lond.) **95**, 38–53 (1961).

Allen, F.W.: Distribution of the fibers originating from the different basal cerebellar nuclei. J. comp. Neurol. **36**, 399–439 (1924).

Allen, G., Fernández, G.: Experimental observations in postural nystagmus. I. Extensive lesions in posterior vermis of the cerebellum. Acta oto-laryng. (Stockh.) **51**, 2–14 (1960).

Alnaes, E., Jansen, J.K.S., Rudjord, T.: Fusimotor activity in the spinal cat. Acta physiol. scand. **63**, 197–212 (1965).

Andersson, S., Gernandt, B.E.: Cortical projection of vestibular nerve in cat. Acta oto-laryng. (Stockh.) Suppl. **116**, 10–18 (1954).

Andersson, A., Gernandt, B.E.: Ventral root discharge in response to vestibular and proprioceptive stimulation. J. Neurophysiol. **19**, 524–543 (1956).

Angaut, P., Brodal, A.: The projection of the "vestibulo-cerebellum" onto the vestibular nuclei in the cat. Arch. ital. Biol. **105**, 441–479 (1967).

Appelberg, B., Bessou, P., Laporte, Y.: Action of static and dynamic fusimotor fibres on secondary endings of cat's spindles. J. Physiol. (Lond.) **185**, 160–171 (1966).

Arduini, A., Pompeiano, O.: Modificazioni dell' attività di unità fastigiali prodotte da stimolazioni cortico-cerebellari e sensitive. Boll. Soc. ital. Biol. sper. **32**, 947–948 (1956a).

Arduini, A., Pompeiano, O.: Influence of cerebellar cortical and sensory volleys on the firing rate of fastigial units. Proc. XX. int. Congr. physiol. Sci. Bruxelles, 32, 1956b.

Arduini, A., Pompeiano, O.: Modificazioni dell'attività di singole unità nel nucleo del tetto per stimolazioni della corteccia cerebellare e della periferia sensitiva. Rend. Accad. naz. Lincei, Cl. Sci. fis., mat. nat., Serie VIII, **22**, 98–100 (1957a).

Arduini, A., Pompeiano, O.: Microelectrode analysis of units of the rostral portion of the nucleus fastigii. Arch. ital. Biol. **95**, 56–70 (1957b).

Aschan, G., Ekvall, L., Grant, G.: Nystagmus following stimulation in the central vestibular pathways using permanently implanted electrodes. Acta oto-laryng. (Stockh.) **58**, Suppl. **192**, 63–77 (1964).

Azzena, G.B., Giretti, M.L.: Responses of the oculomotor units to deep cerebellar stimulation. Brain Res. **6**, 523–534 (1967).

BARRIOS, P., HAASE, J., NASSR-ESFAHANI, H., NOTH, J., ROPTE, H.: Statische und dynamische Aktivitätsänderungen primärer Spindelafferenzen aus den Fussextensoren und prätibialen Flexoren der anaesthesierten und deafferentierten Katze nach intercolliculärer Dezerebrierung, tiefer Spinalisierung und Deefferentierung. Pflügers Arch. ges. Physiol. **299**, 128–148 (1968).

BATINI, C., MORUZZI, G., POMPEIANO, O.: Componenti labirintiche ed extralabirintiche nelle manifestazioni spastiche del gatto decerebrato e decerebellato. Rend .Accad. naz. Lincei, Cl. Sci. fis., mat. nat., Serie VIII, **21**, 328–332 (1956a).

BATINI, C., MORUZZI, G., POMPEIANO, O.: Influenza degli impulsi vestibolari sulla rigidità estensoria dell'arto deafferentato. Boll. Soc. ital. Biol. sper. **32**, 1293–1294 (1956b).

BATINI, C., MORUZZI, G., POMPEIANO, O.: Origine e meccanismi di compensazione dei fenomeni dinamici di Luciani. Rend. Accad. naz. Lincei, Cl. Sci. fis., mat. nat., Serie VIII, **21**, 474–479 (1956c).

BATINI, C., MORUZZI, G., POMPEIANO, O.: Sui meccanismi di compensazione dei fenomeni dinamici di Luciani. Boll. Soc. ital. Biol. sper. **32**, 1291–1292 (1956d).

BATINI, C., MORUZZI, G., POMPEIANO, O.: The release phenomena following cerebellectomy. Proc. XX. int. Congr. physiol. Sci., Bruxelles, 70–71, 1956e.

BATINI, C., MORUZZI, G., POMPEIANO, O.: Cerebellar release phenomena. Arch. ital. Biol. **95**, 71–95 (1957).

BATINI, C., POMPEIANO, O.: Sugli effetti di distruzioni croniche, parziali e totali, del nucleo del tetto nel gatto. Boll. Soc. ital. Biol. sper. **31**, 805–807 (1955).

BATINI, C., POMPEIANO, O.: Effetti di lesioni fastigiali croniche sul tono posturale del gatto. Rend. Accad. naz. Lincei, Cl. Sci. fis., mat. nat., Serie VIII, **20**, 504–507 (1956a).

BATINI, C., POMPEIANO, O.: Opposti effetti esercitati sulla rigidità da decerebrazione dalle porzioni rostro-mediali e rostro-laterali del nucleo del tetto. Boll. Soc. ital. Biol. sper. **32**, 1452–1453 (1956b).

BATINI, C., POMPEIANO, O.: Opposite effects on decerebrate rigidity of rostro-medial and rostro-lateral fastigial lesions. Proc. XX. int. Congr. physiol. Sci. Bruxelles, 71–72, 1956c.

BATINI, C., POMPEIANO, O.: Chronic fastigial lesions and their compensation in the cat. Arch. ital. Biol. **95**, 147–165 (1957).

BATINI, C., POMPEIANO, O.: Opposte influenze esercitate sul tono posturale dalle porzioni rostro-mediale e rostro-laterale del nucleo del tetto. Rend. Accad. naz. Lincei, Cl. Sci. fis., mat. nat., Serie VIII, **24**, 79–82 (1958a).

BATINI, C., POMPEIANO, O.: Effects of rostro-medial and rostro-lateral fastigial lesions on decerebrate rigidity. Arch. ital. Biol. **96**, 315–329 (1958b).

BAUER, J., LEIDLER, R.: Über den Einfluss der Ausschaltung verschiedener Hirnabschnitte auf die vestibulären Augenreflexe. Arb. neurol. Inst. Univ. Wien **19**, 155–225 (1912).

BECHTEREW, W.: Ergebnisse der Durchschneidung des N. acusticus, nebst Erörterung der Bedeutung der semicirculären Canäle für das Körpergleichgewicht. Pflügers Arch. ges. Physiol. **30**, 312–347 (1883).

BERGMANS, J., GRILLNER, S.: Monosynaptic control of static γ-motoneurones from the lower brain stem. Experientia (Basel) **24**, 146–147 (1968).

BILLIA, P.: Importanza dell'intensità dell'eccitamento vestibolare nei riguardi dei riflessi labirintici dopo lesione cerebellare. Boll. Soc. ital. Biol. sper. **28**, 1385–1386 (1952).

BREMER, F.: Contribution à l'étude de la physiologie du cervelet. La fonction inhibitrice du paléocerebellum. Arch. int. Physiol. **19**, 189–226 (1922).

BREMER, F.: Le cervelet. In: G.H. ROGER and L. BINET. Traité de physiologie normale et pathologique. Vol. 10. Paris: Masson 1935.

BRODAL, A.: Anatomical aspects and functional organization of the vestibular nuclei. In: Second symposium on the role of the vestibular organs in space exploration. NASA SP-**115**, 119–141 (1966).

BRODAL, A.: Anatomical studies of cerebellar fibre connections with special reference to problems of functional localization. In: C.A. FOW and R.S. SNIDER: Progress in Brain Research, Vol. 25. The Cerebellum. Amsterdam: Elsevier Publ. Co. 1967a.

BRODAL, A.: Anatomical organization of cerebello-vestibulo-spinal pathways. In: A.V.S. DE REUCK and J. KNIGHT: Myotatic, Kinesthetic and vestibular mechanisms. Ciba Foundation Symposium. London: J. and A. Churchill 1967b.

Brodal, A., Drablos, P.A.: Two types of mossy fiber terminals in the cerebellum and their regional distribution. J. comp. Neurol. **12**, 173–187 (1963).

Brodal, A., Høivik, B.: Site and mode of termination of primary vestibulocerebellar fibres in the cat. An experimental study with silver impregnation methods. Arch. ital. Biol. **102**, 1–21 (1964).

Brodal, A., Pompeiano, O.: The vestibular nuclei in the cat. J. Anat. (Lond.) **91**, 438–454 (1957).

Brodal, A., Pompeiano, O.: The origin of ascending fibres of the medial longitudinal fasciculus from the vestibular nuclei. Acta morph. neerl.-scand. **1**, 306–328 (1958).

Brodal, A., Pompeiano, O., Walberg, F.: The vestibular nuclei and their connections. Anatomy and functional correlations. Edinburgh, London: Oliver and Boyd 1962.

Brodal, A., Torvik, A.: Über den Ursprung des sekundären vestibulocerebellaren Fasern bei der Katze. Eine experimentell anatomische Studie. Arch. Psychiat. Nervenkr. **195**, 550–567 (1957).

Brown, M.C., Engberg, I., Matthews, P.B.C.: Fusimotor stimulation and the dynamic sensitivity of the secondary ending of the muscle spindle. J. Physiol. (Lond.) **189**, 545–550 (1967).

Buchanan, A.R.: Post-rotatory nystagmus following decerebration in guinea pigs with unilateral cerebellar lesions. Proc. Soc. exp. Biol. (N.Y.). **37**, 713–715 (1938).

Busch, H.F.M.: An anatomical analysis of the white matter in the brain stem of the cat. Leiden: Van Gorcum and Co. N.V. – Dr. H.J. Prakke and H.M.G. Prakke 1961.

Cajal, S.R.: Histologie du système nerveux de l'homme et des vertébrés. Tome I et II. Paris: Maloine 1909–1911.

Camis, M.: Le correnti d'azione nel cervelletto per eccitamento del laberinto. Arch. Sci. biol. (Bologna) **1**, 92–119 (1919).

Camis, M.: Nuove osservazioni sui movimenti deambulatori: l'azione delle basse temperature sul cervelletto. Boll. Soc. med. Parma **15**, 54–56 (1922).

Camis, M.: Recherches sur le mécanisme central des mouvements de déambulation. Arch. int. Physiol. **20**, 340–370 (1923).

Camis, M.: La fisiologia dell'apparato vestibolare. Bologna: Zanichelli 1928.

Carli, G., Diete-Spiff, K., Pompeiano, O.: Effetti della stimolazione elettrica del nucleo di Deiters sulla scarica afferente fusale e sulla tensione muscolare nel gastrocnemio di gatto. Boll. Soc. ital. Biol. sper. **42**, 999–1001 (1966a).

Carli, G., Diete-Spiff, K., Pompeiano, O.: Persistenza della risposta di recettori fusali alla stimolazione del nucleo di Deiters dopo blocco periferico dei γ-motoneuroni. Boll. Soc. ital. Biol. sper. **42**, 1001–1003 (1966b).

Carli, G., Diete-Spiff, K., Pompeiano, O.: Skeletomotor and fusimotor control of gastrocnemius muscle from Deiters' nucleus. Experientia (Basel) **22**, 583–584 (1966c).

Carli, G., Diete-Spiff, K., Pompeiano, O.: Responses of the muscle spindle and of the extrafusal fibres in an extensor muscle to stimulation of the lateral vestibular nucleus in the cat. Arch. ital. Biol. **105**, 209–242 (1967a).

Carli, G., Diete-Spiff, K., Pompeiano, O.: Meccanismi attivi e passivi responsabili dell'eccitazione dei recettori fusali. Boll. Soc. ital. Biol. sper. **43**, 275–277 (1967b).

Carli, G., Diete-Spiff, K., Pompeiano, O.: Active and passive factors in muscle spindle excitation. Nature (Lond.) **214**, 838–839 (1967c).

Carli, G., Diete-Spiff, K., Pompeiano, O.: Mechanisms of muscle spindle excitation. Arch. ital. Biol. **105**, 273–289 (1967d).

Carli, G., Pompeiano, O.: Crossed fastigial influence on muscle spindle receptors. Unpublished observations, 1968.

Carpenter, D., Engberg, I., Lundberg, A.: Presynaptic inhibition in the lumbar cord evoked from the brain stem. Experientia (Basel) **18**, 450–451 (1962).

Carpenter, D., Engberg, I., Lundberg, A.: Primary afferent depolarization evoked from the brain stem and the cerebellum. Arch. ital. Biol. **104**, 73–85 (1966).

Carpenter, M.D.: Lesions of the fastigial nuclei in the rhesus monkey. Amer. J. Anat. **104**, 1–25 (1959).

CARPENTER, M.B.: Fiber projections from the descending and lateral vestibular nuclei in the cat. Amer. J. Anat. **107**, 1–22 (1960a).

CARPENTER, M.B.: Experimental anatomical-physiological studies of the vestibular nerve and cerebellar connections. In: G.L. RASMUSSEN and W.F. WINDLE: Neural mechanisms of the auditory and vestibular system. Springfield, Ill.: C.C. Thomas 1960b.

CARPENTER, M.B., ALLING, F.A., BARD, D.S.: Lesions of the descending vestibular nucleus in the cat. J. comp. Neurol. **114**, 39–50 (1960).

CARPENTER, M.B., BARD, D.S., ALLING, F.A.: Anatomical connections between the fastigial nuclei, the labyrinth and the vestibular nuclei in the cat. J. comp. Neurol. **111**, 1–26 (1959a).

CARPENTER, M.B., BRITTIN, G.M., PINES, J.: Isolated lesions of the fastigial nuclei in the cat. J. comp. Neurol. **109**, 65–89 (1958).

CARPENTER, M.B., FABREGA, H., GLINSMANN, W.: Physiological deficits occurring with lesions of labyrinth and fastigial nuclei. J. Neurophysiol. **22**, 222–234 (1959b).

CARPENTER, M.B., STROMINGER, N.L.: Cerebello-oculomotor fibers in the Rhesus monkey. J. comp. Neurol. **123**, 211–229 (1964).

CARREA, R.M.E., METTLER, F.A.: Physiologic consequences following extensive removals of the cerebellar cortex and deep cerebellar nuclei and effect of secondary cerebral ablations in the primate. J. comp. Neurol. **87**, 169–288 (1947).

CARREA, R.M.E., REISSIG, M., METTLER, F.A.: The climbing fibers of the simian and feline cerebellum. Experimental inquiry into their origin by lesions of the inferior olives and deep cerebellar nuclei. J. comp. Neurol. **87**, 321–365 (1947).

CHAMBERS, W.W., SPRAGUE, J.M.: Functional localization in the cerebellum. I. Organization in longitudinal cortico-nuclear zones and their contribution to the control of posture, both extrapyramidal and pyramidal. J. comp. Neurol. **103**, 105–129 (1955a).

CHAMBERS, W.W., SPRAGUE, J.M.: Functional localization in the cerebellum. II. Somatotopic organization in cortex and nuclei. Arch. Neurol. Psychiat. (Chic.) **74**, 653–680 (1955b).

CHANG, H.T., KOSTYUK, P.G.: Discharges of single neurons of the toad's cerebellum evoked by stimulating the vestibular nerve. Sechenov J. Physiol. U.S.S.R. **46**, 926–932 (1960).

COHEN, B., GOTO, K., SHANZER, S., WEISS, A.H.: Eye movements induced by electrical stimulation of the cerebellum in the alert cat. Exp. Neurol. **13**, 145–162 (1965).

COHEN, D., CHAMBERS, W.W., SPRAGUE, J.M.: Experimental study of the efferent projections from the cerebellar nuclei to the brainstem of the cat. J. comp. Neurol. **109**, 233–259 (1958).

CONNOR, G.J.: Functional localization within the anterior cerebellum. Proc. Soc. exp. Biol. (N.Y.) **47**, 205–207 (1941).

CONNOR, G.J., GERMAN, W.J.: Functional localization within the anterior cerebellar lobe. Trans. Amer. neurol. Ass. **67**, 181–186 (1941).

COOK, W.A., JR., CANGIANO, A., POMPEIANO, O.: Vestibular influences on primary afferents in the spinal cord. Pflügers Arch. ges. Physiol. **299**, 334–338 (1968a).

COOK, W.A., JR., CANGIANO, A., POMPEIANO, O.: Vestibular evoked primary afferent depolarization in the lumbar spinal cord. Proc. XXIV int. Congr. physiol. Sci., Washington D.C., **7**, 272 (1968b).

COOK, W.A., JR., CANGIANO, A., POMPEIANO, O.: Vestibular control of transmission in primary afferents to the lumbar spinal cord. Arch. ital. Biol. **107**, 296–320 (1968c).

COOK, W.A., JR., CANGIANO, A., POMPEIANO, O.: Controllo cerebellare sulla trasmissione di impulsi spinali lungo le fibre afferenti muscolari di gruppo I. Boll. Soc. ital. Biol. sper. **44**, fasc. 20 bis, n. 85 (1968d).

CRANMER, R.: Nystagmus related to lesions of the central vestibular apparatus and the cerebellum. Ann. Otol. (St. Louis) **60**, 186–196 (1951).

CURTIS, D.R., WATKINS, J.C.: The pharmacology of amino acids related to gamma-aminobutyric acid. Pharmacol. Rev. **17**, 347–391 (1965).

DEMETRIADES, TH.D., SPIEGEL, E.A.: Zur Frage der Bedeutung des Kleinhirns für die Entwicklung von Spontannystagmus. Z. Hals-, Nas.- u. Ohrenheilk. **19**, 250–257 (1927).

DENNY-BROWN, D.: The cerebral control of movement. Liverpool: Liverpool University Press 1966.

DENNY-BROWN, D., ECCLES, J.C., LIDDELL, E.G.T.: Observation on electrical stimulation of the cerebellar cortex. Proc. roy. Soc. B **104**, 518–536 (1929).

Denny-Brown, D., Gilman, S.: Depression of gamma innervation by cerebellectomy. Trans. Amer. neurol. Ass. **90**, 96–101 (1965).

De Vito, R.V., Brusa, A., Arduini, A.: Cerebellar and vestibular influences on Deitersian units. J. Neurophysiol. **19**, 241–253 (1956).

Diete-Spiff, K., Dodsworth, H., Pascoe, J.E.: An analysis of the effect of ether and ethyl chloride on the discharge frequency of gastrocnemius fusimotor neurones in the rabbit. In: D. Barker, Ed. Symposium on muscle receptors. Hong Kong: Hong Kong University Press 1962.

Diete-Spiff, K., Carli, G., Pompeiano, O.: Analisi delle risposte motorie extra- ed intrafusali prodotte dalla stimolazione elettrica del nervo ottavo e dei nuclei vestibolari nel gastrocnemio di gatto. Boll. Soc. ital. Biol. sper. **42**, fasc. 20 bis, n. 1 (1966).

Diete-Spiff, K., Carli, G., Pompeiano, O.: Spindle responses and extrafusal contraction on stimulation of the VIIIth cranial nerve or the vestibular nuclei in the cat. Pflügers Arch. ges. Physiol. **293**, 276–280 (1967a).

Diete-Spiff, K., Carli, G., Pompeiano, O.: Comparison of the effects of stimulation of the VIIIth cranial nerve, the vestibular nuclei or the reticular formation on the gastrocnemius muscle and its spindles. Arch. ital. Biol. **105**, 243–272 (1967b).

Di Giorgio, A.M.: Comportamento delle reazioni oculari labirintiche nelle lesioni di una metà laterale del cervelletto. Boll. Soc. ital. Biol. sper. **26**, 31–32 (1950a).

Di Giorgio, A.M.: Réflexes vestibulaires et cervelet. Acta oto-rhino-laryng. belg. **4**, 282–294 (1950b).

Di Giorgio, A.M.: Influenza della deviazione degli occhi da lesione cerebellare sui caratteri del nistagmo vestibolare. Boll. Soc. ital. Biol. sper. **26**, 32–34 (1950c).

Di Giorgio, A.M.: Significato della "via finale comune" nel determinismo delle reazioni asimmetriche vestibolari da lesioni del cervelletto. Boll. Soc. ital. Biol. sper. **31**, 31–32 (1955).

Di Giorgio, A.M., Hahn, R.: Azione inibitrice della corteccia cerebellare stricninizzata sui riflessi vestibolari. Boll. Soc. ital. Biol. sper. **27**, 1354–1355 (1951).

Di Giorgio, A.M., Pestellini, G.: Inibizione acquisita dei riflessi vestibolari. Significato degli emisferi cerebrali e del cervelletto. Arch. Fisiol. **48**, 86–110 (1948).

Dohlman, G.F.: Histochemical studies of vestibular mechanisms. In: G.L. Rasmussen and W.F. Windle: Neural mechanisms of the auditory and vestibular systems. Springfield, Ill.: C.C. Thomas 1960.

Dohlman, G., Farkashidy, J., Salonna, F.: Centrifugal nerve fibres to the sensory epithelium of the vestibular labyrinth. J. Laryng. **72**, 984 (1958).

Dow, R.S.: The relation of the paraflocculus to movements of the eyes. Amer. J. Physiol. **113**, 296–298 (1935).

Dow, R.S.: The fiber connections of the posterior parts of the cerebellum in the rat and cat. J. comp. Neurol. **63**, 527–548 (1936).

Dow, R.S.: Efferent connections of the flocculo-nodular lobe in Macaca mulatta. J. comp. Neurol. **68**, 297–305 (1938a).

Dow, R.S.: Effects of lesions in the vestibular part of the cerebellum in primates. Arch. Neurol. Psychiat. (Chic.) **40**, 500–520 (1938b).

Dow, R.S.: Cerebellar action potentials in response to stimulation of various afferent connections. J. Neurophysiol. **2**, 543–555 (1939).

Dow, R.S., Manni, E.: The relationship of the cerebellum to extraocular movements. In: Bender, M.B. The oculomotor system. New York: Harper and Row 1964.

Dow, R.S., Moruzzi, G.: The physiology and pathology of the cerebellum. Minneapolis: The University of Minnesota Press 1958.

Dumont, S.: Effects extralabyrinthiques sur l'activité des cellules des noyaux vestibulaires. J. Physiol. (Paris) **52**, 87–88 (1960).

Dusser de Barenne, J.G.: Die Funktionen des Kleinhirns: Physiologie und allgemeine Neuropathologie. In: G. Alexander und O. Marburg. Handbuch der Neurologie des Ohres. Berlin: Urban und Schwarzenberg **1**, 589–672 (1923).

Dusser de Barenne, J.G.: Experimentelle Physiologie des Kleinhirns. In: O. Bumke und O. Foerster. Handbuch der Neurologie. Berlin: Springer **2**, 235–267 (1937).

EAGER, R.P.: Efferent cortico-nuclear pathways in the cerebellum of the cat. J. comp. Neurol. **120**, 81–104 (1963).

ECCLES, J.C.: The physiology of synapses. Berlin-Göttingen-Heidelberg-New York: Springer 1964.

ECCLES, J.C.: Functional meaning of the patterns of synaptic connections in the cerebellum. Perspect. Biol. Med. **8**, 289–310 (1965).

ECCLES, J.C., ITO, M., SZENTÁGOTHAI, J.: The cerebellum as a neuronal machine. Berlin-Heidelberg-New York: Springer 1967.

ECCLES, J.C., LLINÁS, R., SASAKI, K.: Excitation of cerebellar Purkinje cells by the climbing fibers. Nature (Lond.) **203**, 245–246 (1964).

ECCLES, J.C., LLINÁS, R., SASAKI, K.: The excitatory synaptic action of climbing fibers on the Purkinje cells of the cerebellum. J. Physiol. (Lond.) **182**, 268–296 (1966).

ECCLES, R.M., LUNDBERG, A.: Synaptic actions in motoneurons by afferents which may evoke the flexion reflex. Arch. ital. Biol. **97**, 199–221 (1959).

ELDRED, E., GRANIT, R., MERTON, P.A.: Supraspinal control of the muscle spindles and its significance. J. Physiol. (Lond.) **122**, 498–523 (1953).

ENGSTRÖM, M.: On the double innervation of the sensory epithelia of the inner ear. Acta oto-laryng. (Stockh.) **49**, 109–118 (1958).

ENGSTRÖM, H., WERSÄLL, J.: The ultrastructural organization of the organ of Corti and of the vestibular sensory epithelia. Exp. Cell Res., Suppl. **5**, 460–492 (1958).

ERULKAR, S.D., SPRAGUE, J.M., WHITSEL, B.L., DOGAN, S., JANNETTA, P.J.: Organization of the vestibular projection to the spinal cord of the cat. J. Neurophysiol. **29**, 626–664 (1966).

FADIGA, E., PUPILLI, G.C.: Telesceptive components of the cerebellar function. Physiol. Rev. **44**, 432–486 (1964).

FERNÁNDEZ, C.: Interrelations between flocculonodular lobe and vestibular system. In: G.L. RASMUSSEN and W.F. WINDLE. Neural mechanisms of the auditory and vestibular systems. Springfield, Ill.: C.C. Thomas 1960.

FERNÁNDEZ, C., ALZATE, R., LINDSAY, J.R.: Experimental observation on postural nystagmus. II. Lesions of nodulus. Ann. Otol. (St. Louis) **69**, 94–114 (1960a).

FERNÁNDEZ, C., ALZATE, R., LINDSAY, J.R.: Interrelations between flocculonodular lobe and vestibular system. In: G.L. RASMUSSEN and W.F. WINDLE. Neural mechanisms of the auditory and vestibular systems. Springfield, Ill.: C.C. Thomas 1960b.

FERNÁNDEZ, C., FREDRICKSON, J.M.: Experimental cerebellar lesions and their effects on vestibular function. Acta oto-laryng. (Stockh.) **58**, Suppl. 192, 52–62 (1964).

FERRARO, A., BARRERA, S.E.: Differential features of "cerebellar" and "vestibular" phenomena in Macacus rhesus: Preliminary report based on experiments on 300 monkeys. Arch. Neurol. Psychiat. (Chic.) **39**, 902–918 (1938).

FOX, C.A., HILLMAN, D.E., SIEGESMUND, K.A., DUTTA, C.R.: The primate cerebellar cortex: A Golgi and electron microscopic study. In: C.A. FOX and R.S. SNIDER. Progress in Brain Research. Vol. 25. The cerebellum. Amsterdam: Elsevier Publ. Co. 1967.

FREDRICKSON, J.M., SCHWARZ, D., KORNHUBER, H.H.: Konvergenz und Interaktion vestibulärer und proprioceptiv-somatosensibler Afferenzen an Neuronen der Vestibulariskerne der Katze. Pflügers Arch. ges. Physiol. **291**, 33 (1964).

FREDRICKSON, J.M., SCHWARZ, D., KORNHUBER, H.H.: Convergence and interaction of vestibular and deep somatic afferents upon neurons in the vestibular nuclei of the cat. Acta oto-laryng. (Stockh.) **61**, 168–188 (1966).

FUCHS, A., KORNHUBER, H.H.: Extraocular muscle afferents to the cerebellum of the cat. J. Physiol. (Lond.) **200**, 713–722 (1969).

FULTON, J.F., CONNOR, G.: The physiological basis of three major cerebellar syndromes. Trans. Amer. neurol. Ass. **65**, 53–57 (1939).

GACEK, R.R.: Efferent component of the vestibular nerve. In: G.L. RASMUSSEN and W.F. WINDLE. Neural mechanisms of the auditory and vestibular systems. Springfield, Ill.: C.C. Thomas 1960.

GEREBTZOFF, M.A.: Les bases anatomiques de la physiologie du cervelet. Cellule **49**, 71–166 (1941).

Giaquinto, S., Pompeiano, O., Santini, M.: Risposte di unità deitersiane a stimolazione graduata di nervi cutanei e muscolari in animali decerebrati a cervelletto integro. Boll. Soc. ital. Biol. sper. **39**, 524–527 (1963).

Gidlöf, A.: Intracellular aspects of "release" phenomena in α-extensor motoneurones of the cat. Acta physiol. scand. **68**, Suppl. 277, 58 (1966).

Gilman, S.: A crossed cerebellar influence on muscle spindles primaries. Brain Res. **8**, 216–219 (1968).

Gilman, S., McDonald, W.I.: Cerebellar facilitation of muscle spindle activity. J. Neurophysiol. **30**, 1494–1512 (1967a).

Gilman, S., McDonald, W.J.: Relation of afferent fiber conduction velocity to reactivity of muscle spindle receptors after cerebellectomy. J. Neurophysiol. **30**, 1513–1522 (1967b).

Gilman, S., van der Meulen, J.P.: Muscle spindle activity in dystonic and spastic monkeys. Arch. Neurol. (Chic.) **14**, 553–563 (1966).

Glaser, G.M., Higgins, D.C.: Motor stability, stretch responses and the cerebellum. In: R. Granit, Ed. Nobel Symposium I. Muscle afferents and motor control. Stockholm: Almqvist and Wiksell 1966.

Gleisner, L., Henriksson, N.G.: Efferent and afferent activity pattern in the vestibular nerve of the frog. Acta oto-laryng. (Stockh.) **58**, Suppl. 192, 90–103 (1964).

Goodman, D.C., Hallett, R.E., Welch, R.B.: Patterns of localization in the cerebellar corticonuclear projections of the albino rat. J. comp. Neurol. **121**, 51–67 (1963).

Granit, R.: Receptors and sensory perception. New Haven: Yale University Press 1955.

Granit, R., Holmgren, B., Merton, P.A.: The two routes for excitation of muscle and their subservience to the cerebellum. J. Physiol. (Lond.) **130**, 213–224 (1955).

Granit, R., Kaada, B.: Influence of stimulation of central nervous structures on muscle spindles in cat. Acta physiol. scand. **27**, 130–160 (1952).

Granit, R., Pompeiano, O., Waltman, B.: Fast supraspinal control of mammalian muscle spindles: extra- and intrafusal co-activation. J. Physiol. (Lond.) **147**, 385–398 (1959).

Grant, G.: Projection of the external cuneate nucleus onto the cerebellum in the cat. An experimental study using silver methods. Exp. Neurol. **5**, 179–195 (1962).

Grant, G., Aschan, G., Ekvall, L.: Nystagmus produced by localized cerebellar lesions. Acta oto-laryng. (Stockh.) **58**, Suppl. 192, 78–84 (1964).

Gratscher, S.: Ueber den Einfluss von Reizungen des Kleinhirns auf den vestibulären Nystagmus. Klin. Beitr. Ohrenheilk. Festschrift für Prof. Urbantschisch. Berlin und Wien, **119**, 289–312 (1919).

Grillner, S., Hongo, T., Lund, S.: Interaction between the inhibitory pathways from the Deiters' nucleus and Ia afferents to flexor motoneurones. Acta physiol. scand. **68**, Suppl. 277, 61 (1966).

Groebbels, F.: Zur feineren Analyse der Beziehungen zwischen Labyrinth und Kleinhirn. Klin. Wschr. **6**, 1806–1807 (1927a).

Grobbels, F.: Die Lage und Bewegungsreflexe der Vögel. V. Die physiologische Gruppierung der Lage- und Bewegungsreflexe der Haustaube und ihre weitere Analyse durch Labyrinthentfernung und galvanische Reizung nach Entfernung des Labyrinths und seiner Teile. Pflügers Arch. ges. Physiol. **217**, 631–654 (1927b).

Gualtierotti, T., Passerini, D.: Soglia cerebellare alle accelerazioni rotatorie e sommazione temporale nel piccione viaggiatore. Rend. Accad. naz. Lincei, Cl. Sci. fis., mat. nat., Serie VIII, **25**, 115–118 (1958).

Gualtierotti, T., Passerini, D.: Determinazione delle risposte rotatorie cerebellari dal flocculo-nodulo del gatto curarizzato. Rend. Accad. naz. Lincei, Cl. Sci. fis., mat. nat., Serie VIII, **26**, 79–82 (1959).

Gualtierotti, T., Schreiber, B., Mainardi, D., Passerini, D.: Effect of acceleration on cerebellar potentials in birds and its relation to sense of direction. Amer. J. Physiol. **197**, 469–474 (1959).

Hahn, R.: Eccitabilità vestibolare (stimolazione galvanica) dopo emidecerebellazione e decerebellazione totale. Boll. Soc. ital. Biol. sper. **27**, 27–28 (1951).

Hahn, R.: Influenza delle posizioni compensatorie oculari da riflessi otolitici e del collo sull'attività fasica da stimolazione vestibolare galvanica. Arch. Fisiol. **52**, 20–29 (1952).

Halstead, W.C.: The effect of cerebellar lesions upon habituation of postrotatory nystagmus. Comp. Psychol. Monogr. **12**, 1–130 (1935).

Halstead, W.C., Yacorzynski, G., Fearing, F.: Further evidence of cerebellar influence in the habituation of after-nystagmus in pigeons. Amer. J. Physiol. **120**, 350–355 (1937).

Hámori, J., Szentágothai, J.: Identification under the electron microscope of climbing fibers and their synaptic contacts. Exp. Brain Res. **1**, 65–81 (1966).

Hampson, J.L., Harrison, C.R., Woolsey, C.N.: Somatotopic localization in anterior lobe and lobulus simplex of cerebellum in cat and dog. Fed. Proc. **4**, 31 (1945).

Hampson, J.L., Harrison, C.R., Woolsey, C.N.: Somatotopic localization in the cerebellum. Fed. Proc. **5**, 41 (1946).

Hampson, J.L., Harrison, C.R., Woolsey, C.N.: Cerebro-cerebellar projections and the somatotopic localization of the motor function in the cerebellum. Res. Publ. Ass. nerv. ment. Dis. **30**, 299–316 (1952).

Hauglie-Hanssen, E.: Intrinsic neuronal organization of the vestibular nuclear complex in the cat. A Golgi study. Ergebn. Anat. Entwickl.-Gesch. **40**/5, 1–105 (1968).

Henatsch, H.D., Manni, E., Dow, R.S.: Effects of gamma loop interruption on cerebellar control of individual alpha motoneuron stretch reflexes. J. Neurophysiol. **27**, 193–209 (1964a).

Henatsch, H.D., Manni, E., Wilson, J.H., Dow, R.S.: Linked and independent responses of tonic alpha and gamma hind-limb motoneurons to deep cerebellar stimulation. J. Neurophysiol. **27**, 172–192 (1964b).

Higgins, D.C., Glaser, G.H.: Stretch responses during chronic cerebellar ablation. A study of reflex instability. J. Neurophysiol. **27**, 49–62 (1964).

Hilding, D., Wersäll, J.: Cholinesterase and its relation to the nerve endings in the inner ear. Acta oto-laryng. (Stockh.) **55**, 205–217 (1962).

Holmqvist, B., Lundberg, A., Oscarsson, O.: Supraspinal inhibitory control of transmission to three ascending spinal pathways influenced by the flexion reflex afferents. Arch. ital. Biol. **98**, 60–80 (1960a).

Holmqvist, B., Lundberg, A., Oscarsson, O.: A supraspinal control system monosynaptically connected with an ascending spinal pathway. Arch. ital. Biol. **98**, 402–422 (1960b).

Hoshino, T.: Beiträge zur Funktion des Kleinhirnwurmes beim Kaninchen. Acta oto-laryng. (Stockh.) Suppl. **2**, 1–72 (1921).

Hunt, C.C.: The reflex activity of mammalian small-nerve fibres. J. Physiol. (Lond.) **115**, 456–469 (1951).

Infantellina, F., Riva Sanseverino, E., Urbano, A.: Electroencephalographic changes as a result of labyrinthine stimulation after strychninization of the paraflocculus in the dog. Arch. ital. Biol. **101**, 430–443 (1963).

Ireland, P.E., Farkashidy, J.: Studies on the efferent innervation of the vestibular end organs. Ann. Otol. (St. Louis) **70**, 490–503 (1961).

Ito, M., Hongo, T., Yoshida, M., Okada, Y., Obata, K.: Intracellularly recorded antidromic responses of Deiters neurones. Experientia (Basel) **20**, 295–296 (1964a).

Ito, M., Hongo, T., Yoshida, M., Okada, Y., Obata, K.: Antidromic and trans-synaptic activation of Deiters neurones induced from the spinal cord. Jap. J. Physiol. **14**, 638–658 (1964b).

Ito, M., Kawai, N.: IPSP receptive field in the cerebellum for Deiters neurones. Proc. Jap. Acad. **40**, 762–764 (1964).

Ito, M., Kawai, N., Udo, M.: The origin of cerebellar-induced inhibition and facilitation in the neurones of Deiters and intracerebellar nuclei. Proc. XXIII. int. Congr. physiol. Sci., Tokyo, 997, 1965.

Ito, M., Kawai, N., Udo, M.: The origin of cerebellar-induced inhibition of Deiters neurones. III. Distribution of the inhibitory zone. Exp. Brain Res. **4**, 310–320 (1968).

Ito, M., Obata, K., Ochi, R.: Initiation of IPSP in Deiters and fastigial neurones associated with the activity of cerebellar Purkinje cells. Proc. Jap. Acad. **40**, 765–768 (1964c).

Ito, M., Obata, K., Ochi, R.: The origin of cerebellar-evoked inhibition of Deiters' neurones. II. Temporal correlation between the transsynaptic activation of Purkinje cells and the inhibition of Deiters neurones. Exp. Brain Res. **2**, 350–364 (1966).

Ito, M., Yoshida, M.: The cerebellar-evoked monosynaptic inhibition of Deiters neurones. Experientia (Basel) **20**, 515–516 (1964).

Ito, M., Yoshida, M.: The origin of cerebellar-induced inhibition of Deiters neurones. I. Monosynaptic initiation of the inhibitory postsynaptic potentials. Exp. Brain Res. **2**, 330–349 (1966).

Ito, M., Yoshida, M., Obata, K.: Monosynaptic inhibition of the intracerebellar nuclei induced from the cerebellar cortex. Experientia (Basel) **20**, 575–576 (1964d).

Iurato, S., Taidelli, G.: Relationships and structure of the so-called "much granulated nerve endings" in the crista ampullaris (as studied by means of serial sections). In: M. Titlbach. Electron microscopy. Proc. Third European regional conference, Prague. Czechoslovak Academy of Sciences, Prague, Vol. D, 325–326, 1964.

Jankowska, E., Lund, S., Lundberg, A., Pompeiano, O.: Inibizione postsinaptica dei motoneuroni prodotti dalla stimolazione della formazione reticolare del tronco dell'encefalo. Boll. Soc. ital. Biol. sper. **40**, 1971–1973 (1964a).

Jankowska, E., Lund, S., Lundberg, A., Pompeiano, O.: Postsynaptic inhibition in motoneurones evoked from the lower reticular formation. Experientia (Basel) **20**, 701 (1964b).

Jankowska, E., Lund, S., Lundberg, A., Pompeiano, O.: Inhibitory effects evoked through ventral reticulospinal pathways. Arch. ital. Biol. **106**, 124–140 (1968).

Jansen, J., Brodal, A.: Experimental studies on the intrinsic fibers of the cerebellum. II. The cortico-nuclear projection. J. comp. Neurol. **73**, 267–321 (1940).

Jansen, J., Brodal, A.: Experimental studies on the intrinsic fibers of the cerebellum. The cortico-nuclear projection in the rabbit and the monkey (*Macacus rhesus*). Norske Vid.-Akad. Oslo (Avh.), I, Mat. Naturv. Kl., **3**, 1–50 (1942).

Jansen, J., Brodal, A.: Das Kleinhirn. In: W.v. Möllendorff and W. Bargmann. Handbuch der mikroskopischen Anatomie des Menschen. Vol. 4/8. Nervensystem. Berlin-Göttingen-Heidelberg: Springer 1958.

Jansen, J., Jansen, J.K.S.: On the efferent fibers of the cerebellar nuclei in the cat. J. comp. Neurol. **102**, 607–623 (1955).

Jansen, J.K.S.: On fusimotor reflex activity. In: R. Granit, Ed. Nobel Symposium I. Muscular afferents and motor control. Stockholm: Almqvist and Wiksell 1966.

Jansen, J.K.S., Matthews, P.B.C.: The central control of the dynamic response of muscle spindle receptors. J. Physiol. (Lond.) **161**, 357–378 (1962).

Kasahara, M., Mano, N., Oshima, T., Ozawa, S., Shimazu, H.: Contralateral short latency inhibition of central vestibular neurons in the horizontal canal system. Brain Res. **8**, 376–378 (1968).

Klejin, A. de, Magnus, R.: Ueber die Unabhängigkeit der Labyrinthreflexe vom Kleinhirn und über die Lage der Zentren für die Labyrinthreflexe im Hirnstamm. Pflügers Arch. ges. Physiol. **178**, 124–178 (1920).

Kleyn, A. de: Die reziproke Innervation der Augenmuskeln des Kaninchens bei calorischer Reizung nach totaler Cerebellumexstirpation. Acta oto-laryng. (Stockh.) **8**, 195–198 (1925).

Klimoff, I.A.: Concerning the connections of the cerebellum with the nucleus of the oculomotor nerve (in russian). Vrachebnoe St. Petersburgh **17**, 1013–1014 (1896).

Kobayashi, Y., Oshima, K., Tasaki, I.: Analysis of afferent and efferent systems in the muscle nerve of the toad and cat. J. Physiol. (Lond.) **117**, 152–171 (1952).

Koella, W.: Experimentell-physiologischer Beitrag zum Nystagmusproblem. Helvet. physiol. Acta **5**, 154–168 (1947a).

Koella, W.: Die Beeinflussbarkeit des postrotatorischen Augennystagmus durch propriozeptive Halsreflexe beim Kaninchen. Helvet. physiol. Acta **5**, 430–440 (1947b).

Kuriyama, K., Haber, B., Sisken, B., Roberts, E.: The γ-amino-butyric acid system in rabbit cerebellum. Proc. nat. Acad. Sci. (Wash.) **55**, 846–852 (1966).

Kuzume, G.: Experimentell-anatomische Untersuchungen über die inneren und äusseren Verbindungen des Flocculus und der Kleinhirnkerne (hauptsächlich des Dachkerns). Folia anat. jap. **4**, 75–110 (1926a).

Kuzume, G.: Experimental anatomical studies on the nerve fibers of the flocculus cerebelli and the nucleus cerebelli (mainly nuclei tecti). Jap. med. World (Tokio) **6**, 137–139 (1926b).

Ladpli, R., Brodal, A.: Experimental studies of commissural and reticular formation projections from the vestibular nuclei in the cat. Brain Res. **8**, 65–96 (1968).

LE GROS CLARK, W. E.: The termination of ascending tract in the thalamus of the macaque monkey. J. Anat. (Lond.) **71**, 7–40 (1936).

LEGUIN, J.J., MAGHERINI, P.C. and POMPEIANO, O.: Cholinergic mechanisms related to REM sleep. III. Tonic and phasic inhibition of monosynaptic reflexes induced by an anticholinesterase in the decerebrate cal. Arch. ital. Biol. **111**, 1–23 (1973).

LEIDLER, R.: Kann von der Substanz des Kleinhirns direkt rhythmischer Nystagmus erzeugt werden? Klin. Beitr. Ohrenheilk. Festschrift für Prof. Urbantschisch, Berlin und Wien **119**, 403–412 (1919).

LILJESTRAND, G., MAGNUS, R.: Ueber die Wirkung des Novokains auf den normalen und den tetanusstarren Skelettmuskel und über die Entstehung der lokalen Muskelstarre beim Wundstarrkrampf. Pflügers Arch. ges. Physiol. **176**, 168–208 (1919).

LLINÁS, R.: Mechanisms of supraspinal actions upon spinal cord activities. Differences between reticular and cerebellar inhibitory actions upon alpha extensor motoneurons. J. Neurophysiol. **27**, 1117–1126 (1964).

LLINÁS, R., BLOEDEL, J.: Climbing fibre activation of Purkinje cells in the frog cerebellum. Brain Res. **3**, 299–302 (1966/1967).

LLINÁS, R., BLOEDEL, J.: Frog cerebellum: Absence of long-term inhibition upon Purkinje cells. Science **155**, 601–603 (1967).

LLINÁS, R., PRECHT, W., KITAI, S.T.: Climbing fibre activation of Purkinje cell following primary vestibular afferent stimulation in the frog. Brain Res. **6**, 371–375 (1967).

LLINÁS, R., TERZUOLO, C.A.: Mechanisms of supraspinal actions upon spinal cord activities. Reticular inhibitory mechanisms on alpha extensor motoneurons. J. Neurophysiol. **27**, 579–591 (1964).

LLINÁS, R., TERZUOLO, C.A.: Mechanisms of supraspinal actions upon spinal cord activities. Reticular inhibitory mechanisms upon flexor motoneurones. J. Neurophysiol. **28**, 413–422 (1965).

LORENTE DE NÓ, R.: Ausgewählte Kapitel aus der vergleichenden Physiologie des Labyrinthes: Die Augenmuskelreflexe beim Kaninchen und ihre Grundlagen. Ergebn. Physiol. **32**, 73–242 (1931).

LORENTE DE NÓ, R.: Synaptic stimulation of motoneurons as a local process. J. Neurophysiol. **1**, 195–206 (1938).

LÖWENTHAL, M., HORSLEY, V.: On the relations between the cerebellar and other centers (namely cerebral and spinal) with special reference to the action of antagonistic muscles. Proc. roy. Soc. B **61**, 20–25 (1897).

LÖWY, R.: Über die Faseranatomie und Physiologie der Formatio vermicularis cerebelli. Arb. neurol. Inst. Univ. Wien **21**, 359–382 (1916).

LUND, S., POMPEIANO, O.: Descending pathways with monosynaptic action on motoneurones. Experientia (Basel) **21**, 602–603 (1965).

LUND, S., POMPEIANO, O.: Monosynaptic excitation of alpha motoneurones from supraspinal structures in the cat. Acta physiol. scand. **73**, 1–21 (1968).

LUNDBERG, A.: Ascending spinal hindlimb pathways in the cat. In J.C. ECCLES and J.P. SCHADÉ, Eds. Progress in brain research. Vol. 12. Physiology of spinal neurons. Amsterdam: Elsevier Publ. Co. 1964.

MAFFEI, L., POMPEIANO, O.: Sugli effetti della stimolazione del tegmento mesencefalico dopo interruzione della via rubro-spinale. Boll. Soc. ital. Biol. sper. **37**, 435–437 (1961).

MAFFEI, L., POMPEIANO, O.: Effects of stimulation of the mesencephalic tegmentum following interruption of the rubrospinal tract. Arch. ital. Biol. **100**, 510–525 (1962).

MAGNUS, R.: Welche Teile des Zentralnervensystems müssen für das Zustandekommen des tonischen Hals- und Labyrinthreflexes auf die Körpermuskulatur vorhanden sein? Pflügers Arch. ges. Physiol. **159**, 224–249 (1914).

MAGNUS, R.: Körperstellung. Berlin: Springer 1924.

MAGOUN, H.W., RHINES, R.: Spasticity. The stretch-reflex and extrapyramidal systems. Springfield, Ill.: C.C. Thomas 1947.

MANNI, E.: Localizzazioni cerebellari corticali nella cavia. II. Effetti di lesioni delle "parti vestibolari" del cervelletto. Arch. Fisiol. **50**, 110–123 (1950).

Manni, E., Azzena, G.B., Casey, H., Dow, R.S.: Influence of the labyrinth on the unitary discharge of the oculomotor nucleus and some adjacent formations. Exp. Neurol. **12**, 9–24 (1965a).

Manni, E., Azzena, G.B., Dow, R.S.: Cerebellar influences on the unitary discharge of the oculomotor nucleus and adjacent structures. Exp. Neurol. **13**, 252–263 (1965b).

Manni, E., Dow, R.S.: Some observations on the effects of cerebellectomy in the rat. J. comp. Neurol. **121**, 189–194 (1963).

Manni, E., Henatsch, H.D., Henatsch, E.M., Dow, R.S.: Localization of facilitatory and inhibitory sites in and around the cerebellar nuclei affecting limb posture, alpha and gamma motoneurons. J. Neurophysiol. **27**, 210–228 (1964).

Mano, N., Oshima, T., Shimazu, H.: Inhibitory commissural fibers interconnecting the bilateral vestibular nuclei. Brain Res. **8**, 378–382 (1968).

Marburg, O.: Die Anatomie des Kleinhirns. Dtsch. Z. Nervenheilk. **81**, 8–35 (1924).

Matano, S., Zyo, K., Ban, T.: Experimental studies on the medial longitudinal fasciculus in the rabbit. I. Fibers originating in the vestibular nuclei. Med. J. Osaka Univ. **14**, 339–370 (1964).

Matthews, P.B.C.: The effect of the local application of procaine on the stretch reflex of the soleus muscle of the cat decerebrated by anaemia. J. Physiol. (Lond.) **140**, 408–420 (1958).

Matthews, P.B.C.: The differentiation of two types of fusimotor fibre by their effects on the dynamic response of muscle spindle primary endings. Quart. J. exp. Physiol. **47**, 324–333 (1962).

Matthews, P.B.C.: Muscle spindles and their motor control. Physiol. Rev. **44**, 219–288 (1964).

Matthews, P.B.C., Phillips, C.G., Rushworth, G.: Afferent systems converging upon cerebellar Purkinje cells in the frog. Quart. J. exp. Physiol. **43**, 38–52 (1958).

McMasters, R.E., Weiss, A.H., Carpenter, M.B.: Vestibular projections to the nuclei of the extraocular muscles. Degeneration resulting from discrete partial lesions of the vestibular nuclei in the monkey. Amer. J. Anat. **118**, 163–194 (1966).

Menzio, P.: Riflessi labirintici in animali trattati con streptomicina e significato delle lesioni cerebellari. Boll. Soc. ital. Biol. sper. **26**, 39–41 (1950).

Moruzzi, G.: Effects at different frequencies of cerebellar stimulation upon postural tonus and myotatic reflexes. E.E.G. clin. Neurophysiol. **2**, 463–469 (1950a).

Moruzzi, G.: Problems in cerebellar physiology. Springfield, Ill.: C.C. Thomas 1950b.

Moruzzi, G., Pompeiano, O.: Inversione dell'inibizione paleocerebellare prodotta dalla distruzione parziale del nucleo del tetto. Boll. Soc. ital. Biol. sper. **30**, 493–494 (1954).

Moruzzi, G., Pompeiano, O.: Scomparsa della rigidità da decerebrazione prodotta da lesione della parte caudale del nucleo del tetto contralaterale. Boll. Soc. ital. Biol. sper. **31**, 801–803 (1955a).

Moruzzi, G., Pompeiano, O.: Influenze cerebellari crociate sul tono posturale. Rend. Accad. naz. Lincei, Cl. Sci. fis., mat. nat., Serie VIII, **18**, 420–424 (1955b).

Moruzzi, G., Pompeiano, O.: La inibizione propriocettiva riflessa come causa dell'atonia fastigiale. Rend. Accad. naz. Lincei, Cl. Sci. fis., mat. nat., Serie VIII, **19**, 326–330 (1955c).

Moruzzi, G., Pompeiano, O.: L'inibizione riflessa nel meccanismo dell'atonia fastigiale. Boll. Soc. ital. Biol. sper. **31**, 803–804 (1955d).

Moruzzi, G., Pompeiano, O.: Effetti della sezione intracranica del nervo VIII sull'atonia fastigiale crociata. Boll. Soc. ital. Biol. sper. **31**, 1238–1239 (1955e).

Moruzzi, G., Pompeiano, O.: Soppressione dell'atonia fastigiale del gatto decerebrato mediante sezione del N. VIII contralaterale. Rend. Accad. naz. Lincei, Cl. Sci. fis., mat. nat., Serie VIII, **19**, 471–475 (1955f).

Moruzzi, G., Pompeiano, O.: Effetti di lesioni croniche del nucleo del tetto sulle risposte alla stimolazione elettrica della corteccia cerebellare vermiana del lobus anterior. Rend. Accad. naz. Lincei, Cl. Sci. fis., mat. nat., Serie VIII, **21**, 333–334 (1956a).

Moruzzi, G., Pompeiano, O.: Crossed fastigial atonia. Experientia (Basel) **12**, 35 (1956b).

Moruzzi, G., Pompeiano, O.: Crossed fastigial influence on decerebrate rigidity. J. comp. Neurol. **106**, 371–392 (1956c).

Moruzzi, G., Pompeiano, O.: Effects of vermal stimulation after fastigial lesions. Arch. ital. Biol. **95**, 31–55 (1957a).

MORUZZI, G., POMPEIANO, O.: Inhibitory mechanisms underlying the collapse of decerebrate rigidity after unilateral fastigial lesions. J. comp. Neurol. **107**, 1–25 (1957b).

MUGNAINI, E., WALBERG, F.: An experimental electron microscopical study on the mode of termination of cerebellar corticovestibular fibres in the cat lateral vestibular nucleus (Deiters' nucleus). Exp. Brain Res. **4**, 212–236 (1967).

MUGNAINI, E., WALBERG, F., BRODAL, A.: Mode of termination of primary vestibular fibres in the lateral vestibular nucleus. An experimental electron microscopical study in the cat. Exp. Brain Res. **4**, 187–211 (1967).

NYBERG-HANSEN, R.: Origin and termination of fibers from the vestibular nuclei descending in the medial longitudinal fasciculus. An experimental study with silver impregnation methods in the cat. J. comp. Neurol. **122**, 355–367 (1964).

NYBERG-HANSEN, R., MASCITTI, T.A.: Sites and mode of termination of vestibulo-spinal fibers in the cat. An experimental study with silver methods. J. comp. Neurol. **122**, 369–387 (1964).

OBATA, K.: Pharmacological study on postsynaptic inhibition of Deiters neurones. Proc. XXIII int. Congr. physiol. Sci., Tokyo, 958, 1965.

OBATA, K., ITO, M., OCHI, R., SATO, N.: Pharmacological properties of the postsynaptic inhibition by Purkinje cell axons and the action of γ-aminobutyric acid on Deiters neurones. Exp. Brain Res. **4**, 43–57 (1967).

OSCARSSON, O.: Functional organization of the spino- and cuneocerebellar tracts. Physiol. Rev. **45**, 495–522 (1965).

PETERSON, B.W.: Effect of tilting on the activity of neurons in the vestibular nuclei of the cat. Brain Res. **6**, 606–609 (1967).

PETROFF, A.E.: An experimental investigation of the origin of efferent fiber projections to the vestibular neuro-epithelium. Anat. Rec. **121**, 352–353 (1955).

POLLOCK, L.J., DAVIS, L.: Studies in decerebration. I. A method of decerebration. Arch. Neurol. Psychiat. (Chic.) **10**, 391–398 (1923).

POLLOCK, L.J., DAVIS, L.: The influence of the cerebellum upon the reflex activities of the decerebrate animal. Brain **50**, 277–312 (1927).

POLLOCK, L.J., DAVIS, L.: Studies in decerebration. V. The tonic activities of a decerebrate animal exclusive of the neck and labyrinthine reflexes. Amer. J. Physiol. **92**, 625–629 (1930a).

POLLOCK, L.J., DAVIS, L.: The reflex activities of a decerebrate animal. J. comp. Neurol. **50**, 377–341 (1930b).

POLLOCK, L.J., DAVIS, L.: Studies in decerebration. VI. The effect of deafferentation upon decerebrate rigidity. Amer. J. Physiol. **98**, 47–49 (1931).

POMPEIANO, O.: Responses of electrical stimulation of the intermediate part of the cerebellar anterior lobe in the decerebrate cat. Arch. ital. Biol. **96**, 330–360 (1958).

POMPEIANO, O.: Localizzazione delle risposte posturali alla stimolazione elettrica del nucleo di Deiters nel gatto decerebrato. Boll. Soc. ital. Biol. sper. **36**, 608–609 (1960a).

POMPEIANO, O.: Risposte posturali localizzate alla stimolazione stereotassica del nucleo di Deiters. Rend. Accad. naz. Lincei, Cl. Sci. fis., mat. nat., Serie VIII, **28**, 705–706 (1960b).

POMPEIANO, O.: Organizzazione somatotopica delle risposte posturali alla stimolazione elettrica del nucleo di Deiters nel gatto decerebrato. Arch. Sci. biol. (Bologna) **44**, 497–511 (1960c).

POMPEIANO, O.: Organizzazione somatotopica delle risposte posturali alla stimolazione e alla distruzione della parte caudale del nucleo del tetto. Boll. Soc. ital. Biol. sper. **37**, 916–918 (1961).

POMPEIANO, O.: Somatotopic organization of the postural responses to stimulation and destruction of the caudal part of the fastigial nucleus. Arch. ital. Biol. **100**, 259–271 (1962).

POMPEIANO, O.: Sui rapporti anatomo-funzionali tra cervelletto e midollo spinale. In: V. FLORIS, Ed. Fisiopatologia e clinica del cervelletto. Riv. Pat. nerv. ment. 33–164 (1966a).

POMPEIANO, O.: Discussion of Dr. Shapovalov's paper. Pag. 348. In: R. GRANIT, Ed. Nobel Symposium I. Muscular afferents and motor control. Stockholm: Almqvist and Wiksell 1966b.

Pompeiano, O.: Functional organization of the cerebellar projections to the spinal cord. In: C.A. Fox and R.S. Snider. Progress in Brain Research, Vol. 25. The cerebellum. Amsterdam: Elsevier Publ. Co. 1967.

Pompeiano, O., Brodal, A.: The origin of vestibulospinal fibres in the cat. An experimental-anatomical study, with comments on the descending medial longitudinal fasciculus. Arch. ital. Biol. **95**, 166–195 (1957a).

Pompeiano, O., Brodal, A.: Spino-vestibular fibers in the cat. An experimental study. J. comp. Neurol. **108**, 353–382 (1957b).

Pompeiano, O., Cotti, E.: Risposte di unità deitersiane alla stimolazione galvanica localizzata della corteccia cerebellare vermiana del *lobus anterior*. Boll. Soc. ital. Biol. sper. **35**, 383–384 (1959a).

Pompeiano, O., Cotti, E.: Localizzazione topografica delle risposte deitersiane alla polarizzazione della corteccia cerebellare vermiana del *lobus anterior*. Boll. Soc. ital. Biol. sper. **35**, 385–386 (1959b).

Pompeiano, O., Cotti, E.: Dimostrazione dell'esistenza di proiezioni localizzate cerebello-deitersiane. Rend. Accad. naz. Lincei, Cl. Sci. fis., mat. nat., Serie VIII, **26**, 284–287 (1959c).

Pompeiano, O., Cotti, E.: Modificazione dell'attività di singole unità deitersiane per stimolazioni della periferia sensitiva. Boll. soc. ital. Biol. sper. **35**, 1221–1222 (1959d).

Pompeiano, O., Cotti, E.: Convergenza d'impulsi afferenti su unità deitersiane che rispondono alla stimolazione localizzata del cervelletto. Rend. Accad. naz. Lincei, Cl. Sci. fis., mat. nat., Serie VIII, **27**, 76–79 (1959e).

Pompeiano, O., Cotti, E.: Inibizione cerebellare delle risposte di unità deitersiane a stimolazioni labirintiche. Rend. Accad. naz. Lincei, Cl. Sci. fis., mat. nat., Serie VIII, **27**, 238–241 (1959f).

Pompeiano, O., Cotti, E.: Analisi microelettrodica delle proiezioni cerebello-deitersiane. Arch Sci. biol. (Bologna) **43**, 57–101 (1959g).

Pompeiano, O., Cotti, E.: Effetti della stimolazione corticocerebellare sull'attività di singole unità deitersiane provocata da stimolazioni labirintiche. Boll. Soc. ital. Biol. sper. **36**, 303–304 (1960).

Pompeiano, O., Diete-Spiff, K., Carli, G.: Componenti precoci e tardive nella risposta dei recettori fusali alla stimolazione del nucleo di Deiters. Boll. Soc. ital. Biol. sper. **43**, 273–275 (1967a).

Pompeiano, O., Diete-Spiff, K., Carli, G.: Two pathways transmitting vestibulospinal influences from the lateral vestibular nucleus of Deiters to extensor fusimotor neurones. Pflügers Arch. ges. Physiol. **293**, 272–275 (1967b).

Poppele, R.E.: Response of gamma and alpha motor systems to phasic and tonic vestibular inputs. Brain Res. **6**, 535–547 (1967).

Precht, W., Shimazu, H.: Functional connection of tonic and kinetic vestibular neurons with primary vestibular afferents. J. Neurophysiol. **28**, 1014–1028 (1965).

Precht, W., Shimazu, H., Markham, C.H.: A mechanism of central compensation of vestibular function following hemilabyrinthectomy. J. Neurophysiol. **29**, 996–1010 (1966).

Price, J.B., Spiegel, E.A.: Vestibulo-cerebral pathways. A contribution to the central mechanism of vertigo. Arch. Otolaryng. **26**, 658–667 (1937).

Rademaker, G.G.J.: Das Stehen: Statische Reaktionen, Gleichgewichtsreaktionen und Muskeltonus unter besonderer Berücksichtigung ihres Verhaltens bei kleinhirnlosen Tieren. Berlin: Springer 1931.

Ranson, S.W., Ingram, W.R.: The diencephalic course and termination of the medial lemniscus and brachium conjunctivum. J. comp. Neurol. **56**, 257–275 (1932).

Rasmussen, A.T.: Origin and course of the fasciculus uncinatus (Russel) in the cat, with observation on other fiber tracts arising from the cerebellar nuclei. J. comp. Neurol. **57**, 165–197 (1933).

Rasmussen, G.L., Gacek, R.: Concerning the question of the efferent fiber component of the vestibular nerve of the cat. Anat. Rec. **130**, 361 (1958).

Rexed, B.: A cytoarchitectonic atlas of the spinal cord in the cat. J. comp. Neurol. **100**, 297–380 (1954).

RIVA SANSEVERINO, E., URBANO, A.: Effetti della stimolazione labirintica rotatoria sull'attività elettrica del paraflocculo e di altri lobuli cerebellari, nel gatto. Boll. Soc. ital. Biol. sper. **41**, 89–91 (1965a).

RIVA SANSEVERINO, E., URBANO, A.: Modificazioni dell'attività bioelettrica del paraflocculo e di altri lobuli cerebellari, ottenute nel gatto non anestetizzato mediante stimolazione labirintica rotatoria. Rend. Accad. naz. Lincei, Cl. Sci. fis., mat. nat., Serie VIII, **38**, 933–937 (1965b).

RIVA SANSEVERINO, E., URBANO, A.: Electrical activity of paraflocculus and other cerebellar lobuli following vestibular rotatory stimulation in the cat. Arch. Sci. biol. (Bologna) **49**, 83–96 (1965c).

ROSSI, G.: L'innervation efférente des récepteurs vestibulaires. Acta oto-laryng. (Stockh.) **58**, 230–238 (1964).

ROSSI, G., CORTESINA, G.: Il "sistema efferente colinergico cocleovestibolare". Minerva otorinolaring. **12**, 173–195 (1962).

ROSSI, G., CORTESINA, G.: Research on the efferent innervation of the inner ear. J. Laryng. **77**, 202–233 (1963).

ROSSI, G., CORTESINA, G.: The "efferent cochlear and vestibular system" in *Lepus cuniculus* L. Acta anat. (Basel) **60**, 362–381 (1965).

SACHS, E., FINCHER, E.F.: Anatomical and physiological observations on lesions in the cerebellar nuclei in Macacus rhesus. Brain **50**, 350–356 (1927).

SALA, O.: Modificazioni dell'attività del nervo vestibolare a seguito della stimolazione del sistema vestibolare efferente. Boll. Soc. ital. Biol. sper. **38**, 1048–1050 (1962).

SALA, O.: Modifications of the vestibular nerve activity by stimulation of the efferent vestibular system. Experientia (Basel) **19**, 39 (1963a).

SALA, O.: Effetti della stimolazione ad alta frequenza del sistema vestibolare efferente. Boll. Soc. ital. Biol. sper. **39**, 872–873 (1963b).

SALA, O.: Ricerche elettrofisiologiche sul sistema vestibolare efferente. Valsalva **39**, 9–21 (1963c).

SALA, O.: Modificazioni dei potenziali continui ampollari indotte dalla stimolazione del sistema efferente vestibolare. Boll. Soc. ital. Biol. sper. **40**, 57–59 (1964).

SALA, O.: The efferent vestibular system. Electrophysiological research. Acta oto-laryng. (Stockh.) Suppl. **197**, 34 pp. (1965).

SCHMIDT, R.S.: Frog labyrinthine efferent impulses. Acta oto-laryng. (Stockh.) **56**, 51–64 (1963).

SHAPOVALOV, A.I.: Excitation and inhibition of spinal neurones during supraspinal stimulation. In: R. GRANIT, Ed. Nobel Symposium I. Muscular afferents and motor control. Stockholm: Almqvist and Wiksell 1966.

SHAPOVALOV, A.I., KURCHAVYI, G.G., STROGONOVA, M.P.: Synaptic mechanisms of vestibulospinal influences on alpha-motoneurons. Fiziol. Zh. (Mosk.) **52**, 1401 (1966). Neuroscience Translations **1**, 91–100 (1967/1968).

SHERRINGTON, C.S.: The mammalian spinal cord as an organ of reflex action. Proc. roy. Soc. B **61**, 220–221 (1897).

SHERRINGTON, C.S.: Experiments in examination of the peripheral distribution of the fibers of the posterior roots of some spinal nerves. Phil. Trans. B **190**, 45–286 (1898).

SHIMAZU, H.: Mutual interactions between bilateral vestibular nuclei and their significance in motor regulation. In: M.D. YAHR and D.P. PURPURA, Eds. Neurophysiological basis of normal and abnormal motor activities. Hewlett, New York: Raven Press 1967.

SHIMAZU, H., PRECHT, W.: Tonic and kinetic responses of cat's vestibular neurons to horizontal angular acceleration. J. Neurophysiol. **28**, 991–1013 (1965).

SHIMAZU, H., PRECHT, W.: Inhibition of central vestibular neurons from the contralateral labyrinth and its mediating pathway. J. Neurophysiol. **29**, 467–492 (1966).

Simonelli, G., di Giorgio, A.M.: I rapporti dell'azione cerebellare con alcuni riflessi concernenti l'orientamento e l'equilibrio del corpo. Arch. Fisiol. **24**, 461–535 (1926).

Simonelli, G., di Giorgio, A.M.: Il comportamento del nistagmo spontaneo e provocato nelle lesioni asimmetriche del cervelletto. Boll. Soc. ital. Biol. sper. **6**, 206–211 (1931).

Snider, R.S.: Alterations which occur in mossy terminals of the cerebellum following transection of the brachium pontis. J. comp. Neurol. **64**, 417–435 (1936).

Snider, R.S., McCullock, W.S., Magoun, H.W.: A cerebello-bulbo-reticular pathway for suppression. J. Neurophysiol. **12**, 325–334 (1949).

Snider, R.S., Stowell, S.: Receiving areas of the tactile, auditory and visual systems in the cerebellum. J. Neurophysiol. **7**, 331–357 (1944).

Spiegel, E.A., Demetriades, Th.D.: Die zentrale Kompensation des Labyrinthverlustes. Pflügers Arch. ges. Physiol. **210**, 215–222 (1925).

Spiegel, E.A., Scala, N.P.: Vertical nystagmus following lesions of the cerebellar vermis. Arch. Ophthal. (N.Y.) **26**, 661–669 (1941).

Spiegel, E.A., Scala, N.P.: Positional nystagmus in cerebellar lesions. J. Neurophysiol. **5**, 247–260 (1942).

Sprague, J.M., Chambers, W.W.: Regulation of posture in intact and decerebrate cat. I. Cerebellum, reticular formation, vestibular nuclei. J. Neurophysiol. **16**, 451–463 (1953).

Sprague, J.M., Chambers, W.W.: Control of posture by reticular formation and cerebellum in the intact anesthetized and unanesthetized and in the decerebrate cat. Amer. J. Physiol. **176**, 52–64 (1954).

Sprague, J.M., Ha, H.: The terminal fields of dorsal root fibres in the lumbosacral cord of the cat, and the dendritic organization of the motor nuclei. In: J.C. Eccles and J.P. Schadé, Eds. Progress in Brain Research. Vol. 11. Organization of the spinal cord. Amsterdam: Elsevier Publ. Co. 1964.

Stella, G.: Nuove osservazioni sugli effetti della stimolazione del paleocerebello nell'animale decerebrato. Atti Soc. med.-chir. Padova **23**, 22–24 (1944a).

Stella, G.: Sul meccanismo della rigidità da decerebrazione in arti deafferentati. Atti. Soc. med.-chir. Padova **23**, 5–16 (1944b).

Stella, G.: Influenza del cervelletto sulla rigidità da decerebrazione. Atti Soc. med.-chir. Padova **23**, 17–21 (1944c).

Stella, G.: Nuove osservazioni sull'attività riflessa tonica del cervelletto nell'animale decerebrato. Boll. Soc. ital. Biol. sper. **22**, 78–80 (1946).

Stella, G., Zatti, P., Sperti, L.: Decerebrate rigidity in forelegs after deafferentation and spinal transection in dogs with chronic lesion in different parts of the cerebellum. Amer. J. Physiol. **181**, 230–234 (1955).

Szentágothai, J., Rajkovits, K.: Über den Ursprung der Kletterfasern des Kleinhirns. Z. Anat. Entwickl.-Gesch. **121**, 130–141 (1959).

Terzian, H., Terzuolo, C.: Le componenti automatiche e riflesse del tono posturale. Arch. Fisiol. **54**, 37–61 (1954).

Terzuolo, C.A.: Cerebellar inhibitory and excitatory actions upon spinal extensor motoneurones. Arch. ital. Biol. **97**, 316–339 (1959).

Terzuolo, C.A., Terzian, H.: Sul meccanismo della rigidità da decerebrazione in arti anteriori cronicamente deafferentati. Boll. Soc. ital. Biol. sper. **27**, 1317–1318 (1951a).

Terzuolo, C.A., Terzian, H.: Riflessi di Magnus e tono posturale in arti sottoposti a deafferentazione acuta o cronica. Boll. Soc. ital. Biol. sper. **27**, 1319–1320 (1951b).

Terzuolo, C.A., Terzian, H.: Cerebellar increase of postural tonus after deafferentation and labyrinthectomy. J. Neurophysiol. **16**, 551–561 (1953).

Tyć-Dumont, S.: Contribution à l'étude du contrôle d'origine réticulaire des intégrations sensorimotrices. Thèse à la Faculté des Sciences de l'Université de Paris, 1964.

Vachananda, B.: The major spinal afferent systems to the cerebellum and the cerebellar corticonuclear connection in Macaca mulatta. J. comp. Neurol. **112**, 303–352 (1959).

Van der Meulen, J. P., Gilman, S.: Recovery of muscle spindle activity in cats after cerebellar ablation. J. Neurophysiol. **28**, 943–957 (1965).

Van der Meulen, J. P., Gilman, S., Denny-Brown, D.: Muscle spindle activity in animals with chronic lesions of the central nervous system. In: R. Granit, Ed. Nobel Symposium I. Muscle afferents and motor control. Stockholm: Almqvist and Wiksell 1966.

Voogd, J.: The cerebellum of the cat. Structure and fibre connexions. Leiden: Van Gorcum and Co. N.V., Dr. Prakke, H.J. and H.M.G. Prakke 1964.

Voorhoeve, P.E., van Kanten, R.W.: Reflex behaviour of fusimotor neurones of the cat upon electrical stimulation of various afferent fibres. Acta physiol. pharmacol. neerl. **10**, 391–407 (1962).

Walberg, F., Bowsher, D., Brodal, A.: The termination of primary vestibular fibers in the vestibular nuclei in the cat. An experimental study with silver methods. J. comp. Neurol. **110**, 391–419 (1958).

Walberg, F., Jansen, J.: Cerebellar corticovestibular fibers in the cat. Exp. Neurol. **3**, 32–52 (1961).

Walberg, F., Jansen, J.: Cerebellar corticonuclear projection studied experimentally with silver impregnation methods. J. Hirnforsch. **6**, 338–354 (1964).

Walberg, F., Pompeiano, O., Brodal, A., Jansen, J.: The fastigio-vestibular projection in the cat. An experimental study with silver impregnation methods. J. comp. Neurol. **118**, 49–75 (1962).

Wall, P.D.: Excitability changes in afferent fibre terminations and their relation to slow potentials. J. Physiol. (Lond.) **142**, 1–21 (1958).

Wallenberg, A.: Secundäre Bahnen aus den frontalen sensiblen Trigeminuskernen des Kaninchens. Anat. Anz. **26**, 145–155 (1905).

Wersäll, J.: Studies on the structure and innervation of the sensory epithelium of the cristae ampullares in the guinea pig. A light- and electron-microscopic investigation. Acta otolaryng. (Stockh.). Suppl. **126**, 1–85 (1956).

Wersäll, J.: Electron micrographic studies of vestibular hair cell innervation. In: G.L. Rasmussen and W.L. Windle, Eds. Neural mechanisms of auditory and vestibular systems. Springfield, Ill.: C.C. Thomas 1960.

Wersäll, J., Gleisner, L., Lundquist, P.-G.: Ultrastructure of the vestibular end organs. In: A.V.S. de Reuck and J. Knight. Myotatic, kinesthetic and vestibular mechanisms. Ciba Foundation Symposium. London: J. and A. Churchill 1967.

Wilson, V.J., Kato, M., Thomas, R.C.: Excitation of lateral vestibular neurones. Nature (Lond.) **206**, 96–97 (1965).

Wilson, V.J., Kato, M., Thomas, R.C., Peterson, B.W.: Excitation of lateral vestibular neurons by peripheral afferent fibers. J. Neurophysiol. **29**, 508–529 (1966a).

Wilson, V.J., Kato, M., Peterson, B.W.: Convergence of inputs on Deiters neurones. Nature (Lond.) **211**, 1409–1411 (1966b).

Wilson, V.J., Kato, M., Peterson, B.W., Wylie, R.M.: A single-unit analysis of the organization of Deiters' nucleus. J. Neurophysiol. **30**, 603–619 (1967a).

Wilson, V.J., Wylie, R.M., Marco, L.A.: Projection to the spinal cord from the medial and descending vestibular nuclei of the cat. Nature (Lond.) **215**, 429–430 (1967b).

WILSON, V.J., WYLIE, R.M., MARCO, L.A.: Organization of the medial vestibular nucleus. J. Neurophysiol. **31**, 166–175 (1968a).

WILSON, V.J., WYLIE, R.M., MARCO, L.A.: Synaptic inputs to cells in the medial vestibular nucleus. J. Neurophysiol. **31**, 176–185 (1968b).

WINKLER, C.: Le cervelet. In: Anatomie du Système Nerveux, Haarlem: De Erven F. Bohn **3**, 108–367 (1927).

Chapter IV.

The Vestibulo-Ocular Reflex Arc*

By

B. Cohen, New York (USA)

With 20 Figures

Contents

* Supported by USPHS Research Grant NS-00294 and USPHS Career Research Development Award 1K3 NB-34, 987.

Three topics related to Vestibulo-Ocular Reflexes will be considered in this chapter: (1) The function of eye movements induced by the Vestibulo-Ocular Reflex Arc. (2) The pattern of eye movements induced by various parts of the vestibular apparatus. (3) The central pathways which carry activity responsible for these deviations.[1]

I. The Function of the Vestibulo-Ocular Reflex Arc

Sensory information originating in the labyrinth establishes the relationship of the head in space (Goltz, 1870; Breuer, 1874, 1891; Crum-Brown, 1874; Mach, 1875; Ewald, 1892; Camis and Creed, 1930). Angular head movements are perceived primarily by the semicircular canals (Lowenstein and Sand, 1940a, b; Groen et al., 1952; Lowenstein, 1956; Egmond et al., 1949, 1952; Goldberg and Fernández, 1971a, b; Fernández and Goldberg, 1971). The otolith organs, the utricle and the saccule, sense changes in linear velocity of the head or the static position of the head (Breuer, 1891, De Kleyn, 1920; Magnus, 1924; Benjamins and Huizinga, 1927; Versteegh, 1927; Tait and McNally, 1934; Hasegawa, 1936, 1937; McNally and Stuart, 1942; Lowenstein and Roberts, 1949; Jongkees, 1950; Fujita et al., 1968; Fernández et al., 1972). Eye movements induced by the vestibular apparatus tend to promote vision either with the head stationary or during head movement (Camis and Creed, 1930; Dusser de Barenne, 1934; McNally and Stuart, 1942; Gernandt, 1959). The neural substrate which links the vestibular sensory receptors to the eye muscles is the vestibulo-ocular reflex arc (Lorente de Nó, 1933; Szentágothai, 1950).

Three major types of oculomotor activity occur in response to visual or vestibular stimuli. These are: (1) positions of fixation, (2) slow eye movements, and (3) rapid eye movements. Inspection of stationary objects primarily takes place during periods of fixation. Counter-rolling due to head tilt is an example of a change in fixation due to vestibular stimulation (De Kleyn, 1920; Magnus, 1924; Lorente de Nó, 1928, 1931; Woellner and Graybiel, 1959; Miller, 1962; Krejcova et al., 1971). Slow eye movements include pursuit movements (Dodge, 1900, 1903; Westheimer, 1954b), tonic deviations, slow phases of nystagmus, and convergent movements (Rashbass and Westheimer, 1961. Westheimer and Rashbass, 1961; Zuber, 1971). Slow eye movements are important for perception of targets moving in the visual fields. If the eyes can approximate the velocity of moving targets, then images can be fixed on the

1 The literature on the vestibulo-ocular reflex arc is extensive. Other aspects of this subject are considered in this volume and elsewhere: Magnus, 1924; Camis and Creed, 1930; Dusser de Barenne, 1934; McNally and Stuart, 1942; Spiegel and Sommer, 1944; Wendt, 1951; Egmond et al., 1952; Aschan et al., 1956a; Brodal, 1958; Gernandt, 1959; Whitteridge, 1959; Rasmussen and Windle, 1960; International Symposium on Problems in Otoneurology, 1961; Collegium Oto-Rhino-Laryngologicum, 1961; Brodal et al., 1962; Japan Vestibular Society, 1963; Bender, 1964; Fields and Alford, 1964; International Vestibular Symposium, 1964; International Symposium on Vestibular and Oculomotor Problems, 1965; Role of the Vestibular Organs in the Exploration of Space, 1965; Kornhuber, 1966; Wolfson, 1966; De Reuck and Knight, 1967; Bender, 1969; Cawthorne et al., 1969; Kornhuber, 1970; Bach-y-Rita et al., 1971; Brodal and Pompeiano, 1972; Bizzi and Dichgans, 1972; Wilson, 1973; Uemura and Cohen, 1973.

retina (LUDVIGH and MILLER, 1955; MILLER, 1955; TEUBER, 1960; CRAWFORD, 1960a,b; MELVILL JONES and MILSUM, 1965; ATKIN and BENDER, 1968; YOUNG, 1971). Tonic deviations and slow phases of nystagmus may be induced by the vestibular system either in response to angular or linear head displacements (JONGKEES and PHILIPSZOON, 1964).

Rapid eye movements include saccades, quick phases of nystagmus, microsaccades, and blinks. Perception of the visual scene is reduced during saccades, quick phases, and blinks. Saccades reposition the eyes for new positions of fixation (DODGE, 1903; WESTHEIMER, 1954a; ROBINSON, 1964; YARBUS, 1965; FUCHS, 1967) or cause the eyes to move 'on target' during pursuit movements (WESTHEIMER, 1954a; FENDER and NYE, 1961; RASHBASS, 1961; YOUNG and STARK, 1963; ROBINSON, 1965). Quick phases of nystagmus reset the eyes during continuous pursuit so that tracking can continue during slow phases of nystagmus. Physiological tremor and microsaccades are eye movements of small amplitude which were believed necessary to introduce jitter into positions of fixation (RATLIFF and RIGGS, 1950; RIGGS et al., 1954; DITCHBURN and GINSBORG, 1953; PRITCHARD, 1964; ZUBER et al., 1965). Microsaccades may occur only infrequently in normal vision (STEINMAN et al., 1973). Differences between slow and rapid eye movements have been noted by a number of investigators (WESTHEIMER, 1954a, b; RASHBASS, 1961; ROBINSON, 1964, 1965; FUCHS, 1967; GOTO et al., 1968). Based on these differences RASHBASS (1961) postulated that the neural mechanisms for slow and rapid eye movements are different. This is widely accepted but the neural substrate for this difference is still not entirely clear.

A. Ocular Compensatory Movements Induced by the Vestibular System

For the most part eye movements induced by the vestibular apparatus are compensatory (DODGE, 1903, 1923). That is, they oppose head movements and tend to maintain the angle of vision in space. An example of ocular compensation in a normal individual is shown in Fig. 1A (ATKIN and BENDER, 1968). The top trace is a recording of eye movements (E), and the second trace is a recording of head movements (H). The subject turned his head from side to side while fixing on a stationary target. When the potentials which represent eye and head movement were summed (E+H, upward arrow), they balanced. This indicates that the direction of gaze had remained constant during head movement. Eye movements induced by head turning can compensate for a wide range of head velocities (Fig. 1B).

Compensatory eye movements induced by the vestibular system also occur commonly when turning the head and eyes to view a lateral target. An example in the monkey is shown in Fig. 2A (BIZZI et al., 1971). First the eyes (e) and then the head (h) moved toward the target. As the head began to deviate, the eyes compensated for the head movement by moving in the opposite direction (Fig. 2A, arrow). The compensatory eye movement was largely dependent on vestibular stimulation, and did not occur if the head movement was arrested (Fig. 2B). Activation of neck muscles occurred before activation of eye muscles, but because of the greater mass and inertia of the head, the eyes moved first.

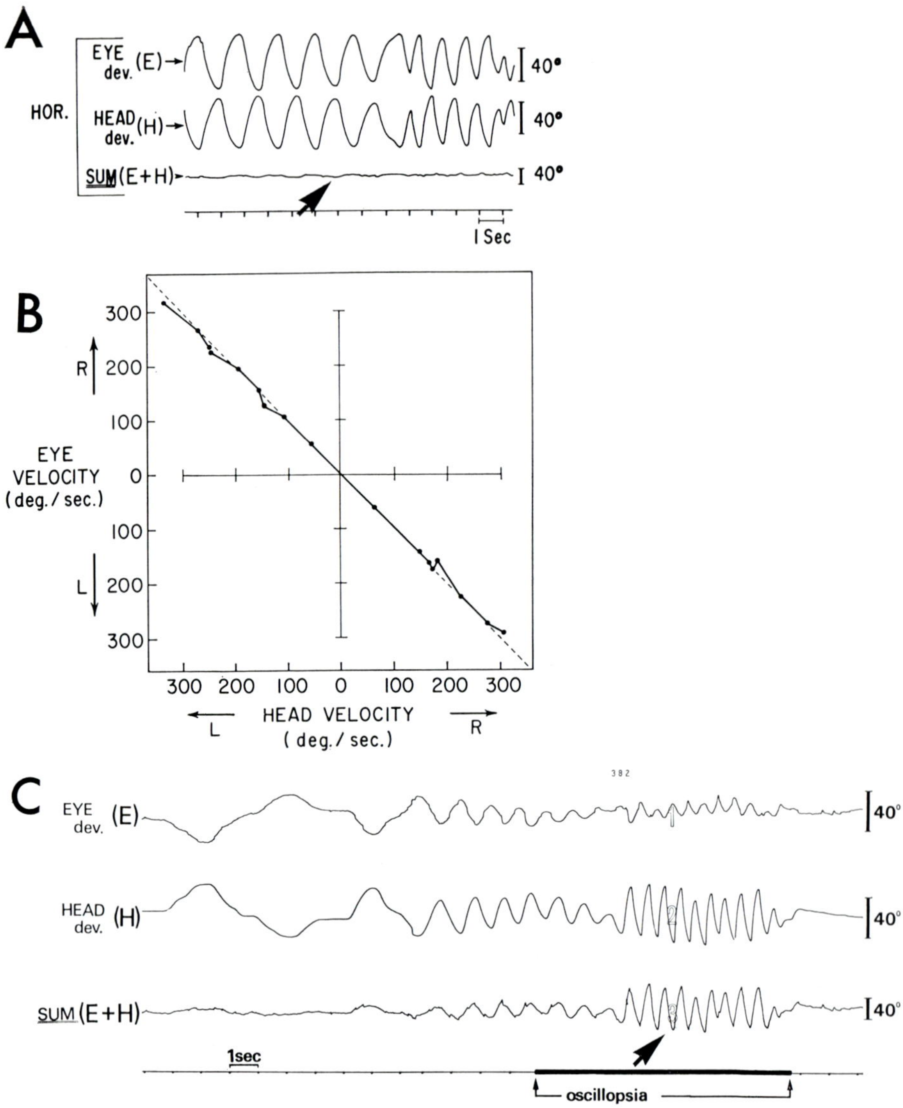

Fig. 1. A. Ocular compensation for head movement. Top trace (E) is electrooculogram recorded with DC-coupling. Second trace (H) is a recording of head movement during head turning from side to side. Deflection of each trace is proportional to the angular deviation of the eyes or head in the horizontal plane. The third trace (E+H) is a summation of the top two traces. The bottom trace is the time base at 1 mark/sec. The vertical bars on the right of the eye and head traces represent 40° of deviation. The subject was in light, fixing on a point in front. As he turned his head from side to side, eye and head movements balanced and the summated trace (E+H, upward arrow) was essentially flat. B. Graph of the relationship between maximum velocity of the eyes and head during head turning as in A. Head velocity is shown on the abscissa and eye velocity on the ordinate. When head velocity was high to the right, eye velocity was high to the left and vice versa. The linearity of the relationship was maintained for head velocities up to 300°/sec. C. Eye and head movements of patient with bilateral labyrinthine disease. As the frequency of head turning increased, the eyes failed to compensate for the head movement and the summated trace (E+H) showed large shifts (upward arrow). During this time the patient had a sensation that the target was moving back and forth. From Atkin and Bender, Arch. Neurol. (Chic.) **18**, 559–566 (1968)

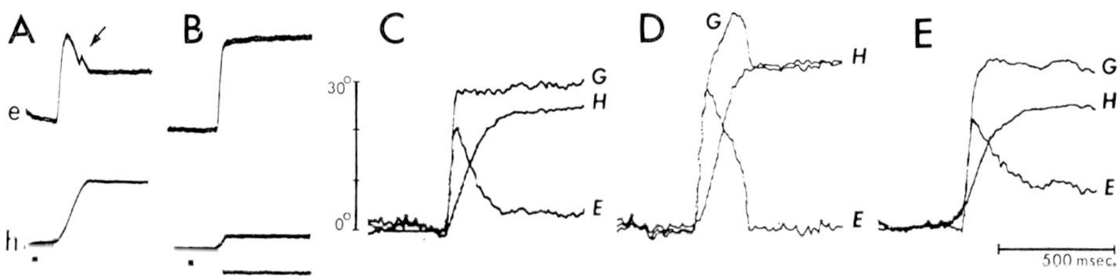

Fig. 2. Eye-head coordination in intact (A–C) and labyrinthectomized (E, F) monkey. Eye movements (E); head movements (H). In C–E gaze movements (G) represent the sum of E+H. A. 30° gaze shift in intact monkey. Compensatory eye movement induced by vestibular system is marked by an arrow. B. Compensatory eye movement does not occur if the head is fixed or braked just after the onset of head movement. C. Normal lateral gaze shift involving head and eyes. D. 40 days after vestibulectomy note gaze overshoot and corrective saccade E. 120 days after vestibulectomy eye-head coordination is similar to A. Note that initial saccade amplitude is smaller than intertarget interval. From Bizzi et al., Science **173**, 452–454 (1971); and Dichgans et al., Exp. Brain Res. **18**, 548–562 (1973)

The role of the vestibular system in maintenance of vision is shown by the defects in vision which may occur after the vestibular apparatus on both sides has been severely damaged or destroyed. Vision may seem normal in such patients when the head is still. However, during either passive or voluntary head movement, there may be apparent movement of the visual surround. This makes fixation or precise vision difficult during locomotion (Ford and Walsh, 1936; Dandy, 1941; Bender, 1965; Bender et al., 1965; Bender and Feldman, 1967; Atkin and Bender, 1968).

Defective compensatory eye movements in a patient with bilateral labyrinthine disease are shown in Fig. 1C. As the head turned at an increasing rate from side to side, the eyes (E) failed to keep pace with the head movement (H), and the summated head and eye movement trace (E+H) showed large shifts (upward arrow). These shifts were accompanied by a subjective report of oscillation or movement of the target. Generally in such patients the target appears to be displaced in the direction opposite to that of the head movement (Bender and Feldman, 1967). However, a variety of subjective complaints can be elicited when these patients are closely questioned, and the direction of target shift cannot always be correlated with the failure of ocular compensation shown in the recording (Bender, 1965).

The interaction between the head and eyes in lateral gaze shifts is changed after labyrinthectomy (Dichgans et al., 1973a). Pre-operative lateral gaze shifts are shown in Fig. 2C. Initially after labyrinthectomy there is an overshoot of gaze when shifting the head and eyes laterally due to the loss of vestibular control of the eyes (Fig. 2D). In time, however, some measure of eye-head coordination is reestablished (Fig. 2E). This is due in part to neck-ocular reflexes, and in part to central "recalibration" of activity responsible for the eye and head movements (Dichgans et al., 1973a).

Eye movements have also been described which are apparently 'anticompensatory' in direction (Melvill Jones, 1964). These are induced by strong sudden impulses of angular acceleration. Melvill Jones proposed that these eye movements lead head displacements so as to prepare for fixation when the head movement has stopped. Similar eye movements called 'return eye movements' have been induced in alert animals by semicircular canal nerve stimulation (Cohen et al., 1967). These movements could also oppose compensatory head movements induced by strong impulses of angular acceleration (Goto et al., 1968).

B. Interaction of Visual and Vestibular Systems

Movement of objects in the visual fields can result either from actual displacement of targets or from eye or head movement relative to these targets. When the head is stationary, eye movements which pursue moving targets are primarily induced by the visual system, although the vestibular system may also participate in their production (see below). When the head moves, the vestibular system responds and acts in concert with neck and visual receptors to produce the induced eye movements (Szentágothai, 1952; Henriksson, 1955a, b; Philipszoon, 1962; Jongkees and Philipszoon, 1964; Takemori and Suzuki, 1969; Bizzi et al., 1971; Suzuki, 1972b; Dichgans et al., 1973a).

There is an intimate relationship between the visual and vestibular systems, and the vestibular system may participate in producing ocular compensatory movements which appear to be predominantly visual in origin. For example, "flash" nystagmus is nystagmus induced by flickering a light in one eye of a rabbit or monkey (Costin et al., 1965, 1966; Pasik et al., 1970). The direction of this nystagmus is dependent on the position of the head in space, indicating that activity of the otolith organs is important for producing this response (Pasik et al., 1973). In accord with this, flash nystagmus disappears after bilateral labyrinthectomy (Pasik et al., 1973).

The labyrinths also play a role in inducing optokinetic nystagmus (OKN) and optokinetic after-nystagmus (OKAN). Monkeys are unable to maintain slow phase velocities of more than 45–60°/sec during OKN after unilateral or bilateral labyrinthectomy (Cohen et al., 1973). Moreover, optokinetic afternystagmus (OKAN) is reduced after unilateral labyrinthectomy and abolished after bilateral labyrinthectomy (Cohen et al., 1973; Uemura and Cohen, 1972, 1973).

Participation of the vestibular system in producing OKN and OKAN is not unreasonable since movement of the entire visual surround (whole field rotation) which induces OKN and OKAN always occurs during head movements in light (Mach, 1875). Suppressive effects of vision on nystagmus induced by the vestibular system were shown by Ohm (1926) and the functional significance of suppressive as well as facilitatory interactions were pointed out by Mowrer (1937), Rademaker and ter Braak (1948), and Jung (1948). The nature of these effects are illustrated in Fig. 3. When optokinetic (Fig. 3B) and per-rotatory nystagmus (Fig. 3A) induced by angular rotation at a constant velocity were summated (Fig. 3C), there was an enhanced per-rotatory response. That is, the velocity of the slow phases of the resultant nystagmus was better maintained at the velocity of rotation. Moreover, post-rotatory nystagmus which was present after rotation in darkness (Fig. 3A) was reduced in Fig. 3C when it was summated with the oppositely-directed OKAN (Fig. 3B). The deflection of the cupula must have been the same in Fig. 3A and C when the rotating platform was suddenly braked.

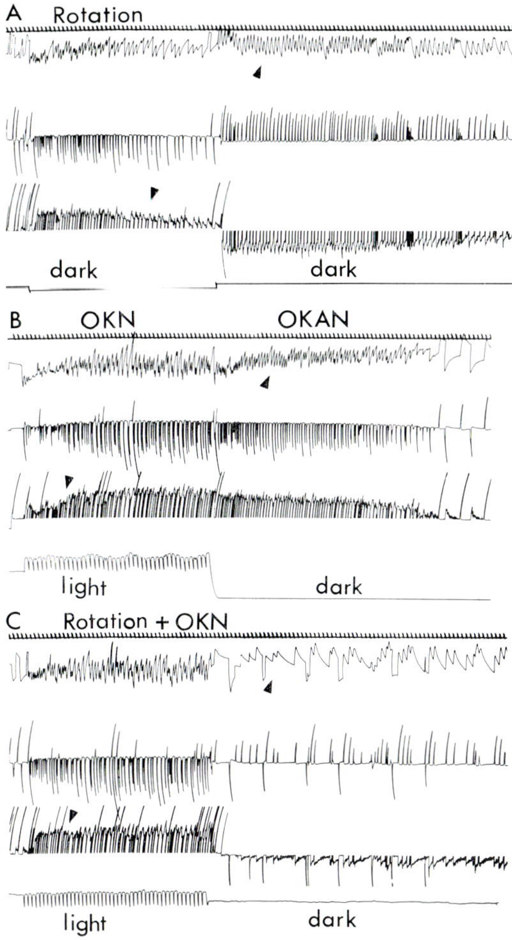

Fig. 3. Nystagmus of intact monkey during constant velocity angular rotation (A), optokinetic stimulation (B), and combined stimulation (C). The top trace in each group is the time base at 1 mark/sec. The second trace is the bitemporal horizontal EOG recorded with DC-coupling. The third trace is the differentiated EOG showing eye velocity and the fourth trace the differentiated rectified EOG showing slow phase velocity. The bottom trace shows the period of rotation in A and the passage of OKN stripes in B and C. Each 45° of OKN drum rotation recorded by a photocell caused a downward pen deflection in B and C. In A the animal was in darkness. Note the steady decline in slow phase velocity during the per-rotatory nystagmus (downward arrow) and the strong post-rotatory response (upward arrow). In B optokinetic nystagmus (OKN) was recorded in light and OKAN in darkness. Note the slow buildup in slow phase velocity during the early part of the response (downward arrow) and the strong OKAN (upward arrow). In C the animal received both rotational and optokinetic stimulation caused by moving the rotating platform and OKN drum in opposite directions simultaneously. At the end of stimulation the lights were extinguished and the post-rotatory response was recorded in darkness. Note the enhanced per-rotatory (downward arrow) and the weak post-rotatory nystagmus (upward arrow) when compared with A. The vertical bars beside A show 10° for the EOG and 100°/sec for the differentiated EOG. From Takemori and Cohen (unpublished data)

However, there was only weak post-rotatory nystagmus if the rotation took place in light and OKN was induced along with the rotatory nystagmus (Fig. 3C). By adjusting the relative intensities of OKN and per-rotatory nystagmus, postrotatory responses could be entirely abolished (TAKEMORI and COHEN, unpublished data). Thus OKN and OKAN reflect processes which enhance compensatory eye movements during head movement and serve to "brake" or suppress unwanted postmovement effects (RADEMAKER and TER BRAAK, 1948).

The interaction of the visual and vestibular systems is also shown by sensation of self-movement (circular vection) caused by whole field rotation in man (BRANDT and DICHGANS, 1972; DICHGANS and BRANDT, 1972). If there is ambiguity as to whether the head or the surround is turning during OKN, the subjective feeling is always that of self-rotation or "circular vection". Even "coriolis-like" sensations, i.e. sensations of movement away from the plane of stimulation, can be induced if the head is tilted during circular vection induced by OKN though the individual is stationary (BRANDT and DICHGANS, 1972). This shows that the brain is responding to the optokinetic stimulus as if the head rather than the surrounding visual field were rotating. Activity originating in the periphery of the visual fields is decisive in inducing circular vection (BRANDT et al., 1973; DICHGANS et al., 1972a, b).

Possible physiological substrates for circular vection and for interactions of OKN and vestibular nystagmus have already been demonstrated in the vestibular nuclei. DUENSING and SCHAEFER (1958) originally showed that eye movements are associated with activity of vestibular nuclei neurons, and KLINKE and SCHMIDT (1970) and SCHMIDT et al. (1972) that this activity is projected to the vestibular end organs by the efferent vestibular system. Recently DICHGANS et al. (1973b) and HENN et al. (1974) demonstrated that activity of neurons responding to rotation in the vestibular nuclei is enhanced when optokinetic stimuli are given which would produce OKN in the same direction as nystagmus induced by rotatory stimuli. Oppositely-directed optokinetic stimuli produced a reduction in the activity of these neurons. Therefore it is clear that at all levels of the vestibular system neuronal activity is affected by ongoing visual stimuli.

Direct pathways from the visual to the vestibular system which might carry visual information are not entirely clear. GILDENBERG and HASSLER (1971) affected vestibular nuclear unit activity by motor cortex stimulation at latencies > 8 msec. There is also evidence that enhancement and suppression of appropriate and inappropriate vestibular compensatory eye movements may be mediated through the accessory optic system and the flocculus. MAEKAWA and SIMPSON (1972) showed that the visual system can activate Purkinje cells in the flocculus via the accessory optic tract and the inferior olive. Axons of these Purkinje cells in turn inhibit cells in the vestibular nuclei (ITO et al., 1970b; HIGHSTEIN and ITO, 1971a, b; BAKER et al., 1972a; FUKUDA et al., 1972; HIGHSTEIN, 1973; ITO et al., 1973c) including cells which mediate horizontal vestibulo-ocular reflexes (ITO et al., 1973c). This provides a mechanism for visual inhibition of direct vestibulo-ocular pathways. LISBERGER and FUCHS (1974) have also shown that activity of flocculus Purkinje cells is closely associated with visual suppression of compensatory movements. In accord with this, TAKEMORI and COHEN (1974b) found that visual suppression of vestibular nystagmus (TAKEMORI and

COHEN, 1974a) is lost after destruction of the flocculus on both sides, and Ito et al. (1974) that compensatory vestibular movements are reduced after flocculus lesions.

Much less is known of how the vestibular system might affect the visual system. HORN and HILL (1969), DENNEY and ADJORANI (1972), HORN et al. (1972), and BISTI et al. (1972) demonstrated that the visual fields of neurons in the visual cortex and superior colliculus are affected by head tilt, although this is disputed by SCHWARTZKROIN (1972). This is a subject for future study. Since the vestibular apparatus reacts to change in position of the head in space, it must respond both during passive and volitional head movement. How peripheral or central vestibular activity might differ during voluntary unexpected head displacement is also not clear.

Study of eye movements during head movement is complicated because vestibular responses may habituate on repeated exposure (HOOD and PFALTZ, 1954; MCCABE, 1960; CRAMPTON, 1962, 1964; GUEDRY, 1964; COLLINS and UPDEGRAFF, 1966; COLLINS, 1966; CHAPTER F.VI.). This occurs when the eye movements are not compensatory (GONSHOR and MELVILL JONES, 1973). Oculomotor reflexes induced by visual stimuli, such as optokinetic nystagmus do not show similar habituation even on prolonged testing (GRÜTTNER, 1939; MACKENSEN and UBER, 1960; KOMATSUZAKI et al., 1969). In addition, not only is there visual and central suppression of vestibular reflexes (COLLINS, 1966; MCCABE, 1960; TAKEMORI and COHEN, 1974a) but the response to repeated stimulation, the 'dynamic or kinetic response', may be just the opposite of the original response (FUKUDA et al., 1958). Finally, interactions between information arising in the otolith organs and the semicircular canals are of considerable importance in determining the form of the oculomotor and postural response to different vestibular stimuli. An example is the potentiation of nystagmus during constant velocity rotation around the long axis of the body, "barbeque rotation" (BENSON and BODIN, 1966). Despite the large body of work on functional aspects of vestibulo-ocular reflexes over the last century, many interesting aspects of vestibular control of the oculomotor system as yet are incompletely understood.

II. Eye Movements Induced by the Vestibular Apparatus: Semicircular Canals

The semicircular canals exert a powerful influence on the ocular muscles. Activity generated in semicircular canal nerves can reach eye muscles at short latencies (TYČ-DUMONT and DELL, 1962; COHEN and SUZUKI, 1963; ITO, F., et al., 1969; ITO, M., et al., 1973a, b), utilizing monosynaptic pathways between the vestibular and oculomotor nuclei (PRECHT et al., 1967; RICHTER and PRECHT, 1968; BAKER et al., 1969a, b; ITO et al., 1970a; HIGHSTEIN, 1971, 1973; HIGHSTEIN and ITO, 1971; FUKUDA et al., 1972; BAKER et al., 1973a, b; SCHWINDT et al., 1973). When the semicircular canal nerves are stimulated, synchronous excitation of eye muscles can be produced at stimulation rates close to the fusion frequency of the fastest eye muscle fibers (COOPER and ECCLES, 1930; COHEN and SUZUKI, 1963; BACH-Y-RITA and ITO, 1966; YAMANAKA and BACH-Y-RITA, 1968). Short latency activation of eye muscles is decreased in drowsiness or by narcosis (COHEN and SUZUKI, 1963). Inhibition of eye muscles is also carried over short latency pathways (COHEN et al., 1964; TYČ-DUMONT, 1966; RICHTER and PRECHT, 1968; BAKER et al., 1969b; ITO et al., 1970a, b; HIGHSTEIN, 1971, 1973; HIGHSTEIN and ITO, 1971; MAEDA et al., 1971a, b; PRECHT and BAKER, 1972; BAKER et al., 1973; ITO et al., 1973b). When the nerves of both canals in the same plane are simultaneously stimulated, inhibition is predominant (COHEN et al., 1964). Analyses of unit activity in the vestibular nuclei and of unit activity in vestibulo-ocular pathways are considered in more detail in this volume by PRECHT and elsewhere by MELVILL JONES and MILSUM (1971), and SKAVENSKI and ROBINSON (1973).

Pathways with longer conduction times also connect eye muscles to the vestibular apparatus (LORENTE DE NÓ, 1933b; SPIEGEL and SOMMER, 1944; SZENTÁGOTHAI, 1950). These pathways are multisynaptic and are at least in part responsible for slow phases of nystagmus and for slow tonic deviations. Both the monosynaptic and multisynaptic pathways will be discussed in more detail subsequently.

Since the semicircular canals respond to changes in angular velocity of the head in every spatial plane, it is not surprising that they induce eye movements which also lie in every spatial plane (SUZUKI et al., 1964). Two semicircular canals, one on each side, lie in each of three planes (QUIX, 1925; CAMIS and CREED, 1930; SPIEGEL and SOMMER, 1944; BLANKS et al., 1972). The ocular reaction induced by excitation of the nerve of one canal is just opposite to that induced by excitation of the nerve of the other canal in the parallel plane (EWALD, 1892; LOWENSTEIN and SAND, 1940a, b; COHEN et al., 1964; SUZUKI et al., 1964). For example, the pattern of eye movement induced by excitation of one posterior canal nerve is similar to that induced by inhibition of the contralateral anterior canal nerve.The same is true for eye movements induced by lateral canal nerves. Rotation in directions which would produce excitation in semicircular canal nerves appears to be somewhat more effective in inducing ocular responses than rotation in the direction which would produce inhibition (EWALD, 1892). There is some controversy as to whether this is true in the normal state (Acta Otolaryngologica Supplement 159, 1961).

Patterns of eye movement induced by stimulation of the individual semicircular canals in fish and birds have been known for many years. Comprehensive reviews of early work have been given by CAMIS and CREED, 1930; DUSSER DE BARENNE, 1934; MCNALLY and STUART, 1942; SPIEGEL and SOMMER, 1944; and GERNANDT, 1959. More recent reviews are included in books or monographs by BENDER, 1964; KORNHUBER, 1966; WOLFSON, 1966.

FLOURENS (1842) originally described that destruction of individual canals in pigeons induced head nystagmus in planes parallel to the plane of the canal which had been destroyed. HÖGYES (1880) destroyed individual canals in rabbits and inferred that one muscle in each eye was primarily activated by each canal. LEE (1893, 1894) compressed individual canals in sharks and showed that the eyes appeared to move in the planes of the canals which had been excited. In classic studies EWALD (1892) induced endolymph currents in individual semicircular canals of pigeons. Oppositely-directed endolymph flow induced oppositely-directed head and eye deviations. These movements were in planes parallel to plane of the canal which had been stimulated.

SZENTÁGOTHAI (1950) was one of the first to show the pattern of activation of eye muscles induced by endolymph flow in individual canals of mammals. In the dog one muscle in each eye was strongly activated by excitation of each canal. FLUUR (1959) stimulated the nerves of individual canals in the cat and found this in most of his experiments. By implanting electrodes close to semicircular canal nerves in cats, dogs, monkeys, and rabbits, it was possible to observe the eye movements and body postural changes induced by stimulation of individual semicircular canal nerves in otherwise intact animals (COHEN and SUZUKI, 1963; SUZUKI et al., 1964; SUZUKI and COHEN, 1964; COHEN et al., 1965a; COHEN et al., 1966; SUZUKI et al., 1969a). These studies will be summarized in the following section.

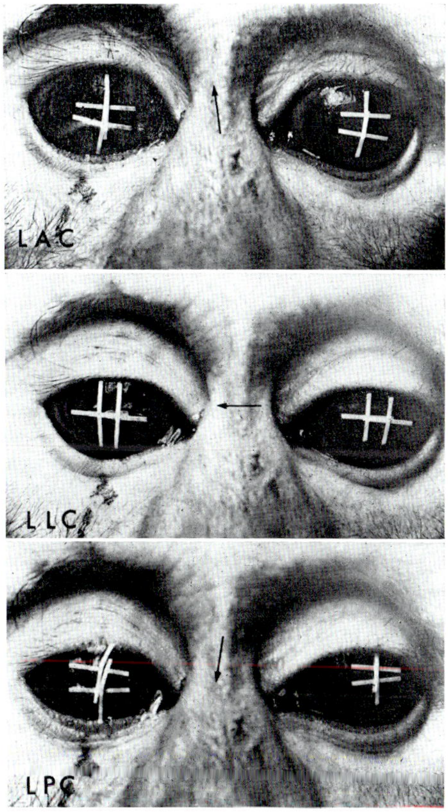

Fig. 4. Eye movements induced by electric stimulation of left anterior canal nerve (LAC), left lateral canal nerve (LLC) and left posterior canal nerve (LPC) in an alert monkey. A white cross on a blackened egg shell membrane covered the locally anesthetized cornea. The stimulus was a 50 msec train of 0.5 msec square waves at an intra-train frequency of 400/sec. Each photograph is a double exposure, one cross showing the position of the eyes at the beginning of stimulation, and the second the position of the eyes shortly after the end of stimulation. The arrows indicate the direction of movement. From the midposition LAC induces upward counterclockwise rotatory eye movements, LLC contralateral horizontal eye movements, and LPC downward counterclockwise rotatory movements. From SUZUKI and COHEN, Exp. Neurol. **10**, 393–405 (1964)

Patterns of eye movement induced by individual semicircular canal nerve stimulation on the left side in an alert monkey are shown in Fig. 4. When the left anterior canal nerve is stimulated (LAC), both eyes elevate, the ipsilateral or left eye intorts, and the contralateral or right eye extorts. When the left lateral canal nerve is stimulated (LLC), both eyes move horizontally to the contralateral side. When the left posterior canal nerve is activated (LPC), the left eye intorts and moves slightly down and the right eye moves down with slight extorsion. Eye movements induced by stimulation of right semicircular canals nerves are mirror images of those in Fig. 4. When both anterior canal nerves are simultaneously activated, both eyes move up without intorsion or extorsion, and when both posterior canal nerves are activated, both eyes move down. When the left anterior and left posterior canal nerves are simultaneously stimulated, the left eye intorts and the right eye extorts. Eye movements in any spatial plane can be induced by summing the eye movements induced by stimulation of several canal nerves.

Since the eyes move in the plane of the canal whose nerve was activated, the actual eye movements themselves must be different in species which have a different relationship between the semicircular canals and the position of the eyes in the head. The semicircular canal planes and the angle of the optic axis of either eye in monkey (m), cat (c), dog (d), and rabbit (r) are shown in the diagrams on the left of Fig. 5. The optic axis is the line between the center of the cornea and the axis of rotation (Johnson, 1900; Imai, 1930). Eye movements in cat (c) and rabbit (r) in planes parallel to the plane of the left anterior semicircular canal are shown in Fig. 5B, in the lower diagram by the oblique arrows.

Actual eye movements induced by stimulation of the left anterior semicircular canal nerve in monkey, cat, dog, and rabbit (Fig. 5C) agree with the predicted patterns (Suzuki et al., 1964). In monkey and man the optic axis makes an angle of about 5° with the midsagittal plane. In the dog this angle is 35°. Therefore, when the anterior canal nerve is stimulated in dog, the ipsilateral eye (E_1) has less rotation and more elevation than in monkey. The converse is true for the contralateral eye (E_r), i.e., there is more rotation and less elevation in dog than in monkey. In the rabbit whose optic axes are 85° from the midsagittal plane, the ipsilateral eye extorts and moves up and the contralateral eye extorts and moves down.

The movements shown in Fig. 5 were induced with the eyes close to the midposition. Changes in initial eye position also affect deviations induced by the semicircular canals. An example of this is shown in Fig. 6 during left posterior canal nerve stimulation (LPC) in a monkey. Its eyes were on the right (rt), in the midposition (mid), and on the left (lt). In Figs. 6B and C are diagrams of the expected intorsion and depression of the left eye during movement in the plane of the left posterior canal. Experimental findings are shown in Fig. 6D. Regardless of the initial position of the eyes in the orbit, the induced eye movements lay in the plane of the left posterior canal (Cohen et al., 1966).

There are two ways in which the nervous system might induce eye movements in planes parallel to canal planes from different initial eye positions. (1) There might be a different pattern of eye muscle activation for each initial eye position. (2) The pattern of activation might be fixed, but the nature of the origin and insertion of the eye muscles is such that they would cause the eyes to move in a

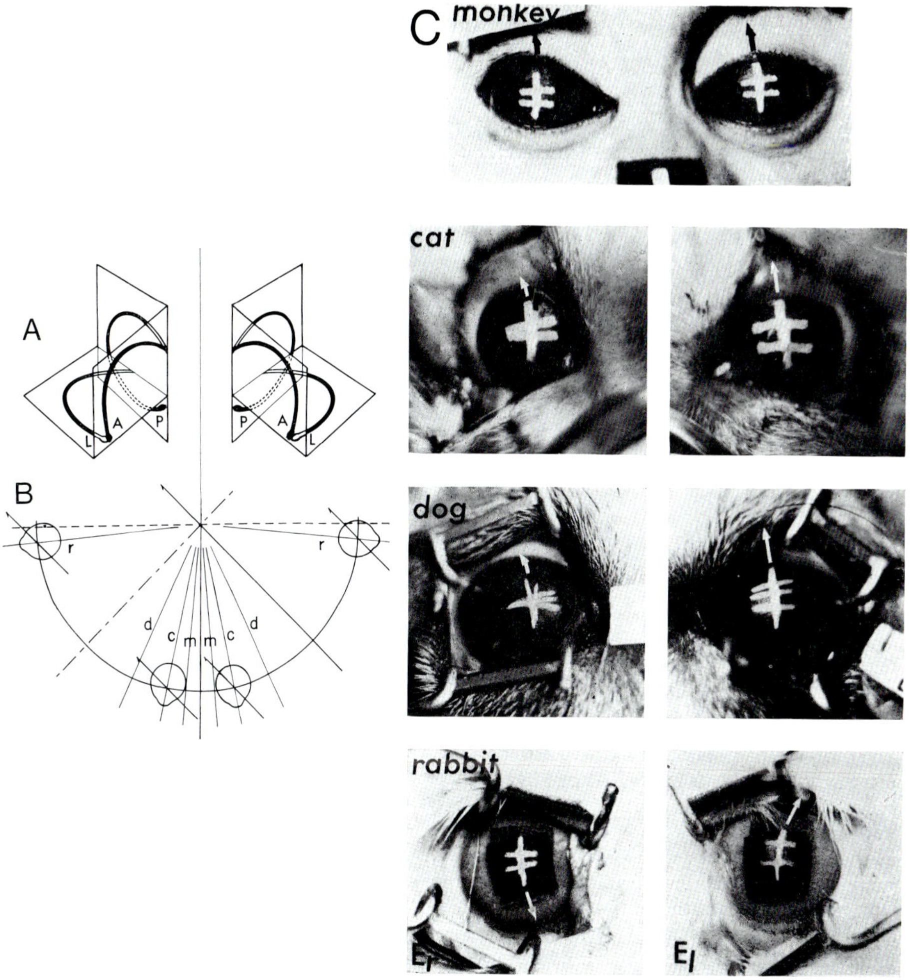

Fig. 5. A. Three dimensional representation of the planes of the semicircular canals. B. Diagram showing the plane of movement of the right and left eyes which would compensate for head movement down and to the left in a plane 45° from the midsagittal plane. This would be an excitatory stimulus for the left anterior canal. The angles which the optic axis makes with the midsagittal plane in each eye in monkey (m), cat (c), dog (d), and rabbit (r) are shown on an idealized head which is viewed from the top. The eyes of cat and rabbit are also drawn. The plane of the compensatory eye movements is shown by oblique arrows up and to the right. The plane of the axis of eye and head movements is perpendicular to the arrows. C. Movements of the right eye (E_r) and left eye (E_l) during left anterior canal nerve stimulation. Eye movements were recorded by the same double-flash technique described in Fig. 4, except in dog where three flashes were used. The arrows above or below the eyes show the direction of the induced eye movements. Note that the direction of rotation of the left eye (E_l) is reversed in monkey and rabbit, and the right eye (E_r) moves up in the monkey and down in the rabbit. From Suzuki et al., Exp. Neurol. **9**, 137–160 (1964)

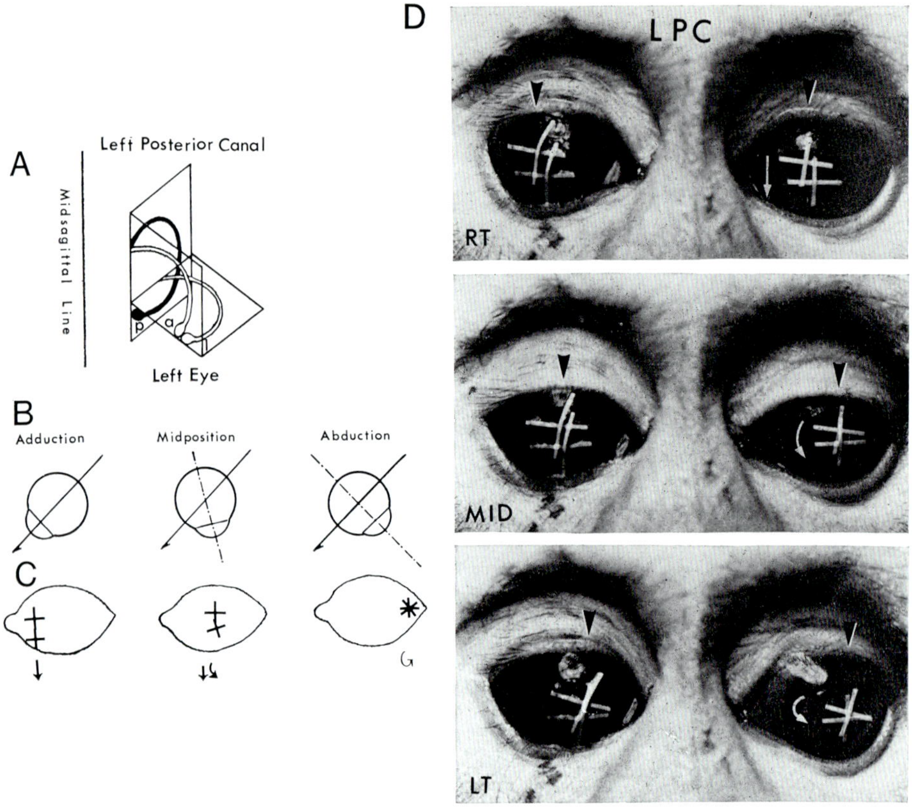

Fig. 6. A–C. Diagrammatic representation of the plane of the left posterior canal and of compensatory movements of the left eye in the plane of the left posterior canal from initial positions of adduction, midposition and abduction. A. Left posterior canal is shown in black. B. Top view of left eye showing optic axis (dashed line) and plane of vertical canal (solid line). Dashed and solid lines coincide when the left eye is adducted. C. Movements of left eye as they would appear from front of animal. Only components of intorsion and depression are shown. One cross represents the initial position and second cross the final position of the eyes. The direction of eye movement is shown by underlying arrows. D. Samples of eye movements induced by stimulation of the left posterior canal nerve in an alert monkey with its eyes to the right (RT), center (MID), and left (LT). The downward arrows show the original position of the center of the cornea. In each case the left eye moved down or intorted, or both. Regardless of initial eye position, eye movements induced by LPC stimulation lay in or close to planes parallel to the plane of the left posterior canal. From COHEN et al., Arch. Ophthal. **76**, 523–531 (1966)

particular plane whatever the initial position of the eyes in the orbit. Activity of individual muscles was sampled during posterior canal nerve stimulation. The amplitude of eye muscle potentials and the tension induced in these muscles did not change significantly when the initial position of the eyes in the orbit shifted (COHEN et al., 1966). Therefore, each canal probably induces a fixed pattern of eye muscle activation, and the eyes move in planes parallel to the planes of the excited canals regardless of initial eye position because of the anatomy of the eye muscles and the orbit.

This is more apparent if movements of the left eye induced by excitation of the left superior oblique muscle (Fig. 7D, TOKUMASU et al., 1965) are compared to movements of the left eye induced by left posterior canal nerve stimulation (Fig. 6D). The left superior oblique is the muscle primarily activated by the left posterior canal (SZENTÁGOTHAI, 1950; FLUUR, 1959; COHEN et al., 1964). Eye movements predicted from the anatomy of the eye are shown in the diagrams in Fig. 7C

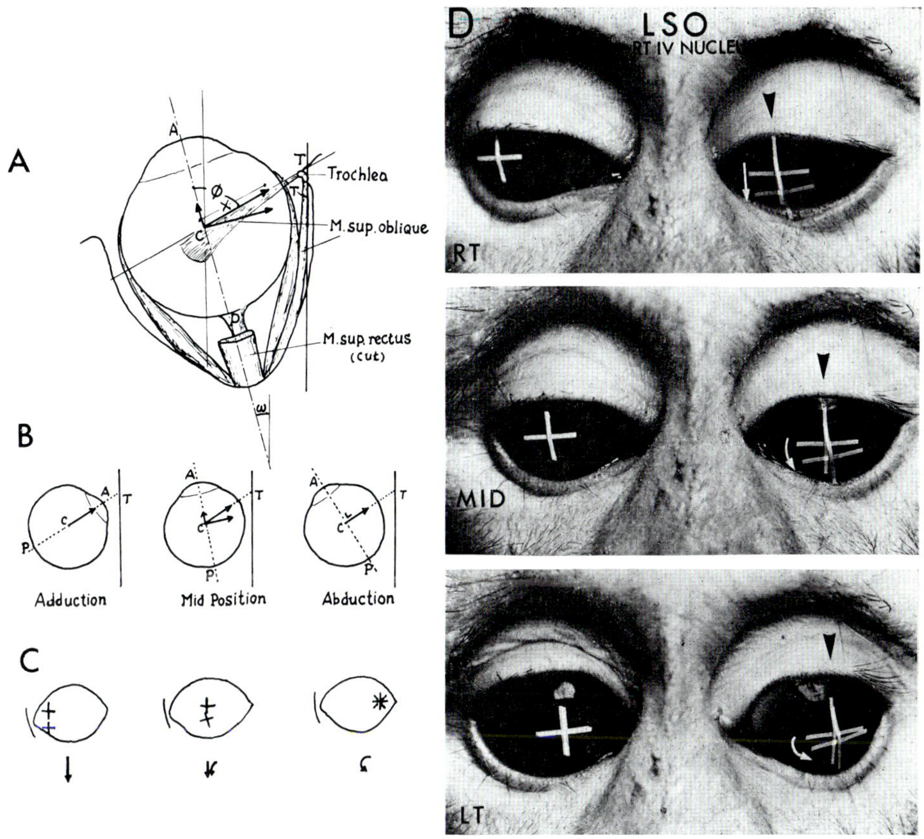

Fig. 7. Left, A, Anatomical relations of the eye, orbit, and superior oblique muscle in monkey. A–P, optic axis; C, point lying on globe above center of rotation; ω, angle between midsagittal plane and optic axis; Φ, angle between optic axis and superior oblique muscle tendon; X, vector of force produced by superior oblique contraction. B. Diagrams showing the vectors of force produced by superior oblique muscle contraction with the left eye in adduction, midposition, or abduction. C. Diagram of movements of the center of the cornea induced by left superior oblique muscle contraction in adduction, midposition, and abduction. First cross shows original eye position and second cross the position to which the eye moved as a result of contraction. D. Movements of left eye induced by stimulation of the right trochlear nucleus and nerve roots in an alert monkey with eyes to the right (RT), center (MID), and left (LT). Double flash techniques as in preceding figures. Arrowheads show the original position of the center of the left cornea. White arrows show the direction of eye movement. Components of intorsion and depression of the left eye are similar to those induced by LPC nerve stimulation (Fig. 6). From TOKUMASU et al., Arch. Ophthal. **73**, 851–862 (1965)

and experimental data in Fig. 7D. As is apparent from Figs. 6 and 7 when the superior oblique muscle contracts, it produces eye movements in planes close to the plane of the posterior canal whatever the initial position of the eye in the orbit.

This implies that the planes of space which are represented in the semicircular canals must have played an important role in the evolution of the anatomy of the eye. If true, then perception of these spatial planes is probably more important for normal functioning of the organism than is commonly appreciated. There is indirect evidence to suggest that these planes of space are probably discretely represented at various places in the nervous system, including the cerebellum (COHEN et al., 1965b) and the vestibular nuclei (TOKUMASU et al., 1969; UEMURA and COHEN, 1973). The data also show that the anatomic connections from individual vertical semicircular canals to eye muscles must vary in different species. For example, in monkey and cat when the left anterior canal nerve is stimulated, the ipsilateral superior oblique and contralateral superior rectus muscles are activated (COHEN et al., 1964). In the rabbit, however, the same stimulus activates the ipsilateral inferior oblique and contralateral inferior rectus muscle (Fig. 5) (ITO et al., 1973a), antagonists of the superior oblique and superior rectus. This requires anatomic connections from anterior canals to portions of the oculomotor nuclei which are quite different in rabbit than in cat or monkey. TARLOV and TARLOV (1971) have shown that the organization of the oculomotor nucleus also varies in different species. Since the optic axis is the same in monkey and man (JOHNSON, 1900; IMAI, 1930) data on monkey are probably applicable to man.

A. Head and Body Movements Induced by Semicircular Canals

If animals are restrained and individual semicircular canals or their nerves are stimulated, only the eyes move. If the head is free, however, both head and eyes move. Head movements induced by semicircular canal nerve stimulation also lie in planes parallel to the plane of the canal whose nerve was excited (SUZUKI and COHEN, 1964). This is true regardless of the initial position of the head on the neck (COHEN et al., 1966). In the cat the ears and whiskers also move in planes parallel to the plane of the excited canals (SUZUKI and COHEN, 1964). Head movements induced by semicircular canal nerve stimulation in the cat are shown diagrammatically in Fig. 8. Head movements have also been induced by caloric stimulation in man (HENRIKSSON et al., 1962). These movements are small and slow compared to those induced by semicircular canal nerve stimulation. Presumably the synchrony and high frequencies induced by electrical stimulation are mainly reponsible for the difference in the induced movements.

Activity induced in the limbs by semicircular canals is organized so as to support the head as it moves to counter angular head deflections in the plane of one or several canals. There is always some ipsilateral forelimb extension and some contralateral forelimb flexion when the canal nerves on one side are stimulated in the cat. In the monkey the postural response may not be striking when the animals are stationary. However, if an ampullary nerve stimulus falls during an ongoing movement, then the postural response is striking. When stimulation of

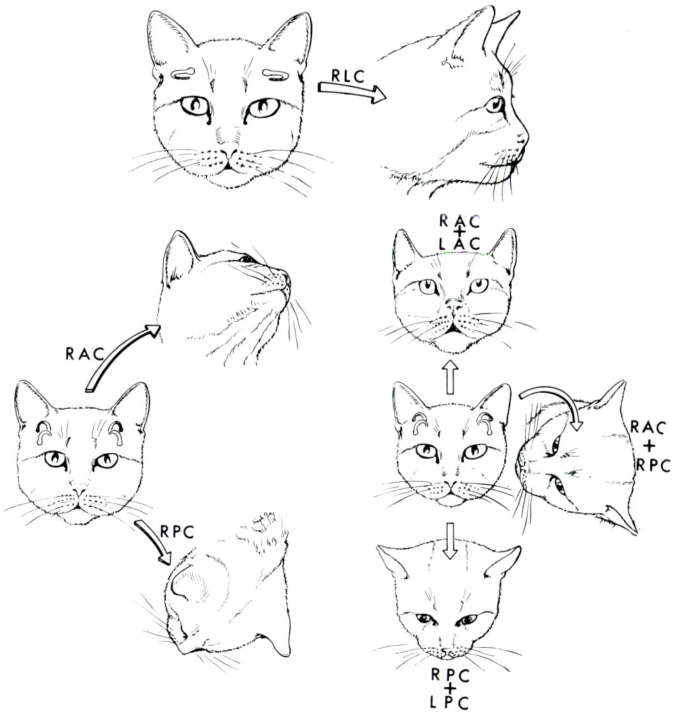

Fig. 8. Schematic drawing of the semicircular canals and of the head movements induced by ampullary nerve stimulation in the cat. The arrows show the direction of induced head movements. RLC, right lateral canal nerve stimulation; RAC, right anterior canal nerve stimulation; RPC, right posterior canal nerve stimulation. In pictures RAC+LAC, RAC+RPC, and RPC+LPC two canal nerves were simultaneously stimulated to produce the head movement. From SUZUKI and COHEN, Exp. Neurol. **10**, 393–405 (1964)

canal nerves is continued, complicated postural changes are induced, and animals attempt to circle in the plane of the canals. This is most easily accomplished in the plane of the lateral canal (Fig. 9, LLC). Similar circling in response to rotation as well as to rotating visual stimuli are found in a wide variety of animals including invertebrates (CAMIS and CREED, 1930; TOKITA et al., 1965; TAUBER and ATKIN, 1968).

When the relationship of the head to the trunk is changed, body movements induced by stimulation of individual canal nerves also change. This is particularly apparent in the cat when both anterior semicircular canal nerves are stimulated (SUZUKI et al., 1964). The natural or adequate stimulus which would cause excitatory activity in both anterior canal nerves would be downward angular movements of the head in the midsagittal plane. The compensatory response is a movement of the head upward and backward in its own midsagittal plane whatever the position of the head on the neck (Fig. 8, RAC+LAC; COHEN et al., 1966). With the head to the left, there will be extension of the left forelimb and flexion of the right forelimb. With the head to the right, there will be extension of the right forelimb and flexion of the left. With the head in the midposition, both forelimbs will extend. These changes in forelimb activity are most probably a manifestation

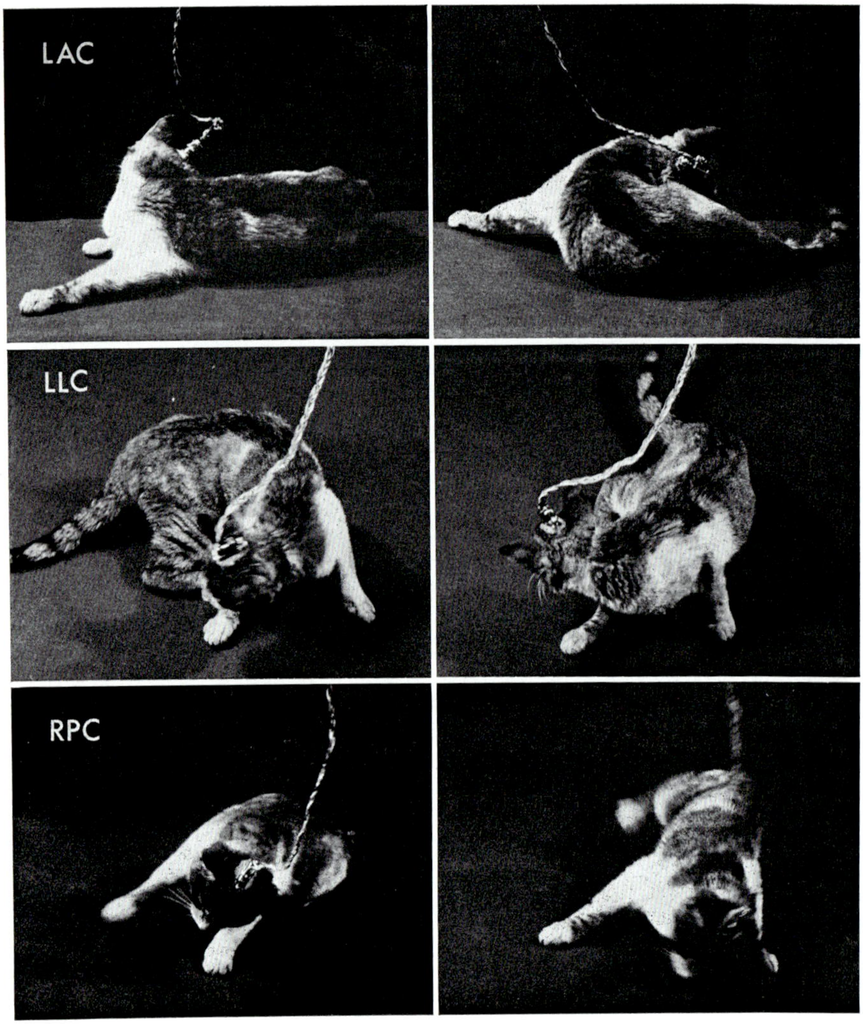

Fig. 9. Head and body movements induced by stimulation of the nerves of the left anterior canal (LAC), left lateral canal (LLC), and right posterior canal (RPC). In each case there was extension of the ipsilateral forelimb and flexion of the contralateral forelimb. The hind limbs were flexed during RAC stimulation and extended during RPC stimulation. Prolonged stimulation produced circling in the plane of the canal whose nerve was excited. This was most easily accomplished during lateral canal nerve stimulation (LLC, picture on right). From SUZUKI and COHEN, Exp. Neurol. **10**, 393–405 (1964)

of the interaction of tonic neck reflexes with vestibulo-spinal reflexes (MAGNUS, 1924). Originally believed to be present only in decerebrate states (MAGNUS, 1924), FUKUDA (1961) has emphasized that tonic neck reflexes are commonly present in many activities of daily life. Vestibulo-spinal activity is considered in detail elsewhere in this volume (Chapter D. V.). It is sufficient to note that the position of the head on the neck, of the eyes in the orbit (GERNANDT, 1968; EASTON, 1971, 1972), of the trunk and limbs, and the time after the start of stimulation are but a few of the variables which probably affect postural responses induced by the vestibular apparatus.

B. Eye Movement Produced by Utricular and Saccular Stimulation

The 'adequate' or natural stimulus for the otolith organs is described elsewhere in this volume. There has been considerable controversy about the oculomotor function of the utricle and saccule, and whether the otolith organs are capable of inducing nystagmus. The older literature is reviewed in detail by CAMIS and CREED (1930), MCNALLY and STUART (1942) and BERGSTEDT (1961). It seems likely that the otolith organs induce compensatory eye movements when the head is in positions other than upright (MILLER, 1962), when the head is tilted (BERTHOZ et al., 1973), or during linear acceleration of the head. In the past considerable attention has been paid to slow tonic deviations induced by the otolith organs in response to changes in static head position (DE KLEYN, 1920; MAGNUS, 1924; BENJAMINS and HUIZINGA, 1927; LORENTE DE NÓ, 1931; MILLER, 1962; KREJCOVA et al., 1971). However, the otolith organs are linear accelerometers, and induce short latency eye movements as well (SUZUKI et al., 1969b; BAKER et al., 1973; SCHWINDT et al., 1973). Varying linear acceleration has been shown to induce or enhance nystagmus in both humans and in animals (BERGSTEDT, 1961; JONGKEES and PHILIPSZOON, 1964; GUEDRY, 1965; BENSON and BODIN, 1966; GRAYBIEL et al., 1972).

1. Counter-Rolling

When the head is tilted the eyes roll in the opposite direction so as to maintain the original angle of the retina in space (HUNTER, 1786). Ocular counter-rolling against lateral head positions is about $\pm 5°$–$7°$ in humans and monkeys (WOELLNER and GRAYBIEL, 1959, 1960; MILLER, 1962; HANNEN et al., 1966; KREJCOVA et al., 1971). Examples of counter-rolling in the monkey are shown in Fig. 10

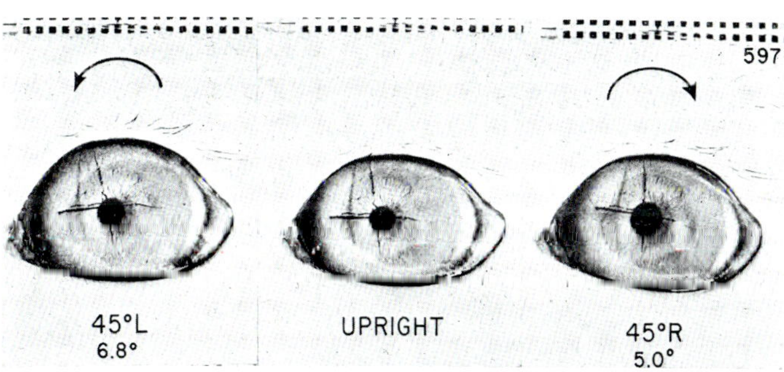

Fig. 10. Compensatory ocular counter-rolling against static head tilt in a monkey. The head and body were tilted together. A black cross tattooed on the cornea was used to indicate the position of the left eye. The center photo (upright) shows the control position. When the animal was 45° to the left (L), the eyes were rotated 6.8° in a counter-clockwise direction. When the animal was 45° to the right (R) the eyes torted 5° in a clockwise direction. From KREJCOVA, HIGHSTEIN and COHEN, Acta oto-laryng. (Stockh.) **72**, 165–171 (1971)

(KREJCOVA et al., 1971). Counter-rolling against lateral head positions (static counter-rolling) is beyond voluntary control and is not much affected by vision (KREJCOVA et al., 1971). It is an imperfect compensatory mechanism since there is little or no ocular torsion against head tilts of 5° and the maximum counter-rolling evoked by head tilts of 45°–90° is not more than 10% of the total angular displacement of the retina. As noted, further adaptation to retinal tilt can probably occur in the visual system, however (HORN and HILL, 1969; BISTI et al., 1972; DENNEY and ADJORANI, 1972; HORN et al., 1972).

The largest part of the activity responsible for static counter-rolling (CR) arises in the otolith organs, with each side contributing activity which produces about half of the response (KREJCOVA et al., 1971; UEMURA and COHEN, 1973). Neck receptors do not induce significant amounts of CR against static head tilt (KREJCOVA et al., 1971; NELSON and COPE, 1971), although activation or destruction of neck roots has been shown to cause positional nystagmus in the rabbit (BIEMOND and DE JONG, 1969), and eye deviations in cat and rabbit (Lorente de Nó, 1931; TAKEMORI and SUZUKI, 1969; SUZUKI, 1972b). HIKOSAKA and MAEDA (1973) recently showed that the pathways from the neck joint receptors to the abducens nucleus are indirect and travel via the medial vestibular nucleus. This might explain why neck-ocular reflexes are subordinate to vestibulo-ocular reflexes, unless the peripheral vestibular system has been damaged or destroyed (DICHGANS et al., 1973a; DE JONG, personal communication). Although static CR is small, dynamic CR can be much larger (MERTON, 1958; MELVILL JONES, 1958; WOELLNER and GRAYBIEL, 1959; HANNEN et al., 1966; COLLEWIJN and NOORDUIN, 1972). Presumably the anterior and posterior semicircular canals and the visual system as well as the otolith organs are activated during rolling head movements. The anterior and posterior canals also cause ocular torsion when they are simultaneously stimulated (SUZUKI et al., 1964).

2. *Utricles*

In the alert cat the excitatory drive of the otolith organs on the eye muscles is strong (SUZUKI et al., 1969b). The latency of eye muscle activation by utricular nerve stimulation is similar to that found after semicircular canal nerve stimulation (SUZUKI et al., 1969b; BERTHOZ et al., 1973; SCHWINDT et al., 1973). It is of interest that increases in stimulation frequency up to 1000 cps can cause an increase in contraction rates of muscles activated by utricular nerves (SUZUKI et al., 1969b). This implies that the utriculo-ocular reflex arc is capable of responding to very high frequencies of stimulation, and that activity at high frequencies may normally be induced in central structures by utricular or saccular stimulation.

Interpretation of eye movements induced by electric stimulation of the nerves of the utricle and saccule is complicated since movement of receptor hairs in different directions on the maculae causes excitation of nerve fibers (Fig. 11A–C) (LOWENSTEIN and ROBERTS, 1949). In contrast there is only one excitatory direction for hair movement on the crista of each semicircular canal (LOWENSTEIN and SAND, 1940a, b; LOWENSTEIN, 1956). The excitatory directions of hair cells in both types of organs agree with the polarization of the kinocilia. The kinocilia have the same orientation on the semicircular canal crista, whereas they are oppositely-directed on various parts of the maculae of the utricle and saccule (Fig. 11A–C; LOWENSTEIN and WERSÄLL, 1959; FLOCK, 1964; SPOENDLIN, 1964).

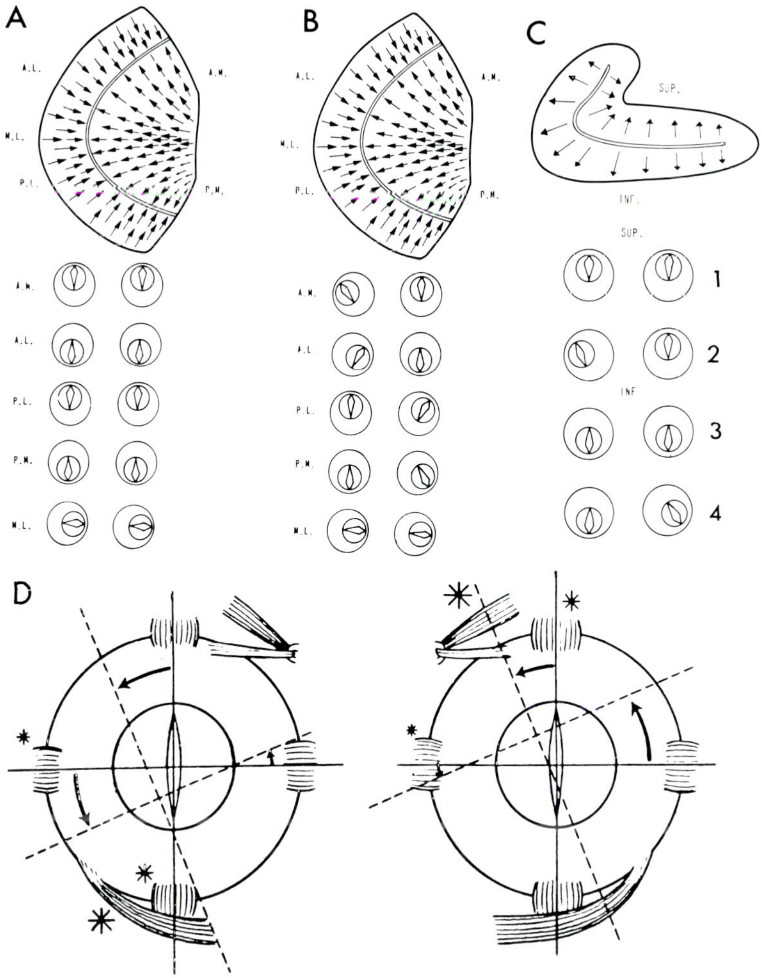

Fig. 11. A–C. Eye movements induced in alert (A, C1, C3) and anesthetized (B, C2, C4) cats from utricular (A, B) and saccular (C) macula stimulation. The directions of polarization of the hair cells on the receptors are shown above. Below are the induced eye movements. Upward movements were induced from antero-median (AM) and posterolateral (PL) stimulation of the utricle, and superior stimulation of the saccule, downward movements from anterolateral (AL) and postero median (PM) utricular and inferior saccular stimulation, and rotatory movements from medial-lateral (ML) utricular stimulation. D. Eye movements and eye muscle contractions induced by left utricular nerve stimulation in the cat. The solid cross is the position of the eyes at the beginning of stimulation and the dashed cross the position of the eyes at the end of the induced movement. The arrows show the direction of movement. Counterclockwise tonic deviations and nystagmus with counter-clockwise slow phases and clockwise quick phases were induced by left utricular nerve stimulation. The muscles most strongly activated (large asterisks) were the left superior oblique and right inferior oblique. The left superior rectus and right inferior rectus muscles also contracted (medium asterisks), and the left medial and right lateral rectus muscles were weakly activated (small asterisks). The other eye muscles were inhibited. Clockwise tonic deviations were not induced by left utricular nerve stimulation. From Fluur and Mellström, Exp. Neurol. **30**, 139–147 (1971) (A–C); and Suzuki et al., Acta oto-laryng. (Stockh.) **68**, 350–362 (1969) (D)

This suggests that different parts of the utricle or saccule might generate eye movements in different directions. Accordingly, SZENTÁGOTHAI (1964) mechanically stimulated the four quadrants of the utricular macula and induced eye movements with oppositely-directed rotatory and vertical components. FLUUR and MELLSTRÖM (1970a, 1971) also induced eye movements with oppositely-directed vertical components by stimulating various parts of the utricle (Fig. 11A, B) and saccule (Fig. 11C). Coordinated eye movements were induced from various parts of the utricle and saccule only in decerebrate alert cats (Fig. 11A, C 1, 3). Disconjugate movements were found under anesthesia (Fig. 11B, C 2, 4).

SUZUKI et al. (1969b) stimulated the utricular macula and nerve in the alert cat. They induced torsional eye movements in only one direction, similar to those which oppose head tilt during counter-rolling. When the left utricular macula and its nerve were stimulated, the predominant induced movement was counterclockwise rotation (Fig. 11D). The ipsilateral eye also moved up slightly and adducted and the contralateral eye moved down and abducted. The vertical or horizontal components of the movements varied somewhat depending on the part of the utricular macula or nerve which was stimulated. The direction of rotation was reversed when the right utricular nerve was stimulated, but clockwise eye movements were not induced by left utricular nerve or macular stimulation nor counterclockwise movements by right-sided stimulation. The muscles activated by left utricular nerve stimulation are marked in Fig. 11D with asterisks. Other muscles were inhibited. Nystagmus in the coronal plane was also induced by utricular nerve stimulation. The quick phases were oppositely-directed to the slow phases.

If each utricule can induce counter-rolling in both directions, then little qualitative change in counter-rolling might be expected after unilateral utricular destruction. However, rolling movements of the eyes were induced by head tilt in only one direction after one utricle was destroyed in the rabbit (VERSTEEGH, 1927). Similarly after unilateral labyrinthectomy in the monkey, counter-rolling was lost only to one side (KREJCOVA et al., 1971). After unilateral labyrinthectomy in humans there was a tendency for counter-rolling to be reduced mainly when the affected side was down (NELSON and HOME, 1971), although in some patients it was reduced but symmetrical to the two sides.

3. *Positional Alcohol Nystagmus*

In regard to the question of whether each utricle can evoke a full gamut of eye movements, it is of interest that oppositely-directed horizontal eye movements can be induced with the head in various positions while under the influence of alcohol. This nystagmus is known as positional alcohol nystagmus (PAN) (BÁRÁNY, 1911; DE KLEYN and VERSTEEGH, 1930; WALTER, 1954; ASCHAN et al., 1956a, b; BERGSTEDT, 1961). Activity responsible for positional alcohol nystagmus arises in the labyrinths, and PAN can no longer be induced after both labyrinths have been destroyed (DE KLEYN and VERSTEEGH, 1930; ASCHAN et al., 1956b, 1964a).

Initially after ingestion of alcohol, the positional nystagmus is geotropic. That is, the slow phases oppose gravity and the quick phases are directed toward the ground. When the first phase (PAN I) passes, it is followed in humans by a second phase (PAN II) in which the nystagmus is apogeotropic, i.e. the quick phases are directed away from the ground. PAN II is absent in many animals, but has been found in the monkey (KOMATSUZAKI et al., 1969). In acute studies in the cat and rabbit, nystagmus was induced in only one direction in the first phase of PAN after unilateral labyrinthectomy (DE KLEYN and VERSTEEGH, 1930; SUZUKI et al., 1968). However, in humans (ASCHAN et al., 1964a) and in monkeys (UEMURA and COHEN, 1973) bidirectional nystagmus was induced during PAN I after unilateral labyrinthectomy if adequate time was allowed for compensation. The intensity of the nystagmus in PAN I (as measured by total deviation of the eyes over a 20 sec period) was reduced by about half after one labyrinth had been destroyed (UEMURA and COHEN, 1973).

Because of the association of PAN with specific head positions, it seems likely that activity responsible for it arises in the otolith organs. OOSTERVELD (1973) has data to support this view. This is in dispute, however, and NITO et al. (1964, 1968), MONEY et al. (1965), SUZUKI et al. (1972a) and MONEY and MYLES (1974) have evidence to suggest that activity responsible for positional alcohol nystagmus originates in the semicircular canals. If PAN does arise in the otolith organs, then the otolith organs on one side can induce horizontal eye movements to either side. However, it has not been clearly demonstrated that oppositely-directed counter-rolling can be induced from the otolith organs on one side.

The physiological basis for the action of alcohol on the vestibular system is not entirely clear. Alcohol appears to reduce the ocular responses to caloric stimulation (SCHROEDER, 1971; COLLINS et al., 1973; TAKEMORI and COHEN, 1974a) and to head tilt (MILLER and GRAYBIEL, 1969) by reducing the sensitivity of the peripheral organ. It is also postulated to cause differences in density between the endolymph of the semicircular canals and the cupula (MONEY and MYLES, 1974). Alcohol acts centrally on the cerebellum and oculomotor system and causes gaze nystagmus and potentiates spontaneous nystagmus (ASCHAN et al., 1956b; BERGSTEDT, 1961). Thus it appears to reduce central inhibition, allowing sensory information which originates in the labyrinths to be expressed as positional nystagmus. In accord with this EIDELBERG et al. (1971) showed that the mean discharge rate of cerebellar units believed to be Purkinje cells and of vestibular units was depressed after small doses of alcohol, while activity of cerebellar interneurons was increased.

4. Saccules

There is little detailed information on eye movements induced by the saccule in mammals. From anatomic considerations and experimental evidence it seems likely that counter-rolling probably arises mainly in the utricles, and that vertical and vertical-rotatory compensatory eye movements originate in the saccules (MAGNUS, 1924; BENJAMINS and HUIZINGA, 1927; HASEGAWA, 1936, 1937; MCNALLY and STUART, 1942; MILLER, 1962). FLUUR and MELLSTRÖM (1970b, 1971) induced upward and downward eye movements by electrical stimulation of various parts of the saccule (Fig. 11C). However, NELSON and HOUSE (1971) noted that counter-rolling was unaffected in humans by section of the superior vestibular nerve. Since the utricle projects through the superior vestibular nerve to the vestibular nuclei, they suggest that the saccule may also participate in production of counter-rolling. This is a subject for further study.

III. Central Pathways for Vestibulo-Ocular Activity

A. The Vestibular Nuclei

Studies of the anatomy of the vestibular nuclei and their central connections are summarized by JANSEN and BRODAL (1954), BRODAL (1958), DOW and MORUZZI (1958), BRODAL et al. (1962), VOOGD (1964), MCMASTERS et al. (1966), HAUGLIE-HANSEN (1968), SADJAPOUR and BRODAL (1968), TARLOV (1970), GACEK (1971). The physiology is summarized by BRODAL et al. (1962), KORNHUBER (1966, 1970), BRODAL and POMPEIANO (1972), WILSON (1973), and PRECHT (this volume). From differences in structure and organization of the vestibular nuclei and from their afferent and efferent connections, BRODAL, POMPEIANO and WALBERG (1962) concluded that the individual vestibular nuclei function quite differently. A wealth of evidence indicates that this is correct (BRODAL and POMPEIANO, 1972). Nevertheless, the exact role of the individual vestibular nuclei in producing oculomotor reflexes is still not entirely clear.

1. Distribution of Afferents from the Semicircular Canals and the Utricle and Saccule

Some insight into the organization of the vestibular nuclei is provided by recent anatomical studies on the termination of first order afferents in the vestibular nuclei. LORENTE DE NÓ (1933a) first showed that there was a partially distinct and partially common central distribution of fibers from the semicircular canals and the otolith organs. More recent studies of STEIN and CARPENTER (1967) and of GACEK (1968, 1969) have confirmed this. Figure 12A–D summarizes the results of STEIN and CARPENTER, and Fig. 12E–F the results of GACEK. There is agreement that neurons from the semicircular canals project heavily to rostral portions of the medial vestibular nucleus (MVN) and to the superior vestibular nucleus (SVN). STEIN and CARPENTER found that few, if any fibers, from the utricle or saccule end in these portions of the vestibular complex (Fig. 12C, D). GACEK is in general agreement with this but also notes a small but distinct projection from the utricle to the medial vestibular nucleus (MVN) (Fig. 12F). Both studies indicate that there are projections from the semicircular canals and otoliths to the ventral part of the lateral vestibular nucleus (LVN), and agree that fibers from the utricle and saccule project to the rostral portion of the descending vestibular nucleus (DVN). STEIN and CARPENTER find that the semicircular canals do not send fibers to DVN, but GACEK noted fine fibers from the canals which project to DVN. SANS et al. (1972) have physiological evidence to support this finding.

Despite some differences these anatomical studies imply that a significant part of the activity which arises in the semicircular canals and otolith organs is processed in separate areas of the vestibular nuclei. In support of this, neurons in SVN and MVN respond to horizontal angular acceleration (ADRIAN, 1943; DUENSING and SCHAEFER, 1958; SHIMAZU and PRECHT, 1965) or to electrical stimulation of the semicircular canals nerves (MARKHAM and CURTHOYS, 1972), while neurons in more caudal portions of the vestibular nuclei respond to head tilt (ADRIAN, 1943; DUENSING and SCHAEFER, 1959; HIEBERT and FERNÁNDEZ. 1965; PETERSON, 1967; FUJITA et al., 1968). In LVN SANS et al. (1972) found a differential distribution of second order cells which were monosynaptically activated by the semicircular canals or the utricle. In some parts of the vestibular nuclei second

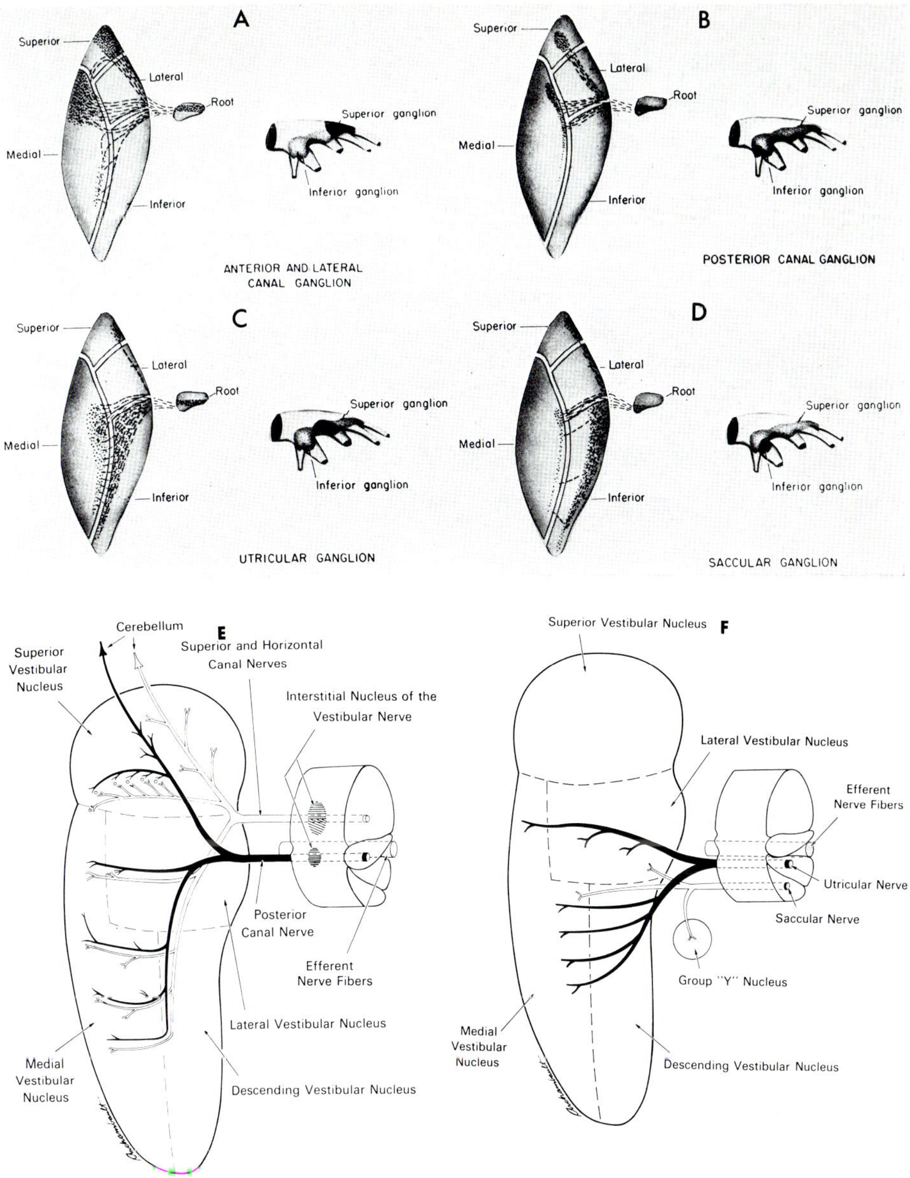

Fig. 12. Diagrammatic representation of the central distribution of degeneration in the vestibular nuclei resulting from lesions of various parts of the vestibular ganglion. In A and E the lesions destroyed cells which innervate the anterior and lateral canals, in B and E the posterior canal, in C and F the utricle, and in D and F the saccule. A–D were taken from the monkey and E and F from the cat. Note that in A, B, and E the most profuse degeneration is present in SVN and in rostral parts of MVN, while in C, D and F central degeneration is most profuse in DVN and in caudal portions of the medial vestibular nucleus. In F Gacek also shows a utricular projection to MVN and to group Y. From Stein and Carpenter, Amer. J. Anat. **120**, 281–318 (1967) (A–D); and Gacek, Acta oto-laryng. (Stockh.) Suppl. **254**, 1–66 (1969) (E, F)

order neurons receive input from only one part of the labyrinths (WILSON and FELPEL, 1972; MARKHAM and CURTHOYS, 1972; KASAHARA and UCHINO, 1971; SANS et al., 1972). In other areas there is convergence from several receptors onto single cells, particularly onto some neurons which could be polysynaptically activated by the receptors (DUENSING and SCHAEFER, 1959; DESOLE and PELESTRINI, 1969; CURTHOYS and MARKHAM, 1971a, b).

Parenthetically, it should be noted that although anatomic and electrophysiological studies generally focus on direct or monosynaptic connections, the possibilities for interaction over polysynaptic paths between various areas of the vestibular nuclei are manifold. For example, anatomically that there are few if any direct projections from the end organs to the dorsal portion of the lateral vestibular nucleus (LVN) (WALBERG et al., 1958). Nevertheless, polysynaptic EPSPs and IPSPs have been recorded throughout the vestibular complex including the dorsal portion of LVN (Deiters' nucleus) when the ipsilateral vestibular nerve is stimulated (WILSON et al., 1966, 1968; ITO et al., 1969; KAWAI et al., 1969).

2. Eye Movements Induced by Vestibular Nucleus Stimulation

There is agreement that eye movements to the contralateral side or nystagmus with contralateral slow phases and ipsilateral quick phases are evoked when the vestibular nuclei are electrically stimulated (INGRAM et al., 1932; CRANMER, 1951). YULES and GAULT (1966) localized the site of stimulation to the lateral vestibular nucleus. TOKUMASU et al. (1969) systematically stimulated the vestibular nuclei in the alert cervically-transected monkey. These results are shown in Fig. 13. The planes of the induced eye movements were roughly similar to the planes of eye movements induced by stimulation of the semicircular canals (SUZUKI et al., 1964; SUZUKI and COHEN, 1964) or of the cerebellum (COHEN et al., 1965b). Upward rotatory eye movements (Fig. 13A) and nystagmus with upward rotatory slow phases were induced by stimulation of SVN. Downward rotatory eye movements were not induced by SVN stimulation. Horizontal movements (Fig. 13B) were primarily induced by stimulation of the midportion of the vestibular complex although upward rotatory and downward rotatory eye movements were also elicited from this region (Fig. 13A, C). Downward rotatory eye movements (Fig. 13C) and nystagmus with downward rotatory slow phases were mainly evoked by activation of the rostral portions of MVN and DVN. These data suggest that there might be a separation of parts of the vestibular nuclei which are responsible for eye movements in various planes of space, but other evidence is necessary to test this hypothesis.

3. Oculomotor Effects of Lesions of the Vestibular Nuclei

The vestibular nuclei are the major sensory receiving area for activity arising in the labyrinth, and changes in eye movements would be expected after vestibular nuclei lesions which reflect the function of the labyrinthine receptors. Lesions of the central vestibular system produce spontaneous nystagmus (FULTON et al., 1930; FERRARO and BARRERA, 1936, 1938; FERRARO et al., 1936, 1940; BUCHANAN, 1940; CRANMER, 1951; SHANZER and BENDER, 1959; CARPENTER et al., 1960; BENDER and SHANZER, 1964; KORNHUBER, 1966; BENDER, 1969; UEMURA and COHEN, 1973) and positional nystagmus (NYLEN, 1931, 1939, 1950; ASCHAN et al., 1956a;

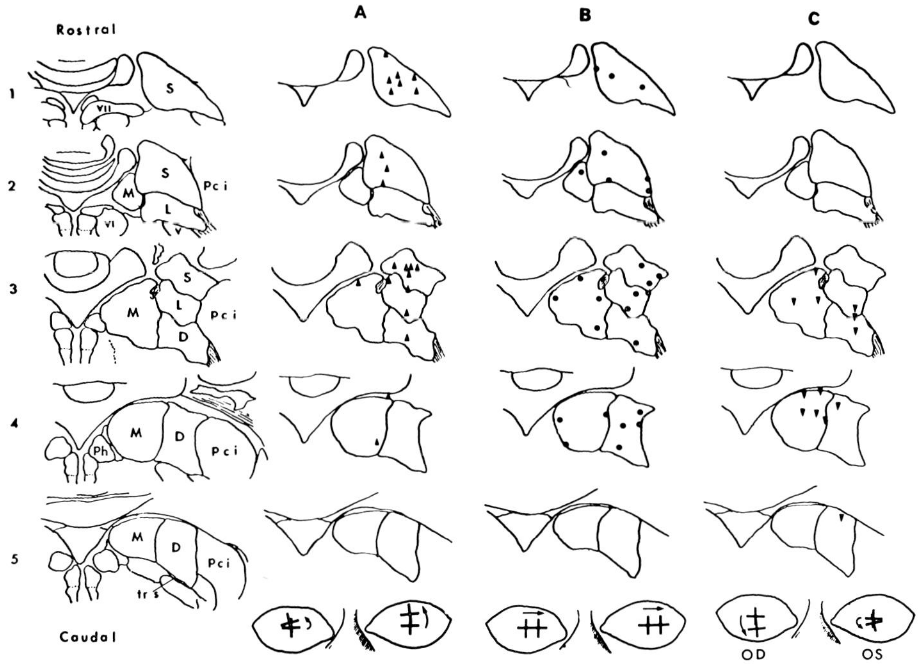

Fig. 13. Sites in the left vestibular nuclei from which eye movements were induced by stimulation with pulse trains. Pulse trains were of 50 msec duration and were composed of 0.5 msec square waves at an intra-train frequency of 500 Hz. Upward rotatory movements are shown in column A, horizontal eye movements in column B, and downward rotatory eye movements in column C. The rotatory component of movements induced by pulse train stimulation of the left side were counter-clockwise. A labelled diagram of these sections is on the left. Each section is 1 mm apart in the 45° stereotaxic plane. Below are shown diagrams of the eye movements referred to by the arrows in columns A–C. When the regions shown in columns A–C were stimulated with repetitive stimuli (0.5 msec pulses at a frequency of 200–250 Hz) nystagmus with slow phases identical to the movement shown in Fig. 13 was induced. The quick phases of nystagmus were opposite to the direction of the slow phases. Abbreviations: S, superior vestibular nucleus; M, medial vestibular nucleus; L, lateral vestibular nucleus; D, descending vestibular nucleus; V, nucleus of spinal tract of trigeminal nerve; VI, abducens nucleus; VII, genu of the facial nerve; tr s, tractus Solitarius; Ph, prepositus hypoglossal nucleus; Pci, inferior cerebellar peduncle. From Tokumasu et al., Ann. Otol. (St. Louis) **78**, 1105–1119 (1969)

Stahle, 1958; Jongkees et al., 1962; Jung and Kornhuber, 1964; Kornhuber, 1966; Uemura and Cohen, 1973). Vestibular nuclei lesions can also affect the response to caloric or rotatory stimulation (Ferraro et al., 1940; Stahle, 1958; Shanzer and Bender, 1959; Jung and Kornhuber, 1964; Kornhuber, 1966; Bender, 1969). Vestibular nuclei lesions undoubtedly also change counter-rolling, nystagmus induced by linear acceleration (Jongkees and Philipszoon, 1964), and more complex aspects of vestibulo-ocular reflex function.

There have been few studies of specific changes in eye movements after lesions of individual vestibular nuclei. Ferraro et al. (1940) and Carpenter (1960) found spontaneous nystagmus to the contralateral side in monkey and cat after MVN lesions. BUCHANAN (1940), however, noted ipsilateral spontaneous nystagmus in the guinea pig after MVN lesions. Spontaneous nystagmus was also ipsilateral when supramedullary portions of the juxta-restiform body were damaged (FERRARO and BARRERA, 1936, 1938; FERRARO et al., 1936). Spontaneous nystagmus is most commonly present to the ipsilateral side after lateral medullary lesions in man (JUNG and KORNHUBER, 1964; KORNHUBER 1966; BENDER, 1969). FERRARO et al. (1940) also noted that there was some change in the response to ipsilateral caloric stimulation after MVN lesions. In contrast, caloric responses were intact when DVN was destroyed in the cat (CARPENTER et al., 1960).

UEMURA and COHEN (1972, 1973) studied ocular and postural changes after small vestibular nuclei lesions in the monkey. Slow phases of spontaneous nystagmus and postural changes were ipsilateral after lateral or caudal lesions of the vestibular nuclei and contralateral after SVN or rostral MVN lesions. Quick phases of nystagmus were not affected by vestibular nuclei lesions, and changes in optokinetic nystagmus (OKN) could generally be attributed to directional preponderance associated with the spontaneous nystagmus. Horizontal components of caloric nystagmus were affected by lesions of parts of the vestibular nerve root which project to ventral parts of LVN. Vertical caloric responses to anterior canal stimulation appeared to be dysinhibited by lesions of SVN and rostral MVN.

Positional nystagmus and PAN were used to test the otolith-ocular reflex arcs. Positional nystagmus was prominent after lesions of SVN and DVN and positional nystagmus and PAN were abolished by a lesion of rostral DVN. These data support the hypotheses that the main primary receiving areas for the otolith organs is in rostral DVN and that activity responsible for otolith-ocular and semicircular canal-ocular reflexes may be processed in different areas of the vestibular nuclei.

B. Vestibulo-Ocular Pathways, General Considerations

There is some indication that direct and multisynaptic vestibulo-ocular pathways have different sites of ending on oculomotor neurons (SZENTÁGOTHAI, 1964). Heavily myelinated axons from vestibular to oculomotor nuclei are carried in the medial longitudinal fasciculus (MLF), and end in large synapses on the soma of oculomotor neurons (SZENTÁGOTHAI, 1964). Multisynaptic pathways through the reticular formation end profusely in axodendritic synapses on these same motoneurons (LORENTE DE NÓ, 1933b). In the fish there are different sites of impulse initiation in oculomotor neurons (KRIEBEL et al., 1969). The vestibular

Fig. 14. Top, Electron micrograph of axodendritic synapses from the oculomotor nucleus of the rhesus monkey. A synaptic ending (A) contains electron lucent vesicles and mitochondria; it forms synapses with a small dendrite (D_2) which contains a multivesicular body (mvb), and with a large dendritic trunk (D_1). Mitochondria are labelled "m". Two arrays of subjunctional bodies (sjb) in the large dendrite are associated with a dense "thickening" of the postsynaptic membrane. The ending and small dendrite are separated from the adjacent neuropil by thin glial lamellae (gl). A myelinated axon (MA) is seen in cross section. × 30,000. Bottom, Axo-axonic synapses from the rhesus monkey oculomotor nucleus. Axonal process A_1 is presynaptic with respect to axon A_2, which, in turn, forms an axodendritic synapse with dendrite D_1. Axon A_3 forms an axo-axonic synapse in which axon A_4 is the postsynaptic element. A_4 is presynaptic with respect to dendrite D_2. ×21,000. From WAXMAN and PAPPAS (unpublished data)

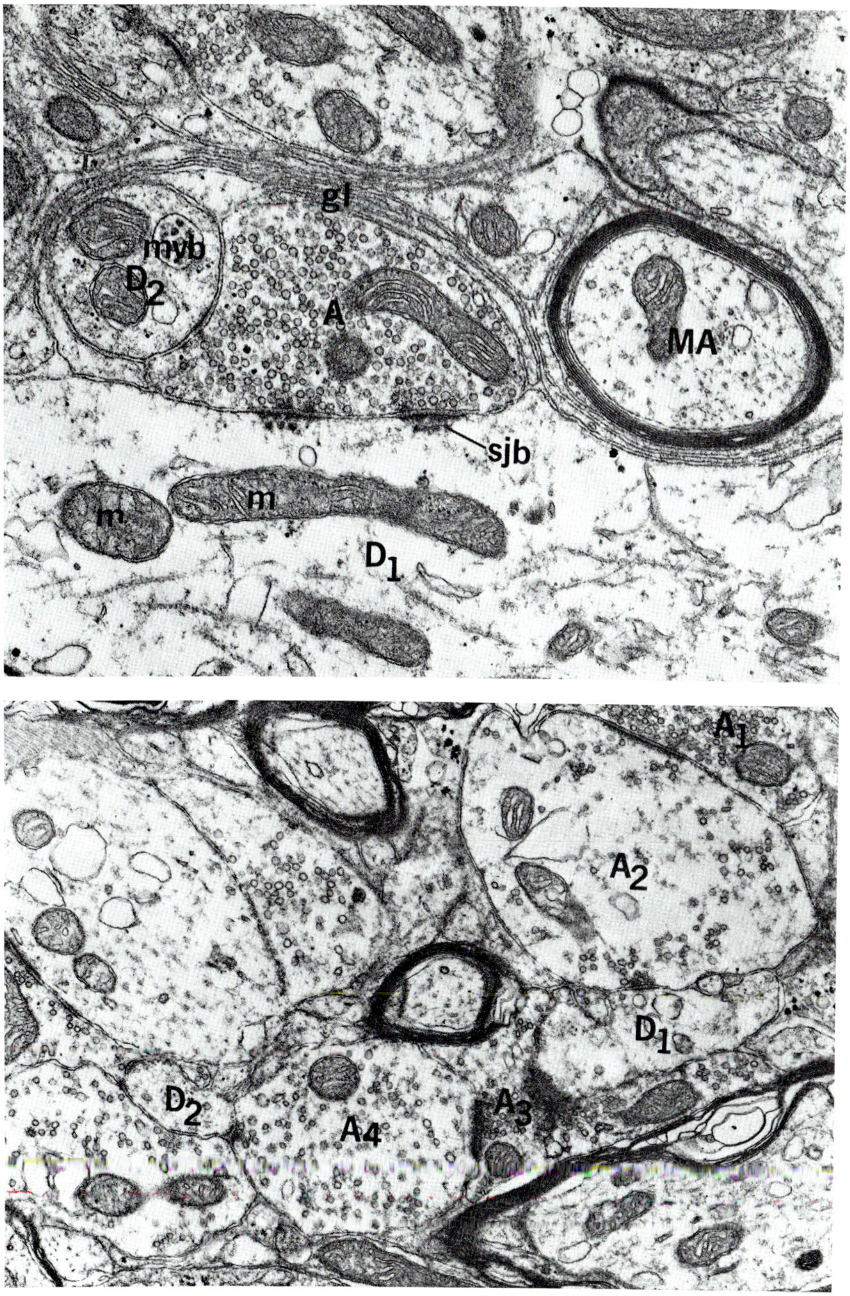

Fig. 14

system acts distal to the cell body, while the visual system causes somatic activation. Axons carrying activity for quick phases of nystagmus have mainly somatic endings (KORN and BENNETT, 1971). Slow phase activity ends primarily in dendritic synapses. Gap junctions provide weak coupling among oculomotor neurons enhancing synchronization (KORN and BENNETT, 1971). In mammals vestibular-initiated activity apparently does not have the same restricted distribution as in fish. However, IPSP's seem generated at or near the soma of motoneurons, while EPSP's are presumed to have a more dendritic origin (PRECHT and BAKER, 1972).

In mammals, synapses on oculomotor neurons appear to be largely if not entirely chemical. In fish, frogs and chameleons, however, oculomotor neurons are activated by both chemical and electrical synapses (KREIBEL et al., 1969; KIDOKORO, 1969; WAXMAN and PAPPAS, 1971). Despite the different types of synapses, the qualitative and quantitative characteristics of eye movements in fish seem similar to those in mammals and man (HERMANN, 1971; EASTER, 1971, 1972). Axoaxonic as well as axodendritic synapses have been found in the oculomotor nuclei of both fish (WAXMAN and PAPPAS, 1971) and cat (Fig. 14, WAXMAN and PAPPAS, 1972). This implies that there may be pre-synaptic inhibition in pathways ending on eye muscle motoneurons. This has been suggested by HORCHOLLE and TYČ-DUMONT (1969), but evidence is not considered conclusive by SHIMAZU (1972) and MAEDA et al. (1972).

There are two potential pathways by which activity generated in the vestibular apparatus might reach the oculomotor nuclei: either through the brainstem or through the cerebellum. Recent experiments on vestibulo-oculomotor reflex pathways indicate that both of these potential pathways are utilized. Areas of MVN and SVN which receive heavy projections from the semicircular canals (STEIN and CARPENTER, 1967; GACEK, 1969) and some fibers from the utricle (GACEK, 1969) project ascending fibers into the MLF and reticular formation (BRODAL and POMPEIANO, 1957; CARPENTER and MCMASTERS, 1963; SZENTÁGOTHAI, 1964; MCMASTERS et al., 1966; LADPLI and BRODAL, 1968; GACEK, 1971). Neither SVN nor MVN are important sources of afferent fibers to the cerebellum (BRODAL, 1964a, b; GACEK, 1972). ITO et al. (1973a) have shown that anterior canal responses in the rabbit synapsing in the Y-group are carried in the brachium conjunctivum. However, semicircular canal-ocular pathways appear to lie mainly within the brainstem, and the cerebellum does not seem to be an essential link in this part of the vestibulo-ocular reflex arc.

On the other hand rostral DVN which receives the bulk of afferent fibers from the otolith organs (STEIN and CARPENTER, 1967; GACEK, 1969) and only a few fibers from the semicircular canals (GACEK, 1969) has only meager direct projections to the oculomotor nuclei through the brainstem (CARPENTER, 1960; BRODAL et al., 1962; MCMASTERS et al., 1966; TARLOV, 1970). Instead it projects mainly into the cerebellum (BRODAL and TORVIK, 1957; CARPENTER et al., 1959; CARPENTER, 1960). From the cerebellum there are direct cerebello-oculomotor fibers which are carried in the brachium conjunctivum (CARPENTER and STROMINGER, 1964; HIGHSTEIN et al., 1971; HIGHSTEIN, 1973). These are noteworthy because they are the only known direct motor connections of the cerebellum. In addition the cerebellum projects into regions of the pontine reticular formation (CARPENTER, 1959; WALBERG et al., 1962) and vestibular nuclei (DOW, 1936, 1938b; JANSEN and BRODAL, 1954; BRODAL et al., 1962; VOOGD, 1964; ANGAUT and BRODAL, 1967; SHIMAZU and SMITH, 1971), which in turn have projections to the oculomotor nuclei. Pathways from vestibular nuclei to eye muscle motor nuclei through the brainstem will be considered first.

1. Direct Pathways through the Brainstem to Eye Muscle Motor Nuclei

When impulses are added to one lateral semicircular canal nerve by electrical stimulation, ampullo-petal angular acceleration, or caloric stimulation, the eyes initially move to the contralateral side (Fig. 1, LLC). Axons from cells in the vestibular nuclei on one side project across the brainstem from rostral portion of MVN to the contralateral abducens nucleus causing the opposite lateral rectus muscle to contract (SCHAEFER, 1965; PRECHT et al., 1967, 1969; BAKER et al., 1969a, b). Ipsilateral lateral rectus motoneurons are concurrently inhibited over a disynaptic pathway by vestibular nerve stimulation or by appropriate angular acceleration (SCHAEFER, 1965; RICHTER and PRECHT, 1968; PRECHT et al., 1969; BAKER et al., 1969b; MAEDA et al., 1971a, b, HIGHSTEIN, 1973). Axons connecting one vestibular nucleus to the contralateral abducens nucleus do not form a discrete bundle but are intermingled in a prominent vestibular commissural system whose function has been investigated by SHIMAZU and PRECHT (1966), KASAHARA et al. (1968), MANO et al. (1968), and MAEDA et al. (1972). These commissural fibers have also been shown to participate in slow and quick phases of nystagmus (MAEDA et al., 1972).

2. Median Longitudinal Fasciculus (MLF)

The other direct pathways from the vestibular nuclei to the eye muscle motor nuclei through the brainstem are carried in the median longitudinal fasciculus (MLF). The MLF is one of the oldest and most prominent structures in the brainstem. Axons which ascend in the MLF from the vestibular system originate largely in MVN, LVN and SVN (BRODAL and POMPEIANO, 1957; CARPENTER and MCMASTERS, 1963; SZENTÁGOTHAI, 1964; MCMASTERS et al., 1966; TARLOV, 1970). The vestibular nuclei also receive descending projections through the MLF from the Interstitial Nucleus of Cajal (POMPEIANO and WALBERG, 1957). The descending fibers excite inhibitory neurons in the vestibular nuclei on the ipsilateral side (MARKHAM et al., 1966). These cells mediate inhibition onto neurons in the horizontal canal system. Descending fibers from the region of the Interstitial Nucleus also excite trochlear motoneurons (SCHWINDT et al., 1974, in press).

Portions of the vestibular nuclei which project through the MLF to the oculomotor trochlear and abducens nuclei in turn receive projections mainly from the semicircular canals (MCMASTERS et al., 1966; STEIN and CARPENTER, 1967; GACEK, 1969, 1972; TARLOV, 1970). When individual semicircular canal nerves or vestibular nerves are stimulated, prominent potential changes are recorded at short latency in the region of the MLF on both sides of the brainstem (COOK et al., 1969). These direct projections would be appropriate for carrying activity during rapid compensatory deviations as would occur during lateral gaze shifts (BIZZI et al., 1971; DICHGANS et al., 1973a).

The distribution and function of the projections from SVN and MVN through the MLF to the oculomotor nuclei are different. Projections in the MLF from SVN are entirely ipsilateral and end in the ipsilateral trochlear and oculomotor nuclei before crossing the brainstem to supply motoneurons in the oculomotor nucleus on the opposite side. ITO et al. (1973c) have emphasized that the projections from SVN to the oculomotor nuclei are entirely inhibitory. There are no known connections of SVN to the abducens nuclei. Projections from MVN are both crossed and uncrossed and provide both excitatory and inhibitory activity to motoneurons. The specific direct vestibulo-ocular connections in the rabbit determined electrophysiologically by HIGHSTEIN et al. (1971) and HIGHSTEIN (1973) are shown in Fig. 15. Thus in the rabbit SVN supplies the entire rostral projecting inhibitory

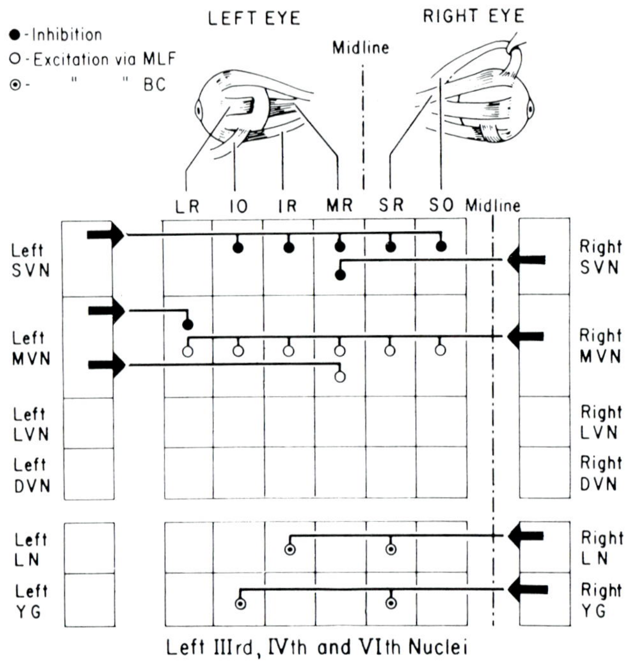

Fig. 15. Vestibulo-ocular connections to the left IIIrd and IVth nuclei in rabbit. Central block of six columns represents the left IIIrd, IVth and VIth nuclei, the long blocks represent relay nuclei of the vestibulo-ocular reflex arcs on both sides. Note that the IO, IR, and MR divisions of the left IIIrd nucleus are ipsilateral to the left eye while the SR and SO innervate the right eye. ● inhibitory connections from the SV; ○ excitatory connections from the MV; ⊙ excitatory connections from the Y-group or LN. LSV, RSV = left and right superior vestibular nuclei, respectively. LMV, RMV = left and right medial vestibular nuclei, respectively. LLN, RLN = left and right Y-groups of the vestibular nuclei, respectively. SO = superior oblique innervated by the IVth nucleus. LN = lateral (dentate) nucleus. From HIGHSTEIN, Mt. Sinai J. Med. **41**, 144–152 (1974)

input to the oculomotor nuclei; while MVN, the Y-group and the dentate (lateral) nucleus provide the rostral projecting excitatory input. As noted, abducens motoneurons are inhibited and excited via MVN.

The inhibitory nature of the ipsilateral projections from SVN is borne out by stimulation and lesion studies. While excitation of trochlear motoneurons causes intorsion and depression, stimulation of SVN which projects to the trochlear nucleus, produces upward rotatory deviations not downward eye movements (TOKUMASU et al., 1969). This suggests that these movements are primarily due to inhibition. After SVN lesions spontaneous nystagmus is present which is oppositely-directed to movements induced by SVN stimulation (UEMURA and COHEN, 1973). Enhancement of contralateral anterior canal responses present after SVN destruction (UEMURA and COHEN, 1973) is also consistent with the proposed inhibitory nature of the projections from this nucleus.

The role which activity carried in the MLF plays in producing horizontal eye movements is still not entirely understood. It seems certain that the MLF is an important output pathway for activity causing adduction of the ipsilateral eye during horizontal eye movements. When one MLF is electrically stimulated, the ipsilateral eye adducts. Lesions of the MLF are followed by paralysis of adduction of the ipsilateral eye (Fig. 16B, D; SPILLER, 1924; BENDER and WEINSTEIN, 1944,

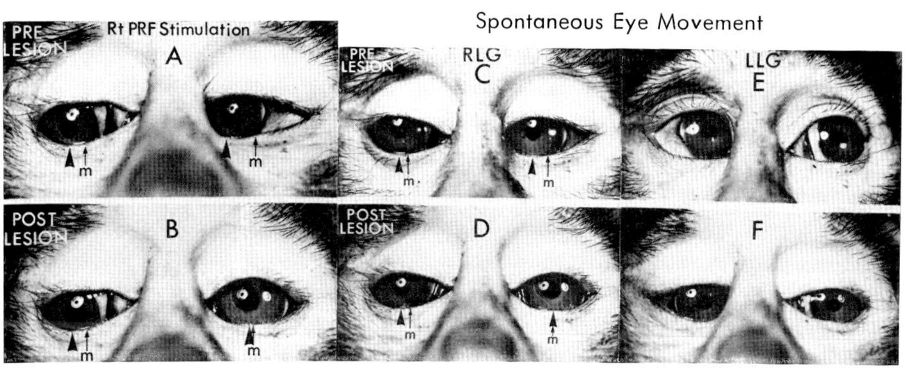

Fig. 16. Induced and spontaneous eye movements before (A, C, E) and after (B, D, F) a left MLF lesion. A, B. Right PRF stimulation. C, D. Right lateral gaze (RLG) and E, F, left lateral gaze (LLG). Notice that the left eye did not cross the midline (M) to the right after lesion either during induced (B) or spontaneous (D) gaze to the right. Movements of both eyes to the left (F) were intact after lesion. The large arrow marks the center of the pupil and the fine arrow (m) the midposition

1950; COGAN, 1948; COGAN et al., 1950; SMITH and COGAN, 1959; SHANZER and BENDER, 1959; CHRISTOFF et al., 1960; CARPENTER and MCMASTERS, 1963; BENDER and SHANZER, 1964; CARPENTER and STROMINGER, 1965; COHEN, 1971). There is also nystagmus in the contralateral eye when it abducts and frequently spontaneous vertical nystagmus is present (SHANZER et al., 1964). Convergence is preserved, showing that the paralysis of adduction is supranuclear. This constellation of signs has been termed anterior inter-nuclear ophthalmoplegia. Except for paralysis of adduction of the ipsilateral eye, patterns of eye movements induced by semicircular canal nerve stimulation are generally maintained after lesions confined to medial parts of the MLF (SHANZER, 1964; SHANZER et al., 1964).

It should be emphasized that the adductive paralysis after MLF lesions is manifest during all types of rapid conjugate horizontal eye movements. These include spontaneous saccades and quick phases of nystagmus, either induced by the visual or vestibular system (Cohen, 1971). The adductive paralysis is also present upon PRF stimulation (Fig. 16B). Thus the MLF not only participates in eye movements induced by the vestibular apparatus but is important for ipsilateral adduction during all types of rapid horizontal eye movements. This makes it unlikely that the paresis of adduction which follows MLF lesions is entirely due to destruction of vestibular fibers. Unless pathways from the visual system were to pass through the vestibular nuclei they could not gain access to neurons located in the vestibular nuclei which project through the MLF to medial rectus motoneurons during quick phases of OKN or during saccades. This seems unlikely for several reasons: (1) No such anatomic projections have been demonstrated. (2) Changes in eye movements similar to those which follow MLF lesions are not caused by vestibular nuclei lesions (McMasters et al., 1966; Uemura and Cohen, 1973). Therefore, it would appear that there must be important extravestibular projections in the MLF or in the region of the MLF which end on oculomotor neurons. It seems likely that destruction of these extravestibular projections is in large part responsible for the paralysis of adduction which has been described both clinically and experimentally. This is a subject for further study.

3. *Multisynaptic Pathways through the Brainstem to Eye Muscle Motor Nuclei*

Multisynaptic pathways from the vestibular nuclei to the eye muscle motor nuclei have been known since the work of Lorente de Nó (1933b) and Szentágothai (1950). These pathways originally project to the pontine reticular formation (Ladpli and Brodal, 1968). From the finding that lesions in the pretectum may affect vertical eye movements but leave horizontal movements intact (Pasik et al., 1969a, b; Jacobs et al., 1972) or vice versa (Bender and Shanzer, 1964; Cohen et al., 1968), it would appear that there is a separation of neural organizations which produce horizontal, vertical and rotatory eye movements at some point along oculomotor pathways. The vestibular organs respond to head movements in every spatial plane and compensatory eye and head movements are also induced in every spatial plane. Therefore, there must be multisynaptic connections from the vestibular nuclei to parts of the brain which induce vertical and rotatory as well as horizontal eye movements. More is known about pathways for horizontal gaze and they will be considered in more detail in the next section.

4. *Paramedian Zone of the Pontine Reticular Formation (PPRF)*

An important part of the neural substrate for horizontal eye movements lies in the tegmentum of the pons in a region designated as the paramedian zone of the pontine reticular formation (PPRF) (Bender and Shanzer, 1964; Cohen et al., 1968; Goebel et al., 1971). The PPRF is not a discrete structure but rather is a region of the pontine reticular formation which has been designated because of its apparent functional specificity. In the monkey it lies in the medial portions of Nucleus Reticularis Magnocellularis. It is bounded medially by the nuclei of the raphe and the MLF, dorsally by the brachium conjunctivum and the gray matter of the floor of the 4th ventricle, and ventrally by the trapezoid body and the roots of the abducens nerve. The lateral extent of this region is between 0.5 and 2 mm from the midline. Antero-posteriorally it extends from the trochlear to the abducens nuclei (Fig. 17A).

The importance of the paramedian zone of the pontine reticular formation in horizontal gaze is suggested by a number of lines of evidence (COHEN and HENN, 1972). Units on both sides of the pons are active before and during quick phases of nystagmus (DUENSING and SCHAEFER, 1957a, b; SPARKS and TRAVIS, 1971; LUSCHEI and FUCHS, 1972; COHEN and HENN, 1972). Gross potential changes are also found in this region which precede every rapid eye movement by 10–20 msec (COHEN and FELDMAN, 1968). PPRF unit activity and gross potential changes associated with eye movements in this region are similar in a number of respects. Frequency changes in units or gross potential changes generally occur between 12 and 20 msec before the onset of quick eye movements. Most neurons have a frequency change before all eye movements, but some units change their activity preferentially before quick eye movements in a particular direction. These directions are predominantly horizontal in many units. Changes in unit activity and gross potential changes are the same regardless of whether quick eye movements are saccades or quick phases of vestibular or optokinetic nystagmus. This supports the contention that saccades and quick phases of nystagmus are generated by common neural mechanism and are similar regardless of whether they are induced by the visual or vestibular systems (COHEN and HENN, 1972). It is postulated that the potential changes in units reflect activity of cells which generate the rapid eye movements. The organization of neural activity in the PPRF responsible for nystagmus and saccades is considered in greater detail elsewhere (HENN and COHEN, 1974). Interneurons in the region of the eye muscle motor nuclei are also important in producing rapid eye movements (HORCHOLLE-BOSSAVIT and TYC-DUMONT, 1968; 1969; GOGAN et al., 1973).

Additional evidence that the PPRF is important for horizontal gaze mechanisms comes from stimulation and lesion studies. All types of horizontal eye movements and positions of fixation are induced by PPRF stimulation (COHEN and KOMATSUZAKI, 1972). Deviations induced by PPRF stimulation tend to be of constant velocity and within limits their size is proportional to the number of pulses used for stimulation. From this it has been inferred that there is integration of neural activity in the PPRF or in the relay between the PPRF and the eye muscle motor nuclei (COHEN and KOMATSUZAKI, 1972).

The latency of PPRF-induced deviations is short and no more than one or two synapses separate it from the eye muscle motor nuclei. Anatomical pathways between the reticular formation to eye motor nuclei were reported by LORENTE DE NÓ (1933b), SCHEIBEL and SCHEIBEL (1958) and SZENTÁGOTHAI (1964), but have not been systematically studied. Nevertheless it is clear from stimulation studies (BENDER and SHANZER, 1964; COHEN and KOMATSUZAKI, 1972) that they exist. Recently electrophysiological studies have confirmed that direct (monosynaptic) pathways extend from the pontine reticular formation to motoneurons in the oculomotor and abducens nuclei (HIGHSTEIN et al., 1974). Occlusion studies showed that at least part of these pathways lay outside the MLF.

The most compelling evidence that the PPRF is intimately involved in generation of horizontal eye movements is from lesion studies. Lesions of the PPRF

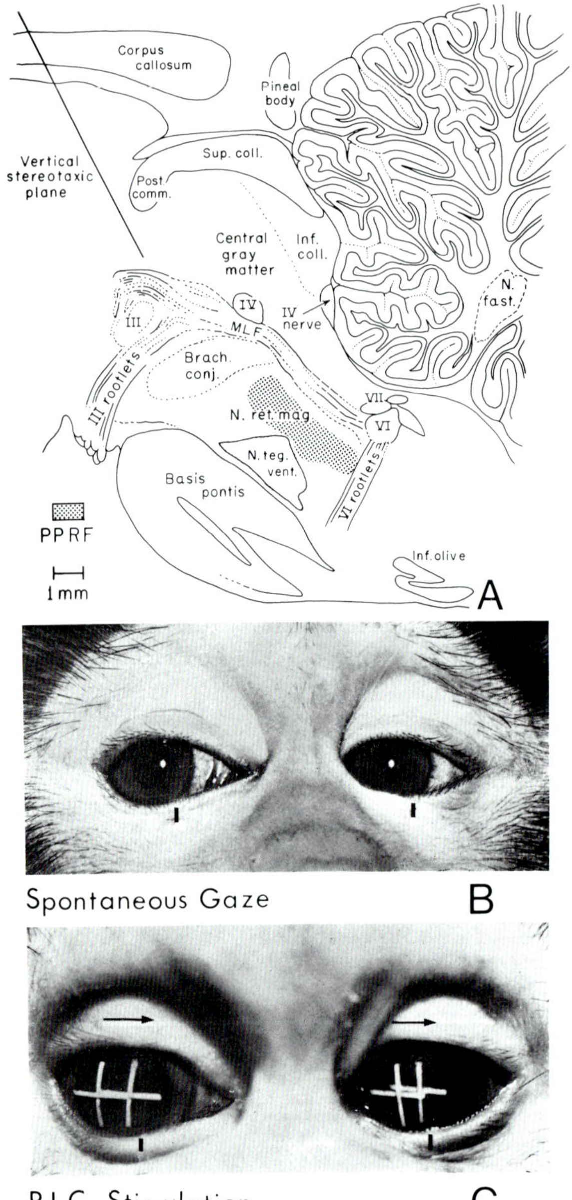

Fig. 17. A. Sagittal section of the brainstem, 0.75 mm from the midline. The PPRF is marked in the cross-hatched region. B, C. Gaze paralysis to left in monkey after left pontine reticular formation lesion. B. Resting position of the eyes. C. Eye movements to left induced by supramaximal stimulation of the right lateral canal nerve (RLC). Pattern of eye movements induced by stimulation of the nerves of the individual canals was not altered by PPRF lesion except that the eyes did not cross the midline to the left. The vertical bars show the approximate midposition of the eye and the arrows the direction of movement induced by the lateral canal stimulus. Double-flash technique described in Fig. 4 was used for the bottom photograph. From Goebel et al., Arch. Neurol. **24**, 431–440 (1971) (A); and Cohen et al., Arch. Neurol. **18**, 78–92 (1968) (B, C)

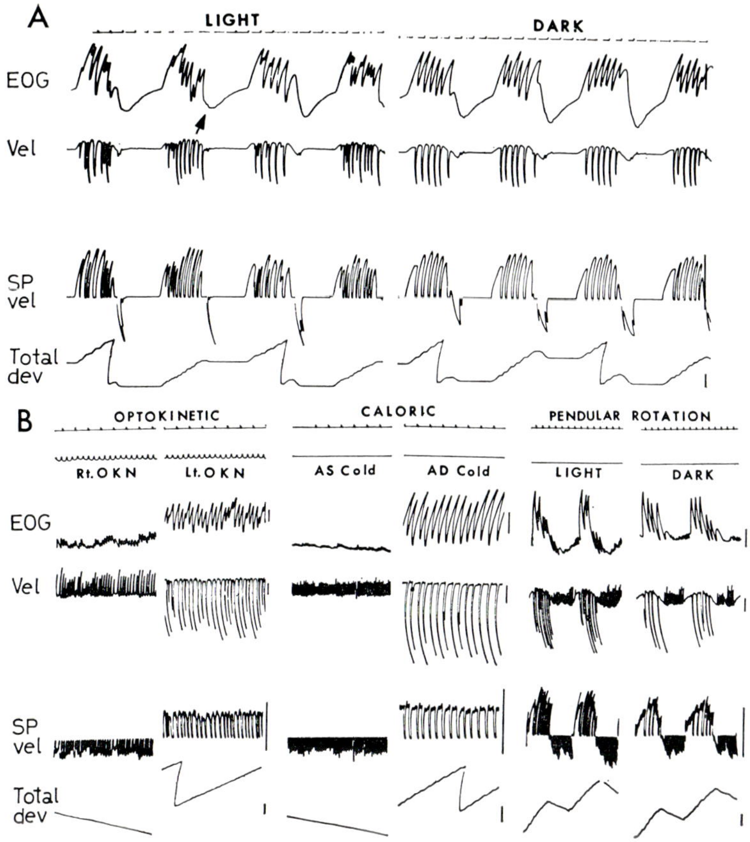

Fig. 18. A. Pendular rotation of a monkey in light and darkness several days after a right PPRF lesion. The eyes moved only in the left hemifield of movement. The stimulus induced nystagmus to the left, but only tonic deviation to the left without quick phases (arrow). B. Comparison of nystagmus induced by optokinetic, caloric, and pendular rotatory stimuli. The eyes moved predominantly in the left field of movement. The eye movements were recorded with a DC-coupling so that the EOG traces show the actual position of the eyes. Optokinetic and vestibular nystagmus were intact to the left. During nystagmus to the right the beats were of high frequency and low amplitude and velocity. The top trace in each series is the time base at 1 mark/sec. The 2nd trace in B shows the photocell which records the passage of optokinetic drum stripes at each 45°. The 3rd trace is the EOG recorded with DC-coupling. The 4th trace is the differentiated EOG showing the velocity of the eye movements. In the 5th trace, the quick phases have been rectified and only slow phase velocity is shown in isolation. The 6th trace shows integrated slow phase velocity indicating total deviation (Total dev.) of the eyes. The vertical bars to the right of the traces are 10° for the EOG, 100°/sec for the differentiated EOG and slow phase velocity traces, and 100° for the total deviation trace. Vel. — Velocity; SP vel. = slow phase velocity; AS cold = left ear cold stimulus; AD cold = right ear cold stimulus. From Cohen and Henn, Bibl. ophthal. (Basel) **82**, 36–55 (1972)

cause profound paralysis of horizontal gaze (Freeman, 1922; Shanzer et al., 1958; Teng et al., 1958; Shanzer and Bender, 1959; Bender and Shanzer, 1964; Cohen et al., 1968; Goebel et al., 1971), and loss of rapid eye movements to the ipsilateral side (COHEN et al., 1968). The region of the brainstem which when destroyed produced paralysis of conjugate gaze is shown in the hatched area of Fig. 17A (GOEBEL et al., 1971). Before the lesions potential changes which preceded rapid eye movements were recorded from this region, and constant velocity eye movements were induced by stimulation. After a lesion on the left side the eyes were constantly on the right of the midline (Fig. 17B). Even supramaximal stimulation of the horizontal canal nerves could not drive the eyes over the midline (Fig. 17C). Vertical eye movements were not impaired.

The main defect after PPRF lesions was in rapid eye movements in the horizontal plane. Just after operation no saccades, or quick phases of nystagmus could be induced toward the side of the lesion (COHEN et al., 1968). Defects in nystagmus to the right after a right PPRF lesion are shown in Fig. 18. The eyes moved mainly in the left hemifield of movement. There was normal nystagmus to the left either in response to optokinetic or to vestibular stimuli. Saccadic eye movements to the left were also intact. On the other hand, during stimuli which would induce nystagmus to the right, the quick phases were either absent or were of small amplitude, high frequency and low maximal velocity. If the nystagmus was absent, there was strong tonic deviation of the eyes to the left in the direction of the slow phases. Saccadic eye movements to the right were similarly affected.

LORENTE DE NÓ (1933b) originally showed that nystagmus was lost after a lesion of the pontine reticular formation. This was disputed by SPIEGEL and PRICE (1939), but was corroborated by BENDER and SHANZER (1964), MCCABE (1965) and COHEN et al. (1968). CROSBY (1953) postulated the presence of a para-abducens nucleus whose destruction was responsible for horizontal gaze paralysis. However, the separate existence of this nucleus has not been accepted by other anatomists (BRODAL, 1958; CARPENTER et al., 1963) and gaze palsy is produced by lesions which are several millimeters distant from the abducens nucleus (COHEN, 1971; GOEBEL et al., 1971). It seems likely that this nucleus is actually part of the adjacent reticular formation. CARPENTER et al. (1963) produced gaze paralysis after lesions in the region of the abducens nuclei. They noted that it was unlikely that this paralysis was produced by destruction of motoneurons in the abducens nuclei, but rather was probably due to interruption of axons which passed through this region (CARPENTER et al., 1963). Vertical eye movements are usually normal after small lesions of the pons. Larger bilateral lesions, however, can abolish eye movements in all directions (FREEMAN, 1922; BENDER, 1960; BENDER and SHANZER, 1964).

Lesions of similar size also in the nervous system do not cause conjugate gaze paralysis (PASIK et al., 1959, 1960, 1966; BENDER and SHANZER, 1964; PASIK and PASIK, 1964; WAGMAN, 1964; COHEN et al., 1968; KOMATSUZAKI et al., 1972). Only after much larger lesions such as hemispherectomy (PASIK et al., 1960; PASIK and PASIK, 1964), or in patients with larger expanding cerebral tumors can a similar type of gaze defect be produced and it is usually temporary. Instead after cerebral lesions, gaze preference rather than gaze paralysis is more often found (PASIK and PASIK, 1964; BENDER and SHANZER, 1964). During gaze preference associated with cerebral lesions, the eyes are usually deviated to the same side but can cross the midline in response to a vestibular or auditory stimulus (PASIK et al., 1960; JUNG and KORNHUBER, 1964; KOMATSUZAKI et al., 1971). After mesencephalic reticular formation (MRF) lesions the amplitude and velocity of quick phases can be equal in both directions and caloric nystagmus may be entirely normal. However, the slow phases of OKN and quick phases to the opposite side may be permanently impaired (KOMATSUZAKI et al., 1972). Similar oculomotor impairment does not occur after superior colliculus (PASIK et al., 1966) or cerebral peduncle destruction (BENDER and SHANZER, 1964).

Based on the effects of stimulation and lesions MONNIER (1946), BENDER (1962), and BENDER and SHANZER (1964) have shown that there is a physiological decussation of pathways which carry descending activity responsible for horizontal eye movements. Evidence from stimulation and lesion studies indicates that this decussation is at the level of the IIIrd nerve nucleus. Stimulation above the decussation causes contralateral deviations, below it ipsilateral deviations are induced. Lesions above the decussation produce defective optokinetic nystagmus with quick phases to the contralateral side, below it lesions cause defective optokinetic and caloric nystagmus with quick phases to the ipsilateral side. Spontaneous nystagmus is to the ipsilateral side after lesions above the decussation (KOMATSUZAKI et al., 1971), to the contralateral side after lesions below it (COHEN et al., 1968). Positional nystagmus is generally not produced by lesions of either the pontine or mesencephalic reticular formation (COHEN et al., 1968). The anatomical basis for the oculomotor decussation is still lacking.

5. *Rotatory and Vertical Eye Movements*

The organization of central pathways for rotatory and vertical eye movements is still unclear. Direct pathways for downward or for rotatory eye movements probably lie in the region of the MLF particularly in its lateral aspects and project to the mesencephalon (SZENTÁGOTHAI, 1964; MCMASTERS et al., 1966; TARLOV, 1970; GACEK, 1972; COOK et al., 1969). POTTHOFF et al. (1967) have shown that there is a direct projection from the vestibular nuclei to the mesencephalon, and SCHWINDT et al. (1974) that the region of the Interstitial Nucleus sends projections to trochlear motoneurons. The location of multisynaptic pathways for rotatory or vertical rotatory eye movements is largely unknown. Pathways for downward or for rotatory eye movements probably terminate in the mesencephalon (SZENTÁGOTHAI, 1943; HESS et al., 1946; HASSLER and HESS, 1954; HESS, 1957; HYDE and TOCZEK, 1962, PASIK et al., 1969). However, HYDE and TOCZEK (1962) have shown that rotatory eye movements persist after destruction of the brainstem in the region of the Nuclei of Darkschewitch and Cajal.

Recently PASIK et al. (1966a, 1969a, b) have shown that after bilateral lesions limited to the pretectum in the region of the Nucleus Interstitialis of the posterior commissure, monkeys are unable to look up above the horizontal meridian. More extensive lesions in the pretectal region may also be associated with paralysis of downward gaze, pupillary abnormalities, abnormalities in posture, and lightning eye movements (ATKIN and BENDER, 1964; PASIK et al., 1966a, 1969a, b). CARPENTER has confirmed this (1971). Horizontal eye movements appear normal after pretectal lesions and downward eye movements below the horizontal meridian may also be preserved after small pretectal lesions. Lesions of the pretectum probably are responsible for the paralysis of upward gaze which may accompany pineal tumors. This was originally believed to be due to destruction of the superior colliculi. However, after complete destruction of the superior colliculi, upward gaze is normal (PASIK et al., 1966b).

Motor organizations which control gaze movements and nystagmus below the horizontal meridian also appear to be located in the midbrain (MUSKENS, 1934, 1936; ANGELERGUES et al., 1957; PASIK et al., 1966, 1969a, b; JACOBS et al., 1972), but their precise location is not clear from experimental studies. An interesting aspect of vertical eye movement organization has been noted by BENDER (1960). He pointed out that movements in the vertical (midsagittal) plane are induced only by bilateral stimulation. Moreover, he noted that pathological vertical nystagmus only follows lesions which extend across the midline. This hypothesis is consistent with the findings of WAGMAN (1964), PASIK and PASIK (1964) and COHEN et al. (1964, 1965b).

C. Vestibulo-Ocular Reflex Arc, Cerebellum

Primary afferent fibers from the labyrinth reach the dentate and fastigial nuclei and the cortex of the nodulus and flocculus directly (DOW, 1936; BRODAL and HOIVIK, 1964; PRECHT and LLINÁS, 1969a, b; LLINÁS et al., 1971; CARPENTER et al., 1972; WILSON et al., 1974). In addition, DVN which receives saccular, utricular and some semicircular canal projections (STEIN and CARPENTER, 1967; GACEK, 1969), projects heavily into the cerebellum, reaching the dentate, interpositus, and fastigial nuclei as well as the flocculus and nodulus (BRODAL and TORVIK, 1957; CARPENTER et al., 1959; CARPENTER, 1960). These projections are shown in Fig. 19A. Areas of DVN which receive primary afferents from the labyrinth are not coexistent with portions from which cerebellar projections originate, but are adjacent (Fig. 19B, C).

It seems clear that the cerebellum has strong representation of vestibular activity allowing for modulation or modification of vestibular reflexes. Many recent findings suggest that the cerebellum plays an active role in producing saccadic eye movements, in modulating or transmitting activity responsible for utriculo-ocular and/or sacculo-ocular reflexes, and in controlling reflexes from the semicircular canals. Aspects of this subject have recently been reviewed elsewhere (COHEN and HIGHSTEIN, 1972).

1. Cerebello-Oculomotor Connections

CARPENTER and STROMINGER (1964) have shown that there are direct cerebello-oculomotor fibers in the brachium conjunctivum of the monkey. These fibers originate in the dentate nucleus and project to the IIIrd nerve nuclei. HIGHSTEIN et al. (1971) also find direct cerebello-oculomotor connections in the rabbit. In mammals direct cerebello-oculomotor fibers do not originate in the cerebellar cortex although in fish Purkinje cell axons project directly onto oculomotor axons, mediating inhibition (KIDOKORO, 1968).

Eye muscle motor nuclei which receive direct cerebellar projections in the monkey would cause the eye to move up and rotate (WARWICK, 1964). Similarly in the rabbit the lateral nucleus of the cerebellum sends direct projections to the portions of the oculomotor nucleus which innervate the inferior and superior rectus muscles (HIGHSTEIN, 1973). Therefore direct cerebello-oculomotor projections are

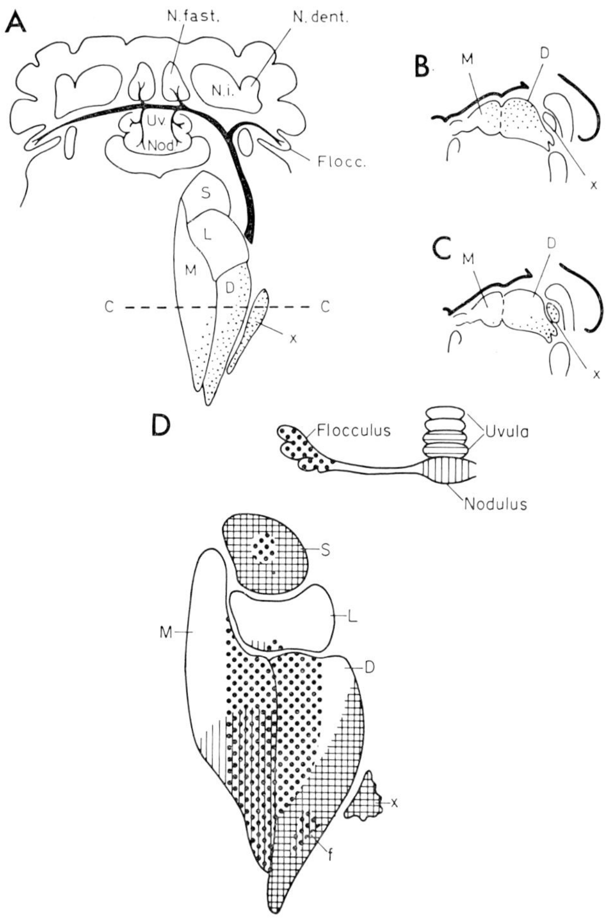

Fig. 19. A. Diagram showing the origin of secondary vestibulo-cerebellar fibers projected on a horizontal section through the vestibular nuclei of the cat. Sites of termination of the fibers are shown according to Dow (1936). B, C. Section through dotted lines shown in A (C---C). B shows sites of termination of primary vestibular afferents and C sites of origin of vestibulo-cerebellar projections in this portion of the vestibular nuclei. The two areas are not identical. D. Diagram of the distribution within the vestibular nuclei of fibers from the flocculus, nodulus and uvula. Note the overlap of portions of DVN and MVN which receive and send fibers to the cerebellum. From Brodal, Progr. Brain Res., Vol. 37, 1972 (A–C); and Angaut and Brodal, Arch. ital. Biol. **105**, 441–479 (1967) (D)

related to eye movements in planes of space other than horizontal. There are also cerebellar projections of the fastigial nuclei through the uncinate fasciculus and juxtarestiform body to regions of the pontine reticular formation (Carpenter et al., 1958; Carpenter, 1959; Walberg et al., 1962b) and vestibular nuclei (Dow, 1936; Jansen and Brodal, 1954; Brodal et al., 1962; Walberg et al., 1962a; Voogd, 1964; Angaut and Brodal, 1967) which project to the oculomotor nuclei (McMasters et al., 1966; Tarlov, 1970; Gacek, 1972). These regions particularly

of the pontine tegmentum (BENDER and SHANZER, 1964; COHEN et al., 1968; GOEBEL et al., 1971; COHEN, 1971; COHEN and KOMATSUZAKI, 1972) could cause the eyes to move horizontally.

2. Stimulation Studies

FERRIER (1876) was the first to demonstrate that electrical stimulation of the cerebellar cortex induces eye and body movements in a wide range of species. Other stimulation studies include those of BÁRÁNY (1914), HOSHINO (1921), MUSSEN (1934), KOELLA (1955, 1962), COHEN et al. (1965b) and RON and ROBINSON (1973). In cats horizontal eye movements were induced at short latencies by stimulation of the region of the fastigial nuclei and the vermis overlying the fastigial nuclei (COHEN et al., 1965b). Stimulation in the region of the juxtarestiform body and uncinate fasciculus at the lateral margins of the 4th ventricle also induced strong ipsilateral horizontal eye movements. Efferent pathways from the cerebellum which carry activity responsible for horizontal eye movements probably lie in these regions.

Horizontal eye movements were not induced by stimulation of the lateral cerebellum or of the dentate or interpositus nuclei. Rather stimulation of the dentate nuclei or of the ansate lobes induced upward rotatory eye movements in planes roughly parallel to the plane of the anterior semicircular canal on the same side. Nodulus, uvula or interpositus nucleus stimulation induced downward rotatory eye movements in planes parallel to the plane of the posterior canals. Rotatory eye movements in the coronal plane were induced from the region of the brachium conjunctivum. Thus eye movements in different spatial planes, similar to those induced by semicircular canal nerve or vestibular nuclei stimulation were induced from discrete regions of the cerebellum.

There is a complex intercrossing of pathways in the region of the cerebellar nuclei (ANGAUT and BRODAL, 1967), and some ambiguity in results might be expected in stimulation studies. RON and ROBINSON (1973) stimulated the cerebellum of alert monkeys. The spatial planes of the induced movements were somewhat different than those found by COHEN et al. (1965b) in the cat. They suggest that different types of eye movements, i.e. saccades, smooth movements or pursuit movements are separately represented in different areas of the cortex.

In many species (monkeys, cats, dogs, rabbits) it has been shown that stimulation of the fastigial nuclei or of the vermis which overlies the fastigial nuclei mainly induces eye movements in the horizontal plane (FERRIER, 1876; HOSHINO, 1921; MUSSEN, 1934; COHEN et al., 1965b). These include animals in which the position of the eyes in the head varies widely. This suggests that the function of parts of the fastigial nuclei and overlying vermis may in some way be concerned with eye movements in the horizontal plane. It raises the question of whether eye movements in other planes of space may not be represented in homologous areas of the cerebellum in different species.

3. Role of the Cerebellum in Saccadic Eye Movements

Electrophysiological studies indicate that parts of the vermis including Larsell's lobules 5, 6, 7A and 7B may participate in generation of saccadic eye movements. These do not receive direct afferent projections from the vestibular system, but are activated by stimulation of the primary visual, auditory and sensory motor cortex as well as by the frontal eye fields (SNIDER and STOWELL, 1944; HAMPSON et al., 1952; SNIDER and ELDRED, 1952). Stimulation of this region produces saccadic eye movements (COHEN et al., 1965b; RON and ROBINSON, 1973). Recently it has been shown that Purkinje cells in Larsell's lobules 5, 6 and 7 are activated by eye muscle stretch (FUCHS and KORNHUBER, 1969) over both mossy and climbing fiber inputs (BAKER et al., 1972b). Earliest activation after eye muscle stretch occurred at a latency of approximately 4 msec and individual eye muscles did not have a unique projection. WOLFE (1971) has also demonstrated that gross potential changes are recorded in the vermis during saccadic eye movements and he and LLINÁS (LLINÁS, 1974) that units in the cerebellar cortex are activated when the eyes move.

Lesion studies also provide support for the hypothesis that the cerebellum is involved in generation of saccadic eye movements. KORNHUBER (1971) has shown that there is an inability to generate saccadic eye movements of large amplitude in patients with diffuse cerebellar cortical atrophy. When these patients move to lateral targets they do so in a series of smaller jumps which considerably prolong the duration of the fixation shift. COLLEWIJN (1970) reported that rabbits do not recenter their eyes during OKN after cerebellectomy. ASCHOFF and COHEN (1971) showed that when parts of the vermis and adjacent paravermis including Larsell's lobules 6 and 7A were ablated, the eyes moved most often from the midline into the contralateral hemifield. Saccades to the contralateral side were generally larger than to the ipsilateral side after one-sided vermian and paravermian lesions.

4. *Cerebellar Participation in Vestibulo-Ocular Reflexes*

MAGNUS (1924) noted that compensatory eye movements induced by changes in head position or by rotational stimuli were preserved after cerebellectomy. He concluded that the cerebellum is not essential for production of either otolith-ocular or semicircular canal-ocular reflexes. DOW (1938a) and FERRARO and BARRERA (1936, 1938) also reported that cerebellar lesions had little effect on caloric nystagmus. Nevertheless, there is evidence to suggest that the cerebellum may be important in processing activity in otolith-ocular reflex arcs and may also control semicircular canal-induced ocular reflexes.

As noted the labyrinth sends direct primary afferents to each part of the vestibulo-cerebellum and to the dentate nucleus (CARPENTER et al., 1972). The direct primary afferents end as mossy fibers in the cerebellum (PRECHT and LLINÁS, 1969a) although some climbing fibers may also be activated by adequate stimulation of the labyrinthine receptors (FERIN et al., 1971). Fastigial and dentate nuclei also receive primary vestibular input (PRECHT and LLINÁS, 1969b). Thus the vestibulo-cerebellar cortex as well as the dentate and fastigial nuclei receive considerable information from the labyrinth which would enable them to monitor incoming vestibular activity.

a) *Otolith-Ocular Reflexes*

The saccule and the utricle project into the descending vestibular nuclei (DVN) (STEIN and CARPENTER, 1967; GACEK, 1969) and DVN projects mainly into the cerebellum (BRODAL and TORVIK, 1957; CARPENTER et al., 1959; CARPENTER,

1960). As noted, projections from DVN through the brainstem to the oculomotor nuclei are relatively minor or are absent (POMPEIANO and WALBERG, 1957; CARPENTER et al., 1960; BRODAL et al., 1962; MCMASTERS et al., 1966; TARLOV, 1970; GACEK, 1972). The presence of direct cerebello-oculomotor connections suggest that a vestibulo-cerebello-oculomotor loop exists which may subserve otolith reflexes.

Evidence that the cerebellum may be important in mediating otolith-ocular reflexes comes from a number of sources. MANNI (1950) reported that compensatory eye movements for head tilt were defective after cerebellar lesions in the guinea pig. Positional nystagmus was produced by cerebellar lesions in cat, monkey, rabbit and man (NYLÉN, 1931, 1950; SPIEGEL and SCALA, 1941, 1942; DIX and HALLPIKE, 1952; ALLEN and FERNÁNDEZ, 1960; FERNÁNDEZ and FREDRICKSON, 1964; ASCHAN et al., 1964b; GRANT et al., 1964; COHEN et al., 1969; GRAND, 1971). Positional nystagmus is nystagmus which appears after a particular head position is assumed (BÁRÁNY, 1913; NYLÉN, 1924), and is a common symptom of damage of the otolith organs or dysfunction in otolith-ocular reflex arcs (BÁRÁNY, 1913; NYLÉN, 1924, 1950; DIX and HALLPIKE, 1952; ASCHAN et al., 1956b; JONGKEES, 1961; ASCHAN, 1960; JONGKEES and PHILIPSZOON, 1964). Tests for positional nystagmus were not conducted in most of the early studies on effects of cerebellar lesions (FERRARO and BARRERA, 1936, 1938; DOW, 1938a; DOW and MORUZZI, 1958).

After cerebellar nuclear lesions positional nystagmus can persist for long periods of time and vertigo and positional nystagmus in patients with cerebellar tumors can be persistent and severe. Positional nystagmus is not produced by mesencephalic or brainstem reticular formation lesions or by lesions rostral to the mesencephalon (COHEN et al., 1968). It is present, however, after lesions of the posterior fossa (NYLÉN, 1931) particularly when lesions involve the vestibular nuclei (ASCHAN et al., 1956; STAHLE, 1958; JONGKEES et al., 1962; JUNG and KORNHUBER, 1964; UEMURA and COHEN, 1972). To the extent that positional nystagmus represents a disorder of sensing position of the head in space, the cerebellum participates either primarily or indirectly in controlling these reflexes.

Recent research in the rabbit (HIGHSTEIN, 1971) has shown that in addition to the dentate nucleus, the Y-group of the vestibular nuclei (BRODAL et al., 1962) also contributes to activity carried in the brachium conjunctivum which directly influences IIIrd nucleus motoneurons. The Y-group sends monosynaptic excitatory projections through the brachium conjunctivum of the rabbit to motor nuclei of the inferior oblique and superior rectus muscles. It has been shown that the Y-group receives primary vestibular afferents of saccular origin (GACEK, 1969) and that stimulation of the saccule can produce patterned eye movements (FLUUR and MELLSTRÖM, 1970) associated with ocular counter-rolling (JONGKEES, 1950). Thus eye movements induced by the saccule may be mediated at least in part by the Y-group.

b) Flocculus and Nodulus Control of Semicircular Canal-Ocular Reflexes

The flocculus and nodulus receive heavy projections from the vestibular system and in turn project heavily to SVN, MVN, and DVN (Fig. 19B). This provides a medium for floccular and nodular control of vestibulo-ocular reflexes. BÁRÁNY (1914) reported changes in post-rotatory nystagmus after lesions of the flocculus. It is clear, however, that horizontal caloric nystagmus is not primarily affected by lesions of the cerebellum (MAGNUS, 1924; FERRARO and BARRERA, 1936, 1938; DOW, 1938a; CARPENTER et al., 1960), although some directional preponderance of caloric nystagmus can be produced by cerebellar nuclear lesions (JUNG and KORNHUBER, 1964) or flocculus lesions (TAKEMORI and COHEN, 1974b).

It has been suggested that the caloric nystagmus is enhanced or prolonged by cerebellectomy (BAUER and LEIDLER, 1912) or by cerebellar lesions (FERRARO and BARRERA, 1938; FERNÁNDEZ and FREDRICKSON, 1964; SINGLETON, 1967). FERNÁNDEZ and FREDRICKSON (1964) suggest that this is due to lesions of the nodulus. They found that caloric nystagmus was inhibited by electrical stimulation of the nodulus and postulate that this region mediates inhibition onto semicircular canal-ocular reflexes. Nevertheless, FUKUDA et al. (1972) were unable to find intracellular evidence of dysfacilitation or direct inhibition of the disynaptic vestibulo-ocular reflex when the nodulus was electrically stimulated.

As noted in the section on visual-vestibular interactions there is reason to believe that visual inhibition of vestibular reflexes is mediated through the flocculus. Similar studies have not been done for the nodulus. ITO et al. (1970b), FUKUDA et al. (1972), BAKER et al. (1972b) and HIGHSTEIN (1973) have shown that SVN neurons which project through the MLF are inhibited by Purkinje cell axons from the flocculus. Thus flocculus stimulation causes dysinhibition of oculomotor and trochlear motor neurons and would facilitate some semicircular canal-ocular pathways ending in these motor nuclei (PRECHT, 1972). Floccular stimulation can also inhibit direct vestibulo-ocular pathways carrying excitation (FUKUDA et al., 1972). Thus the flocculus can either inhibit inhibitory or excitatory pathways in the direct vestibulo-ocular reflex arc. The specific excitatory and inhibitory pathways which are controlled in the rabbit have been determined by ITO et al. (1973c, Fig. 20). Consistent with the patterned nature of the flocculus control, either the excitatory or the inhibitory pathway to motoneurons of any single muscle were affected, but not both. Anterior and lateral, but not posterior canal induced activity was affected by flocculus stimulation. Repetitive activity produced by vestibular nerve stimulation also disappears after flocculus ablation (BAKER et al. 1973).

An interesting aspect of vestibulo-visual interactions has been noted in an earlier section, namely that the visual system is able to activate Purkinje cells of the flocculus (MAEKAWA and SIMPSON, 1973). Since the Purkinje cells are themselves inhibitory, this provides a medium for the visual system to activate flocculus control of vestibular reflexes. Accordingly TAKEMORI and COHEN (1974a, b) ablated the flocculus and tested visual suppression of vestibular nystagmus. After bilateral flocculus ablation visual suppression disappeared or was markedly attenuated. OKN was also affected but aside from slight directional preponderance caloric nystagmus in darkness was normal. ITO et al. (1974) found a similar loss of effects of vision on compensatory eye movements in rabbits after flocculus ablation and LISBERGER and FUCHS (1974) have recently demonstrated that Purkinje cell activity in the flocculus is strongly affected during suppression of compensatory movements in light. Thus evidence indicates that the flocculus supports ocular

Abbreviations: i-, ipsilateral; c-, contralateral; SR, superior rectus; IO, inferior oblique; MR, medial rectus; LR, lateral rectus; SO, superior oblique; IR, inferior rectus; +, present; —, absent.

Reflex action	*Vestibulo-ocular pathways*				*Inhibition from*	
	No.	*Receptor canal*	*Relay nucleus*	*Effector muscle*	*Flocculus*	*OX, AOT*
Excitatory	E_1	anterior	y group	i-SR	+	—
	E_2			c-IO	+	—
	E_3	horizontal	medial	i-MR	+	+
	E_4			c-LR	—	—
	E_5	posterior	medial	i-SO	—	—
	E_6			c-IR	—	—
Inhibitory	I_1	anterior	superior	i-IR	+	—
	I_2			c-SO	+	—
	I_3	horizontal	medial	i-LR	+	+
	I_4		superior	c-MR	—	—
	I_5	posterior	superior	i-IO	—	—
	I_6			c-SR	—	—

Fig. 20. Table of flocculus, optic tract (OT), and accessory optic tract (AOT) control of excitation and inhibition in vestibulo-ocular reflexes. Flocculus stimulation caused inhibition of lateral and anterior canal pathways but had no effect on posterior canal pathways. OT and AOT stimulation mainly affected horizontal eye movers. From ITO et al., Brain Res. **69**, 238–243 (1973)

compensatory movements, while damping inappropriate vestibular activity which could lead to disorientation or vertigo.

The cerebellum may also be important for habituation of caloric nystagmus. If caloric stimulations are given repetitively there is a decrease in duration of maximum slow phase velocity of the nystagmus which is induced. HALSTEAD (1935, 1937) first demonstrated that head nystagmus in pigeons would not habituate after cerebellectomy. This habituation can be studied only if the state of alertness is carefully controlled and is present for stimulation of single canals and for nystagmus induced in specific directions (CRAMPTON, 1962, 1964; GUEDRY, 1964; COLLINS and UPDEGRAFF, 1966; COLLINS, 1969). More recently SINGLETON (1967) destroyed the nodulus and indicated that there was no habituation of caloric nystagmus after operation. WOLFE (1968) has reached similar conclusions. However this would still appear to be a matter for further study.

IV. Summary

(1) The vestibulo-ocular reflex arcs are the neural substrate which links the vestibular sensory receptors to the eye muscles. They induce eye movements whose primary function is to promote vision. These eye movements lie in all spatial

planes and are commonly compensatory. That is, they tend to oppose head deviations and maintain the angle of vision. There is an intimate interaction between the visual and vestibular system in producing or suppressing various types of compensatory eye movements. Part of this interaction is mediated through the flocculus.

(2) Eye movements induced by semicircular canals have been described in detail. When one canal or its nerves are activated, the eyes and head move in planes parallel to the plane of the excited canal regardless of the position of the eyes in the orbit or of the head on the neck. Eye movements induced by natural stimulation of the utricle and saccule are not entirely clear, and there are differences in results of studies of electrical stimulation of the utricular and saccular maculae. When utricular nerves are stimulated, conjugate rotatory eye movements are induced with intorsion of the ipsilateral eye and extorsion of the contralateral eye, similar to eye movements which occur during compensatory counter-rolling.

(3) The course of various pathways between the vestibular apparatus and the oculomotor nuclei has been considered. Many of the projections from the semicircular canals and the otolith organs end in different parts of the vestibular nuclei. This suggests that reflexes from these receptors may be separately processed. Lesion studies provide support for this hypothesis. Eye movements in different planes of space induced by stimulation of the vestibular nuclei were also described.

(4) There are two potential pathways over which activity from the vestibular nuclei can reach the motor nuclei of eye muscles. One lies in the brainstem, the other in the cerebellum. The brainstem pathways extend through commissural fibers, the MLF and the pontine reticular formation, and the cerebellar pathways through the brachium conjunctivum and probably through the uncinate fasciculus and the juxtarestiform body. Activity from the semicircular canals appears to project mainly through the brainstem. Activity from otolith organs also utilizes brainstem pathways, but evidence suggests that part of this activity may go through the cerebellum as well.

(5) Beyond the vestibular nuclei there is some separation of pathways which mediate activity for horizontal and vertical rotatory eye movements. Pathways which carry activity for horizontal movements from vestibular nuclei can reach appropriate oculomotor nuclei via commissural fibers, the MLF, or through the pontine reticular formation. Direct pathways for vertical and rotatory gaze lie in the MLF, but the location of multisynaptic pathways is still obscure.

(6) Effects of brainstem lesions on horizontal eye movements have been described. MLF lesions produce paralysis of ipsilateral adduction. After lesions of the paramedian zone of the pontine reticular formation there is paralysis of conjugate horizontal gaze and all ipsilateral rapid eye movements including saccades and quick phases of nystagmus are affected. Mesencephalic reticular formation lesions produce gaze preference, but not gaze palsy. Vestibulo-ocular reflexes are not much affected by MRF lesions. Paralysis of upward eye movements is produced by lesions of the pretectum. It appears that rapid eye movements in the horizontal plane are generated in the pontine reticular formation and vertical movements in the pretectum. The location of central neural organizations which produce rotatory eye movements is not known for certain, but probably lie in the midbrain in the region of the interstitial nucleus of Cajal.

(7) Eye movements in various spatial planes are induced by stimulation of regions of the cerebellum which appear to be partially separate from each other. There is evidence that the cerebellum participates in producing saccadic eye movements, is associated with mediation or modulation of otolith-ocular reflexes, and is a medium through which the visual system can enhance or suppress vestibular reflexes.

References

ADRIAN, E.D.: Discharge from vestibular receptors in the cat. J. Physiol. (Lond.) **101**, 389–407 (1943).

ALLEN, G., FERNÁNDEZ, C.: Experimental observations in postural nystagmus. I. Extensive lesions in posterior vermis of the cerebellum. Acta oto-laryng. (Stockh.) **51**, 2–14 (1960).

ANGAUT, P., BRODAL, A.: The projection of the "vestibulocerebellum" onto the vestibular nuclei in the cat. Arch. ital. Biol. **105**, 441–479 (1967).

ANGELERGUES, R., DE AJURIAGUERRA, J., HÉCAEN, H.: Paralysie de la verticalité du regard d'origine vasculaire. Étude anatomoclinique. Rev. neurol. **96**, 301–319 (1957).

ASCHAN, G., BERGSTEDT, M., STAHLE, J.: Nystagmography. Acta oto-laryng. (Stockh.) Suppl. **129**, 1–103 (1956a).

ASCHAN, G., BERGSTEDT, M., GOLDBERG, L., LAURELL, L.: Positional nystagmus in man during and after alcohol intoxication. Quart. J. Stud. Alcohol **17**, 381–405 (1956b).

ASCHAN, G.: The pathogenesis of positional nystagmus. Acta oto-laryng. (Stockh.) Suppl. **159**, 90–93 (1960).

ASCHAN, G., BERGSTEDT, M., GOLDBERG, L.: Positional alcohol nystagmus in patients with unilateral and bilateral labyrinthine destructions. Confin. neurol. (Basel) **24**, 80–102 (1964a).

ASCHAN, G., EKVALL, L., GRANT, G.: Nystagmus following stimulation in the central vestibular pathways using permanently implanted electrodes. Acta oto-laryng. (Stockh.) Suppl. **192**, 63–77 (1964b).

ASCHOFF, J.C., COHEN, B.: Changes in saccadic eye movements produced by cerebellar cortical lesions. Exp. Neurol. **32**, 123–133 (1971).

ATKIN, A., BENDER, M.B.: "Lightning eye movements" (ocular myoclonus). J. neurol. Sci. **1**, 2–12 (1964).

ATKIN, A., BENDER, M.B.: Ocular stabilization during oscillatory head movements. Vestibular system dysfunction and the relation between head and eye velocities. Arch. Neurol. (Chic.) **19**, 559–566 (1968).

BACH-Y-RITA, P., ITO, F.: In vivo studies on fast and slow muscle fibers in cat extraocular muscles. J. gen. Physiol. **49**, 1177–1198 (1966).

BAKER, R.G., MANO, N., SHIMAZU, H.: Intracellular recording of antidromic responses from abducens motoneurons in the cat. Brain Res. **15**, 573–576 (1969a).

BAKER, R.G., MANO, N., SHIMAZU, H.: Postsynaptic potentials in abducens motoneurons induced by vestibular stimulation. Brain Res. **15**, 577–580 (1969b).

BAKER, R., PRECHT, W., LLINÁS, R.: Cerebellar modulatory action on the vestibulo-trochlear pathway in the cat. Exp. Brain Res. **16**, 364–385 (1972a).

BAKER, R., PRECHT, W., LLINÁS, R.: Mossy and climbing fiber projections of extraocular muscle afferents to the cerebellum. Brain Res. **38**, 440–445 (1972b).

BAKER, R., PRECHT, W., BERTHOZ, A.: Synaptic connections to trochlear motoneurons determined by individual vestibular nerve branch stimulation in the cat. Brain Res. **64**, 402–406 (1973).

BÁRÁNY, R.: Experimentelle Alkohol intoxication. Mschr. Ohrenheilk. **45**, 959–962 (1911).

BÁRÁNY, R.: Dauernde Veränderung des spontanen Nystagmus bei Veränderung der Kopflage. Mschr. Ohrenheilk. **47**, 481–483 (1913).

BÁRÁNY, R.: Untersuchungen über die Funktion des Flocculus am Kaninchen. Jb. Psychiat. Neurol. **26**, 631–651 (1914).

Bauer, J., Leidler, R.: Über den Einfluß der Ausschaltung verschiedener Hirnabschnitte auf die vestibulären Augenreflexe. Arb. neurol. Inst. Univ. Wien **19**, 155–226 (1912).

Bender, M.B., Weinstein, E.A.: Effects of stimulation and lesion of the median longitudinal fasciculus in the monkey. Arch. Neurol. Psychiat. (Chic.) **52**, 106–113 (1944).

Bender, M.B., Weinstein, E.A.: The syndrome of the median longitudinal fasciculus. Proc. Ass. Res. Nerv. Ment. Dis. **28**, 414–420 (1950).

Bender, M.B.: Comments on the physiology and pathology of eye movements in the vertical plane. J. nerv. ment. Dis. **130**, 456–466 (1960).

Bender, M.B.: The oculomotor decussation. Amer. J. Ophthal. **54**, 591–596 (1962).

Bender, M.B.: (Ed.) The oculomotor system. New York: Harper and Row (Hoeber) 1964.

Bender, M.B., Shanzer, S.: Oculomotor pathways defined by electric stimulation and lesions in the brainstem of monkey. In: The oculomotor system. p. 81–140. New York: Harper and Row (Hoeber) 1964.

Bender, M.B.: Oscillopsia. Arch. Neurol. (Chic.) **13**, 204–213 (1965).

Bender, M.B., Feldman, M., Atkin, A.: Optic illusions in lesions of the vestibular system. In: Proc. Int. Symposium on Vestibular and Oculomotor Problems. Tokyo: Nippon Hoechst 1965.

Bender, M.B., Feldman, M.: Visual illusions during head movement in lesions of the brain stem. Arch. Neurol. (Chic.) **17**, 354–364 (1967).

Bender, M.B.: Disorders of eye movements. In: Handbook of clinical neurology. p. 574–630. Amsterdam: North-Holland Publishing Company 1969.

Benjamins, C.E., Hiuzinga, E.: Untersuchungen über die Funktion des Vestibularapparates bei der Taube. Pflügers Arch. ges. Physiol. **217**, 105–123 (1927).

Benson, A.J., Bodin, M.A.: Interaction of linear and angular accelerations on vestibular receptors in man. Aerospace Med. **37**, 144–154 (1966).

Bergstedt, M.: Studies of positional nystagmus in the human centrifuge. Acta oto-laryng. (Stockh.) Suppl. **165**, 1–144 (1961).

Berthoz, A., Baker, R., Precht, W.: Labyrinthine control of interior oblique motoneurons. Exp. Brain Res. **18**, 225–241 (1973).

Biemond, A., de Jong, J.M.B.V.: On cervical nystagmus and related disorders. Brain **92**, 437–458 (1969).

Bisti, S., Maffei, L., Piccolino, M.: Variations of the visual responses of the superior colliculus in relation to body roll. Science **175**, 456–457 (1972).

Bizzi, E., Kalil, R.E., Tagliasco, V.: Eye-head coordination in monkeys: Evidence for centrally patterned organization. Science **173**, 452–454 (1971).

Blanks, R.H.I., Curthoys, I.S., Markham, C.H.: Planar relationships of semicircular canals in the cat. Amer. J. Physiol. **223**, 55–62 (1972).

Brandt, Th., Dichgans, J.: Circularvektion, optische Pseudocoriolis-Effekte und optokinetischer Nachnystagmus. Eine vergleichende Untersuchung subjektiver und objektiver optokinetischer Nacheffekte. Albrecht v. Graefes Arch. klin. exp. Ophthal. **184**, 42–57 (1972).

Brandt, Th., Dichgans, J., Koenig, E.: Differential effects of central versus peripheral vision on egocentric and exocentric motion perception. Exp. Brain Res. **16**, 476–491 (1973).

Breuer, J.: Über die Funktion der Bogengänge des Ohrlabyrinths. Med. Jahrb. **4**, 72–124 (1874).

Breuer, J.: Über die Funktion der Otolithen-Apparate. Pflügers Arch. ges. Physiol. **48**, 195–306 (1891).

Brodal, A., Pompeiano, O.: The origin of ascending fibres of the medial longitudinal fasciculus from the vestibular nuclei. An experimental study in the cat. Acta morph. neerl.-scand. **1**, 306–328 (1957).

Brodal, A., Torvik, A.: Über den Ursprung der sekundären vestibulocerebellaren Fasern bei der Katze. Eine experimentell-anatomische Studie. Arch. Psychiat. Nervenkr. **195**, 550–567 (1957).

Brodal, A.: The reticular formation of the brainstem. Anatomical aspects and functional correlations. Springfield/Ill.: C.C. Thomas 1958.

Brodal, A., Pompeiano, O., Walberg, F.: The vestibular nuclei and their connections: anatomy and functional correlations. Springfield/Ill.: C.C. Thomas 1962.

Brodal, A.: Anatomical organization and fiber connections of the vestibular nuclei. In: Neurological aspects of auditory and vestibular disorders. p. 107–145. Springfield/Ill. C.C. Thomas 1964a.

Brodal, A.: Anatomical observations on the vestibular nuclei with special reference to their relations to the spinal cord and cerebellum. Acta oto-laryng. (Stockh.) Suppl. **192**, 24–51 (1964b).

Brodal, A., Høivik, B.: Site and mode of termination of primary vestibulo-cerebellar fibres in the cat. Arch. ital. Biol. **102**, 1–21 (1964).

Brodal, A., Pompeiano, O.: (Eds.) Basic aspects of central vestibular mechanisms. Prog. Brain Res. Vol. 37. Amsterdam: Elsevier 1972.

Buchanan, A.R.: Nystagmus and eye deviations in guinea pigs with lesions in the brainstem. Laryngoscope (St. Louis) **50**, 1002–1011 (1940).

Camis, M., Creed, R.S.: The physiology of the vestibular apparatus. London: Oxford University Press (Clarendon) 1930.

Carpenter, M.B., Brittin, G.M., Pines, J.: Isolated lesions of the fastigial nuclei in the cat. J. comp. Neurol. **109**, 65–90 (1958).

Carpenter, M.B.: Lesions of the fastigial nuclei in the rhesus monkey. Amer. J. Anat. **104**, 1–34 (1959).

Carpenter, M.B., Bard, D.S., Alling, F.A.: Anatomical connections between the fastigial nuclei, the labyrinth and the vestibular nuclei in the cat. J. comp. Neurol. **111**, 1–26 (1959).

Carpenter, M.B.: Fiber projections from the descending and lateral vestibular nuclei in the cat. Amer. J. Anat. **107**, 1–22 (1960).

Carpenter, M.B., Alling, F.A., Bard, D.S.: Lesions of the descending vestibular nucleus in the cat. J. comp. Neurol. **114**, 39–50 (1960).

Carpenter, M.B., McMasters, R.E., Hanna, G.R.: Disturbances of conjugate horizontal eye movements in the monkey. I. Physiological effects and anatomical degeneration resulting from lesions of the abducens nucleus and nerve. Arch. Neurol. (Chic.) **8**, 231–247 (1963).

Carpenter, M.B., McMasters, R.E.: Disturbances of conjugate horizontal eye movements in the monkey. II. Physiological effects and anatomical degeneration resulting from lesions of the medial longitudinal fasciculus. Arch. Neurol. (Chic.) **8**, 347–368 (1963).

Carpenter, M.B., Strominger, N.L.: Cerebello-oculomotor fibers in the rhesus monkey. J. comp. Neurol. **123**, 211–230 (1964).

Carpenter, M.B., Strominger, N.L.: The medial longitudinal fasciculus and disturbances of conjugate horizontal eye movements in the monkey. J. comp. Neurol. **125**, 41–66 (1965).

Carpenter, M.B.: Central oculomotor pathways. In: The control of eye movements. p. 67–103. New York: Academic Press 1971.

Carpenter, M.B., Stein, B.M., Peter, P.: Primary vestibulo-cerebellar fibers in the monkey: Distribution of fibers arising from distinctive cell groups of the vestibular ganglia. Amer. J. Anat. **135**, 221–250 (1972).

Christoff, N., Anderson, P., Nathanson, M., Bender, M.B.: Problems in anatomic analysis of lesions of the median longitudinal fasciculus. Arch. Neurol. (Chic.) **2**, 293–304 (1960).

Cogan, D.G.: Neurologic significance of lateral conjugate deviation of the eyes on forced closure of the lids. Arch. Ophthal. (Chic.) **39**, 37–42 (1948).

Cogan, D.G., Kubik, C.S., Smith, W.L.: Unilateral internuclear ophthalmoplegia. Report of eight clinical cases with one postmortem study. Arch. Ophthal. (Chic.) **44**, 783–796 (1960).

Cohen, B., Suzuki, J.: Eye movements induced by ampullary nerve stimulation. Amer. J. Physiol. **204**, 347–351 (1963).

Cohen, B., Suzuki, J., Bender, M.B.: Eye movements from semicircular canal nerve stimulation in the cat. Ann. Otol. (St. Louis) **73**, 153–169 (1964).

Cohen, B., Suzuki, J., Bender, M.B.: Nystagmus induced by electric stimulation of ampullary nerves. Acta oto-laryng. (Stockh.) **60**, 422–436 (1965a).

Cohen, B., Goto, K., Shanzer, S., Weiss, A.H.: Eye movements induced by electric stimulation of the cerebellum in the alert cat. Exp. Neurol. **13**, 145–162 (1965b).

COHEN, B., TOKUMASU, K., GOTO, K.: Semicircular canal nerve, eye and head movements: The effect of changes in initial eye and head position on the plane of the induced movement. Arch. Ophthal. (Chic.) **76**, 523–531 (1966).

COHEN, B., GOTO, K., TOKUMASU, K.: Return eye movements, an ocular compensatory reflex in the alert cat and monkey. Exp. Neurol. **17**, 172–185 (1967).

COHEN, B., FELDMAN, M.: Relationship of electrical activity in pontine reticular formation and lateral geniculate body to rapid eye movements. J. Neurophysiol. **31**, 806–817 (1968).

COHEN, B., KOMATSUZAKI, A., BENDER, M.B.: Electro-oculographic syndrome in monkeys after pontine reticular formation lesions. Arch. Neurol. (Chic.) **18**, 78–92 (1968).

COHEN, B., KOMATSUZAKI, A., ALPERT, J.: Positional nystagmus after lesions of the cerebellum. Proc. 9th Int. Congr. Neurol. **93**, 198–199 (1969).

COHEN, B.: Vestibulo-ocular relations. In: The control of eye movements. p. 105–148. New York: Academic Press 1971.

COHEN, B., HIGHSTEIN, S.M.: Cerebellar control of the vestibular pathways to oculomotor neurons. In: Basic aspects of central vestibular mechanisms. Progr. Brain Res., Vol. 37, p. 411–425. Amsterdam: Elsevier 1972.

COHEN, B., KOMATSUZAKI, A.: Eye movements induced by stimulation of the pontine reticular formation: Evidence for integration in oculomotor pathways. Exp. Neurol. **36**, 101–117 (1972).

COHEN, B., HENN, V.: The origin of quick phases of nystagmus in the horizontal plane. In: Cerebral control of eye movements and motion perception. Bibl. ophthal. Vol. 82, p. 36–55. Basel: Karger 1972.

COHEN, B., UEMURA, T., TAKEMORI, S.: Effects of labyrinthectomy on optokinetic nystagmus (OKN) and optokinetic after-nystagmus (OKAN). Equil. Res. **3**, 80–93 (1973).

COLLEWIJN, H.: Dysmetria of fast phase of optokinetic nystagmus in cerebellectomized rabbits. Exp. Neurol. **28**, 144–154 (1970).

COLLEWIJN, H., NOORDUIN, H.: Vertical and torsional optokinetic eye movements in the rabbit. Pflügers Arch. **332**, 87–95 (1972).

COLLINS, W.E.: Vestibular responses from figure skaters. Aerospace Med. **37**, 1098–1104 (1966).

COLLINS, W.E., UPDEGRAFF, B.P.: A comparison of nystagmus habituation in the cat and the dog. Acta oto-laryng. (Stockh.) **62**, 19–26 (1966).

COLLINS, W.E.: Influence of head position on the habituation of vertical vestibular nystagmus in the cat. J. comp. physiol. Psychol. **67**, 156–159 (1969).

COLLINS, W.E., SCHROEDER, D.H., HILL, R.J.: Some effects of alcohol on vestibular responses. Advanc. Oto-rhino-laryng. **19**, 295–303 (1973).

COOK, W.A., JR., CANGIANO, A., POMPEIANO, O.: An electrical investigation of the efferent pathway from the vestibular nuclei. Arch. ital. Biol. **107**, 235–271 (1969).

COOPER, S., ECCLES, J.C.: The isometric response of mammalian muscle. J. Physiol. (Lond.) **69**, 377–385 (1930).

COSTIN, A., CHAIMOVITZ, M., BERGMANN, F.: Nystagmus evoked by intermittent photic stimulation of the rabbit's eye. Experientia (Basel) **21**, 167–171 (1965).

COSTIN, A., BERGMANN, F., CHAIMOVITZ, M.: Influence of side position of the head on central and flash nystagmus in the rabbit. Acta oto-laryng. (Stockh.) **61**, 323–331 (1966).

CRAMPTON, G.H.: Directional imbalance of vestibular nystagmus in cat following repeated unidirectional angular acceleration. Acta oto-laryng. (Stockh.) **55**, 41–48 (1962).

CRAMPTON, G.H.: Habituation of ocular nystagmus of vestibular origin. In: The oculomotor system. p. 332–346. New York: Harper and Row (Hoeber) 1964.

CRANMER, R.: Nystagmus related to lesions of the central vestibular apparatus and the cerebellum. Ann. Otol. (St. Louis) **60**, 186–196 (1951).

CRAWFORD, W.A.: The perception of mining objects: ability and visual acuity. Gt. Brit. Fly. Personnel Res. Comm. **150**, 1–10 (1960a).

CRAWFORD, W.A.: The perception of mining objects: eye movements. Gt. Brit. Fly. Personnel Res. Comm. **150**, 10–24 (1960b).

CROSBY, E.C.: Relations of brain centers to normal and abnormal eye movements in the horizontal plane. J. comp. Neurol. **99**, 437–480 (1953).

CRUM-BROWN, A.: On the sense of rotation and the anatomy and physiology of the semicircular canals of the inner ear. J. Anat. Physiol. (Lond.) **8**, 327–331 (1874).

CURTHOYS, I.S., MARKHAM, C.H.: Convergence of labyrinthine influences on units in the vestibular nuclei of the cat. I. Natural stimulation. Brain Res. **35**, 469–490 (1971).

DANDY, W.E.: The surgical treatment of Ménière's Disease. Surg. Gynec. Obstet. **72**, 421–425 (1941).

DENNEY, D., ADORJANI, C.: Orientation specificity of visual cortical neurons after head tilt. Exp. Brain Res. **14**, 312–317 (1972).

DESOLE, C., PALLESTRINI, E.A.: Responses of vestibular units to stimulation of individual semicircular canals. Exp. Neurol. **24**, 310–324 (1969).

DICHGANS, J., BRANDT, TH.: Visual-vestibular interaction and motion perception. In: Cerebral control of eye movements and motion perception. Bibl. ophthal. Vol. 82, p. 327–338. Basel: Karger 1972.

DICHGANS, J., SCHMIDT, C.L., WIST, E.R.: Frequency modulation of afferent and efferent unit activity in the vestibular nerve by oculomotor impulses. In: Basic aspects of central vestibular mechanisms. Progr. Brain Res. Vol. 37, p. 449–456. Amsterdam: Elsevier 1972a.

DICHGANS, J., HELD, R., YOUNG, L.R., BRANDT, TH.: Moving visual scenes influence the apparent direction of gravity. Science **178**, 1217–1219 (1972b).

DICHGANS, J., BIZZI, E., MORASSO, P., TAGLIASCO, V.: Mechanisms underlying recovery of eye-head coordination following bilateral labyrinthectomy in monkeys. Exp. Brain Res. **18**, 548–562 (1973a).

DICHGANS, J., SCHMIDT, C.L., GRAF, W.: Visual input improves the speedometer functions of the vestibular nuclei in the goldfish. Exp. Brain Res. **18**, 319–322 (1973b).

DITCHBURN, R.W., GINSBORG, B.L.: Involuntary eye movements during fixation. J. Physiol. (Lond.) **119**, 1–17 (1953).

DIX, M.R., HALLPIKE, C.S.: The pathology, symptomatology, and diagnosis of certain common disorders of the vestibular system. Proc. roy. Soc. Med. **45**, 341–354 (1952).

DODGE, R.: Visual perception during eye movement. Psychol. Rev. **7**, 454–465 (1900).

DODGE, R.: Five types of eye movements in the horizontal meridian plane of the field of regard. Amer. J. Physiol. **8**, 307–329 (1903).

DODGE, R.: Adequacy of reflex compensatory eye-movements including the effects of neural rivalry and competition. J. exp. Psychol. **6**, 169–181 (1923).

DOW, R.S.: The fiber connections of the posterior parts of the cerebellum in the cat and rat. J. comp. Neurol. **63**, 527–548 (1936).

DOW, R.S.: Effect of lesions in the vestibular part of the cerebellum in primates. Arch. Neurol. Psychiat. (Chic.) **40**, 500–520 (1938a).

DOW, R.S.: Efferent connections of the flocculo-nodular lobe in Macaca mulatta. J. comp. Neurol. **68**, 297–305 (1938b).

DOW, R.S., MORUZZI, G.: The physiology and pathology of the cerebellum. Minneapolis: The University of Minnesota Press 1958.

DUENSING, F., SCHAEFER, K.P.: Die Neuronenaktivität in der Formatio reticularis des Rhombencephalons beim vestibulären Nystagmus. Arch. Psychiat. Nervenkr. **196**, 265–290 (1957a).

DUENSING, F., SCHAEFER, K.P.: Die "locker gekoppelten" Neurone der Formatio reticularis des Rhombencephalons beim vestibulären Nystagmus. Arch. Psychiat. Nervenkr. **196**, 402–420 (1957b).

DUENSING, F., SCHAEFER, K.P.: Die Aktivität einzelner Neurone im Bereich der Vestibulariskerne bei Horizontalbeschleunigungen unter besonderer Berücksichtigung des vestibulären Nystagmus. Arch. Psychiat. Nervenkr. **198**, 225–252 (1958).

DUENSING, F., SCHAEFER, K.P.: Über die Konvergenz verschiedener labyrinthärer Afferenzen auf einzelne Neurone des Vestibulariskerngebietes. Arch. Psychiat. Nervenkr. **199**, 345–371 (1959).

DUSSER DE BARENNE, J.G.: The labyrinthine and postural mechanisms. In: A handbook of general experimental psychology. p. 204–246. Worcester, Mass.: Clark University Press 1934.

EASTER, S.: Spontaneous eye movements in restrained goldfish. Vision Res. **11**, 333–342 (1971).

EASTER, S.: Pursuit eye movements in goldfish (Carassius auratus). Vision Res. **12**, 673–688 (1972).

EASTON, T.A.: Patterned inhibition from horizontal eye movement in cat. Exp. Neurol. **31**, 419–430 (1971).

EASTON, T.A.: Patterned inhibition from single eye muscle stretch in the cat. Exp. Neurol. **34**, 497–510 (1972).

EGMOND, A.A.J. VAN, GROEN, J.J., JONGKEES, L.B.W.: The mechanism of the semicircular canal. J. Physiol. (Lond.) **110**, 1–17 (1949).

EGMOND, A.A.J. VAN, GROEN, J.J., JONGKEES, L.B.W.: The function of the vestibular organ. Basel: Karger 1952.

EIDELBERG, E., BOND, M.L., KELTER, A.: Effects of alcohol on cerebellar and vestibular neurones. Arch. int. Pharmacodyn. **192**, 213–219 (1971).

EWALD, J.R.: Physiologische Untersuchungen über das Endorgan des Nervus Octavus. Wiesbaden: Bergmann 1892.

FENDER, D.H., NYE, P.W.: An investigation of the mechanisms of eye movement control. Kybernetik **1**, 81–88 (1961).

FERIN, M., GRIGORIAN, R.A., STRATA, P.: Mossy and climbing fiber activation in the cat cerebellum by stimulation of the labyrinth. Exp. Brain Res. **12**, 1–17 (1971).

FERNÁNDEZ, C.: Interrelations between flocculonodular lobe and vestibular system. In: Neural mechanisms of the auditory and vestibular systems. p. 285–296. Springfield: Thomas 1960.

FERNÁNDEZ, C., FREDRICKSON, J.M.: Experimental cerebellar lesions and their effect on vestibular function. Acta oto-laryng. (Stockh.) Suppl. **192**, 52–62 (1964).

FERNÁNDEZ, C., GOLDBERG, J.M.: Physiology of peripheral neurons innervating semicircular canals of the squirrel monkey. II. Response to sinusoidal stimulation and dynamics of peripheral vestibular system. J. Neurophysiol. **34**, 661–675 (1971).

FERNÁNDEZ, C., GOLDBERG, J.M., ABEND, W.K.: Response to static tilts of peripheral neurons innervating otolith organs of the squirrel monkey. J. Neurophysiol. **35**, 978–997 (1972).

FERRARO, A., BARRERA, S.E.: Effects of lesions of the juxta-restiform body (I.A.K. Bundle) in Macacus rhesus monkeys. Arch. Neurol. Psychiat. (Chic.) **35**, 13–29 (1936).

FERRARO, A., BARRERA, S.E., BLAKESLEE, G.A.: Vestibular phenomena of central origin. Brain **59**, 466–482 (1936).

FERRARO, A., BARRERA, S.E.: Differential features of "cerebellar" and "vestibular" phenomena in Macacus rhesus. Preliminary report based on experiments on 300 monkeys. Arch. Neurol. Psychiat. (Chic.) **39**, 902–918 (1938).

FERRARO, A., PACELLA, B.L., BARRERA, S.E.: Effects of lesions of the medial vestibular nucleus. An anatomical and physiological study in Macacus rhesus monkeys. J. comp. Neurol. **73**, 7–36 (1940).

FERRIER, D.: The functions of the brain. New York: Putnam and Sons 1876.

FLOCK, A.: Structure of the macula utriculi with special reference to directional interplay of sensory responses as revealed by morphological polarization. J. Cell Biol. **22**, 413–432 (1964).

FLOURENS, P.: Recherches experimentales sur les propriétés et les fonctions du système nerveux dans les animaux vertébrés. Paris: Crevot 1842.

FLUUR, E.: Influences of semicircular ducts on extraocular muscles. Acta oto-laryng. (Stockh.) Suppl. **149**, 1–46 (1959).

FLUUR, E., MELLSTRÖM, A.: Utricular stimulation and oculomotor reactions. Laryngoscope (St. Louis) **80**, 1701–1712 (1970a).

FLUUR, E., MELLSTRÖM, A.: Saccular stimulation and oculomotor reactions. Laryngoscope (St. Louis) **80**, 1713–1721 (1970b).

FLUUR, E., MELLSTRÖM, A.: The otolith organs and their influence on oculomotor movements. Exp. Neurol. **30**, 139–147 (1971).

FORD, F.R., WALSH, F.B.: Clinical observations upon the importance of vestibular reflexes on ocular movements: Effects of section of one or both vestibular nerves. Bull. Johns Hopk. Hosp. **58**, 80–88 (1936).

FREEMAN, W.: Paralysis of associated lateral movements of the eyes. A symptom of intrapontile lesion. Arch. Neurol. Psychiat. (Chic.) **7**, 454–487 (1922).

Fuchs, A.F.: Saccadic and smooth pursuit eye movements in the monkey. J. Physiol. (Lond.) **191**, 609–631 (1967).

Fuchs, A.F., Kornhuber, H.H.: Extraocular muscle afferents to the cerebellum of the cat. J. Physiol. (Lond.) **200**, 713–722 (1969).

Fujita, Y., Rosenberg, J., Segundo, J.P.: Activity of cells in the lateral vestibular nucleus as a function of head position. J. Physiol. (Lond.) **196**, 1–18 (1968).

Fukuda, T., Hinoki, M., Tokita, T.: Static and kinetic labyrinthine reflex. Acta oto-laryng. (Stockh.) **49**, 467–477 (1958).

Fukuda, T.: Studies on human dynamic postures from the view point of postural reflexes. Acta oto-laryng. (Stockh.) Suppl. **161** (1961).

Fukuda, J., Highstein, S.M., Ito, M.: Cerebellar inhibitory control of the vestibulo-ocular reflex investigated in rabbit IIIrd nucleus. Exp. Brain Res. **14**, 511–526 (1972).

Fulton, J.R., Liddell, E.G.T., Rioch, D. McK.: The influence of unilateral destruction of the vestibular nuclei upon posture and the knee-jerk. Brain **53**, 327–343 (1930).

Gacek, R.R.: The innervation of the vestibular labyrinth. Ann. Otol. (St. Louis) **77**, 676–685 (1968).

Gacek, R.R.: The course and central termination of first order neurons supplying vestibular end organs in the cat. Acta oto-laryng. (Stockh.) Suppl. **254**, 1–66 (1969).

Gacek, R.R.: Anatomical demonstration of the vestibulo-ocular projections in the cat. Acta oto-laryng. (Stockh.) Suppl. **293**, 1–63 (1971).

Gernandt, B.E.: Vestibular mechanisms. In: Handbook of physiology. p. 549–564. Washington, D.C.: American Physiological Society 1959.

Gernandt, B.E.: Interactions between extraocular myotatic and ascending vestibular activities. Exp. Neurol. **20**, 120–134 (1968).

Gildenberg, P.L., Hassler, R.: Influence of stimulation of the cerebral cortex on vestibular nuclei units in the cat. Exp. Brain Res. **14**, 77–94 (1971).

Goebel, H.H., Komatsuzaki, A., Bender, M.B., Cohen, B.: Lesions of the pontine tegmentum and conjugate gaze paralysis. Arch. Neurol. (Chic.) **24**, 431–440 (1971).

Gogan, P., Gueritaud, J.P., Horcholle-Bossavit, G., Tyč-Dumont, S.: Inhibitory nystagmic interneurons. Physiological and anatomical identification within the abducens nucleus. Brain Res. **59**, 410–416 (1973).

Goldberg, J.M., Fernández, C.: Physiology of peripheral neurons innervating semicircular canals of the squirrel monkey. I. Resting discharge and response to constant angular accelerations. J. Neurophysiol. **34**, 635–660 (1971a).

Goldberg, J.M., Fernández, C.: Physiology of peripheral neurons innervating semicircular canals of the squirrel monkey. III. Variations among units in their discharge properties. J. Neurophysiol. **34**, 676–684 (1971b).

Goltz, F.: Über die physiologische Bedeutung der Bogengänge des Ohrlabyrinths. Pflügers Arch. ges. Physiol. **3**, 172–192 (1870).

Gonshor, A., Melvill Jones, G.: Changes of human vestibulo-ocular response induced by vision-reversal during head rotation. J. Physiol. (Lond.) **234**, P102–P103 (1973).

Goto, K., Tokumasu, K., Cohen, B.: Return eye movements, saccadic movements, and the quick phase of nystagmus. Acta oto-laryng. (Stockh.) **65**, 426–440 (1968).

Grand, W.: Positional nystagmus: An early sign in medulloblastoma. Neurology (Minneap.) **21**, 1157–1159 (1971).

Grant, G., Aschan, G., Ekvall, L.: Nystagmus produced by cerebellar lesions. Acta oto-laryng. (Stockh.) Suppl. **192**, 78–84 (1964).

Graybiel, A., Stockwell, C.W., Guedry, F.E., Jr.: Evidence for a test of dynamic otolith function considered in relation to responses from a patient with idiopathic progressive vestibular degeneration. Acta oto-laryng. (Stockh.) **73**, 1–3 (1972).

Groen, J.J., Lowenstein, O., Vendrik, A.J.H.: The mechanical analysis of the responses from the end organs of the horizontal semicircular canal in the isolated elasmobranch labyrinth. J. Physiol. (Lond.) **117**, 329–346 (1952).

Grüttner, R.: Experimentelle Untersuchungen über den optokinetischen Nystagmus. Z. Sinnesphysiol. **68**, 1–48 (1939).

Guedry, F.E., Jr.: Visual control of habituation to complex vestibular stimulation in man. Acta oto-laryng. (Stockh.) **58**, 377–389 (1964).

GUEDRY, F.E., JR.: Orientation of the rotation-axis relative to gravity: Its influence on nystagmus and the sensation of rotation. Acta oto-laryng. (Stockh.) **60**, 30–48 (1965).

HALSTEAD, W.C.: The effects of cerebellar lesions upon the habituation of postrotatory nystagmus. Comp. Psychol. Monogr. **42**, 1–130 (1935).

HALSTEAD, W.C., YACORZYNSKI, G., FEARING, F.: Further evidence of cerebellar influence in the habituation of after-nystagmus in pigeons. Amer. J. Physiol. **120**, 350–355 (1937).

HAMPSON, J.L., HARRISON, C.R., WOOLSEY, C.N.: Cerebrocerebellar projections and the somatotopic localization of motor function in the cerebellum. A. Res. Nerv. Ment. Dis. Proc. **30**, 299–316 (1952).

HANNEN, R.A., KABRISKY, M., REPLOGLE, C.R., HARTZLER, V.L., ROCCAFORTE, P.A.: Experimental determination of a portion of the human vestibular system response through measurement of eyeball counterroll. IEEE Trans. Biomed. Engin. **13**, 65–70 (1966).

HASEGAWA, T.: Labyrinthreflexe nach Abschleuderung der Otolithen-membranen. Pflügers Arch. ges. Physiol. **236**, 589–593 (1936).

HASEGAWA, T.: Die stato-kinetische Funktion des Sacculus. Z. Hals-, Nas.- u. Ohrenheilk. **43**, 129–132 (1937).

HASSLER, R., HESS, W.R.: Experimentelle und anatomische Befunde über die Drehbewegungen und ihre nervösen Apparate. Arch. Psychiat. Z. Neurol. **192**, 488–526 (1954).

HAUGLIE-HANSSEN, E.: Intrinsic neuronal organization of the vestibular nuclear complex in the cat. Ergebn. Anat. Entwickl.-Gesch. **40**, 1–105 (1968).

HENN, V., COHEN, B.: Activity in eye motoneurons and brain stem units during eye movements. In: Basic mechanisms of ocular motility and their clinical implications. Stockholm 1974 (in press).

HENN, V., YOUNG, L.R.. FINLEY, C.: Vestibular nucleus units in alert monkeys are also influenced by moving visual fields. Brain Res. **71**, 144–149 (1974).

HENRIKSSON, N.G.: An electrical method for registration and analysis of the movements of the eyes in nystagmus. Acta oto-laryng. (Stockh.) **45**, 25–41 (1955a).

HENRIKSSON, N.G.: The correlation between the speed of the eye in the slow phase of nystagmus and vestibular stimulus. Acta oto-laryng. (Stockh.) **45**, 120–136 (1955b).

HENRIKSSON, N.G., DOLOWITZ, D.A., FORSSMAN, B.: Studies of cristospinal reflexes (Laterotorsion). I. A method for objective recording of cristospinal reflexes. Acta oto-laryng. (Stockh.) **55**, 33–40 (1962).

HERMANN, H.T.: Eye movements in goldfish. Vision Res. **11**, 313–331 (1971).

HESS, W.R., BURGI, S., BUCHER, V.: Motorische Funktion des Tektal- und Tegmentalgebietes. Mschr. Psychiat. Neurol. **112**, 1–52 (1946).

HESS, W.R.: The functional organization of the diencephalon. New York: Grune and Stratton 1957.

HIEBERT, T.G., FERNÁNDEZ, C.: Deitersian unit response to tilt. Acta oto-laryng. (Stockh.) **60**, 180–190 (1965).

HIGHSTEIN, S.M.: Organization of the inhibitory and excitatory vestibulo-ocular reflex pathways to the IIIrd and IVth nuclei in rabbit. Brain Res. **32**, 218–224 (1971).

HIGHSTEIN, S.M., ITO, M.: Differential localization within the vestibular nuclear complex of the inhibitory and excitatory cells innervating IIIrd nucleus oculomotor neurons in rabbit. Brain Res. **29**, 358–362 (1971).

HIGHSTEIN, S.M., ITO, M., TSUCHIYA, T.: Synaptic linkage in the vestibulo-ocular reflex pathway of rabbit. Exp. Brain Res. **13**, 306–326 (1971).

HIGHSTEIN, S.M.: Electrophysiological investigation of the organization of the vestibulo-ocular pathways in rabbit. Bibl. ophthal. (Basel) **82**, 89–98 (1972).

HIGHSTEIN, S.M.: The organization of the vestibulo-oculomotor and trochlear reflex pathways in the rabbit. Exp. Brain Res. **17**, 285–300 (1973a).

HIGHSTEIN, S.M.: Synaptic linkage in the vestibulo-ocular and cerebello-vestibular pathways to the VIth nucleus in the rabbit. Exp. Brain Res. **17**, 301–314 (1973b).

HIGHSTEIN, S.M.: Synaptic linkage of the vestibulo-ocular reflex pathways in the rabbit. Mt. Sinai J. Med. **41**, 144–152 (1974).

HIGHSTEIN, S.M., COHEN, B., MATSUNAMI, K.: Monosynaptic projections from the pontine reticular formation to the IIIrd nucleus in the cat. Brain Res. (1974) (in press).

HIKOSAKA, O., MAEDA, M.: Cervical effects on abducens motoneurons and their interaction with vestibulo-ocular reflex. Exp. Brain Res. **18**, 512–530 (1973).

HÖGYES, A.: On the nervous mechanism of the involuntary associated movements of the eyes. Orv. Hetil. **23**, 17–29 (1880).

HOOD, J.D., PFALTZ, C.R.: Observations upon the effects of repeated stimulation upon rotational and caloric nystagmus. J. Physiol. (Lond.) **124**, 130–144 (1954).

HORCHOLLE, G., TYČ-DUMONT, S.: Activités unitaires des neurones vestibulaires et oculomoteurs au cours du nystagmus. Exp. Brain Res. **5**, 16–31 (1968).

HORCHOLLE-BOSSAVIT, G., TYČ-DUMONT, S.: Phénomènes synaptiques du nystagmus. Exp. Brain Res. **8**, 201–218 (1969).

HORN, G., HILL, R.M.: Modifications of receptive fields of cells in the visual cortex occurring spontaneously and associated with bodily tilt. Nature (Lond.) **221**, 186–188 (1969).

HORN, G., STECHLER, G., HILL, R.M.: Receptive fields of units in the visual cortex of the cat in the presence or absence of bodily tilt. Exp. Brain Res. **15**, 113–132 (1972).

HOSHINO, T.: Beiträge zur Funktion des Kleinhirnwurmes beim Kaninchen. Acta oto-laryng. (Stockh.) Suppl. **2**, 1–72 (1921).

HUNTER, J.: The use of the oblique muscles. In: Observations on certain parts of the animal oeconomy. p. 209–212. London 1786.

HYDE, J., TOCZEK, S.: Functional relation of interstitial nucleus to rotatory movements evoked from zona incerta stimulation. J. Neurophysiol. **25**, 455–466 (1962).

IMAI, R.: Studies on the angle gamma of the eye. Acta Soc. Ophthal. Jap. **34**, 117–210 (1930).

INGRAM, W.R., RANSON, S.W., HANNETT, F.I., ZEISS, F.R., TERWILLIGER, E.H.: Results of stimulation of the tegmentum with the Horsley-Clarke stereotaxic apparatus. Arch. Neurol. Psychiat. (Chic.) **28**, 513–541 (1932).

ITO, F., BACH-Y-RITA, P., YAMANAKA, Y.: Extraocular muscle intracellular and motor nerve responses to semicircular canal stimulation. Exp. Neurol. **24**, 438–449 (1969).

ITO, M., HIGHSTEIN, S.M., TSUCHIYA, T.: The postsynaptic inhibition of rabbit oculomotor neurones by secondary vestibular impulses and its blockage by picrotoxin. Brain Res. **17**, 520–523 (1970a).

ITO, M., HIGHSTEIN, S.M., FUKUDA, J.: Cerebellar inhibition of the vestibulo-ocular reflex in rabbit and cat and its blockage by picrotoxin. Brain Res. **17**, 524–526 (1970b).

ITO, M., NISIMARU, N., YAMAMOTO, M.: The neural pathways mediating reflex contraction of extraocular muscles during semicircular canal stimulation in rabbits. Brain Res. **55**, 183–188 (1973a).

ITO, M., NISIMARU, N., YAMAMOTO, M.: The neural pathways relaying reflex inhibition from semicircular canals to extraocular muscles of rabbits. Brain Res. **55**, 189–193 (1973b).

ITO, M., NISIMARU, N., YAMAMOTO, M.: Specific neural connections for the cerebellar control of vestibulo-ocular reflexes. Brain Res. **60**, 238–243 (1973c).

ITO, M., SHIIDA, T., YAGI, N., YAMAMOTO, M.: Visual influence on rabbit horizontal vestibulo-ocular reflex presumably effected via the cerebellar flocculus. Brain Res. **65**, 170–174 (1974).

JACOBS, L., ANDERSON, P.F., BENDER, M.B.: The lesions producing paralysis of downward but not upward gaze. Trans. Amer. neurol. Ass. (1972).

JANSEN, J., BRODAL, A.: Aspects of cerebellar anatomy. Oslo: Johan Frundt Tanum Vorlag 1954.

JOHNSON, G.L.: Contributions to the comparative anatomy of the mammalian eye, chiefly based on ophthalmoscopic examination. Phil. Trans. B **194**, 1–82 (1900).

JONGKEES, L.B.W.: On the function of the saccule. Acta oto-laryng. (Stockh.) Suppl. **38**, 18–26 (1950).

JONGKEES, L.B.W.: On positional nystagmus. Acta oto-laryng. (Stockh.) Suppl. **159**, 78–83 (1961).

JONGKEES, L.B.W., MAAS, J.P.M., PHILIPSZOON, A.J.: Clinical nystagmography. A detailed study of electronystagmography in 341 patients with vertigo. Pract. oto-rhino-laryng. (Basel) **24**, 65–93 (1962).

JONGKEES, L.B.W., PHILIPSZOON, A.J.: Electro-nystagmography. Acta oto-laryng. (Stockh.) Suppl. **189**, 1–111 (1964).

JUNG, R.: Die Registrierung des postrotatorischen und optokinetischen Nystagmus und die optisch-vestibuläre Integration beim Menschen. Acta oto-laryng. (Stockh.) **36**, 199–202 (1948).

JUNG, R., KORNHUBER, H.H.: Results of electronystagmography in man: The value of optokinetic, vestibular, and spontaneous nystagmus for neurologic diagnosis and research. In: The oculomotor system. p. 428–482. New York: Harper and Row (Hoeber) 1964.

KASAHARA, M., MANO, N., OSHIMA, T., OZAWA, S., SHIMAZU, H.: Contralateral short latency inhibition of central vestibular neurons in the horizontal canal system. Brain Res. **8**, 376–378 (1968).

KASAHARA, M., UCHINO, Y.: Selective mode of commissural inhibition induced by semicircular canal afferents on secondary vestibular neurons in the cat. Brain Res. **34**, 366–369 (1971).

KAWAI, N., ITO, M., NOZUE, M.: Postsynaptic influences on the vestibular non-Deiters nuclei from primary vestibular nerve. Exp. Brain Res. **8**, 190–200 (1969).

KIDOKORO, Y.: Direct inhibitory innervation of teleost oculomotor neurons by cerebellar Purkinje cells. Brain Res. **10**, 453–456 (1968).

KIDOKORO, Y.: Cerebellar and vestibular control of fish oculomotor neurons. In: Neurobiology of cerebellar evolution and development. p. 257–272. Chicago: American Medical Association 1969.

DE KLEYN, A.: Tonischer Labyrinthreflex auf die Augenmuskeln. Arch. ges. Physiol. **178**, 179–192 (1920).

DE KLEYN, A., VERSTEEGH, C.: Experimentelle Untersuchungen über den sogenannten Lagennystagmus während akuter Alkoholvergiftung beim Kaninchen. Acta oto-laryng. (Stockh.) **14**, 356–377 (1930).

KLINKE, R., SCHMIDT, C.L.: Efferent influence on the vestibular organ during active movement of the body. Pflügers Arch. **318**, 325–332 (1970).

KOELLA, W.P.: Motor effects from electrical stimulation of basal cerebellum in the unrestrained cat. J. Neurophysiol. **18**, 559–573 (1955).

KOELLA, W.P.: Organizational aspects of some subcortical motor areas. Int. Rev. Neurobiol. **4**, 71–116 (1962).

KOMATSUZAKI, A., HARRIS, H.E., ALPERT, J., COHEN, B.: Horizontal nystagmus of rhesus monkeys. Acta oto-laryng. (Stockh.) **67**, 535–551 (1969).

KOMATSUZAKI, A., ALPERT, J., HARRIS, H.E., COHEN, B.: Effects of mesencephalic reticular formation lesions on optokinetic nystagmus. Exp. Neurol. **34**, 522–534 (1972).

KORN, H., BENNETT, M.V.L.: Dendritic and somatic impulse initiation in fish oculomotor neurons during vestibular nystagmus. Brain Res. **27**, 169–175 (1971).

KORNHUBER, H.H.: Physiologie und Klinik des zentral-vestibulären Systems (Blick- und Stützmotorik). Hals-Nasen-Ohren-Heilkunde **3**, 2150–2351 (1966).

KORNHUBER, H.H.: Motor functions of cerebellum and basal ganglia: The cerebellocortical saccadic (ballistic) clock, the cerebellonuclear hold regulator, and the basal ganglia ramp (voluntary speed smooth movement) generator. Kybernetik **8**, 157–162 (1971).

KREJCOVA, H., HIGHSTEIN, S., COHEN, B.: Labyrinthine and extra-labyrinthine effects on ocular counter-rolling. Acta oto-laryng. (Stockh.) **72**, 165–171 (1971).

KRIEBEL, M.E., BENNETT, M.V.L., WAXMAN, S.G., PAPPAS, G.D.: Oculomotor neurons in fish: Electrotonic coupling and multiple sites of impulse initiation. Science **166**, 520–524 (1969).

LADPLI, R., BRODAL, A.: Experimental studies of commissural and reticular formation projections from the vestibular nuclei in the cat. Brain Res. **8**, 65–96 (1968).

LEE, F.S.: A study of the sense of equilibrium in fishes. I. J. Physiol. (Lond.) **15**, 311–348 (1893).

LEE, F.S.: A study of the sense of equilibrium in fishes. II. J. Physiol. (Lond.) **17**, 192–210 (1895).

LISBERGER, S.G., FUCHS, A.F.: Response of flocculus Purkinje cells to adequate vestibular stimulation in the alert monkey: fixation vs. compensatory eye movements. Brain Res. **69**, 347–353 (1974).

LLINÁS, R., PRECHT, W., CLARKE, M.: Cerebellar Purkinje cell responses to physiological stimulation of the vestibular system. Exp. Brain Res. **13**, 408–431 (1971).

LLINÁS, R.: Motor aspects of cerebellar control. Physiologist **17**, 19–46 (1974).

Lorente de Nó, R.: Labyrinthreflexe auf die Augenmuskeln. Vienna: Urban 1928.

Lorente de Nó, R.: Ausgewählte Kapital aus der vergleichenden Physiologie des Labyrinths. Die Augenmuskel-reflexe bei dem Kaninchen und ihre Grundlagen. Ergebn. Physiol. **32**, 73–242 (1931).

Lorente de Nó, R.: Anatomy of the eighth nerve. Laryngoscope (St. Louis) **63**, 1–38 (1933a).

Lorente de Nó, R.: Vestibulo-ocular reflex arc. Arch. Neurol. Psychiat. (Chic.) **30**, 245–291 (1933b).

Lowenstein, O., Sand, A.: The mechanism of the semicircular canal: A study of the responses of single fibre preparation to angular acceleration and to rotation at constant speed. Proc. roy. Soc. B **129**, 256–275 (1940a).

Lowenstein, O., Sand, A.: The individual and integrated activity of the semicircular canals of the elasmobranch labyrinth. J. Physiol. (Lond.) **99**, 89–101 (1940b).

Lowenstein, O., Roberts, T.D.M.: The equilibrium function of the otolith organs of the thornback ray (Raja clavata). J. Physiol. (Lond.) **110**, 392–415 (1949).

Lowenstein, O.: Peripheral mechanism of equilibrium. Brit. med. Bull. **12**, 114–118 (1956).

Lowenstein, O., Wersäll, J.: A functional interpretation of the electron-microscopic structure of the sensory hairs in the cristae of the elasmobranch Raja clavata in terms of directional sensitivity. Nature (Lond.) **184**, 1807–1808 (1959).

Ludvigh, E., Miller, J.W.: Study of visual acuity during the ocular pursuit of moving test objects. I. Introduction. J. Opt. Soc. Amer. **48**, 799–802 (1955).

Luschei, E.S., Fuchs, A.F.: Activity of brain stem neurons during eye movements of alert monkeys. J. Neurophysiol. **35**, 445–461 (1972).

Mach, E.: Grundlinien der Lehre von den Bewegungsempfindungen. Leipzig: Engelman 1875.

Mackensen, G., Uber, J.: Untersuchungen zur Physiologie des optokinetischen Nystagmus. Das Verhalten des optokinetischen Nystagmus bei langer Reizdauer. Albrecht v. Graefes Arch. Ophthal. **161**, 599–604 (1960).

Maeda, M., Shimazu, H., Shinoda, Y.: Inhibitory postsynaptic potentials in the abducens motoneurons associated with the quick relaxation phase of vestibular nystagmus. Brain Res. **26**, 420–424 (1971a).

Maeda, M., Shimazu, H., Shinoda, Y.: Rhythmic activity of secondary vestibular efferent fibers recorded within the abducens nucleus during vestibular nystagmus. Brain Res. **34**, 361–365 (1971b).

Maeda, M., Shimazu, H., Shinoda, Y.: Nature of synaptic events in cat abducens motoneurons at slow and quick phase of vestibular nystagmus. J. Neurophysiol. **35**, 279–296 (1972).

Maekawa, K., Simpson, J.I.: Climbing fiber activation of Purkinje cells in the flocculus by impulses transferred through the visual pathway. Brain Res. **35**, 245–251 (1972).

Maekawa, K., Simpson, J.I.: Climbing fiber responses evoked in vestibulo-cerebellum of rabbit from visual system. J. Neurophysiol. **36**, 649–666 (1973).

Magnus, R.: Körperstellung. Berlin: Springer 1924.

Manni, E.: Localizzazioni cerebellari corticali nella cavia. II. Effetti di lesioni delle "parti vestibolari" del cervelletto. Arch. Fisiol. **50**, 110–123 (1950).

Mano, N., Oshima, R., Shimazu, H.: Inhibitory commissural fibers interconnecting the bilateral vestibular nuclei. Brain Res. **8**, 378–382 (1968).

Markham, C.H., Curthoys, I.S.: Labyrinthine convergence on vestibular nuclear neurons using natural and electrical stimulation. In: Basic aspects of central vestibular mechanisms. Progr. Brain Res. Vol. **37**, p. 121–137. Amsterdam: Elsevier 1972.

Markham, C.H., Precht, W., Shimazu, H.: Effect of stimulation of interstitial Nucleus of Cajal on vestibular unit activity in the cat. J. Neurophysiol. **29**, 493–507 (1966).

Melvill Jones, G.: Vestibular interference with vision in flight. Proc. roy. Soc. Med. **52**, 185–186 (1958).

Melvill Jones, G.: Predominance of anti-compensatory oculomotor response during rapid head rotation. Aerospace Med. **35**, 965–968 (1964).

Melvill Jones, G.M., Milsum, J.H.: Spatial and dynamic aspects of visual fixation. IEEE Trans. Biomed. Engin. **12**, 54–62 (1965).

MELVILL JONES, G., MILSUM, J.H.: Frequency-response analysis of central vestibular unit activity resulting from rotational stimulation of the semicircular canals. J. Physiol. (Lond.) **219**, 191–215 (1971).

MERTON, P.A.: Compensatory rolling movements of the eye. J. Physiol. (Lond.) **132**, 25–27P (1956).

MILLER, E.F.: Counterrolling of the human eyes produced by head tilt with respect to gravity. Acta oto-laryng. (Stockh.) **54**, 479–501 (1962).

MILLER, E.F., GRAYBIEL, A.: Effect of drugs on ocular counter-rolling. Clin. Pharmacol. Ther. **10**, 92–99 (1969).

MILLER, J.W.: Study of visual acuity during the ocular pursuit of moving test objects. J. Opt. Soc. Amer. **48**, 803–818 (1955).

MONEY, K.E., JOHNSON, W.H., CORLETT, B.M.A.: Role of semicircular canals in positional alcohol nystagmus. Amer. J. Physiol. **208**, 1065–1070 (1965).

MONEY, K.E., MYLES, W.S.: Heavy water nystagmus and effects of alcohol. Nature **247**, 404–405 (1974).

MONNIER, M.: Les formations reticulées tegmentales; équilibrium des postures du regard de la tête et du tronc. Rev. neurol. **78**, 422–452 (1946).

MOWRER, O.H.: The influence of vision during bodily rotation upon the duration of post-rotational vestibular nystagmus. Acta oto-laryng. (Stockh.) **25**, 351–364 (1937).

MUSKENS, L.J.J.: Das supra-vestibulare System. Amsterdam: N.V. Noord-Hollandsche Uitgeversmaatschappij 1934.

MUSKENS, L.J.J.: Die loco- (und oculo-) motorische Funktion der Kerne der hinteren Commissur und Kerne des zentralen Höhlengraus des Mesencephalons. Jb. Psychiat. Neurol. **53**, 117 (1936).

MUSSEN, A.T.: Cerebellum and red nucleus. Arch. Neurol. Psychiat. (Chic.) **31**, 110–126 (1934).

MCCABE, B.F.: Vestibular suppression in figure skaters. Trans. Amer. Acad. Ophthal. Otolaryng. **64**, 264–268 (1960).

MCCABE, B.F.: The quick component of nystagmus. Laryngoscope (St. Louis) **75**, 1619–1646 (1965).

MCMASTERS, R.E., WEISS, A.H., CARPENTER, M.B.: Vestibular projections to the nuclei of the extraocular muscles: Degeneration resulting from discrete partial lesions of the vestibular nuclei in the monkey. Amer. J. Anat. **118**, 163–194 (1966).

MCNALLY, W.J., STUART, E.A.: Physiology of the labyrinth reviewed in relation to sea sickness and other forms of motion sickness. War Med. (Chic.) **2**, 683–771 (1942).

NELSON, J.R., COPE, D.: The otoliths and the ocular counter torsion reflex. Arch. Otolaryngol. (Chic.) **94**, 40–50 (1971).

NELSON, J.R., HOUSE, W.F.: Ocular counter torsion as an indicator of otolith function: Effects of unilateral vestibular lesions. Trans. Amer. Acad. Ophthal. Otolaryng. **75**, 1313–1321 (1971).

NITO, Y., JOHNSON, W.H., MORREY, K.E., IRELAND, P.E.: The non-auditory labyrinth and positional alcohol nystagmus. Acta oto-laryng. (Stockh.) **58**, 65–67 (1964).

NITO, Y., JOHNSON, W.H., IRELAND, P.E.: Positional alcohol nystagmus in the cat. Ann. Otol. (St. Louis) **77**, 111–125 (1968).

NYLÉN, C.O.: Some cases of ocular nystagmus due to certain position of the head. Acta oto-laryng. (Stockh.) **6**, 106–137 (1924).

NYLÉN, C.O.: Clinical study on positional nystagmus in cases of brain tumor. Acta oto-laryng. (Stockh.) Suppl. **15**, 1–113 (1931).

NYLÉN, C.O.: Oto-neurologic diagnosis of tumors of the brain. Acta oto-laryng. (Stockh.) Suppl. **33**, 1–151 (1939).

NYLÉN, C.O.: Positional nystagmus: A review and future prospects. J. Laryng. **64**, 295–318 (1950).

OHM, J.: Über den Einfluß des Sehens auf den vestibulären Drehnystagmus und Nachnystagmus. Z. Hals-, Nas.- u. Ohrenheilk. **16**, 521–540 (1926).

OOSTERVELD, W.J.: On the origin of positional alcohol nystagmus. Acta oto laryng. (Stockh.) **75**, 252–258 (1973).

PASIK, P., PASIK, T., KRIEGER, H.P.: Effects of cerebral lesions upon optokinetic nystagmus in monkeys. J. Neurophysiol. **22**, 297–304 (1959).

Pasik, P., Pasik, T., Bender, M.B.: Oculomotor function following cerebral hemidecortication in the monkey: A study with special reference to optokinetic and vestibular nystagmus. Arch. Neurol. (Chic.) **3**, 298–305 (1960).

Pasik, P., Pasik, T.: Oculomotor functions in monkeys with lesions of the cerebrum and the superior colliculi. In: The oculomor system. p. 40–80. New York: Harper and Row (Hoeber) 1964.

Pasik, T., Pasik, P., Bender, M.B.: The superior colliculi and eye movements. Arch. Neurol. (Chic.) **15**, 420–436 (1966).

Pasik, P., Pasik, T., Bender, M.B.: The pretectal syndrom in monkeys. I. Disturbances of gaze and body posture. Brain **92**, 521–534 (1969a).

Pasik, T., Pasik, P., Bender, M.B.: The pretectal syndrome in monkeys. II. Spontaneous and induced nystagmus and "lightning" eye movements. Brain **92**, 871–884 (1969b).

Pasik, T., Pasik, P., Valciukas, J.A.: Nystagmus induced by stationary repetitive light flashes in monkeys. Brain Res. **19**, 313–317 (1970).

Pasik, P., Valciukas, J.A., Pasik, T.: Effect of head and body tilt on flicker-induced nystagmus in monkeys. Exp. Neurol. **41**, 15–28 (1973).

Peterson, B.W.: Effect of tilting on the activity of neurones in the vestibular nuclei of the cat. Brain Res. **6**, 606–609 (1967).

Philipszoon, A.J.: Compensatory eye movements and nystagmus provoked by stimulation of the vestibular organ and the cervical nerve roots. Pract. oto-rhino-laryng. (Basel) **24**, 193–202 (1962).

Pompeiano, O., Walberg, F.: Descending connections to the vestibular nuclei. An experimental study in cat. J. comp. Neurol. **108**, 465–503 (1957).

Potthoff, P.C., Burandt, H.R., Richter, H.P.: Neuronale Reaktionen in Pons und Mesencephalon der Katze nach galvanischer Labyrinthpolarisation. Arch. klin. exp. Ohr.-, Nas.-, u. Kehlk.-Heilk. **189**, 262–280 (1967).

Precht, W., Grippo, J., Richter, A.: Effect of horizontal angular acceleration on neurons in the abducens nucleus. Brain Res. **5**, 527–531 (1967).

Precht, W., Llinás, R.: Functional organization of the vestibular afferents to the cerebellar cortex of frog and cat. Exp. Brain Res. **9**, 30–52 (1969a).

Precht, W., Llinás, R.: Comparative aspects of the vestibular input to the cerebellum. In: Neurobiology of cerebellar evolution and development. p. 677–702. Chicago: A.M.A. Education and Research Foundation 1969b.

Precht, W., Richter, A., Grippo, J.: Responses of neurones in cat's abducens nuclei to horizontal angular acceleration. Pflügers Arch. **309**, 285–309 (1969).

Precht, W.: Vestibular and cerebellar control of oculomotor functions. In: Cerebral control of eye movements and motion perception. Bibl. ophthal., Vol. 82, p. 71–88. Basel: Karger 1972.

Precht, W., Baker, R.: Synaptic organization of the vestibulo-trochlear pathway. Exp. Brain Res. **14**, 158–184 (1972).

Pritchard, R.M.: Physiological nystagmus and vision. In: The oculomotor system. p. 321–331. New York: Harper and Row (Hoeber) 1964.

Quix, F.H.: The function of the vestibular organ and the clinical examination of the otolithic apparatus. J. Laryng. **40**, 425–443 (1925).

Rademaker, G.G.J., Ter Braak, J.W.G.: On the central mechanism of some optic reactions. Brain **71**, 48–76 (1948).

Rashbass, C.: The relationship between saccadic and smooth tracking eye movements. J. Physiol. (Lond.) **159**, 326–338 (1961).

Rashbass, C., Westheimer, G.: Disjunctive eye movements. J. Physiol. (Lond.) **159**, 339–360 (1961).

Ratliff, F., Riggs, L.A.: Involuntary movements of the eye during monocular fixation. J. exp. Psychol. **40**, 687–701 (1950).

Richter, A., Precht, W.: Inhibition of abducens motoneurons by vestibular nerve stimulation. Brain Res. **11**, 701–705 (1968).

Riggs, L.A., Armington, J.C., Ratliff, F.: Motions of the retinal image during fixation. J. Opt. Soc. Amer. **44**, 315–321 (1954).

ROBINSON, D.A.: The mechanics of human saccadic eye movement. J. Physiol. (Lond.) **174**, 245–264 (1964).

ROBINSON, D.A.: The mechanics of human smooth pursuit eye movement. J. Physiol. (Lond.) **180**, 569–591 (1965).

RON, S., ROBINSON, D.A.: Eye movements evoked by cerebellar stimulation in the alert monkey. J. Neurophysiol. **36**, 1004–1022 (1973).

SADJADPOUR, K., BRODAL, A.: The vestibular nuclei in man: A morphological study in the light of experimental findings in the cat. J. Hirnforsch. **10**, 299–323 (1968).

SANS, A., RAYMOND, J., MARTY, R.: Projections des crêtes ampullaires et de l'utricle dans les noyaux vestibulaires primaires. Étude microphysiologique et corrélations anatomo-fonctionnelles. Brain Res. **44**, 337–356 (1972).

SCHAEFER, K.P.: Die Erregungsmuster einzelner Neurone des Abducens-Kernes beim Kaninchen. Pflügers Arch. ges. Physiol. **284**, 31–52 (1965).

SCHEIBEL, M.E., SCHEIBEL, A.B.: Structural substrates for integrative patterns in the brain stem reticular core. In: Reticular formation of the brain. p. 31–55. Boston: Little, Brown and Co. 1958.

SCHMIDT, C.L., WIST, E.R., DICHGANS, J.: Efferent frequency modulation in the vestibular nerve of goldfish correlated with saccadic eye movements. Exp. Brain Res. **15**, 1–14 (1972).

SCHROEDER, D.J.: Influence of alcohol on vestibular responses to angular accelerations. Aerospace Med. **42**, 959–970 (1971).

SCHWARZKROIN, P.A.: The effect of body tilt on the directionality of units in cat visual cortex. Exp. Neurol. **36**, 498–506 (1972).

SCHWINDT, P.C., RICHTER, A., PRECHT, W.: Short latency utricular and canal input to ipsilateral abducens motoneurons. Brain Res. **60**, 259–262 (1973).

SCHWINDT, P.C., PRECHT, W., RICHTER, A.: Monosynaptic excitatory and inhibitory pathways from medial midbrain nuclei to trochlear motoneurons. Exp. Brain Res. **71**, (1974) (in press).

SHANZER, S., TENG, P., KRIEGER, H.P., BENDER, M.B.: Defects in optokinetic after-nystagmus in lesions of the brain stem. Amer. J. Physiol. **194**, 419–422 (1958).

SHANZER, S., BENDER, M.B.: Oculomotor responses on vestibular stimulation of monkeys with lesions of the brain stem. Brain **82**, 669–682 (1959).

SHANZER, S.: Effects of semicircular canal stimulation in monkeys with lesions of the median longitudinal fasciculus. Fed. Proc. **23**, 414 (1964).

SHANZER, S., GOTO, K., COHEN, B., BENDER, M.B.: Median longitudinal fasciculus and vertical eye movements. Trans. Amer. neurol. Ass. **89**, 225–226 (1964).

SHIMAZU, H., PRECHT, W.: Tonic and kinetic responses of cat's vestibular neurons to horizontal angular acceleration. J. Neurophysiol. **28**, 991–1013 (1965).

SHIMAZU, H., PRECHT, W.: Inhibition of central vestibular neurons from the contralateral labyrinth and its mediating pathway. J. Neurophysiol. **29**, 467–492 (1966).

SHIMAZU, H., SMITH, C.M.: Cerebellar and labyrinthine influences on single vestibular neurons identified by natural stimuli. J. Neurophysiol. **34**, 493–508 (1971).

SHIMAZU, H.: Vestibulo-oculomotor relations: Dynamic responses. In: Basic aspects of central vestibular mechanisms. Progr. Brain Res., Vol. 37, p. 493–506. Amsterdam: Elsevier 1972.

SINGLETON, G.T.: Relationships of the cerebellar nodulus to vestibular function: A study of the effects of nodulectomy on habituation. Laryngoscope (St. Louis) **77**, 1579–1620 (1967).

SKAVENSKI, A.A., ROBINSON, D.A.: Role of abducens neurons in vestibulo-ocular reflex. J. Neurophysiol. **36**, 724–738 (1973).

SMITH, J.L., COGAN, D.G.: Internuclear ophthalmoplegia. Arch. Ophthal. (Chic.) **61**, 687–691 (1959).

SNIDER, R.S., STOWELL, A.: Receiving areas of the tactile, auditory, and visual systems in the cerebellum. J. Neurophysiol. **7**, 331–357 (1944).

SNIDER, R.S., ELDRED, E.: Cerebrocerebellar relationships in the monkey. J. Neurophysiol. **15**, 27–40 (1952).

SPARKS, D.L., TRAVIS, R.P., JR.: Firing patterns of reticular formation neurons during horizontal eye movements. Brain Res. **33**, 477–481 (1971).

SPIEGEL, E.A., PRICE, J.B.: Origin of the quick component of labyrinthine nystagmus. Arch. Otolaryng. (Chic.) **20**, 576–588 (1939).

SPIEGEL, E.A., SCALA, N.P.: Vertical nystagmus following lesions of the cerebellar vermis. Arch. Ophthal. (Chic.) **26**, 661–669 (1941).

SPIEGEL, E.A., SCALA, N.P.: Positional nystagmus in cerebellar lesions. J. Neurophysiol. **5**, 247–260 (1942).

SPIEGEL, E.A., SOMMER, I.: Neurology of eye, ear, nose and throat. New York: Grune and Stratton 1944.

SPILLER, W.G.: Ophthalmoplegia internuclearis anterior: A case with necropsy. Brain **47**, 345–357 (1924).

SPOENDLIN, H.H.: Organization of the sensory hairs in the gravity receptors in utricle and saccule of the squirrel monkey. Z. Zellforsch. **62**, 701–716 (1964).

STAHLE, J.: Electro-nystagmography in the caloric and rotatory test. Acta oto-laryng. (Stockh.) Suppl. **137**, 1–83 (1958).

STEIN, B.M., CARPENTER, M.B.: Central projections of portions of the vestibular ganglia innervating specific parts of the labyrinth in the rhesus monkey. Amer. J. Anat. **120**, 281–318 (1967).

STEINMAN, R.M., HADDAD, G.M., SKAVENSKI, A.A., WYMAN, D.: Miniature eye movement. Science **181**, 810–819 (1973).

SUZUKI, J., COHEN, B.: Head, eye, body and limb movements from semicircular canal nerves. Exp. Neurol. **10**, 395–405 (1964).

SUZUKI, J., COHEN, B., BENDER, M.B.: Compensatory eye movements induced by vertical semicircular canal stimulation. Exp. Neurol. **9**, 137–160 (1964).

SUZUKI, J., GOTO, K., KOMATSUZAKI, A., NOZUE, M.: Otolithic influences on tonus changes of the extra ocular muscles. Ann. Otol. (St. Louis) **77**, 959–970 (1968).

SUZUKI, J., GOTO, K., TOKUMASU, K., COHEN, B.: Implantation of electrodes near individual nerve branches in mammals. Ann. Otol. (St. Louis) **78**, 815–826 (1969a).

SUZUKI, J., TOKUMASU, K., GOTO, K.: Eye movements from single utricular nerve stimulation in the cat. Acta oto-laryng. (Stockh.) **68**, 350–362 (1969b).

SUZUKI, J., TAKEMORI, S.: Eye movements induced from the spinal nerves. Equil. Res. Suppl. **2**, 33–40 (1971).

SUZUKI, J.: Vestibulo-oculomotor relations: Static responses. In: Basic aspects of central vestibular mechanisms. Progr. Brain Res., Vol. 37, p. 507–514. Amsterdam: Elsevier 1972a.

SUZUKI, J.: Vestibular and spinal control of eye movements. In: Cerebral control of eye movements and motion perception. Bibl. ophthal., Vol. **82**, p. 109–115. Basel: Karger 1972b.

SZENTÁGOTHAI, J.: Die zentrale Innervation der Augenbewegungen. Arch. Psychiat. Nervenkr. **116**, 721–760 (1943).

SZENTÁGOTHAI, J.: The elementary vestibulo-ocular reflex arc. J. Neurophysiol. **13**, 395–407 (1950).

SZENTÁGOTHAI, J.: Die Rolle der einzelnen Labyrinthrezeptoren bei der Orientation von Augen und Kopf in Raume. Budapest: Akademiai Kiado 1952.

SZENTÁGOTHAI, J.: Pathways and synaptic articulation patterns connecting vestibular receptors and oculomotor nuclei. In: The oculomotor system. p. 205–223. New York: Harper and Row (Hoeber) 1964.

TAIT, J., MCNALLY, W.J.: Some features of the action of the utricular maculae (and of the associated action of the semicircular canals) of the frog. Phil. Trans. B **224**, 241–286 (1934).

TAKEMORI, S., SUZUKI, J.: Influences of neck torsion on otolithogenic eye deviations in the rabbit. Ann. Otol. (St. Louis) **78**, 640–647 (1969).

TAKEMORI, S., COHEN, B.: Visual suppression of vestibular nystagmus in rhesus monkeys. Brain Res. **72**, 203–212 (1974a).

TAKEMORI, S., COHEN, B.: Loss of visual suppression of vestibular nystagmus after flocculus lesions. Brain Res. **72**, 213–224 (1974b).

TARLOV, E.: Organization of vestibulo-oculomotor projections in the cat. Brain Res. **20**, 159–179 (1970).

TARLOV, E., TARLOV, R.S.: The representation of extraocular muscles in the oculomotor nuclei: Experimental studies in the cat. Brain Res. **34**, 37–52 (1971).

TAUBER, E.S., ATKIN, A.: Optomotor responses to monocular stimulation. Relation to visual system organization. Science **160**, 1365–1367 (1968).

TENG, P., SHANZER, S., BENDER, M.B.: Effects of brainstem lesions on optokinetic nystagmus in monkeys. Neurology (Minneap.) **8**, 22–26 (1958).

TEUBER, H.: Perception. In: Handbook of physiology, p. 1595–1668. Washington, D.C.: American Physiological Society 1960.

TOKITA, T., AOKI, S., FUKUDA, T.: The evolution of nystagmus, experimental studies on reflex pattern. In: Proc. Internat. Symposium on Vestibular and Oculomotor Problems, p. 195–200. Tokyo: Nippon Hoechst 1965.

TOKUMASU, K., GOTO, K., COHEN, B.: Eye movements produced by the superior oblique muscle. Arch. Ophthal. (Chic.) **73**, 851–862 (1965).

TOKUMASU, K., GOTO, K., COHEN, B.: Eye movements from vestibular nuclei stimulation in monkeys. Ann. Otol. (St. Louis) **78**, 1105–1119 (1969).

TYČ-DUMONT, S., DELL, P.: Composantes facilitatrices et inhibitrices du reflexe vestibulo-oculaire. J. Physiol. (Paris) **54**, 331–332 (1962).

TYČ-DUMONT, S.: Reticular control of a vestibulo-ocular reflex. In: Cortico-subcortical relationship in sensory regulation. Havana, Cuba: Academy of Sciences 1966.

UEMURA, T., COHEN, B.: Vestibulo-ocular reflexes: Effects of vestibular nuclear lesions. In: Basic aspects of central vestibular mechanisms. Progr. Brain Res., Vol. 37, p. 515–528. Amsterdam: Elsevier 1972.

UEMURA, T., COHEN, B.: Effects of vestibular nuclei lesions on vestibulo-ocular reflexes and posture in monkeys. Acta oto-laryng. (Stockh.) Suppl. **315**, 1–71 (1973).

VERSTEEGH, C.: Ergebnisse partieller Labyrinthexstirpation bei Kaninchen. Acta oto-laryng. (Stockh.) **11**, 393–408 (1927).

VOOGD, J.: The cerebellum of the cat. Structure and fibre connexions. Assen: Van Gorcum and Co., thesis, 1964.

WAGMAN, I.H.: Eye movements induced by electric stimulation of cerebrum in monkeys and their relationship to bodily movements. In: The oculomotor system. p. 18–39. New York: Harper and Row (Hoeber) 1964.

WALBERG, F., BOWSHER, D., BRODAL, A.: The termination of primary vestibular fibers in the vestibular nuclei in the cat. An experimental study with silver methods. J. comp. Neurol. **110**, 391–419 (1958).

WALBERG, F., POMPEIANO, O., WESTRUM, L.E., HAUGLIE-HANSSEN, E.: Fastigio-reticular fibers in the cat. J. comp. Neurol. **119**, 187–199 (1962).

WALTER, H.W.: Alkoholmißbrauch und Alkohollagenystagmus. Dtsch. Z. ges. gerichtl. Med. **43**, 232–241 (1954).

WARWICK, R.: Oculomotor organization. In: The oculomotor system, p. 173–204. New York: Harper and Row (Hoeber) 1964.

WAXMAN, S.G., PAPPAS, G.D.: An electron microscopic study of synaptic morphology in the oculomotor nuclei of three inframammalian species. J. comp. Neurol. **143**, 41–72 (1971).

WESTHEIMER, G.: Mechanism of saccadic eye movements. Arch. Ophthal. (Chic.) **52**, 710–724 (1954a).

WESTHEIMER, G.: Eye movement responses to a horizontally moving visual stimulus. Arch. Ophthal. (Chic.) **52**, 932–941 (1954b).

WESTHEIMER, G., RASHBASS, C.: Barbiturates and eye vergence. Nature (Lond.) **191**, 833–834 (1961).

WILSON, V.J., KATO, M., THOMAS, R.C., PETERSON, B.W.: Excitation of lateral vestibular neurones by peripheral afferent fibers. J. Neurophysiol. **29**, 508–529 (1966).

WILSON, V.J., WYLIE, R.M., MARCO, L.A.: Synaptic inputs to cells in the medial vestibular nucleus. J. Neurophysiol. **31**, 176–185 (1968).

WILSON, V.J.: Physiological pathways through the vestibular nuclei. In: International review of neurobiology, p. 27–81. New York: Academic Press 1972.

WILSON, V.J., FELPEL, L.P.: Specificity of semicircular canal input to neurones in the pigeon vestibular nuclei. J. Neurophysiol. **35**, 253–264 (1972).

WILSON, V.J., ANDERSON, J.A., FELIX, D.: Unit and field potential activity evoked in the pigeon vestibulo-cerebellum by stimulation of individual semicircular canals. Exp. Brain Res. **19**, 142–157 (1974).

WOELLNER, R.C., GRAYBIEL, A.: Counter rolling of the eyes and its dependence on the magnitude of gravitational or inertial force acting laterally on the body. J. appl. Physiol. **14**, 632–634 (1959).

WOELLNER, R.C., GRAYBIEL, A.: The loss of counter-rolling of the eyes in three persons presumably without functional otolith organs. Ann. Otol. (St. Louis) **69**, 1006–1012 (1960).

WOLFE, J.W.: Evidence for control of nystagmic habituation by folium-tuber vermis and fastigial nuclei. Acta oto-laryng. (Stockh.) **231**, 1–48 (1968).

WOLFE, J.W.: Relationship of cerebellar potentials to saccadic eye movements. Brain Res. **30**, 204–206 (1971).

WOLFSON, R.J.: (Ed.): The vestibular system and its diseases. Philadelphia: University of Pennsylvania Press 1966.

YAMANAKA, Y., BACH-Y-RITA, P.: Conduction velocities in the abducens nerve correlated with vestibular nystagmus in cats. Exp. Neurol. **20**, 143–155 (1968).

YARBUS, A.L.: Eye movements and vision. New York: Plenum Press 1967.

YOUNG, L.R., STARK, L.: A discrete model for eye tracking movements. IEEE Trans. Mil. Electr. **7**, 2–3 (1963).

YOUNG, L.R.: Pursuit eye tracking movements. In: The control of eye movements, p. 429–446. New York: Academic Press 1971.

YULES, R.B., GAULT, F.P.: The relationship of nystagmus to lateral vestibular nucleus stimulation. Exp. Neurol. **15**, 475–483 (1966).

ZUBER, B.L., STARK, L., COOK, G.: Micro-saccades and the velocity-amplitude relationship for saccadic eye movements. Science **150**, 1459–1460 (1965).

ZUBER, B.L.: Control of vergence eye movements. In: The control of eye movements. p. 447–471. New York: Academic Press 1971.

Chapter V.

Vestibulo-Spinal Mechanisms*

By

B. E. Gernandt, Pensacola, Florida (USA)

With 10 Figures

Contents

I. Introduction

Descriptive and analytical aspects of our knowledge of the vestibular system have changed considerably during the last decade as a result of a sudden interest being focused on the system and the fact that it has been the target of a steadily increasing number of experimental studies. Previously, only a small number of anatomists and physiologists were concerned with the vestibular system and, in comparison with the vigor by which other sensory systems were studied, one had the feeling that it was regarded as being of less significance to the welfare of the organism; some kind of exorbitant organ, frustratingly concealed and bioeconomically dispensable.

The vestibular system is now looked upon as an example of a highly specific organization, and evidence to this effect is given by recent contributions to the literature which emphasize the topographical arrangements, the cellular mechanisms of vestibular synaptic influences, and the wealth of inhibitory effects which can be observed at all levels along the vestibular pathways. There is a continued interest in the centrifugal control of vestibular inflow, and the role of a

* Submitted July 29, 1968.

specific gating mechanism is now being investigated and compared, or even contrasted, to the unspecific reticular control which had been previously studied (GERNANDT, 1967a).

The large variety of methods now being tried for studying the vestibular system, and the fact that the investigator who uses even one of them is likely to become entangled in the technical and theoretical problems common to all methods, have suddenly given rise to a voluminous amount of literature. History of science has shown again and again that the development of an important new method is followed by crucial and often epoch-making discoveries. The histochemical approach, the use of the electronmicroscope for obtaining better insight into the anatomical structure of the vestibular organ at a cellular level, and the application of the microelectrode technique for recording from within single nerve cells are the most recent examples of such methodological advances employed in vestibular research. Because of speed, sensitivity, and relative high resolution, electrophysiological technique continues to be productive in studying spatial and temporal patterning of vestibular firing set amidst the ever oscillating spontaneous background activity of the nervous system, and the questions asked are how as well as where.

The enormous increase in knowledge regarding the anatomy of the vestibular system (BRODAL et al., 1962; CARPENTER, 1967; WERSÄLL, 1966; NYBERG-HANSEN, 1964, 1965) offers impetus, authority, and a sound foundation to the growing accumulation of facts which emphasize the functional properties of the system. The present chapter concerns primarily vestibulo-spinal activity and the interaction at spinal levels among vestibular, segmental and intersegmental propriospinal, and pyramidal activities.

II. Methods Employed in Functional Studies of the Vestibular System

Activity in central neurons is determined, supported, and controlled by different influences, but none is more unanimously accepted and analyzed than that initiated by receptor activation. The process responsible for generation of impulses in the vestibular receptors is a specific transducer effect by which mechanical energy evokes depolarization of vestibular nerve terminals. While the response of the receptors is a local potential change which spreads electrotonically into the fibers, the generated afferent impulses are a propagated phenomenon. In the majority of vestibular fibers there is always an afferent firing that goese on in the absence of any overt or intentionally provoked stimulation (ADRIAN, 1943; GERNANDT, 1949; RUPERT et al., 1963). These neurons, designated as the "tonic" type, respond along flat slopes to application or cessation of angular stimulation. Some neurons do not discharge in the resting condition, but increase or decrease their firing rate along steep slopes during angular stimulation or at cessation of stimulation. They have been termed "kinetic" neurons (SHIMAZU and PRECHT, 1965).

Thus, the afferent firing can be strongly influenced by applying angular and linear acceleration or deceleration, or by caloric and galvanic stimulation. These kinds of stimuli, which are not easily graded or measured in the precise manner which characterizes studies of audition and vision, are not brief enough for evoking synchronized volleys of impulses that can be traced throughout the central nervous system. In order to obtain short-lasting potential changes, electrical square wave pulses have been applied to the peripheral vestibular axons equipped with stimulating electrodes (ANDERSSON and GERNANDT, 1954), and these sensory evoked potentials, more or less predictable and reproducible both from time to time and from animal to animal, have been used to map the central representation of the vestibular system. Direct electrical stimulation of the different vestibular nuclei (especially Deiters' nucleus) has been used frequently, but this method is very hazardous since there is always the issue of whether the results obtained are due to stimulation of the target structure or are caused by spread of current to adjacent structures.

III. Efferent Connections of the Vestibular Nuclei

The connections of the vestibular system consist of numerous chains of neurons, reciprocally linked in many ways and having their synapses in various anatomical nuclei. All the neural chains work in intimate collaboration, and the final pattern of reflex responses is attributable largely to the highly complex activity of the center; in addition, the vestibular system is directly and indirectly related to and dependent upon interconnections with other sensory systems. A reduction of the normal number of such interconnections interferes with the amount and pattern of vestibular information input, the ascending and descending vestibulofugal impulse traffic, and alters the basis for maintenance of equilibrium and spatial orientation with respect to the terrestrial environment. To keep the body upright and in equilibrium we have to rely on information transmitted by a number of sensory organs under the influence of various stimuli. Postural reflexes are in operation but changing all the time. Sometimes, when a particularly striking change occurs, it is described as a definite kind of postural reflex. The neuronal network of posture, however, has not suddenly become active when the reflex is observed; it has been active all along but has now altered its activity under the new conditions in order to go on doing what it has been doing all along – adjusting the body to the best mechanical advantage. Merely to ascertain a fixed position of our limbs we are not to the same degree dependent on the composite pattern of impressions received from the receptors in the labyrinth, muscle, joints, skin, and eyes as we are in respect of posture and equilibrium. The labyrinth is the sensory organ which is especially adapted to provide us with the necessary information for such purposes. Deflection of the cupulae under the impact of angular acceleration in the appropriate plane of space represents the stimulus to which we react with the well-known dynamic effector reflexes in the form of compensatory movements of neck, trunk, limbs, and eyes.

The vestibular nuclei, the cerebellum, and the reticular formation together form a close-knit functional unit primarily concerned with the maintenance of equilibrium and locomotion. The application of electrical stimulation to the peripheral branches of the vestibular nerve evokes an orthodromic, synchronized volley of impulses which then reaches the ipsilateral vestibular nuclei, the cerebellum, and rather extensive regions of the reticular formation. Furthermore, each Deiters' nucleus projects to its fellow nucleus on the opposite side (DE VITO et al., 1956; PRECHT and SHIMAZU, 1965). Experimental evidence indicates that the synapses between vestibular primary neurons and cells within the vestibular nuclear complex are powerful ones, and the input-output relation of vestibular neurons is quite different from that of spinal motoneurons (PRECHT and SHIMAZU, 1965; WILSON et al., 1968b). Because of the strategic position of the vestibular nuclei at the beginning of the various vestibular reflex arcs, they probably constitute the most important way-station of the executive system. Here the stream of vestibular impulses can be controlled by the influence of tonic and phasic central commands, the spatial and temporal pattern can be remodeled, and the input-output relation drastically changed (GERNANDT, 1967a). Such a station for programming and distributing vestibular signals through higher order neurons must constitute a link of utmost importance in amalgamating and adjusting activities so that the body is maintained at the best possible position to respond to the necessities imposed by the often changing environment.

In addition to primary vestibular neurons projecting onto the vestibular nuclei, there are fibers from the mesencephalon (POMPEIANO and WALBERG, 1957; MARKHAM et al., 1966), the cerebellar nuclei (WALBERG and JANSEN, 1961; WALBERG et al., 1963), and spinovestibular fibers (POMPEIANO and BRODAL, 1957; WILSON et al., 1968b). Anatomical (COHEN et al., 1958) and physiological (SNIDER et al., 1949; DE VITO et al., 1956) studies elaborate on the multitudinous cerebello-reticular, cerebello-vestibular, and cerebello-reticulo-vestibular connections. The dorsal neurons of Deiters' nucleus receive Purkinje cell axons directly and, in turn, innervate some spinal neurons monosynaptically (ITO, 1965). The anatomical and functional association of the cerebellum with those parts of the vestibular system projecting to the spinal cord has been summarized (DOW and MORUZZI, 1958; BRODAL, POMPEIANO and WALBERG, 1962). The importance of the vestibular nuclei as an excitatory source for the spinal cord is well established. Sectioning of the brain stem just below the level of the vestibular nuclei destroys the rigidity of a decerebrate cat and changes the status of the preparation to that of a spinal animal. The means by which the nuclei modulate the tonic properties of spinal motoneurons have been investigated (BACH and MAGOUN, 1947; WARD, 1947; KEMPINSKY and WARD, 1950; GERNANDT and THULIN, 1953; ANDERSSON and GERNANDT, 1956).

The neuronal tracts by which vestibular stimulation can activate the spinal cord are several, some relatively direct and others more complex and involving multisynaptic connections. By three descending pathways, the *vestibulospinal*, the *reticulospinal*, and the *medial longitudinal fasciculus* spinal motor cells are placed under the reflex control of the vestibular apparatus. Considerable attention has been devoted to the sites of origin and anatomical characteristics of these vestibulofugal pathways (BRODAL et al., 1962; NYBERG-HANSEN, 1964, 1965). The fact that at least three different tracts may serve vestibulospinal transmission and that they have both crossed and uncrossed fractions complicates an analysis of the specificity of these different connections. The spinal termination of these descending tracts are predominately on interneurons, but the interneurons in cervical segments receive a denser synaptic impingement than do those in lumbar segments. The functional properties of the vestibulospinal and descending medial longitudinal fasciculus are easier to investigate and comprehend than those of the reticulospinal tract. One of the most significant disclosures has been that of the governing role of the reticular formation in the coordination of posture and locomotion – this through the interplay of facilitatory and inhibitory effects on both spinal neurons and on those of the cerebral cortex. The nonspecific brain stem reticular system belongs to the visceral as well as to the somatic spheres of activity. It is affected by exteroceptive and interoceptive afferent impulses and its continuous tonic activity is dependent directly upon crucial components of the milieu intérieur (MAGOUN, 1964). This convergence of impulses from a multitude of different sensory receptors and central structures onto the reticular formation through abundant collaterals is now well established. It has been shown that vestibular stimulation leads to a gross activation of the bulbar reticular formation (GERNANDT and THULIN, 1953; GERNANDT, IRANYI and LIVINGSTON, 1959) that is known to control not only the amplitude and pattern of motor reflex phenomena but also to gate incoming sensory activity. Microelectrode recordings from individual units in the reticular formation have demonstrated a wide variability in the afferent fields of such units; some respond to a wide range of stimulation and modalities while others can be influenced by a much smaller range of stimulation, almost to the extent that it appears that some units might be differentially responsive to specific sensory inputs. The spatial and temporal patterns of vestibular impulses conducted eventually through reticulospinal connections are remodeled at this internuncial relay station that constitutes such a fundamental element of the vestibular reflex arc, as pointed out by LORENTE DE NÓ (1933).

In addition, it has been shown by MEGIRIAN and TROTH (1964) that vestibular stimulation evokes discharge of the pyramidal neurons, indicating vestibulo-pyramidal connections. Since the cerebellum, the spinal cord, and the cortical vestibular receiving areas are not essential for the generation of this pyramidal tract discharge, ascending vestibular activity is probably channeled through some subcortical relay nuclei. Thus, the vestibular organ can influence spinal motor outflow via "direct" descending vestibulofugal tracts, the vestibulospinal and medial longitudinal fasciculus, and via "indirect" channels, the reticulospinal and pyramidal tracts, including the cerebellum, the reticular formation, and some unidentified subcortical relay stations.

IV. Bulbospinal Correlation System

A stimulating electrode placed in the floor of the fourth ventricle will evoke activity in a number of descending fiber tracts which occupy the white matter of the ventral half of the feline spinal cord (LLOYD, 1941; WILLIS et al., 1967). The most prominent among these are the reticulospinal tracts, the vestibulospinal tract, the propriospinal system (TOWER, 1937; SZENTÁGOTHAI, 1951, 1964), and the descending portion of the medial longitudinal fasciculus. Only the first three tracts mentioned will conduct activity as far down as the lumbosacral levels of the cord; the medial longitudinal fasciculus is of no importance below a mid-thoracic level (GERNANDT, 1968).

LLOYD (1941) compared the effectiveness of the volleys in evoking ventral root discharges, interneuronal activity, and facilitation of monosynaptic reflexes when applying electrical shocks to the floor of the fourth ventricle and to the ventrolateral columns of the spinal cord. Since the results of stimulating these different regions were the same, he placed these tracts in a single descriptive category which was termed "the bulbospinal correlation system". This system, however, may be divided into two fiber groups, the long fibers represented by the reticulospinal, vestibulospinal, and long propriospinal tracts and the short fibers represented by short propriospinal tracts. Impulses from the long fibers reach the spinal motoneurons directly and by the appropriate short propriospinal relays. These tract impulses also activate local interneuron pools of the ventral horn region, which in turn deliver impulses to the motoneurons. The excitatory action of ventral cord volleys upon motoneurons was greatly enhanced by repetitive stimulation, and the summation of impulses in the short propriospinal relays with local internuncial impulses from the ventral motor pools controls the timing of firing of the earliest motoneuron volleys. The direct tract impulses, arriving at the motoneurons approximately 1 msec earlier than the propriospinal relays, are ineffective. For the direct impulses to become effective the dorsal interneuron pools must be active under the control of primary afferents. Since it is now known that vestibulospinal and reticulospinal activity may exert different effects upon particular motoneurons, the concept of a bulbospinal correlation system has been an over-simplification.

WILLIS et al. (1967) have more recently studied the synaptic actions upon lumbosacral motoneurons elicited by volleys conducted in pathways located in the ventral spinal cord. They also described a monosynaptic excitation of motoneurons, thus confirming the findings of LLOYD (1941) and of SASAKI et al. (1962). By intracellular recording, monosynaptic excitatory postsynaptic potentials (EPSPs) were observed in motoneurons of both extensor and flexor muscles. A number of motoneurons generated disynaptic EPSPs, which substantiates LLOYD's (1941) observation that motoneurons were excited both directly and indirectly via an interneuronal relay. Some of the motoneurons generated inhibitory postsynaptic potentials (IPSPs) in response to ventral cord stimulation. A few of the evoked IPSPs were disynaptic but the majority had latencies which suggested more complicated pathways. LLOYD (1941) described these descending tracts as having the conduction velocity of alpha fibers, and according to WILLIS et al. (1967), the speed of conduction ranged from 62 to 117 m/sec, with a mean value of 84 m/sec.

V. Vestibular Responses Recorded from Motor Nerves of Cervical and Lumbosacral Levels

Input-output curves for ascending vestibular activity, as revealed by recording evoked slow wave potentials at the orbital and anterior temporal surfaces of the cortex and in the pyramidal tracts, and descending vestibular activity, recorded from lumbosacral ventral roots, ipsilateral vagus (GERNANDT, 1964), and splanchnic nerves, show that as vestibular input increases, the ascending vestibular activity reaches a virtual maximum before overt descending vestibular activity is detected. These findings suggest that the low threshold vestibular afferent fibers functionally activate the ascending vestibular system, whereas the high

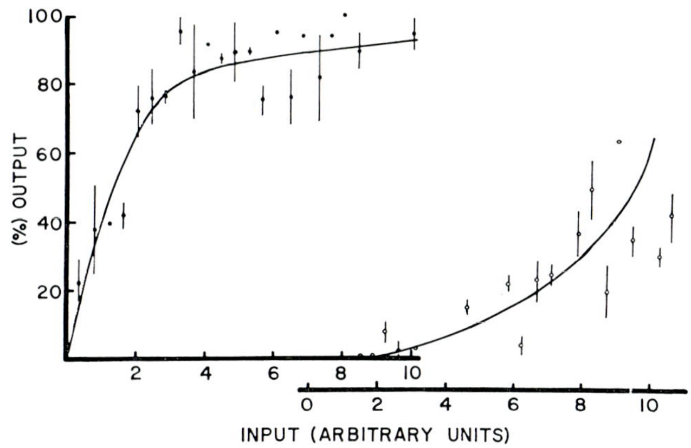

Fig. 1. Abscissa, size, in arbitrary units, of compound action potentials recorded from eighth nerve entry zone. Ordinate, vestibular evoked responses, expressed as per cent of maximum. Average of ascending vestibular evoked responses, as recorded from orbital and anterior temporal surfaces of cerebral cortex and from pyramidal tract (dots), and average descending vestibular evoked responses, as recorded from lumbosacral ventral roots bilaterally, vagus, and splanchnic nerves (circles) plotted as a function of input (MEGIRIAN and MANNING, 1967)

threshold fibers activate the descending vestibular system (Fig. 1; MEGIRIAN and MANNING, 1967).

Single shock electrical stimulation applied to the peripheral branches of the vestibular nerve will at least evoke activity in the vestibulospinal tract, reticulospinal tract, and the medial longitudinal fasciculus, i.e., tracts belonging to LLOYD's (1941) bulbospinal correlation system. The evoked responses can be recorded from both ipsilateral and contralateral motor nerves of cervicothoracic and lumbosacral levels (GERNANDT et al., 1957; GERNANDT, 1967b). Hemisection of the spinal cord two or three segments above the level of recording obliterates the vestibular responses on the side of the section but does not alter those in the opposite motor nerves. Dorsal quadrant section does not affect the responses, whereas ventral quadrant section completely obliterates them. The ventral quadrant alone is sufficient for the transmission of vestibular responses inasmuch as contralateral hemisection and ipsilateral dorsal quadrant section in the same animal still leave an apparently intact response to vestibular stimulation (GERNANDT et al., 1957). Thus, it is not surprising that the results obtained by activating the bulbospinal correlation system through stimulation of the ventral quadrant of the cord are more or less the same as when the peripheral branches of the vestibular nerve are stimulated.

The high spinal segmental discharge to vestibular stimulation shows an early bilateral spikelike response which immediately precedes or slightly overlaps a double wave response. At the lumbar level only the double wave responses are seen (Fig. 2). The evidence indicates that there must be some stronger connections influencing the cervical level which are not distributed down as far as the lumbar region (GERNANDT and GILMAN, 1959; ERULKAR et al., 1966; WILSON et al., 1968b). Ten per second or higher frequency stimulation of the vestibular nerve

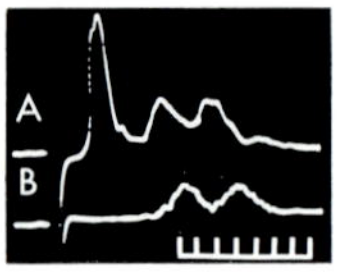

Fig. 2. Responses to single shock vestibular stimulation recorded from ipsilateral deep radial nerve (upper beam) and ventral root L7 (lower beam). Time scale in 1 msec intervals (GERNANDT, 1964)

causes a small reduction in amplitude of the spikelike portion of the cervical response and a steplike augmentation of the first wave at both levels.

Relay through the contralateral vestibular nuclei is not essential to the spinal motor responses. This was shown unequivocally by removing those nuclei or by a mid-line longitudinal splitting of the pontine and bulbar brain stem. In both instances the ipsilateral and contralateral ventral root responses remained intact. Paths descending from the ipsilateral bulb (from the region of the vestibular nuclei and reticular formation) are therefore sufficient to account for both ipsilateral and contralateral motor responses. The contralateral vestibular effects must depend upon crossings which take place below the level of the obex. Since the lumbar responses are still present bilaterally after a mid-line split of the lumbar region of the spinal cord, in the same animals whose brain stem was split throughout the pontine and bulbar levels, there must be sufficient crossings in the cervical and thoracic regions (GERNANDT et al., 1959).

VI. The Effect of Vestibular Activity upon Alpha and Gamma Motoneurons

There are two routes leading to muscular contraction; one is direct activation of alpha motoneurons, and the other indirect by way of gamma fibers (about one third of the ventral root axons), muscle spindles, and afferent fibers. Therefore, in considering the influence of the vestibular system on myotatic reflexes and tonus, one must think of the two ways in which such reflexes can be influenced: (a) by facilitation or inhibition of the large alpha motoneurons which innervate the extrafusal muscle fibers; (b) by facilitation or inhibition of the small gamma motoneurons which cause contraction of the intrafusal fibers of the muscle spindles, thereby increasing the rate of spindle firing, which in turn influences the amount of the alpha motoneuron firing.

Descending vestibular volleys culminate in the activation of alpha and gamma motoneurons. The functional relationship between the vestibular system and alpha motoneuron discharge combined with the excitatory effect of vestibular stimulation on muscle spindles discharge is well established (ANDERSSON and GERNANDT, 1956; GERNANDT, IRANYI and LIVINGSTON, 1959). The importance of the direct excitation exerted by descending vestibulofugal connections upon motoneurons versus the indirect activation of motoneurons through the gamma loop has been investigated (GERNANDT, 1967b; CARLI et al., 1967). In the experiments of ANDERSSON and GERNANDT (1956) it was shown that a weak, descending vestibular volley activated the gamma fibers alone before an increase in stimulus strength activated in parallel the alpha and gamma motoneurons. This indicates that muscle spindles are activated before stronger stimulation evokes alpha discharge, causing muscular contraction. DIETE-SPIFF et al. (1967) applied stimulation to the vestibular nerve and recorded the response of a gastrocnemius muscle spindle receptor. As the frequency of vestibular stimulation increased the response of the receptor increased but without being accompanied by an extrafusal contraction until the stimulus frequency reached 16 pulses/sec. The spindle discharge outlasted the stimulus and the extrafusal contraction, if this was also induced, by several seconds.

Simultaneous recording of the response to single shock vestibular stimulation from a filament of a lumbosacral ventral root and from the parent root itself demonstrates that the typical two-wave response represents the firing of gamma fibers, grouped into two clusters (GERNANDT et al., 1959). As mentioned, vestibular stimulation at 10 pulses/sec results in a two-stage augmentation of the first wave. The filament recording shows a more dense gamma firing during the first stage and a gradually increasing negative potential shift in the baseline. In the second stage the negative potential shift becomes stronger, and finally large amplitude alpha spikes appear on top of it. There are characteristic changes in the responses recorded from the parent root which correspond to these two stages. The first wave grows slightly in amplitude during the increased gamma firing and then abruptly jumps to a greater height at the instant when the large alpha spikes appear in the root filament.

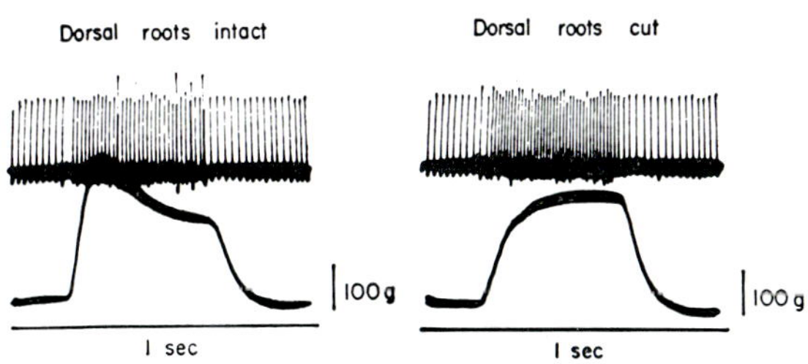

Fig. 3. Effect of dorsal root section on a gastrocnemius muscle spindle receptor, and on extrafusal tension following stimulation of Deiters' nucleus. Initial tension of muscle 10 mm. Stimulation with 7 V, 0.5 msec pulses at 500/sec before and after section of ipsilateral dorsal roots L6 to S2 (CARLI, DIETE-SPIFF and POMPEIANO, 1967)

After the gamma loop had been interrupted by cutting the dorsal roots, it was not surprising that the rise of tension in the gastrocnemius muscle caused by vestibular stimulation was only slightly reduced because of abolition of the input from spindle afferents to motoneurons. However, the rate of rise of tension to a final peak value was slower (Fig. 3; CARLI et al., 1966, 1967). The whole spectrum of facilitatory, inhibitory, or diphasic modulations evoked by vestibular impulses upon the alpha discharges, with intact gamma loops, could similarly be obtained after the elimination of the loops, although the amount of available gamma support determines the threshold at which the alpha effects are manifested. Thus, as far as vestibular motor effects are concerned, the gamma loop does not provide the alpha motoneurons with an input that is essential for extrafusal contraction. However, it is often the case that the nervous system solves problems by both of two alternative approaches and does not rely on either approach exclusively, and it is dangerous to state questions that require the acceptance of one mode of functional organization to the total exclusion of the other.

The vestibulospinal impingement is monosynaptic and will inevitably discharge its cells directly in advance of impulses that have to make a double journey back to the muscle fibers (Lund and Pompeiano, 1965). Further evidence, obtained with dorsal roots intact, was the demonstration of an extrafusal motor response to vestibular stimulation while the spindles were deactivated during the brief period preceding the full recovery of intrafusal motor end plates from an injection of a curarizing agent (Carli et al., 1967). As far as the muscular contraction elicited by Deiters' nucleus stimulation is concerned, the gamma loop seems to function as a sensitizing or priming device in concert with the direct monosynaptic vestibulomotor coupling and not as a triggering mechanism (Lund and Pompeiano, 1965). Alpha control is probably employed when speed is essential, whereas gamma signals ensure a smoother, continuous control.

VII. Interaction between Vestibular and Intersegmental Propriospinal Reflex Activities

Each motoneuron of the spinal cord is subjected to a multitude of influences, some reinforcing and some antagonistic, and the balance of these influences at any time determines the membrane potential and hence the excitability level of the cell. Therefore, the effect of descending vestibular impulses upon spinal motor pools is influenced by simultaneous convergent afferent bombardment from other receptors and the motor outflow will change from moment to moment and thus, the participation of different motoneurons and their subservient muscles in reflex actions will display an infinite variety of behavioral patterns.

Two distinguishable systems coordinate and amalgamate spinal reflex activities. One system, the propriospinal, with bilateral projections which frequently cross and recross, is restricted within the extent of the cord and is relatively direct. The long propriospinal neurons have their cell bodies in the central gray matter and send their axons into the adjacent white matter where the fibers run up or down for variable distances before reentering the gray matter itself. A second system involves projections from the spinal cord going up to the brain stem and returning to influence spinal motor pool activity (Gernandt and Megirian, 1961; Gernandt and Shimamura, 1961; Shimamura and Livingston, 1963). The central nervous system is constantly receiving information over the proprioceptive pathways. These two longitudinal sensorimotor coordinating systems together with the vestibular system are presumed to contribute to the over-all organization of postural and locomotive reflexes.

Some insight into the complex interaction between activity conducted in the propriospinal, spino-bulbo-spinal, and vestibular systems can be obtained by stimulating these systems in a controlled temporal sequence while recording the

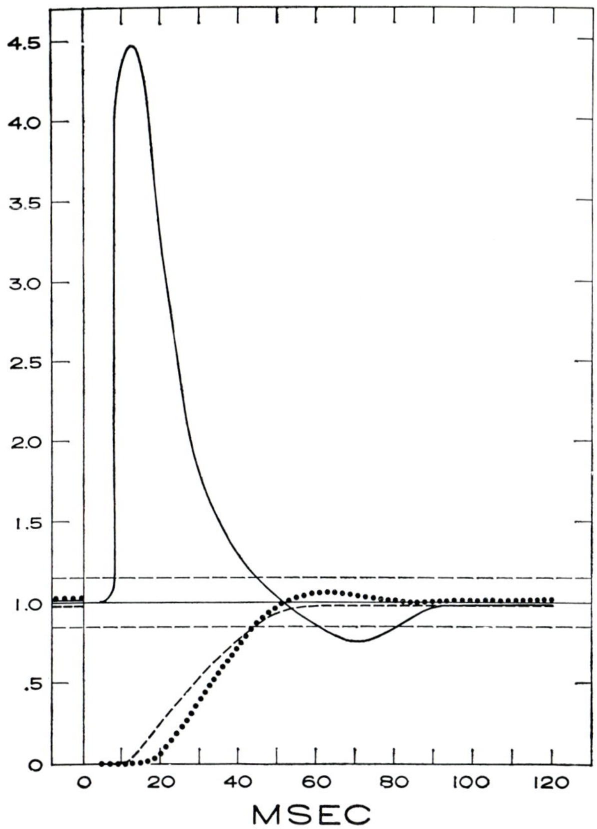

Fig. 4. Amplitude variations of vestibular response when conditioned by single brachial plexus shocks at increasing intervals, recorded from ipsilateral ventral root L7 (solid line). Supramaximal L7 dorsal root shocks preceding vestibular responses recorded from corresponding ventral root at increasing intervals (dotted line). Effects upon brachial plexus response when conditioned by single vestibular shocks, recorded from ipsilateral ventral root L7 at increasing intervals (dashed line). Amplitude variations of tests responses relative to control = 1.0 plotted against time in msec (Gernandt and Gilman, 1960a)

average discharge activity from different spinal motor nerves (Gernandt and Gilman, 1960a). The brachial plexus is utilized as an input lead to activate the intersegmental and spino-bulbo-spinal systems. The reflex responses of the longitudinal sensorimotor coordination systems, recorded from lumbosacral ventral roots, are markedly reduced in amplitude or totally obliterated by a preceding vestibular volley when the two shocks are delivered in close succession (Fig. 4, dashed line). As the interval between stimuli is gradually widened, the tail of the response reappears and successively earlier portions are added until the entire response is restored at an interval between stimuli of about 60 msec. When a volley of impulses conducted in the longitudinal coordination system reaches lumbosacral levels before the vestibular activity, the first wave of the vestibular reflex response is enhanced four to ten times, and the second wave is abolished for an interval of about 50 msec (Fig. 4, solid line).

VIII. Interactions between Vestibular and Segmental Propriospinal Reflex Activities

Stimulation of the gastrocnemius extensor nerve at an intensity subthreshold for its ventral root response yields a clearly discernible monosynaptic response in those roots when preceded by vestibular stimulation (Fig. 5, A, B). If the strength of gastrocnemius nerve stimulation is increased to a just discernible ventral root response (C) and is preceded by vestibular stimulation (D), an obvious facilitation of the gastrocnemius nerve response is seen. Between E and F can be noted a fourfold increase of the monosynaptic component. In another experiment

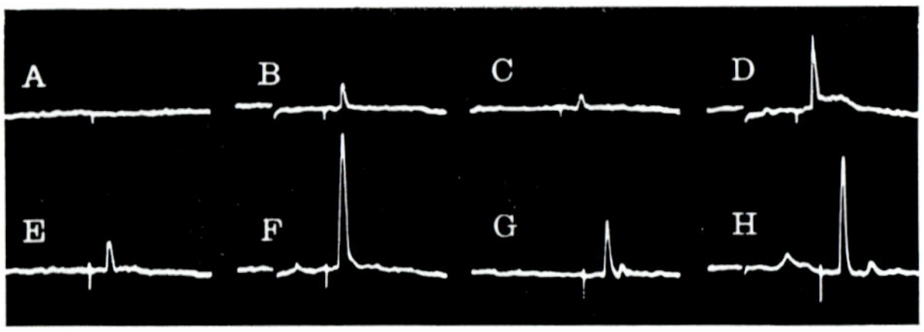

Fig. 5. Vestibular effects on spinal segmental reflexes. A shows ventral root L7 inactivity following a subthreshold gastrocnemius shock stimulation, and B illustrates facilitatory influence of prior vestibular nerve stimulation; C and D show same influence on a just suprathreshold gastrocnemius response; E and F ditto on stronger gastrocnemius stimulation; G and H show vestibular influence on response evoked by supramaximal gastrocnemius stimulation (Gernandt, Katsuki and Livingston, 1957)

the response to gastrocnemius stimulation at supramaximal intensity (G) still is clearly facilitated by the preceding vestibular excitation (H). These facilitatory effects are of more than 25-msec duration. This finding is consistent with Lloyd's (1941) observation concerning the duration of bulbospinal facilitatory effects when stimulation is applied directly to the bulb. Although the tibialis anticus nerve is a functional antagonist of the gastrocnemius, the segmental reflex response evoked by tibialis anticus stimulation is clearly facilitated by a preceding vestibular stimulation.

The influence of local reflex activity upon vestibular outflow is the opposite, i.e., a strong inhibition (Fig. 4, dotted line). The response to single shock vestibular stimulation is obliterated for a period of about 15 msec by a preceding supramaximal shock to a motor, mixed, our cutaneous nerve. This demonstrates that although a muscle contraction may be initiated by vestibular stimulation, its subsequent control comes into being mainly through the muscles themselves. This self-regulation of the muscle influences both alpha and gamma activity. If impulses are recorded from an alpha fiber whose cell is in contact with both the descending vestibular path and the segmental proprioceptive connections, a muscular contraction gives rise to an inhibition of the vestibular response, however strong it may be. This closed loop that regulates the activity of each muscle individually is the basic control mechanisms of the motor system.

IX. Interaction between Vestibular and Pyramidal Activities

Posture can be assumed, modified, and shifted so that the instant obedience of a muscle to pyramidal demands can be met. During potent vestibular stimulation, however, the spinal keyboard does not receive the commands from the motor cortex as a docile instrument ready to transmit, blindly and faithfully, carefully prepared orders to the muscles. The cord interprets the orders that it receives and transmits them only as a function of an ever-changing state of receptivity.

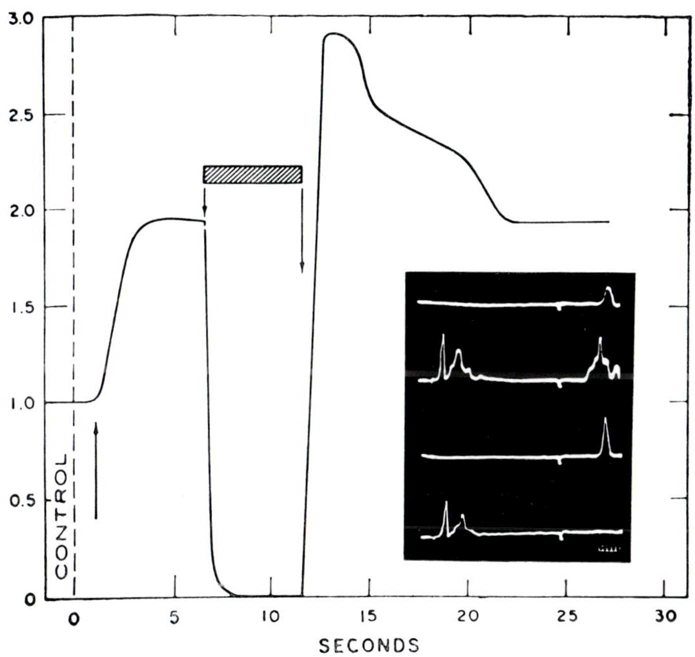

Fig. 6. Insert depicts control response to single shock pericruciate cortical stimulation recorded from contralateral deep radial nerve and when conditioned by vestibular volley (upper pair). Response to 3 pulses/sec cortical stimulation and when preceded at this frequency by conditioning vestibular volleys (lower pair). Time scale in msec. Curve represents amplitude of original response at 1 and 3 pulses/sec (first arrow), during (marked by bar), and after conditioning vestibular stimulation (GERNANDT and GILMAN, 1960b)

The response to single-shock electrical stimulation of the pericruciate cortex recorded from a contralateral motor nerve of cervicothoracic or lumbosacral spinal origin is strongly augmented in amplitude when preceded by a vestibular volley of impulses within a time lapse of about 30 msec (Gernandt and Gilman, 1960b). If the two shocks are delivered at progressively shorter intervals, the corticospinal response is completely obliterated at an interval of 10 to 15 msec. The increase in size of the response to motor cortex stimulation (1 pulse/sec) by a conditioning vestibular volley applied at a suitable interval is demonstrated in the oscilloscopic tracing of Fig. 6, upper pair.

If the evoked corticospinal response is augmented by an increase in stimulation frequency to 3 shocks per second and the vestibular conditioning response is delivered at the same interval and frequency, the test response is abolished (lower pair). If the conditioning vestibular stimulation is discontinued, the corticospinal response reappears, showing a rebound. The entire sequence of effect of vestibular stimulation upon cortically evoked responses is demonstrated by the curve of Fig. 6.

X. Synaptic Mechanisms of Vestibulofugal Influences on Spinal Interneurons and Motoneurons

Recently the understanding of the spinal mechanisms of vestibular control has been essentially improved through analysis carried out by intracellular investigation of synaptic events in spinal neurons. The synaptic articulations of fibers belonging to the vestibulospinal tract, the reticulospinal tract, and the medial longitudinal fasciculus have been studied, and an analysis of the mechanisms through which motoneuron excitability is altered by volleys of vestibular impulses descending in these pathways reveals that the motoneurons can be activated monosynaptically as well as via interneuronal relays. By activating these tracts selectively or collectively it has been possible to obtain insight into the effectiveness of the volleys in eliciting interneuronal activity, membrane potential changes in motoneurons as recorded intracellularly, facilitation and inhibition of monosynaptic reflexes, and ventral root discharge. This section deals with the membrane shifts evoked by vestibulofugal volleys.

Erulkar et al. (1966) showed by intracellular recordings that, in the cat, there exist well-defined vestibular projections to interneurons at all levels of the spinal cord. The configuration of the synaptic potentials in response to peripheral vestibular nerve activation indicates that some interneurons receive either excitatory or inhibitory inputs or both. At the cervical level the majority of interneurons responded with a multiple spike discharge superimposed on a depolarizing wave, but at the lumbar level the interneurons responded only with a single spike followed by a depolarizing after potential (Fig. 7). This difference may be related to a stronger synaptic impingement of the tracts onto the neurons at cervical levels and also to the distribution of input onto the receptor surfaces of the interneurons. Those investigations were also able to demonstrate that vestibular stimulation could elicit antidromic discharge from dorsal roots. It thus appears as if the vestibular system exerts a presynaptic inhibitory control via the interneurons upon activity of afferent fibers to the spinal cord.

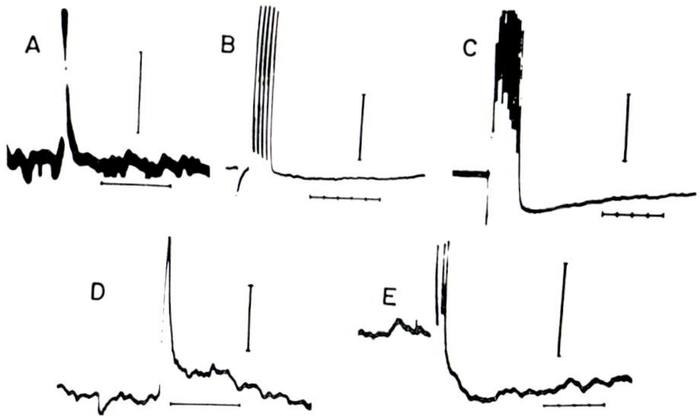

Fig. 7. Spike discharge of interneurons in response to ipsilateral vestibular nerve stimulation and recorded from cervical (A–C), and lumbar (D, E) levels. Each complete time line represents 10 msec. Calibrations: A, B, and D = 20 mV; C and E = 5 mV (ERULKAR, SPRAGUE, WHITSEL, DOGAN and JANNETTA, 1966)

A. Vestibulospinal Tract

This tract is poorly developed in man but is prominent in monkey and cat and can easily be traced as far as lumbar and sacral spinal levels. The fibers rigionate in the lateral vestibular nucleus according to a somatotopic arrangement and descend homolaterally (BRODAL et al., 1962). Although the tract is primarily uncrossed, a small component of the pathway reaches the contralateral gray matter via the spinal ventral gray commisure. Silver impregnation studies of terminal fiber degeneration following destruction of the lateral nucleus indicate a termination of the tract throughout the length of the cord in lamina VIII and the medial part of lamina VII among interneurons which project most densely to motoneurons of the axial and proximal limb musculature (REXED, 1964; NYBERG-HANSEN and MASCITTI, 1964). Some sparse degenerations among motoneurons were described, and this finding is supported by functional studies (GERNANDT et al., 1957).

There have been several reports in the literature concerning monosynaptic excitation of motoneurons by vestibular fibers descending in the spinal cord. LUND and POMPEIANO (1965) found that the extensor, but not the flexor, motoneurons generate monosynaptic excitatory postsynaptic potentials (EPSPs) in response to activation of the vestibulospinal tract. In flexor motoneurons there is a disynaptic inhibition. SASAKI et al. (1962) and SHAPOVALOV et al. (1967) have described this fast excitatory postsynaptic potential arising after a latency of 3 to 4 msec in response to stimulation of Deiters' nucleus. The amplitude of this component varied from 1 to 4 mV, and the time course was similar to that of the monosynaptic EPSP evoked by group Ia afferent volley (ECCLES, 1964). A later wave of postsynaptic depolarization appears immediately after the first component and is the result of polysynaptic excitation. Higher frequency stimulation gives rise to a marked potentiation of the monosynaptic vestibulospinal EPSPs. Stimulation of Deiters' nucleus also produced inhibitory postsynaptic potentials (IPSPs), but they appeared after a latency of 6 to 7 msec indicating a more elaborate polysynaptic relay.

B. Reticulospinal Tract

Inasmuch as vestibular impulses definitely activate the bulbar reticular formation, descending crossed and uncrossed reticulospinal components may contribute substantially to both ipsilateral and contralateral motor responses along the spinal cord. Anatomical findings concerning reticulospinal neurons have been reviewed by BRODAL (1957) and ROSSI and ZANCHETTI (1957), and a study of retrograde degeneration showed that 50% or more of the neurons in the pontile and medullary reticular formation send fibers into the spinal cord (TORVIK and BRODAL, 1957). The tract ends in laminae VII and VIII according to REXED'S (1952) nomenclature. The sites and mode of termination of the reticulospinal fibers in the cat have been studied by NYBERG-HANSEN (1965). A wide range of conduction velocities, between 20 and 138 m/sec, was described by WOLSTENCROFT (1964) but according to WILLIS and MAGNI (1964), who used intracellular recording, the great majority of reticulospinal axons conduct at a speed of 90 to 130 m/sec.

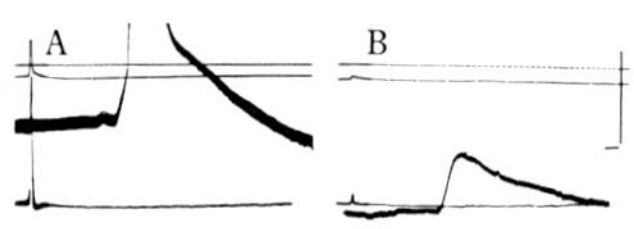

Fig. 8. Effects on alpha extensor motoneurons by stimulation of bulbar inhibitory reticular formation. Control record to quadriceps nerve stimulation (A). Impulse activity in impaled cell (second trace at low gain and sweep speed, and third trace at higher gain and faster sweep speed). Monosynaptic reflex response recorded simultaneously from ventral root (fourth trace) at same sweep speed as for second trace. Impulse activity in impaled cell prevented, and monosynaptic reflex response inhibited by reticular formation stimulation (B). Resulting sustained increase of membrane potential can be seen in both low- and high-gain intracellular recordings using the first trace as a reference line. Calibrations (0.5 msec; 10 mV) apply only to intracellular high-gain record (LLINÁS and TERZUOLO, 1964)

Stimulation of the caudal pontine reticular formation can give rise to a monosynaptic impingement upon flexor motoneurons (GRILLNER and LUND, 1966). A sustained depolarization of the motoneuron's membrane, enabling an otherwise subthreshold monosynaptic EPSP to initiate impulse activity and simultaneously facilitating the monosynaptic reflex discharge, recorded from ventral lumbar roots, followed repetitive stimulation of the appropriate region of the reticular stimulation (TERZUOLO et al., 1965).

Llinás and Terzuolo (1964, 1965) studied the inhibitory effect of reticular formation stimulation upon the monosynaptic extensor reflex in the absence of the gamma loop (Fig. 8). This postsynaptic inhibitory influence is due to a sustained synaptic impingement causing a hyperpolarization of the membrane. IPSPs produced in both extensor and flexor motoneurons have been reported (Jankowska et al., 1964; Llinás and Terzuolo, 1964).

C. Medial Longitudinal Fasciculus (MLF)

The fibers originate in the medial vestibular nucleus (Brodal et al., 1962) and terminate at a mid-thoracic level (Massopoust, 1957; Nyberg-Hansen,

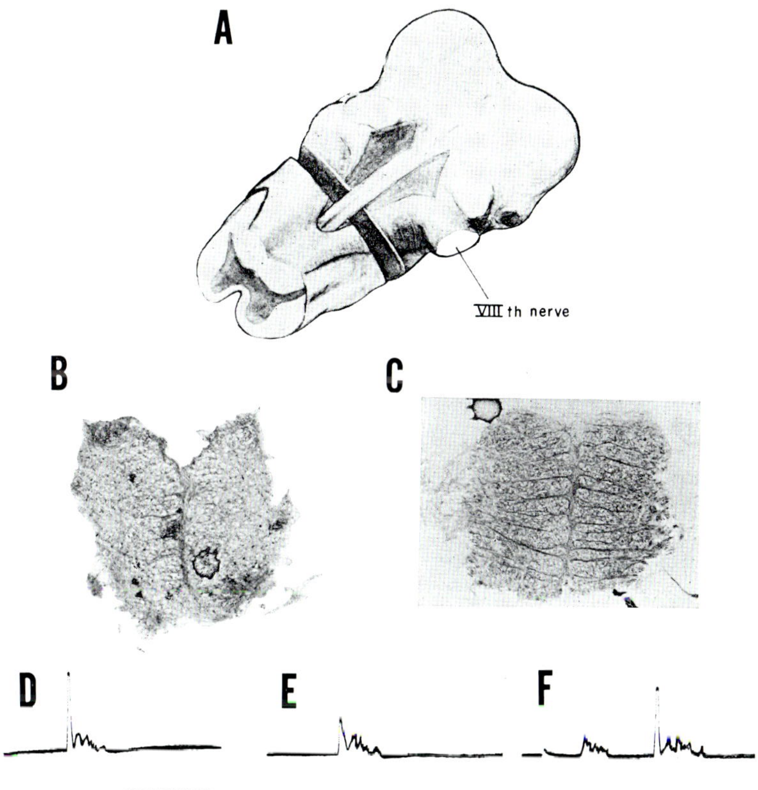

Fig. 9. Drawing of brain stem showing medial longitudinal fasciculi bridging gap (A). Histological controls upon hematoxylin-eosin (B) and Weil-Weigert (C) stained microscopic cross sections of bridge containing main group of fibers constituting medial longitudinal fasciculi. Amplification 15 ×. Segmental response to DRC5 stimulation and deep radial nerve recording before (D) and after (E) creating bridge according to drawing. Segmental response preceded by vestibular activity exclusively funneled through MLF (F). Time scale in msec (Gernandt, 1968)

1964; Wilson et al., 1968a). No monosynaptic connections have been found between the MLF and spinal motoneurons.

The functional importance of the MLF in carrying vestibular impulses into the spinal cord has been studied in cats (Gernandt, 1968). In evaluating the hierarchical importance of the three descending vestibulofugal pathways it becomes obvious that the MLF offers a much weaker link than the connections represented by the vestibulospinal and reticulospinal tracts. By sectioning all pathways other than the MLF in the brain stem at the cerebellopontine angle, this tract could be investigated in anatomical isolation from adjacent vestibular connections (Fig. 9A). In B and C are shown histological cross sections through the MLF bridge. In addition to a more or less transient depression of reflexes induced by transection of the brain stem, the vestibular facilitatory influx to the cord is reduced due to the elimination of the two other vestibulofugal pathways and thus, the excitability level of the motor pools is lowered when the cells are impinged upon by the evoked activity funneled through the MLF exclusively. In order to obtain some insight into changes in spinal excitability level after the creation of the bridge and the elimination of all but one channel for exerting vestibular control, cervical segmental reflex testing was utilized (Fig. 9, D to F). Vestibular stimulation applied to this "MLF animal" preparation evoked motor responses which could be recorded as far down as the mid-thoracic levels. No sign of activity was ever recorded from lumbosacral levels. Judged by the response, the MLF seems to have a homogenous fiber spectrum, and the mean speed of conduction of the neurons is about 63 m/sec. Single MLF axon recordings demonstrated that the discharge frequency in response to vestibular stimulation may reach values that are more than twice the value of ventral root alpha fiber discharge in response to identical stimulation and that the synaptic transmission across the vestibular nuclei occurs with a considerable safety factor. Excitatory and inhibitory postsynaptic potentials evoked by vestibular activity conducted in the MLF have been recorded

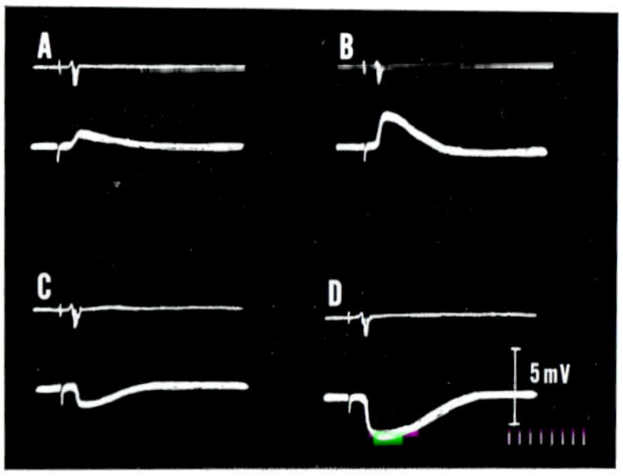

Fig. 10. Upper traces indicate arrival of MLF volley in spinal cord at the level of microelectrode penetration. Lower traces intracellular records of postsynaptic potentials in deep radial motoneurons. EPSPs evoked by 1 pulse/sec (A) and 50 pulses/sec (B) vestibular stimulation. IPSPs elicited by 1 pulse/sec (C) and 50 pulses/sec (D) vestibular stimulation. Time scale in 5 msec-intervals (Gernandt, 1968)

intracellularly from flexor and extensor motoneurons at cervical levels (Fig. 10). The relative amounts of excitatory and inhibitory action on a test motoneuron are variable. Pure EPSPs or IPSPs can be recorded but the majority of motoneurons showed EPSPs. The long latencies of the EPSPs and IPSPs were approximately the same and indicate that spinal interneurons are involved in the transmission. These depolarizing and hyperpolarizing effects could be recorded in a random fashion from flexor and extensor neurons as identified by antidromic stimulation. No consistent sign of reciprocity was obtained when recording from neurons with antagonistic function.

XI. Vestibular Stimulation and Muscular Activity

Balance is maintained by associated reflexes that cause flexion or extension of neck, trunk, and limbs. This muscular control is managed by a hierarchy of feedback systems. KOELLA et al. (1956) studied the quantitative interrelation between the degree of imposed muscle stretch, position of the head in space, and the resulting muscle tension. The tension increment produced by a particular stretch increases as the position changes from prone to supine around the longitudinal axis. The greater the initially imposed stretch, the greater will be the vestibular influence; stretch afferents and vestibular receptors exert their influence upon motoneuron excitability in a quantitatively interdependent fashion. The effects of labyrinthine stimulation and stimulation of the skin by touch and pressure on the motor discharge to cervical muscles have been investigated by NAKAYAMA (1957). Reciprocal effects were demonstrated in ipsi- and contra-lateral muscles, and it was further shown that the effect of pressure summated algebraically with that of tilting and rotation. The result give a picture of the activity patterns in muscles that take part in reflexes designated as "body righting reflexes acting upon the head".

A decerebrate and decerebellate cat with the spinal cord sectioned at the Th 12 level shows responses to head rotation that are not reciprocally organized; both extremities are extended in response to head movements. A longitudinal, midsagittal section through the medulla and pons, however, immediately permits the reciprocal response to rotation to appear. Subsequent unilateral labyrinthectomy gives rise to a postural asymmetry due to the lowering of the homolateral extensor tonus, but the reciprocal response to rotation is still present. As a result of bilateral labyrinthectomy, all responses are eliminated and a symmetrical position is obtained. These findings by AJALA and POPPELE (1967) made them draw the following conclusions: (1) Each labyrinth exerts a bilateral influence on the forelimbs in response to angular stimulation since both limbs respond when only one labyrinth is functioning, even after a mid-line section through the brain stem. (2) Each labyrinth exerts a unilateral influence on postural tonus in the split brain stem preparation, since changes in tonus occur only in the limb ipsilateral to the side of labyrinthectomy. (3) The connections and mechanisms responsible for the mutual interactions between vestibular inputs reside in the pons and medulla.

Among the objective manifestations of vestibular activity evoked by stronger stimulation and funneled into the spinal cord are the falling reaction and past-pointing. Some recent findings may contribute to our understanding of the neuronal events behind the falling reaction. During high-frequency vestibular stimulation (30 to 50 pulses/sec) the spinal segmental flexor or extensor reflexes become greatly augmented, but subsequently there is an enduring, powerful inhibition of the same motoneurons which outlasts the cessation of stimulation by 2 to 3 min (GERNANDT, KATSUKI and LIVINGSTON, 1957; GERNANDT and GILMAN, 1960a). This prolonged inhibition of the test responses is not a result of ordinary post-excitatory refractoriness, but is due to an active, inhibitory process which continues during the entire period of depression. The source of the enduring inhibition has been localized to the reticular formation within the brain stem. LLINÁS and TERZUOLO (1964) were able to show that the synaptic inhibitory impingement obtained by reticular formation activation was due to a sustained, postsynaptic hyperpolarization of the motoneuron membrane. A more comprehensive picture and discussion of this long-lasting inhibitory process of spinal activity have been presented more recently (GERNANDT, 1967b).

It is well known that vestibular input is essential to decerebrate rigidity and the alpha-type rigidity following cerebellar ablation. BATINI, MORUZZI and POMPEIANO (1957) performed unilateral and bilateral eighth nerve sections in decerebrate cats and found that ipsilateral alpha rigidity was greatly reduced by nerve section after a post-brachial cord transection (Schiff-Sherrington phenomenon). If the contralateral eighth nerve was sectioned in addition, extensor tone reappeared in the flaccid forelimb, although the alpha rigidity was somewhat less after bilateral nerve section than in the decerebellate-decerebrate state. In decerebrate and decerebellate nonanesthetized cats, the dorsal Deiters' neurons are found to be discharging tonically with a regular rhythm of 10 to 80 impulses per sec (WILSON et al., 1966).

Since part of the cerebellar effect on the stretch reflex is carried over descending vestibulofugal pathways, HIGGINS (1968) studied the frequency characteristics of this reflex after removal of the labyrinthine input. Sinusoidal stretch was applied to the tendon of triceps surae in acutely decerebrate cats following unilateral or bilateral section of the eighth nerve. It appeared that the ipsilateral labyrinthine afferents primarily affect those brain stem circuits which regulate the gain of the stretch reflex (output force per increment of length change). The spontaneous firing of the contralateral eighth nerve chiefly influences brain stem function which operates on the timing of stretch responses, although there is some effect on gain, as well. Either eighth nerve may affect the magnitude of tension responses in stretch cycles initiating motion.

The effects of vestibular activation on posture have been studied by stimulation of the ampullary nerve of each semicircular canal in unrestrained, chronic monkeys and cats. The resultant motor effects were confined to rather stereotyped postural movements in which ipsilateral extension of the forelimb was accompanied contralateral by curvature of the trunk and contralateral forelimb flexion (SUZUKI and COHEN, 1964).

References

ADRIAN, E. D.: Discharges from the vestibular receptors in the cat. J. Physiol. (Lond.) **101**, 389–407 (1943).

AJALA, G. F., POPPELE, R. E.: Some problems in the central action of vestibular inputs. In: Neurophysiological Basis of Normal and Abnormal Motor Activities, M. D. YAHR and D. P. PURPURA, Eds., pp. 141–154. Hewlett, New York: Raven Press 1967.

ANDERSSON, S., GERNANDT, B. E.: Cortical projection of vestibular nerve in cat. Acta oto-laryng. (Stockh.) Suppl. **116**, 10–18 (1954).

ANDERSSON, S., GERNANDT, B. E.: Ventral root discharge in response to vestibular and proprioceptive stimulation. J. Neurophysiol. **19**, 524–543 (1956).

BACH, L. M. N., MAGOUN, H. W.: The vestibular nuclei as an excitatory mechanism for the cord. J. Neurophysiol. **10**, 331–337 (1947).

BATINI, C., MORUZZI, G., POMPEIANO, O.: Cerebellar release phenomena. Arch. ital. Biol. **95**, 71–95 (1957).

BRODAL, A.: The Reticular Formation of the Brain Stem. Anatomical Aspects and Functional Correlations. Edinburgh: Oliver & Boyd 1957.

BRODAL, A., POMPEIANO, O., WALBERG, F.: The Vestibular Nuclei and Their Connections, Anatomy and Functional Correlations. Springfield, Ill.: C. C. Thomas 1962.

CARLI, G., DIETE-SPIFF, K., POMPEIANO, O.: Skeletomotor and fusimotor control of gastrocnemius muscle from Deiter's nucleus. Experientia (Basel) **22**, 583–584 (1966).

CARLI, G., DIETE-SPIFF, K., POMPEIANO, O.: Responses of the muscle spindles and of the extrafusal fibres in an extensor muscle to stimulation of the lateral vestibular nucleus in the cat. Arch. ital. Biol. **105**, 209–242 (1967).

CARPENTER, M. B.: Central connections of the vestibular system. Arch. Otolaryng. **85**, 517–520 (1967).

COHEN, D., CHAMBERS, W. W., SPRAGUE, J. M.: Experimental study of the efferent projections from the cerebellar nuclei to the brain stem of the cat. J. comp. Neurol. **109**, 233–259 (1958).

DEVITO, R. V., BRUSA, A., ARDUINI, A.: Cerebellar and vestibular influences on deitersian units. J. Neurophysiol. **19**, 241–253 (1956).

DIETE-SPIFF, K., CARLI, G., POMPEIANO, O.: Comparison of the effects of stimulation of the VIIIth cranial nerve, the vestibular nuclei or the reticular formation on the gastrocnemius muscle and its spindles. Arch. ital. Biol. **105**, 243–272 (1967).

DOW, R. S., MORUZZI, G.: The Physiology and Pathology of the Cerebellum. Minneapolis: University of Minnesota Press 1958.

ECCLES, J. C.: The Physiology of Synapses. Berlin-Göttingen-Heidelberg-New York: Springer 1964.

ERULKAR, S. D., SPRAGUE, J. M., WHITSEL, B. L., DOGAN, S., JANNETTA, P. J.: Organization of the vestibular projection to the spinal cord of the cat. J. Neurophysiol. **29**, 626–664 (1966).

GERNANDT, B. E.: Response of mammalian vestibular neurons to horizontal rotation and caloric stimulation. J. Neurophysiol. **12**, 173–184 (1949).

GERNANDT, B. E.: Somatic and Autonomic Motor Outflow to Vestibular Stimulation. In: Neurological Aspects of Auditory and Vestibular Disorders, W. S. FIELDS and B. R. ALFORD, pp. Eds., 194–215. Springfield, Ill.: C. C. Thomas 1964.

GERNANDT, B. E.: Central regulation of the vestibular system. Arch. Otolaryng. **85**, 521–528 (1967a).

GERNANDT, B. E.: Vestibular influence upon spinal reflex activity. In: Ciba Foundation Symposium on Myotatic, Kinesthetic and Vestibular Mechanisms, A. V. S. DE REUCK and J. KNIGHT, Eds., pp. 170–183. London: J. and A. Churchill Ltd. 1967b.

GERNANDT, B. E.: Functional properties of the descending medial longitudinal fasciculus. Exp. Neurol. **22**, 326–341 (1968).

GERNANDT, B. E., GILMAN, S.: Descending vestibular activity and its modulation by proprioceptive, cerebellar, and reticular influences. Exp. Neurol. **1**, 274–304 (1959).

Gernandt, B. E., Gilman, S.: Vestibular and propriospinal interactions and protracted spinal inhibition by brain stem activation. J. Neurophysiol. **23**, 269–287 (1960a).

Gernandt, B.E., Gilman, S.: Interaction between vestibular, pyramidal, and cortically evoked extrapyramidal activities. J. Neurophysiol. **23**, 516–533 (1960b).

Gernandt, B.E., Iranyi, M., Livingston, R.B.: Vestibular influences on spinal mechanisms. Exp. Neurol. **1**, 248–273 (1959).

Gernandt, B.E., Katsuki, Y., Livingston, R.B.: Functional organization of descending vestibular influences. J. Neurophysiol. **20**, 453–469 (1957).

Gernandt, B.E., Megirian, D.: Ascending propriospinal mechanisms. J. Neurophysiol. **24**, 364–376 (1961).

Gernandt, B.E., Shimamura, M.: Mechanisms of interlimb reflexes in cat. J. Neurophysiol. **24**, 665–676 (1961).

Gernandt, B.E., Thulin, C.-A.: Vestibular connections of the brain stem. Amer. J. Physiol. **171**, 121–127 (1953).

Grillner, S., Lund, S.: A descending pathway with monosynaptic action on flexor motoneurons. Experientia (Basel) **22**, 390 (1966).

Higgins, D.C.: Vestibular component in dynamic muscle stretch. Amer. J. Physiol. **214**, 482–487 (1968).

Ito, M.: The Origin of Cerebellar Inhibition on Deiters' and Intracerebellar Nuclei. In: Studies in Physiology, D. R. Curtis and A. K. McIntyre, Eds., pp. 100–106. New York: Springer 1965.

Janowska, E., Lund, S., Lundberg, A., Pompeiano, O.: Postsynaptic inhibition in motoneurones evoked from the lower reticular formation. Experientia (Basel) **20**, 701–702 (1964).

Kempinsky, W.H., Ward, A.A., Jr.: Effect of section of vestibular nerve upon cortically induced movement in cat. J. Neurophysiol. **13**, 295–304 (1950).

Koella, W.P., Nakao, H., Evans, R.L., Wada, J.: Interaction of vestibular and proprioceptive reflexes in the decerebrate cat. Amer. J. Physiol. **185**, 607–613 (1956).

Llinás, R., Terzuolo, C.A.: Mechanisms of supraspinal actions upon spinal cord activities. Reticular inhibitory mechanisms on alpha-extensor motoneurons. J. Neurophysiol. **27**, 579–591 (1964).

Llinás, R., Terzuolo, C.A.: Mechanisms of supraspinal actions upon spinal cord activities. Reticular inhibitory mechanisms upon flexor motoneurons. J. Neurophysiol. **28**, 413–422 (1965).

Lloyd, D.P.C.: Activity in neurons of the bulbospinal correlation system. J. Neurophysiol. **4**, 115–134 (1941).

Lorente de Nó, R.: Vestibulo-ocular reflex arc. Arch. Neurol. Psychiat. (Chic.) **30**, 245–291 (1933).

Lund, S., Pompeiano, O.: Descending pathways with monosynaptic action and motoneurons. Experientia (Basel) **21**, 602–603 (1965).

Magoun, H. W.: The Waking Brain, 2nd ed., p. 188. Springfield, Ill.: C. C. Thomas 1964.

Markham, C.H., Precht, W., Shimazu, H.: Effect of stimulation of interstitial nucleus of Cajal on vestibular unit activity in the cat. J. Neurophysiol. **29**. 493–507 (1966).

Massopust, L.C.: Terminal degeneration study of the spinal component of the medial longitudinal fasciculus. Anat. Rec. **127**, 330 (1957).

Megirian, D., Manning, J.W.: Input-output relations of the vestibular system. Arch. ital. Biol. **105**, 15–30 (1967).

Megirian, D., Troth, R.: Vestibular and muscle nerve connections to pyramidal tract neurons of cat. J. Neurophysiol. **27**, 481–492 (1964).

Nakayama, T.: Behaviors of cervical muscles in labyrinthine and skin-pressure reflexes. Jap. J. Physiol. **7**, 99–112 (1957).

Nyberg-Hansen, R.: Origin and termination of fibers from the the vestibular nuclei descending in the medial longitudinal fasciculus. An experimental study with silver impregnation methods in the cat. J. comp. Neurol. **122**, 355–367 (1964).

NYBERG-HANSEN, R.: Sites and mode of termination of reticulospinal fibers in the cat. An experimental study with silver impregnation methods. J. comp. Neurol. **124**, 71–100 (1965).

NYBERG-HANSEN, R., MASCITTI, T. A.: Sites and mode of termination of fibers of the vestibulospinal tract in the cat. J. comp. Neurol. **122**, 369–387 (1964).

POMPEIANO, O., BRODAL, A.: The origin of vestibulospinal fibres in the cat. An experimental-anatomical study with comments on the descending medial longitudinal fasciculus. Arch. ital. Biol. **95**, 166–195 (1957).

POMPEIANO, O., WALBERG, F.: Descending connections to the vestibular nuclei. An experimental study in the cat. J. comp. Neurol. **108**, 465–503 (1957).

PRECHT, W., SHIMAZU, H.: Functional connections of tonic and kinetic vestibular neurons with primary vestibular afferents. J. Neurophysiol. **28**, 1014–1028 (1965).

REXED, B.: The cytoarchitectonic organization of the spinal cord in the cat. J. comp. Neurol. **96**, 415–495 (1952).

REXED, B.: Some aspects of the cytoarchitectonics and synaptology of the spinal cord. In: Progress in Brain Research, Vol. 11, pp. 58–90. Amsterdam: Elsevier 1964.

ROSSI, G. F., ZANCHETTI, A.: The Brain Stem Reticular Formation. Anatomy and Physiology. Arch. ital. Biol. **95**, 199–435 (1957).

RUPERT, A., MOUSHEGIAN, G., GALAMBOS, R.: Microelectrode studies of primary vestibular neurons in cat. Exp. Neurol. **5**, 100–112 (1962).

SASAKI, K., TANAKA, T., MORI, K.: Effects of stimulation of pontine and bulbar reticular formation upon spinal motoneurons of the cat. Jap. J. Physiol. **12**, 45–62 (1962).

SHAPOVALOV, A. I., KURCHAVYI, G. G., STROGONOVA, M. P.: Synaptic mechanisms of vestibulospinal influences on alpha-motoneurons. Neuroscience Translations **1**, 91–100 (1967–68).

SHIMAMURA, M., LIVINGSTON, R. B.: Longitudinal conduction systems serving spinal and brain stem coordination. J. Neurophysiol. **26**, 258–272 (1963).

SHIMAZU, H., PRECHT, W.: Tonic and kinetic responses of cat's vestibular neurons to horizontal angular acceleration. J. Neurophysiol. **28**, 991–1013 (1965).

SNIDER, R. S., MCCULLOCH, W. S., MAGOUN, H. W.: A cerebello-bulbo-reticular pathway for suppression. J. Neurophysiol. **12**, 325–334 (1949).

SUZUKI, J. T., COHEN, B.: Head, eye, body and limb movements from semicircular canal nerves. Exp. Neurol. **10**, 393–405 (1964).

SZENTÁGOTHAI, J.: Short propriospinal neurons and intrinsic connections of the spinal gray matter. Acta morph. Sci. hung. **1**, 81–94 (1951).

SZENTÁGOTHAI, J.: Propriospinal pathways and their synapses. In: Progress in Brain Research: Organization of the Spinal Cord, J. C. ECCLES and J. P. SCHADÉ, Eds., Vol. 11, pp. 155–174. New York: Elsevier 1964.

TERZUOLO, C. A., LLINÁS, R., GREEN, K. T.: Mechanisms of supraspinal actions upon spinal cord activities: distribution of reticular and segmental inputs in cat's alpha-motoneurons. Arch. ital. Biol. **103**, 635–651 (1965).

TORVIK, A., BRODAL, A.: The origin of reticulospinal fibers in the cat. An experimental study. Anat. Rec. **128**, 113–137 (1957).

TOWER, S. S.: Function and structure in the chronically isolated lumbo-sacral spinal cord of the dog. J. comp. Neurol. **67**, 109–131 (1937).

WALBERG, F., JANSEN, J.: Cerebellar corticovestibular fibers in the cat. Exp. Neurol. **3**, 32–52 (1961).

WALBERG, F., POMPEIANO, O., BRODAL, A., JANSEN, J.: Fastigiovestibular fibers in the cat. An experimental study with silver methods. J. comp. Neurol. **118**, 49–75 (1963).

WARD, A. A., JR.: Decerebrate rigidity. J. Neurophysiol. **10**, 89–103 (1947).

WERSÄLL, J.: Vestibular Nerve. Submicroscopic Structure of the Inner Ear. S. IURATO, Eds., pp. 245–248. London: Pergamon Press 1966.

WILLIS, W. D., MAGNI, F.: The properties of reticulospinal neurons. In: Progress in Brain Research: Physiology of Spinal Neurons, J. C. ECCLES and J. P. SCHADÉ, Eds., Vol. 12, pp. 56–64. New York: Elsevier 1964.

WILLIS, W. D., WILLIS, J. C., THOMPSON, W. M.: Synaptic actions of fibers in the ventral spinal cord upon lumbosacral motoneurons. J. Neurophysiol. **30**, 382–397 (1967).

WILSON, V.J., KATO, M., THOMAS, R.C., PETERSON, B.W.: Excitation of lateral vestibular neurons by peripheral afferent fibers. J. Neurophysiol. **29**, 508–529 (1966).

WILSON, V.J., WYLIE, R.M., MARCO, L.A.: Organization of the medial vestibular nucleus. J. Neurophysiol. **31**, 166–175 (1968a).

WILSON, V.J., WYLIE, R.M., MARCO, L.A.: Synaptic inputs to cells in the medial vestibular nucleus. J. Neurophysiol. **31**, 176–185 (1968b).

WOLSTENCROFT, J.H.: Reticulospinal neurons. J. Physiol. (Lond.) **174**, 91–108 (1964).

Chapter VI.

Cortical Projections of the Vestibular Nerve

By

J. M. Fredrickson, Toronto, H. H. Kornhuber, Ulm,
and D.W.F. Schwarz, Toronto

With 10 Figures

Contents

I. Introduction

The existence of a cortical representation of vestibular function has been questioned (e.g. Griffith, 1922). On the other hand, a cortical representation has been postulated with the argument that there is true vestibular sensation and that vestibular signals might be also useful for higher motor mechanisms (Spitzer, 1924). Information concerning the vestibular sensory systems has been gathered relatively recently.

II. Earlier Views about Cortical Vestibular Function

Since the early thirties of this century a vestibular projection to the temporal lobe near the auditory area has been conjectured (Spiegel, 1932 and 1934; Gerebtzoff, 1940). This view was seemingly supported by the finding of a directional preponderance of the caloric nystagmus in temporal lobe lesions (Carmichael et al., 1954) and by sensations of vertigo on stimulation of the temporal lobe (Penfield and Jasper, 1954). However, the directional preponderance of caloric nystagmus was later shown to result from subcortical hemispheric lesions of the cortico-fugal efferents to the brainstem and not from cortical lesions in the temporal lobe (BADER and KORNHUBER, 1965; cf. KORNHUBER's chapter on otoneurology in volume VI/2). With respect to the vertigo of labyrinthine type reported by seven out of 108 patients during temporal lobe stimulation, PENFIELD himself (1957) wrote: "Dizziness is a word patients use not infrequently to describe the effect of stimulation. It is often associated with eye movement or pupillary change. But it occurs in many areas of the cortex that I could never be sure that it was related to vestibular sensation. Even in those (7) cases of dizziness from stimulation in the temporal lobe... I only assume that we are dealing with the direct sensory connection from the vestibular system because of the evidence from animal experimentation". The animal experiments referred to were those of WALZL and MOUNTCASTLE (1949) in the cat. But with respect to them PENFIELD (1957) commented: "WALZL and MOUNTCASTLE showed in laboratory animals that evoked potentials from the stimulation of the labyrinths could be recorded in the cerebral cortex between the auditory area, the Rolandic somatic sensory area, and the second somatic sensory area. It is difficult to pass from animal localisation to man, by extrapolation, and I shall not attempt it." LENNOX (1960) wrote: "The term vertigenous... is associated with symptoms not of vertigo, but of brief episodes of unreality, disorientation, confusion or dizziness, possibly with associated automatic movements. Episodes are brief... They represent temporal lobe rather than vestibular disturbances." – In our experience, typical vestibular sensations of being rotated or tilted are very rare in temporal lobe epilepsy.

III. The Parietal Cortical Projection in the Cat

A cortical vestibular area was first clearly identified in the cat by WALZL and MOUNTCASTLE (1949) with the evoked potential method in barbiturate anesthesia. This field is located in the anterior suprasylvian sulcus, posterior to the face zone of the first somatosensory field, medial to the second somatosensory field, and just anterior to the auditory area. The projection is bilateral (KORNHUBER and FONSECA, 1964), but the ipsilateral projection is somewhat weaker and more easily suppressed by deep barbiturate anesthesia. In the experiments of WALZL and MOUNTCASTLE (1949) and of MICKLE and ADES (1952), the latency of the response on electrical stimulation of the vestibular nerve during barbiturate anesthesia was found to be 6–8 msec. KORNHUBER and FONSECA (1964), in the unanesthetized cat, found a latency of 4 msec on galvanic labyrinthine polarisation with single unit recording. This difference may be explained by the barbiturate anesthesia.

In this suprasylvian cortical vestibular representation an overlap with somatic afferents has been found by MICKLE and ADES (1952). More specifically the toes of the foreleg and hindleg of S II seem to overlap with the vestibular area (BERMAN, 1961).

The juxtaposition of the vestibular and auditory cortical areas was taken by some authors as confirmation of the temporal lobe hypothesis. However, it is in this region between the second somatic and the auditory fields where the sylvian fissure has evolved in primates because of the large development of the associa-

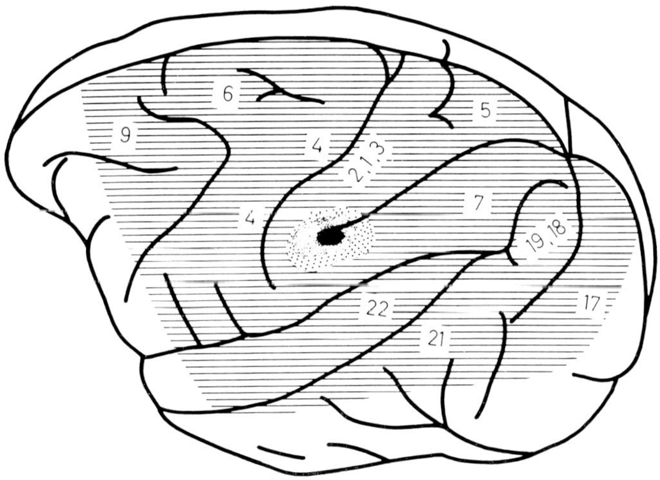

Fig. 1. Location of the primary vestibular area in the Rhesus monkey at the lower end of the intraparietal sulcus according to evoked responses following electrical stimulation of the contralateral vestibular nerve in barbiturate anesthesia. Response amplitudes are divided into: 600–500 μV (dark), 300–600 μV (medium) and 0–300 μV (light). Numbers show approximate location of Brodmann's cytoarchitectonic areas. Striped zone represents the extent of cortical exploration. The evoked response consists of a surface positive wave with a latency of 5–6 msec. From FREDRICKSON, FIGGE, SCHEID and KORNHUBER, Exp. Brain Res. **2** (1966)

tion cortex. An extrapolation from the cat to the primate brain was therefore not possible, since it was uncertain whether the vestibular projection went with the auditory to the temporal or with the somatosensory to the parietal lobe. A study of the vestibular cortical projection in the Rhesus monkey solved this problem (KORNHUBER et al., 1965; FREDRICKSON et al., 1966).

IV. The Vestibular Representation in Area 2v of the Rhesus Monkey

In the Rhesus monkey, the primary cortical projection area of the vestibular nerve was discovered in the postcentral gyrus at the lower end of the intraparietal sulcus, at the face level of the first somatosensory field. It does not extend into Brodmann's area 1 which borders the central sulcus, but it is mainly located within the lower bank of the intraparietal sulcus at it's tip (Fig. 3).

V. Cytoarchitectonic Structure of Area 2v

Originally, this vestibular representation in the monkey's postcentral gyrus was thought to belong to Brodmann's area 2 because according to VOGT (1919) and to ROBERTS and AKERT (1963) the stripe of cortex above and below the end of the intraparietal sulcus was included in area 2. There are, indeed, functional similarities with the somatosensory area 2 as will be pointed out. However, subsequent analysis showed that the vestibular field is different from area 2 in its

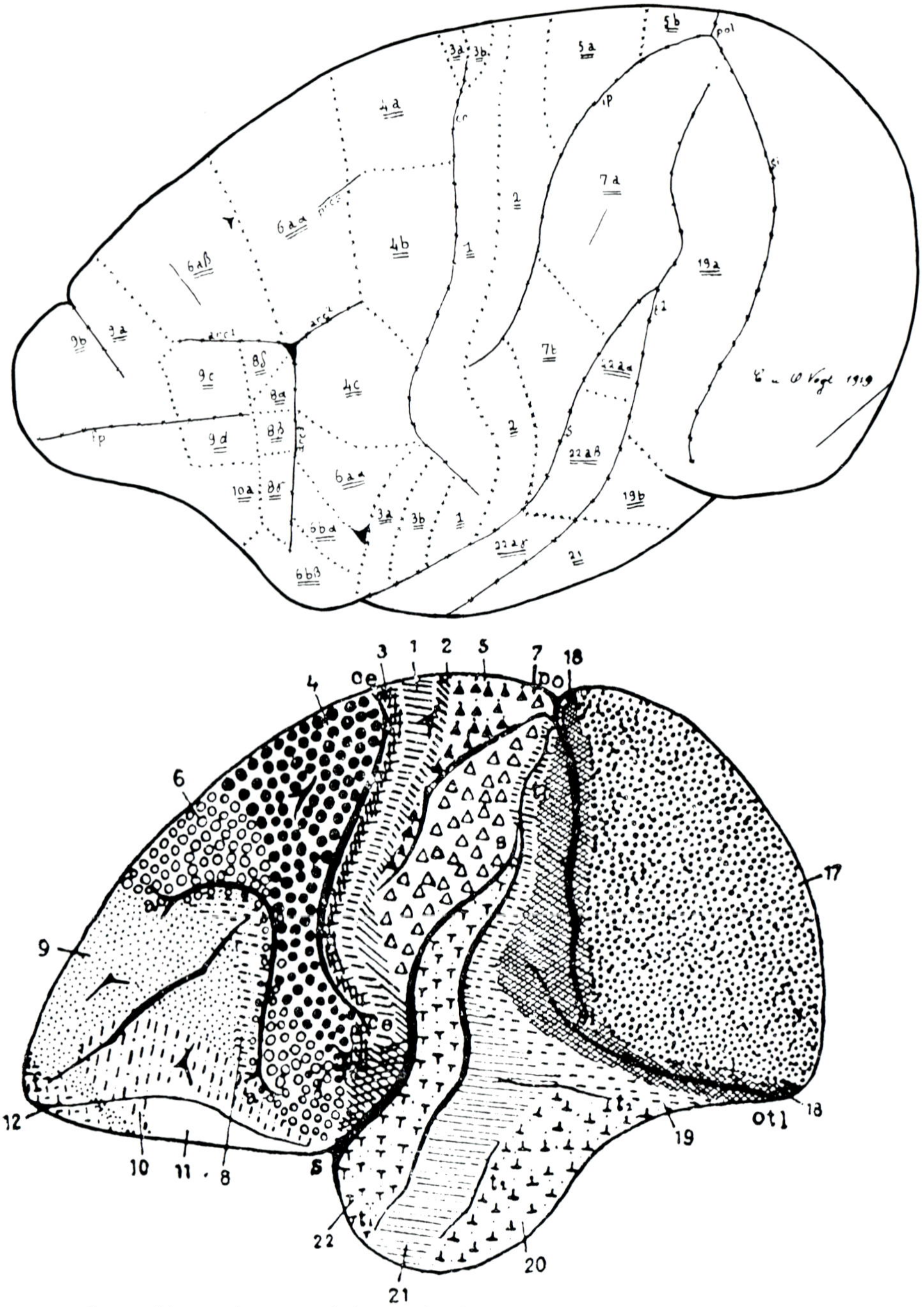

Fig. 2. Cytoarchitectonic maps of the monkey's cortex according to C. and O. VOGT (1919) (above) and BRODMANN (1909) (below). According to BRODMANN, area 5 has a small strip going down to the tip of the intraparietal sulcus whereas according to the VOGTS this tissue belongs to area 2. The maps of POWELL and MOUNTCASTLE (1959) and ROBERTS and AKERT (1963) agree with the opinion of the VOGTS in this respect. The cortex below the tip of the intraparietal sulcus belongs to area 2 according to the VOGTS, and ROBERTS and AKERT agree with them. See also the juxtaposition of the vestibular cortex with areas 2 and 5 in Fig. 8

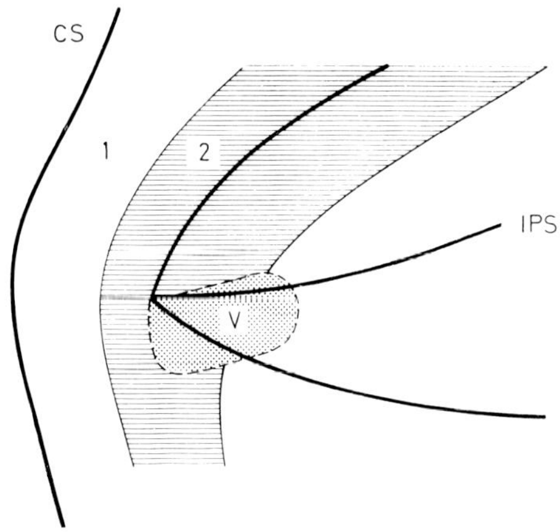

Fig. 3. Location of the vestibular field at the tip of the intraparietal sulcus in the left hemisphere of the Rhesus monkey. Frontal is left, occipital is right. CS central sulcus. The intraparietal sulcus (IPS) is unfolded. The vestibular field is located mainly on the lower lip in the sulcus and extends only slightly to the surface. 1 = area 1 of BRODMANN, 2 = area 2, v = vestibular field (area 2v)

cytoarchitectonic structure (Fig. 4). For this reason and because of the different senses represented in the somatic area 2 and in the vestibular area, we like to call this vestibular field area 2v.

VI. Responses of Single Neurons in Area 2v

So far, there has been no microelectrode investigation of the neuronal responses in area 2v to adequate rotatory and positional stimuli. However, it has been shown in the cat that single neurone in 2v respond strongly to caloric and galvanic labyrinthine stimulation (KORNHUBER and FONSECA, 1964). There are several types of response to galvanic polarisation of the labyrinths; the response of most neurons is of the specific type according to the criteria of KORNHUBER and FONSECA (1964), which are based upon responses to vestibular and other sensory stimuli of 575 neurons in different sensory, association and motor areas of the cat's cortex. There is no significant relationship between the side of the stimulated labyrinth and the direction-dependence of the responses, which probably means that both labyrinths inform the cerebral hemispheres about the direction of acceleration to the same extent (KORNHUBER and FONSECA, 1964). This is contrary to the situation in the vestibular nuclei as well as in the motor cortex. In the motor cortex most neurons responding to labyrinthine polarisation are cathodally activated and anodally inhibited by the ipsilateral labyrinth, and anodally activated and cathodally inhibited by the contralateral labyrinth (KORNHUBER and ASCHOFF, 1964). Another difference is the latency: in the primary vestibular cortex the majority of neurons show a short latency (down to 4 msec in the cat). In the motor cortex most neurons show a longer latency to labyrinthine stimulation. However, in one respect there is full agreement between the neuronal responses in both areas: in the motor cortex (KORNHUBER and

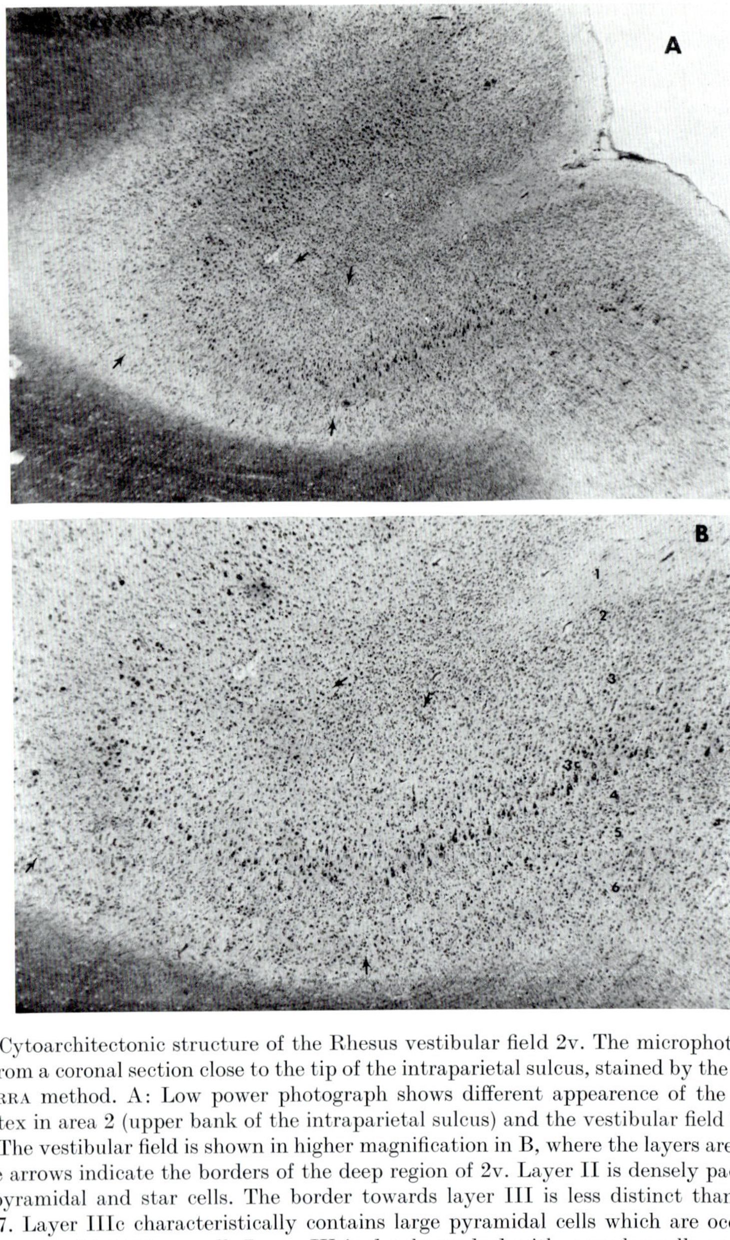

Fig. 4. Cytoarchitectonic structure of the Rhesus vestibular field 2v. The microphotograph is taken from a coronal section close to the tip of the intraparietal sulcus, stained by the KLÜVER-BARRERRA method. A: Low power photograph shows different appearence of the layers of the cortex in area 2 (upper bank of the intraparietal sulcus) and the vestibular field 2v (lower bank). The vestibular field is shown in higher magnification in B, where the layers are numbered. The arrows indicate the borders of the deep region of 2v. Layer II is densely packed with small pyramidal and star cells. The border towards layer III is less distinct than in areas 2,5 or 7. Layer IIIc characteristically contains large pyramidal cells which are occasionally found in superficial IV as well. Layer IV is densly packed with granular cells and sharply defined from Layer V which contains only single small and medium sized cells in Vb close to the fundus, whereas, in the more superficial regions medium sized pyramidal cells are somewhat more prominent in Va. Layer VI is very narrow throughout. In the fundal region it is clearly devisable into VIa containing a few small fusiform and star cells and VIb which is almost cell free. This border becomes somewhat blurred close to the surface where VI is thicker and the cell density increases

Aschoff, 1964) as well as in area 2v (Schwarz and Fredrickson, 1971) many neurons showing vestibular responses also receive deep somatic afferents. This convergence of vestibular and deep somatic messages has also been found in the vestibular nuclei (Fredrickson et al., 1965). Furthermore, there is agreement between the neurons in 2v and somatic area 2 (Powell and Mountcastle, 1959) regarding their somatic inputs: in both fields the neurons predominantly respond to deep somatic stimuli carrying messages from position sense and kinesthesis.

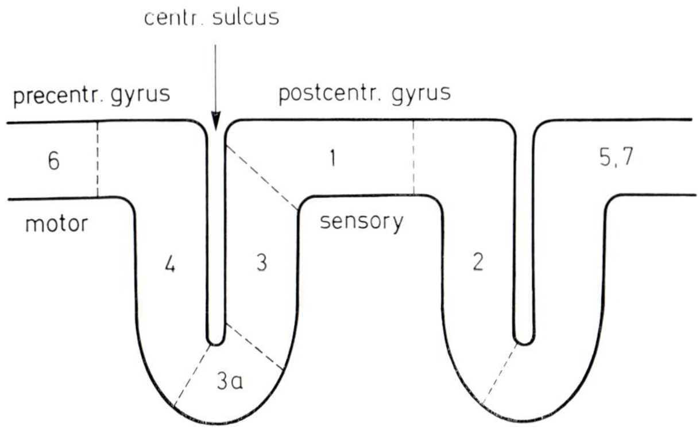

Fig. 5. Scheme of the subdivisions of motor and sensory cortex on a fronto-occipital section through the hand projection of the Rhesus cortex

The somatic area 2 is, in comparison to areas 1 and 3, a more complex somatic cortex. Neuronal responses in area 2 are more easily depressed by barbiturate anesthesia and in addition to joint afferents signalling position and movement there are also some messages related to movement on the skin (Werner and Whitsel, 1970). Area 5 is a still more complex somatic association cortex, in which neurons often respond to movements of several different joints, even from both sides of the body (Duffy and Burchfiel, 1971; Sakata, 1974). In some respect, the vestibular field 2v is similar to somatic area 5 for the deep somatic afferents in 2v often come from several joints and may be bilateral (Schwarz and Fredrickson, 1971). However, although the somatic responses of some neurons in the vestibular field might seem more characteristic of area 5 than area 2, the vestibular field certainly does not belong to area 5 since it's thalamic input comes from the ventroposterior thalamic nucleus (Deecke et al., 1974).

VII. Speculations about the Location of the Vestibular Sensory Area in Man

The most likely location of the vestibular sensory area in the human brain is in the cortex buried in the anterior portion of the intraparietal sulcus where (similar to the location of 2v in the monkey and in the cat) the lower end of area 5 borders area 2. Foerster (1936) found with electrical stimulation of the upper

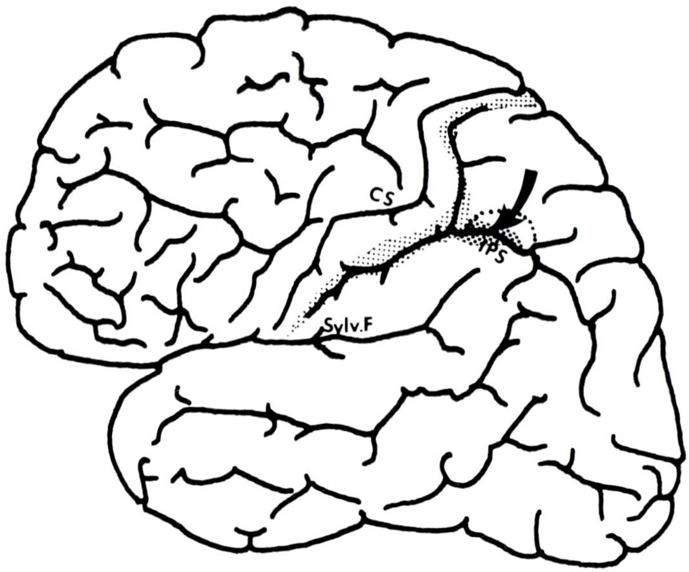

Fig. 6. Hypothetic localisation of the vestibular field in the human cortex in the upper lip of the intraparietal sulcus according to O. FOERSTER. BRODMANN's area 2 is stippled. The coarser stippling indicates the extension of area 2 into the intraparietal sulcus which in the Chimpanzee, according to GERHARDT, differs from area 2. The arrow points at the depth of the intraparietal sulcus, where FOERSTER described the location of vestibular sensation upon electrical stimulation of the human cortex. The dotted line indicates FLECHSIG's area 13, an area myelinated earlier than the rest of the parietal cortex. Note the juxtaposition of the vestibular field to areas 2 and 5 which corresponds to a similar situation in the monkey (Fig. 2, BRODMANN's view) and in the cat (Fig. 8)

lip of the intraparietal sulcus in patients typical vestibular sensations of being rolled with apparent motion of the visual surroundings. FOERSTER (1936) and MORSIER (1938) reported several cases with focal lesions in the region of the intraparietal sulcus, who had epileptic fits starting with typical vestibular sensation. Even PENFIELD (1957) inspite of his temporal lobe hypothesis admitted: "Electrical stimulation in the parietal lobe may at times result in a sense of rotation or bodily displacement, and seizure discharge here may produce an epileptic aura of that type." – FOERSTER (1936) called attention to FLECHSIG's finding that a small field juxtaposed to the intraparietal sulcus undergoes myelination earlier than the surrounding parietal cortex (FLECHSIG's area 13, see FLECHSIG (1905) and Fig. 6), and to SMITH's (1907) finding, that the cortex buried in the intraparietal sulcus shows a special structure. Furthermore, it seems suggestive of this location that there is a caudal extension of what seemed to be area 2 into the lips of the intraparietal sulcus in man and Chimpanzee. This extension of postcentral cortex into the intraparietal sulcus was subsequently clearly separated from area 2 in the Chimpanzee (GERHARDT, 1938: her area 75). According to HASSLER (personal communication), GERHARDT's area 75 is, however, a special subdivision of area 2 and not a cortex of area 5 type.

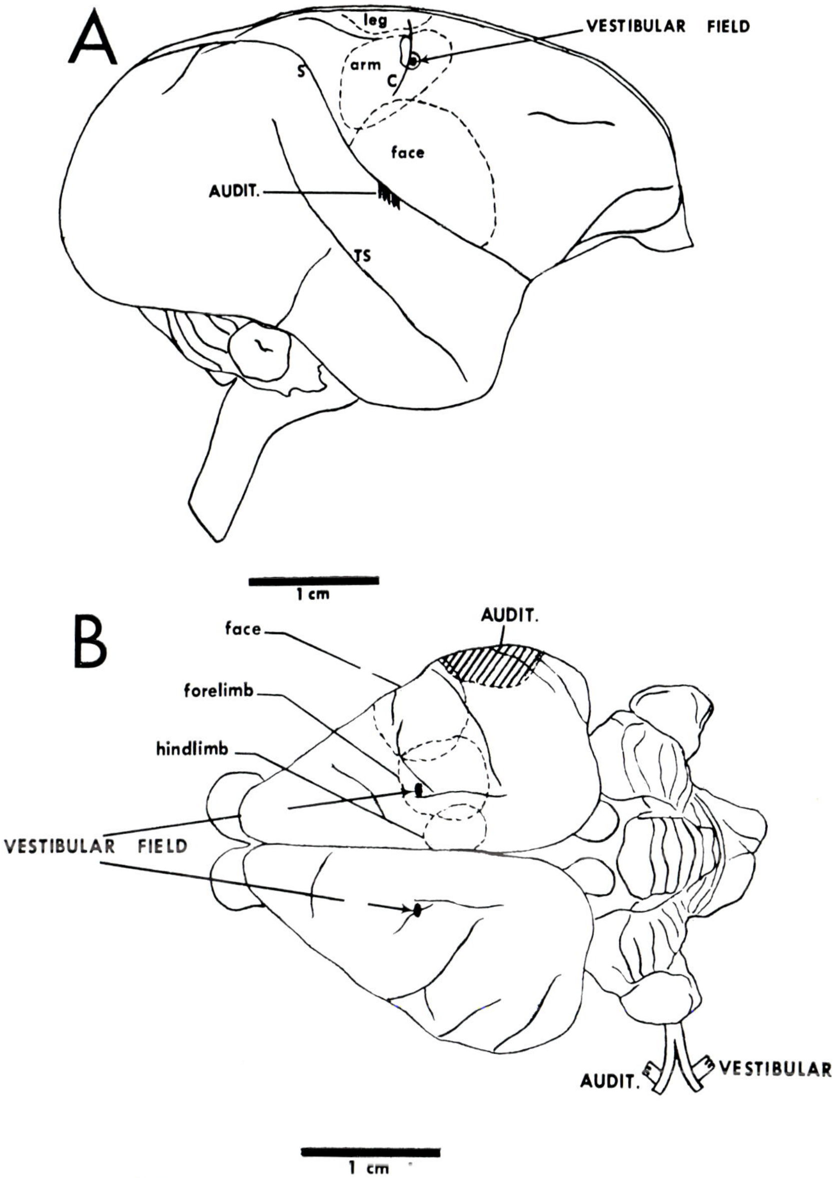

Fig. 7. The vestibular projection to area 3a somatosensory arm field in the squirrel monkey (A) and in the rabbit (B). In A, the smooth line circumscribes the zone where surface positive potentials were obtained after electrical stimulation of the vestibular nerve. However, the real projection is more restricted: it is the small field where a reversal to negativity occurs in the middle cortical layers, indicated by the black dot. The somatosensory and auditory areas outlined in this map are those yielding surface positive evoked potentials irrespective of reversal within the cortex. C = central sulcus, S = Sylvian sulcus, TS = temporal sulcus. – B: A similar diagram for the Rabbit's cortex. The dots labelled "vestibular field" represent zones yielding depth negativity, while the hindlimb, forelimb, face, and auditory areas represent fields of surface positive evoked potentials under pentobarbital anesthesia. A: From Ödkvist, Schwarz, Fredrickson and Hassler, Experimental Brain Research 1974, B: From Ödkvist, Rubin, Schwarz and Fredrickson, J. comp. Neurol. **149**

VIII. The Vestibular Projection to Area 3a

In four species, guinea pig (ÖDKVIST et al., 1973b), rabbit (ÖDKVIST et al., 1973a), squirrel monkey (ÖDKVIST et al., 1974) and cat (SANS et al., 1970), a vestibular projection has been found to area 3a which belongs to S1 and borders the motor cortex (area 4). In the Rhesus monkey there is probably also a projection to area 3a, for a short latency (5–6 msec) positive-negative potential (distinct from the evoked potential in 2v) has been recorded in area 4 (KORNHUBER et al., 1965) which probably reflects activity in area 3a buried in the depth of the central sulcus. The shape of this potential was shown in KORNHUBER (1966) Fig. 51. In the rabbit (ÖDKVIST et al., 1973a) and in the guinea pig (ÖDKVIST et al., 1973b) there are almost no sulci and therefore the total upper hemispheric surface of these lisencephalic animals is exposed. Only one vestibular projection was found, namely that to the rostral part of the somatosensory arm field which probably corresponds to area 3a. In the squirrel monkey the location in 3a is clear. It seems likely that there is only one vestibular projection in rodents while there are two in carnivores and primates. A vestibular projection to area 3a has been predicted by HASSLER (1948).

IX. The Common Denominator of the Areas 2v and 3a

is the convergence of vestibular and deep somatic afferents, in 2v predominantly from the joints (but probably also from muscle, see SILFVENIUS 1968, BURCHFIEL and DUFFY 1972), in 3a from muscles spindles. The predominance of joint afferents in area 2 was found in the classical study of POWELL and MOUNTCASTLE (1959), the projection of fast (group I) muscle afferents to area 3a has been found in the cat by AMASSIAN and BERLIN (1958) and OSCARSSON and ROSÉN (1963), in the monkey by PHILLIPS et al. (1971). This cortical convergence of vestibular and proprioceptive somatic messages is not surprising in the view of vestibular function. A similar convergence is well established in the motor cortex (KORNHUBER, 1962; KORNHUBER and ASCHOFF, 1964), in the vestibular nuclei (FREDRICKSON et al., 1966) and in the thalamic vestibular nucleus (DEECKE et al., 1973b).

X. General Cortical Arousal Effects Following Vestibular Stimuli

There is ample evidence suggesting that vestibularly evoked cortical activity in areas other than 2v and 3a is mediated via long polysynaptic pathways, including the arousal system of the brainstem reticular formation and medial thalamus (GEREBTZOFF, 1940; ROGER et al., 1956; MOLNAR, 1959, and others). Vestibular stimuli cause more arousal reactions than other sensory stimuli, except for pain.

After investigating several hundred neurons in different sensory, association and motor areas of the cat under a variety of sensory stimuli, KORNHUBER and FONSECA (1964) concluded that vestibular stimuli tend to produce non-specific

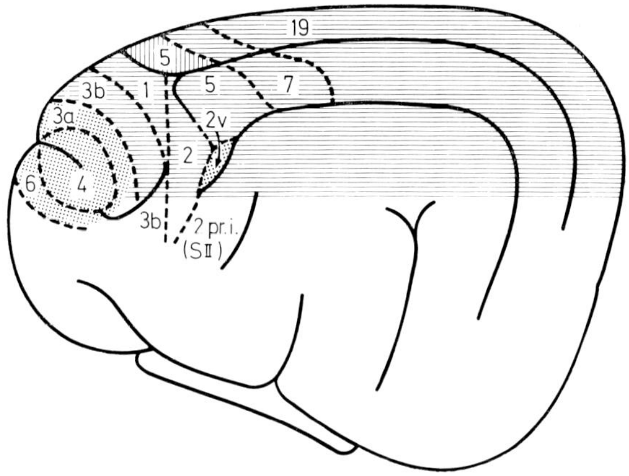

Fig. 8. Specific responses of single neurons in the upper convolutions of the cat's cortex to galvanic polarisation of the labyrinth are concentrated in area 2v on the one hand and in areas 3a, 4 and 6 on the other hand. The other fields of the upper convolutions of the cat's cortex including visual, auditory, temporal, and parietal association areas show non-specific activation by vestibular stimulation. In area 5 occurs neuronal inhibition classified as non-specific. Specific responses of neurons to vestibular stimuli stippled, non-specific activation horizontal hatching, non-specific inhibition vertical hatching. Neuronal responses redrawn from KORNHUBER, Habilitationsschrift, Freiburg i. Br. 1962. Cytoarchitectonic fields according to HASSLER and MUHS-CLEMENT, J. Hirnforsch. **6** (1964)

responses in all cortical areas (see Fig. 8). Specific responses have a constant and short latency, maximal primary reaction and strict dependence on the duration of the stimulus; non-specific responses have a variable, long latency, they begin with slow increase and often persist for a long time after the end of the stimulus. Most neuronal responses to vestibular stimuli outside the primary vestibular and motor cortical areas, are of this non-specific type.

Non-specific changes in the animal's alertness, perhaps in connection with a size constancy mechanism (MARG and ADAMAS, 1970), seem also to be the most likely explanation for the effects of body tilt on the receptive fields of a few neurons in the cat's visual cortex observed by HORN and HILL (1969), SPINELLI (1970) and DENNY and ADORJANI (1972), since changes in size, shape and direction of visual receptive fields of neurons in area 17 and 18 occur also spontaneously (SCHWARTZKROIN, 1972) even after bilateral labyrinthectomy or cervical spinal cord section (HORN et al., 1972). However, see contrary opinion of BROOKS and JUNG, this handbook, vol. VII/3, p. 408.

XI. Sensory Function of the Vestibular Cortical Representation

Of the two vestibular fields in the cortex, it seems more likely that area 2v has the perceptive function. At least, the fast muscle afferents in area 3a are not used as discriminative messages for operant conditioning of cats, even when the muscle afferents give rise to a cortical evoked potential (SWETT and BOURASSA, 1967) while joint afferents projecting to area 2 are certainly an easily discriminable cue. The inferiority of muscle afferents in kinesthesia has not yet been ruled out by the studies of Goodwin et al. (1972).

Area 2v, like the rest of area 2, presumably has direct or indirect (via area 5) connections with area 7, where messages from all spatial senses converge (Pandya and Kuypers, 1969; Jones and Powell, 1970) in order to form a unified representation of the spatial situation. Lesions in this parietal region (especially bilateral lesions or lesions in the minor hemisphere) result in disturbances of spatial orientation (Head, 1920; Kleist, 1934; McFie et al., 1950; Semmes et al., 1955; Hecaen, 1962).

Vestibular participation in this general spatial orientation probably exists because experiments with passive motion (blindfolded) show a disturbance of conscious spatial orientation and memory after bilateral labyrinthine loss (Beritachvili, 1963). Furthermore, parietal lesions result in the acute stage in a tilt of the subjective optical vertical (Bender and Jung, 1948). In experiments with reversing spectacles, vestibular and somatosensory afferents determine what is up and down in vision (Stratton, 1897; Kohler, 1951).

XII. Motor Function of the Cortical Vestibular Representation

Both of the deep somatic areas of SI (2 and 3a) have strong direct fiber connections to the motor area 4 (Jones and Powell, 1968, 1969, for details see Jones and Powell, this handbook, vol. II, p. 593–596). Although this has not been investigated explicitly, it is likely that the corresponding vestibular areas, 2v and the vestibular parts of 3a, have the same direct connections to area 4. In any case, about 65% of the neurons of the cat's motor cortex show responses to somatosensory stimuli and about 50% to vestibular stimuli (Kornhuber and Aschoff, 1964). Although there are many neurons in the motor cortex receiving somatosensory afferents from the skin, only neurons with deep somatic afferents receive direction specific vestibular afferents (Kornhuber and Aschoff, 1964).

What is the function of the vestibular afferents in the motor cortex? Are they related to eye movements or vestibular nystagmus? As discussed in more detail in another chapter of this handbook (VI/2 G. II.) the motor cortex is not the master of all movements but only of those which need sophisticated somatosensory regulation. These are, in primates, especially foot, hand, finger, lip and tongue movements, but not eye movements. Electrical stimulation of the vestibular cortical areas, of the somatosensory and motor cortex does not yield eye movements (see Fig. 9). However, in order to be able to carry out skilled goal directed movements of the limbs, safe postural adjustments are a prerequisite. Therefore, vestibular messages are needed in the motor cortex in addition to somatosensory input. Besides the well known loss of higher reflexes induced by somatosensory stimuli (the tactile placing and hopping reactions of Bard (1938) and the grasping reaction of Denny-Brown, 1960) the vestibular placing reaction of the contralateral foreleg is lost after unilateral exstirpation of the motor cortex while the visual placing reaction remains intact (Bard and Orias, 1933). Detailed in-

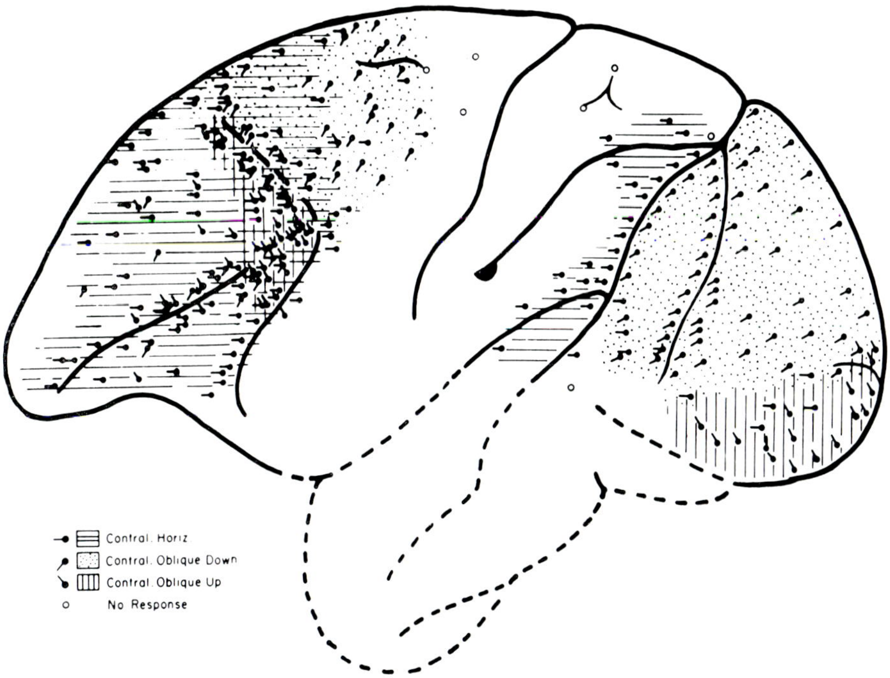

Fig. 9. Eye movements are elicited by electrical stimulation (according to Wagman, 1964) from extensive fields in occipital, posterior parietal, temporal, and frontal regions of the Rhesus monkey's cerebral cortex, but the vestibular field and the other somatosensory and motor cortical areas on either side of the central sulcus do not yield eye movements. The Rhesus vestibular area of Fredrickson and Kornhuber is inserted in the original diagram (arrow) of Wagman, published in Bender: The oculomotor system, Hoeber, New York 1964

vestigations of the defects following lesions in the vestibular cortical areas have not been published.

XIII. The Ascending Pathway to the Cortex

Although numerous articles are available concerning the vestibulo-thalamic projection, only one study has identified a thalamic cell group which is both activated by vestibular input and projects directly to a primary cortical vestibular area (Deecke et al., 1973a, 1974). Short latency (2.5 msec) field potentials were recorded in the Rhesus monkey thalamus under barbiturate anesthesia in a cell group located in the lower ventroposterior region of the thalamus, close to the VPL and VPM nuclei. Olszewski (1952) included this cell group within the borders of the VPI (nucleus ventralis posterior inferior). It has been demonstrated by antidromic stimulation that the axons of these thalamic vestibular neurons project directly to the Rhesus cortical vestibular field 2v. They also have the same type of bimodal input, that is 80% of the vestibular units also respond to joint input (Deecke et al., 1973b). Maximal vestibular field potentials in the Rhesus thalamus were recorded in the upper (dorsal) part of the VPI which, as previously

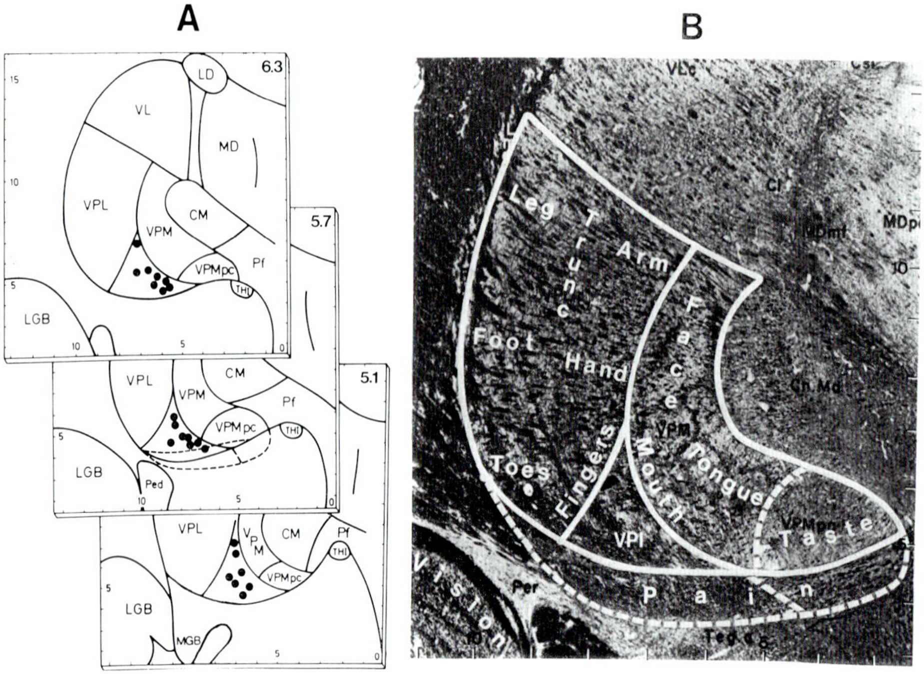

Fig. 10. Location of electrolytic lesions in the ventroposterior thalamus at places of maximal short latency response to electrical stimulation of the vestibular nerve in the Rhesus monkey. A: 23 lesions were localized by microprojection onto 3 subsequent frontal sections according to OLSZEWSKI's atlas. Four lesions best fitting plate + 6.9 have been included in +6.3, and 4 lesions fitting plate +4.5 were plotted into +5.1. The dotted lines of plate 5.7 indicate HASSLER's V.c.pc. B: Thalamic nuclei surrounding VPI and their function. Dotted: HASSLER's V.C.pc. where pain is represented. Dorsolateral of VPI, hand representation; dorsomedial, perioral face representation, paralleling neighborhood relations of vestibular cortex. From DEECKE, SCHWARZ and FREDRICKSON, Exp. Brain Res. **20** (1974)

mentioned, is closely related to the VPL and VPM. Contrary to the lower, parvocellular part (HASSLER's Vc.pc. – see HASSLER, 1959) which contains a pain representation, the upper (i.e. VPI) has medium sized cells similar to VPM cells. Furthermore, it contains the horizontal fiber bundles also found in VPL and VPM which are the lemniscal endings.

Field potentials to vestibular stimuli were also observed in other areas of the thalamus including the magnocellular medial geniculate nucleus. Their latency of 5 msec, however, is too long to consider them as a direct thalamo-cortical relay to areas 3a or 2v since the cortical latency is just 5 to 6 msec; furthermore, these nuclei do not project to SI.

Evidence concerning the path between the vestibular nuclei and the thalamus is incomplete. The medial longitudinal fasciculus has been ruled out since in 4 Rhesus monkeys the cortical potential remained unaltered following bilateral MLF transection at the level of the oculomotor nuclei (SCHWARZ and ÖDKVIST, unpublished). In fact, when three quarters of the brainstem was transected at that level leaving only the contralateral ventral quarter intact, the contralateral cortical response to vestibular nerve stimulation remained intact. At the level of the meso-diencephalic junction, a large potential of 2 msec latency has been recorded in the narrow space between the medial and lateral lemnisci (DEECKE et al., 1973). This fits perfectly with the 2.5 msec latency vestibular response found in the VPI thalamic nucleus (DEECKE et al., 1974). These electrophysiological data suggest that there is a direct projection from the vestibular nuclei to the thalamus and that the findings of CARPENTER and STROMINGER (1965), who reported degeneration in the VPI following lesions of the vestibular nuclei, are not due to unwanted lesions of other ascending fiber systems (as was suspected by TARLOV, 1969).

Stimulation in the thalamus of conscious man evoked vestibular sensations (sensation of being tilted or whirled or falling) from an area immediately adjacent to the somatic mouth representation of the ventrocaudal nuclei (TASKER and ORGAN, 1971). This location most probably corresponds to the monkey VPI and may shed light on the functional significance of the short latency vestibulo-VPI-2v projection: conscious vestibular perception. Furthermore, vestibular sensation could be elicited by stimuli near the magnocellular medial geniculate where the afferent vestibular fibres pass to the VPI.

The vestibulo-cortical pathway terminating within the area 3a arm field has not yet been identified. HASSLER (1948) predicted that the V.im., situated between the VL and VPL transmits vestibular impulses to area 3a. The main afferents of the V.im., however, come not from the labyrinths, they come from muscle spindles (ROSÉN, 1969).

It was suggested, that the late thalamic vestibular responses (5 msec) might pass through the cerebellum. However, vestibular potentials with similar latencies have been recorded following cerebellectomy (DEECKE et al., 1974).

XIV. Summary

In summary, vestibular representations in thalamus and cerebral cortex show that labyrinthine messages join somatic proprioception. From the functional point of view this is meaningful, since both of them signal the position and movements of the body. The cortical vestibular representation is in the Rolandic sensorimotor area, not in the temporal lobe. It belongs to the first somatosensory area (SI). It serves conscious orientation in space and higher motor regulations of the limbs. It has nothing to do with eye movements.

References

AMASSIAN, V.E., BERLIN, L.: Early cortical projection of group I afferents in the forelimb muscle nerves of cat. J. Physiol. (Lond.) **143**, 61P (1958).

BADER, W., KORNHUBER, H.H.: Großhirnläsionen und vestibulärer Nystagmus. Vergleichende elektronystagmographische Untersuchungen bei geschlossenen Augen und mit visueller Fixation. Acta oto-laryng. (Stockh.) **60**, 197–206 (1965).

BARD, P.: Studies in the cortical representation of somatic sensibility. Harvey Lect. **33**, 143–169 (1938).

BARD, P., ORIAS, O.: Localized cortical management of visual and labyrinthine placing reactions. Amer. J. Physiol. **105**, 2–3 (1933).

BENDER, M., JUNG, R.: Abweichungen der subjektiven optischen Vertikalen und Horizontalen bei Gesunden und Hirnverletzten. Arch. Psychiat. Nervenkr. **181**, 193–212 (1948).

BERITACHVILI (BERITOFF), J.S.: Les méchanismes nerveux de l'orientation spatiale chez l'homme. Neuropsychologia **1**, 233–249 (1963).

BERMAN, A.L.: Overlap of somatic and auditory cortical response fields in anterior ectosylvian gyrus of cat. J. Neurophysiol. **24**, 595 (1961).

BRODMANN, K.: Vergleichende Lokalisationslehre der Großhirnrinde, in ihren Prinzipien dargestellt auf Grund des Zellenbaues. Leipzig: J. A. Barth 1909.

BURCHFIEL, J.L., DUFFY, F.H.: Muscle afferent input to single cells in primate somatosensory cortex. Brain Res. **45**, 241–246 (1972).

CARMICHAEL, E.A., DIX, M.R., HALLPIKE, C.S.: Lesions of the cerebral hemispheres and their effects upon optokinetical and caloric nystagmus. Brain **77**, 345–372 (1954).

CARPENTER, M.B., STROMINGER, N.L.: The medial longitudinal fasciculus and disturbance of conjugate horizontal eye movements in the monkey. J. comp. Neurol. **125**, 41–66 (1965).

DEECKE, L., SCHWARZ, D.W.F., FREDRICKSON, J.M.: The vestibular thalamus in the rhesus monkey. Adv. Oto-Rhino-Laryng. (Basel: Karger) **19**, 210–219 (1973a).

DEECKE, L., SCHWARZ, D.W.F., FREDRICKSON, J.M.: Single unit recordings in the vestibular thalamus (VPI area) of the macaque. Pflügers Arch. **339**, Suppl. R 79 (1973b).

DEECKE, L., SCHWARZ, D.W.F., FREDRICKSON, J.M.: Nucleus ventroposterior inferior (VPI) as the vestibular thalamic relay in the Rhesus monkey. I. Field potential investigation. Exp. Brain Res. **20**, 88–100 (1974).

DENNEY, D., ADORJANI, C.: Orientation specifity of visual cortical neurons after head tilt. Exp. Brain Res. **14**, 312–317 (1972).

DENNY-BROWN, D.: The general principles of motor integration. In: J. FIELD, H.W. MAGOUN, V.E. HALL, Eds. Handbook of Physiology, Sect. I: Neurophysiology. Washington: Amer. Physiol. Society 1960.

DUFFY, F.H., BURCHFIEL, J.L.: Somatosensory system: organizational hierarchy from single units in monkey area 5. Science **172**, 273–275 (1971).

FLECHSIG, P.: Einige Bemerkungen über die Untersuchungsmethoden der Großhirnrinde, insbesondere des Menschen. Arch. Anat. u. Physiol., Anat. Abtlg. **1905**, 337–444.

FOERSTER, O.: Motorische Felder und Bahnen. In: O. BUMKE, O. FOERSTER, Hrsg. Handbuch der Neurologie, Vol. 6, pp. 1–357. Berlin: Springer 1936.

FOERSTER, O.: Sensible corticale Felder. In: O. BUMKE, O. FOERSTER, Hrsg. Handbuch der Neurologie, Vol. 6, pp. 358–448. Berlin: Springer 1936.

FREDRICKSON, J.M., FIGGE, U., SCHEID, P., KORNHUBER, H.H.: Vestibular nerve projection to the cerebral cortex of the rhesus monkey. Exp. Brain Res. **2**, 318–327 (1966).

FREDRICKSON, J.M., SCHWARZ, D., KORNHUBER, H.H.: Convergence and interaction of vestibular and deep somatic afferents upon neurons in the vestibular nuclei of the cat. Acta otolaryng. (Stockh.) **61**, 168–188 (1965).

GEREBTZOFF, M.A.: Recherches sur la projection corticale du labyrinthe: des effects de la stimulation labyrinthique sur l'activité électrique de l'écorce cérébrale. Arch. int. Physiol. **50**, 59–99 (1940).

GERHARDT, E.: Der Isocortex parietalis beim Schimpansen. J. Psychol. Neurol. (Lpz.) **48**, 329–386 (1938).

GOODWIN, G.M., MCCLOSKEY, D.I., MATTHEWS, P.B.C.: The contribution of muscle afferents to kinaesthesia found by vibration induced illussions of movement and by the effects of paralysing joint afferents. Brain **95**, 705–748 (1972).

GRIFFITH, C.R.: An historical survey of vestibular equilibration. Univ. Illinois Bull. **20**, 7—178 (1922).

HASSLER, R.: Forels Haubenfaszikel als vestibuläre Empfindungsbahn mit Bemerkungen über einige andere sekundäre Bahnen des Vestibularis und Trigeminus. Arch. Psychiat. Nervenkr. **180**, 23 (1948).

HASSLER, R.: Anatomy of the thalamus. In: G. SCHALTENBRAND, P. BAILEY, Eds. Introduction to stereotaxis with an atlas of the human brain, Vol. 1, pp. 230–290. Stuttgart: Thieme 1959.

HASSLER, R., MUHS-CLEMENT, K.: Architektonischer Aufbau des sensomotorischen und parietalen Cortex der Katze. J. Hirnforsch. **6**, 377–420 (1964).

HEAD, H.: Studies in Neurology, Vol. 2. London: Oxford Medical Publ. 1920.
HECAEN, H.: Clinical symptomatology in right and left hemispheric lesions. In: Interhemispheric lesions and cerebral dominance. V.B. MOUNTCASTLE, Ed., pp. 215–243. Baltimore: Johns Hopkins Press 1962.
HORN, G., HILL, R.M.: Modifications of receptive fields of cells in the visual cortex occuring spontaneously and associated with body tilt. Nature (Lond.) **221**, 186–188 (1969).
HORN, G., STECHLER, G., HILL, R.M.: Receptive fields of units in the visual cortex of the cat in the presence and absence of bodily tilt. Exp. Brain Res. **15**, 113–132 (1972).
JONES, E.G., POWELL, T.P.S.: The ipsilateral cortical connections of the somatic sensory areas in the cat. Brain Res. **9**, 71–84 (1968).
JONES, E.G., POWELL, T.P.S.: Connections of the somatic sensory cortex of the rhesus monkey. I. Ipsilateral cortical connections. Brain **92**, 504–531 (1969).
JONES, E.G., POWELL, T.P.S.: An anatomical study of converging sensory pathways within the cerebral cortex of the monkey. Brain **93**, 793–820 (1970).
KLEIST, K.: Gehirnpathologie. Leipzig: J. A. Barth 1934.
KOHLER, I.: Über Aufbau und Wandlungen der Wahrnehmungswelt. Sitz Ber. Österr. Akad. Wiss., Wien, Phil-hist. Kl. **227**, 1 (1951).
KORNHUBER, H.H.: Optisch-vestibuläre und somatisch-vestibuläre Integration an Neuronen der Großhirnrinde: ein Beitrag zur multimodalen Koordination der Sinnesafferenzen. Habilitationsschrift, Med. Fak. Universität Freiburg/Br. 1962.
KORNHUBER, H.H.: Physiologie und Klinik des zentral-vestibulären Systems (Blick- und Stützmotorik). In: J. BERENDES et al.: Hals-, Nasen-, Ohrenheilkunde, Bd. III/3, S. 2150–2351, 1966. Stuttgart: G. Thieme
KORNHUBER, H.H., ASCHOFF, J.C.: Somatisch-vestibuläre Integration an Neuronen des motorischen Cortex. Naturwissenschaften **51**, 62–63 (1964).
KORNHUBER, H.H., DA FONSECA, J.S.: Optovestibular integration in the cats cortex: A study of sensory convergence on cortical neurons. In: M. B. BENDER, Ed. The oculomotor system, p. 239–279. New York: Hoeber 1964.
KORNHUBER, H.H., FREDRICKSON, J.M., FIGGE, U.: Die korticale Projektion der vestibulären Afferenz beim Rhesusaffen. Pflügers Arch. ges. Physiol. **283**, 20 (1965).
LENNOX, W.G.: Epilepsy and related disorders. Boston: Little, Brown 1960.
MARG, E., ADAMS, J.E.: Evidence for a neurological zoom system in vision from angular changes in some receptive fields of single neurons with changes in fixation distance in the human visual cortex. Experientia (Basel) **26**, 270–271 (1970).
MCFIE, G., PIERCY, M.F., ZANGWILL, O.L.: Visual-spatial agnosia associated with lesions of the right cerebral hemisphere. Brain **73**, 167–190 (1950).
MICKLE, W.A., ADES, H.W.: A composite sensory projection area in the cerebral cortex of the cat. Amer. J. Physiol. **170**, 682–689 (1952).
MOLNAR, L.: Die Bedeutung der Labyrinthimpulse in der Spontan- und Krampftätigkeit der Hirnrinde. Arch. Psychiat. Nervenkr. **198**, 554–573 (1959).
DE MORSIER, J.: Contribution a l'étude des centres vestibulaires corticaux et des hallucinations lilliputiennes. Encéphale **33**, 57–73 (1938).
ÖDKVIST, L.M., RUBIN, A.M., SCHWARZ, D.W.F., FREDRICKSON, J.M.: Vestibular cortical projection in the rabbit. J. comp. Neurol. **149**, 117–120 (1973a).
ÖDKVIST, L.M., RUBIN, A.M., SCHWARZ, D.W.F., FREDRICKSON, J.M.: Vestibular and auditory cortical projection in the guinea pig (Cavia porcellum). Exp. Brain Res. **18**, 279–286 (1973b).
ÖDKVIST, L.M., SCHWARZ, D.W.F., FREDRICKSON, J.M., HASSLER, R.: Projection of the vestibular nerve to the area 3a arm field in the squirrel monkey (Saimiri sciureus). Exp. Brain Res. (1974).
OLSZEWSKI, I.: The thalamus of the macaca mulatta. Basel: Karger 1952.
OSCARSSON, O., ROSÉN, I.: Projection to cerebral cortex of large muscle-spindle afferents in forelimb nerves of the cat. J. Physiol. (Lond.) **169**, 924 (1963).
PANDYA, D.N., KUYPERS, H.G.J.M.: Cortico-cortical connections in the Rhesus monkey. Brain Res. **13**, 13–36 (1969).
PENFIELD, W.: Vestibular sensation and the cerebral cortex. Ann. Otol. (St. Louis) **66**, 691–698 (1957).

PENFIELD, W., JASPER, H.H.: Epilepsy and the functional anatomy of the brain. London 1954.

PHILLIPS, C.G., POWELL, T.P.S., WIESENDANGER, M.: Projection from low-threshold muscle afferents of hand forearm to area 3a of baboon's cortex. J. Physiol. (Lond.) **217**, 419–446 (1971).

POWELL, T.P.S., MOUNTCASTLE, V.B.: Some aspects of the functional organisation of the cortex of the postcentral gyrus of the monkey: a correlation of findings obtained in single unit analysis with cyto-architecture. Bull. Johns Hopk. Hosp. **105**, 133 (1959).

ROBERTS, T.S., AKERT, K.: Insular and opercular cortex and its thalamic projection in Macaca mulatta. Schweiz. Arch. Neurol. Psychiat. **92**, 1–43 (1963).

ROGER, A., ROSSI, G.F., ZIRONDOLI, A.: Le Role des afferences des nerves craniens dans le maintien de l'état vigile de la preparation 'encéphale isolé'. Electroenceph. clin. Neurophysiol. **8**, 1–13 (1956).

ROSÉN, I.: Excitation of group I activated thalamocortical relay neurons in the cat. J. Physiol. (Lond.) **205**, 237–255 (1969).

SAKATA, H.: Somatic sensory responses of neurons in the parietal association area (area 5) of monkeys. In: H. H. KORNHUBER, Ed. The somatosensory system. Stuttgart: Thieme 1974.

SANS, A., RAYMOND, J., MARTY, R.: Responses thalamiques et corticales a la stimulation électrique du nerf vestibulaire chez le Chat. Exp. Brain Res. **10**, 265–275 (1970).

SCHWARZ, D.W.F., FREDRICKSON, J.M.: Rhesus monkey vestibular cortex: a bimodal primary projection field. Science **172**, 289–291 (1971).

SCHWARTZKROIN, P.A.: The effect of body tilt on the directionality of units in cat visual cortex. Exp. Neurol. **36**, 498–506 (1972).

SEMMES, J., WEINSTEIN, S., GHENT, L., TEUBER, H.-L.: Spatial orientation in man after cerebral injury: 1. analysis by locus of lesion. J. Psychol. **39**. 227–244 (1955).

SILFVENIUS, H.: Cortical projections of large muscle afferents from the cat's forelimb. Acta physiol. scand. **74**, 25A–26A (1968).

SMITH, G.E.: A new topographical survey of the human cerebral cortex, being an account of the distribution of the anatomical distinct cortical areas and their relation to the cerebral sulci. J. Anat. Physiol. **41**, 237–257 (1907).

SPIEGEL, E.A.: Cortical centers of the labyrinth. J. nerv. ment. Dis. **75**, 504–512 (1932).

SPIEGEL, E.A.: Labyrinth and cortex. The electroencephalogram of the cortex in stimulation of the labyrinth. Arch. Neurol. Psychiat. (Chic.) **31**, 469–482 (1934).

SPINELLI, D.N.: Recognition of visual patterns. In: D. A. HAMBURG, Ed. Perception and its disorders, p. 139–149. Baltimore: Williams & Wilkins 1970.

SPITZER, A.: Anatomie und Physiologie der zentralen Bahnen des Vestibularis. Arb. neurol. Inst. Univ. Wien **25**, 454 (1924).

STRATTON, G.M.: Vision without inversion of the retinal image. Psychol. Rev. **4**, 341, 463 (1897).

SWETT, I.E., BOURASSA, C.M.: Comparison of sensory discrimination thresholds with muscle and cutaneous nerve volleys in the cat. J. Neurophysiol. **30**, 530–545 (1967).

TARLOV, E.: The rostral projections of the primate vestibular nuclei: An experimental study in macaque, baboon and chimpanzee. J. comp. Neurol. **135**, 27–56 (1969).

TASKER, R.R., ORGAN, L.W.: Mapping of somatosensory and auditory pathways in upper midbrain and thalamus of man. Internat. Congr. Ser. 253: Neurophysiology studied in man, p. 169–187. Amsterdam: Excerpta medica 1971.

VOGT, C., VOGT, O.: Allgemeinere Ergebnisse unserer Hirnforschung. 3. Mitteilung: Die architektonische Rindenfelderung im Lichte unserer neuesten Forschungen. J. Psychol. Neurol. (Lpz.) **25**, 361–398 (1919).

WAGMAN, J.H.: Eye movements induced by electric stimulation of cerebrum in monkeys and their relationship to bodily movements. pp. 18—39.In: M.BENDER, Ed. The oculomotor system. New York: Hoeber 1964.

WALZL, E.M., MOUNTCASTLE, V.B.: Projection of vestibular nerve to cerebral cortex of cat. Amer. J. Physiol. **159**, 595 (1949).

WERNER, G., WHITSEL, B.L.: Stimulus feature detection by neurons in somatosensory areas I and II of primates. IEEE Trans. MMS-11, p. 36, 1970.

Chapter VII.

Vestibular Influences during Sleep[1]

By

O. POMPEIANO, Pisa (Italy)

With 10 Figures

Contents

1 The manuscript of this article was sent to the Editor in June, 1968. New contributions to the subject have recently appeared (POMPEIANO, 1969, 1970, 1972, 1973; MAGHERINI et al., 1972; SEGUIN et al., 1973; THODEN et al., 1972).

I. Introduction

Recent experiments indicate that sleep is not a passive event but an active phenomenon involving several brain structures (cf. Moruzzi, 1963; Jouvet, 1967). Physiological sleep of mammals consists of a synchronized phase, or light sleep, characterized by large-amplitude, slow electroencephalogram (EEG) waves, frequently grouped in spindles (cf. Moruzzi, 1963) and a desynchronized phase, or deep sleep, characterized by low voltage, fast cortical waves (Dement, 1958, 1964), and a great reduction of the tonic electromyographic (EMG) activity recorded from the postural neck muscles (Jouvet, 1962, 1967). One typical feature of desynchronized sleep is the sudden appearance from time to time of bursts of rapid eye movements, REM (Aserinsky and Kleitman, 1953, 1955; Dement, 1958, 1964; Jouvet, 1962, 1967), often associated with a typical motor pattern, characterized by the occurrence of quick muscular contractions (cf. Gassel et al., 1964c). Independent but mutually related mechanisms are responsible for the two phases of sleep.

Investigation of the central mechanisms responsible for the occurrence of the rapid eye movements indicated that during this phase of sleep there are phasic increases in the vestibular activity (Bizzi, Pompeiano and Somogyi, 1964a, b, c). During wakefulness the activity of the second-order vestibular neurons depends upon *external* labyrinthine input, while during desynchronized sleep the increase in the activity of the vestibular neurons depends upon *internal* extralabyrinthine input. It has been suggested that pontine structures, which are active during desynchronized sleep (cf. Jouvet, 1962, 1967), contribute to the appearance of the outbursts of vestibular discharge (cf. Morrison and Pompeiano, 1966d). Experiments were then performed to determine whether the occurrence of large phasic increases in the vestibular discharge during desynchronized sleep were responsible not only for the REM, but also for all the physiological events related in time with them. While most of the electrophysiological investigations performed thus far on the vestibular system utilized anesthetized or decerebrate preparations, REM periods of desynchronized sleep could be used to study vestibular mechanisms in unrestrained, unanesthetized animals with intact, whole brains.

It will be shown here that vestibular activity controls somatic and vegetative functions during sleep (cf. Pompeiano, 1966a, 1967b, c, 1968a). During the REM phase of sleep in particular, the vestibular system affects not only the oculomotor neurons, but also the spinal motoneurons through both their ascending and descending projections. Muscle contractions which affect the somatic musculature during the bursts of REM are actually associated with both pyramidal and extrapyramidal discharges, which are triggered by ascending vestibular volleys. Moreover the appearance of a typical motor pattern during the periods of REM permits the study of how sensory communication to the brain is processed during motor activities induced under strictly physiological conditions by vestibular volleys. The main finding from such investigations was that the flow of sensory information into the nervous system from different receptor organs is controlled at different relay stations of several sensory pathways by active mechanisms, which are triggered by vestibular activity during the REM phase of sleep. In addition, new mechanisms of sensory control which depend upon vestibular activity were discovered, and a neural model of sensorimotor integration was proposed, which could account for the sensory mechanisms associated with the motor activities related in time with the REM. It was concluded that just at the time when both spinal and ocular motoneurons are excited, the transmission of sensory volleys along different sensory pathways is partially blocked by active inhibitory processes which operate at both presynaptic and postsynaptic levels (cf. POMPEIANO, 1966a, 1967b, c, 1968a). On the other hand, a facilitation of the sensory-evoked responses occurs at both thalamic and cortical levels (cf. POMPEIANO, 1968a).

The arrival of corticipetal volleys originating from or triggered by the vestibular system at the time of the REM bursts is of particular relevance not only from the standpoint of the vestibular physiology but also from that of the sleep physiology. In man, in whom this phase of sleep also occurs, a striking relation has been found between eye movements and dream activity (ASERINSKY and KLEITMAN, 1953, 1955; DEMENT and KLEITMAN, 1957a, b; DEMENT, 1964). This aspect of the problem is mentioned here simply to show the large sphere of influence of the vestibular system during natural sleep.

All the results summarized in the following chapters were obtained in unrestrained, unanesthetized cats, with permanently implanted electrodes. Further experiments are required to determine whether the vestibular mechanisms described during the deepest phase of sleep are also operative during the motor activities produced by natural labyrinthine stimulations.

II. Postural and Motor Activities during REM

A. Activity of Spinal Motoneurons

A slight depression of the neck muscular activity occurs during synchronized sleep, while further striking depression of the antigravity tonus, frequently reaching electromyographic silence, is present throughout the desynchronized phase of sleep (JOUVET, 1962). The abolition of tonic muscular activities during this phase of sleep involves not only the posterior cervical muscles, but also several other extensor and flexor muscles of the hindlimbs (POMPEIANO and SWETT, 1962; GASSEL et al., 1964c).

In some instances, however, the abolition of the spontaneous muscular activity is not complete. In these cases the residual muscular activity disappears completely during the bursts of REM (GASSEL et al., 1964c). This striking phenomenon was obviously missed when the electromyographic activity was tonically abolished throughout the desynchronized phase.

There are therefore two suppressive processes during desynchronized sleep: i) a *tonic* depression which lasts as long as the sleep episode, and ii) a *phasic* depression that occurs synchronously with the bursts of REM.

This article will not contain a discussion of the evidence summarized in previous reports (POMPEIANO, 1965, 1966a, 1967b) indicating that the *tonic* abolition of the muscular activity during desynchronized sleep (Fig. 1A, B) is due to reduced excitability of the α motoneurons. This phenomenon can be attributed to supraspinal descending volleys running along the ventral quadrants of the spinal cord and exerting postsynaptic inhibitory influences on these spinal neurons. Suffice is to say that these volleys probably originate from the inhibitory area of the medul-

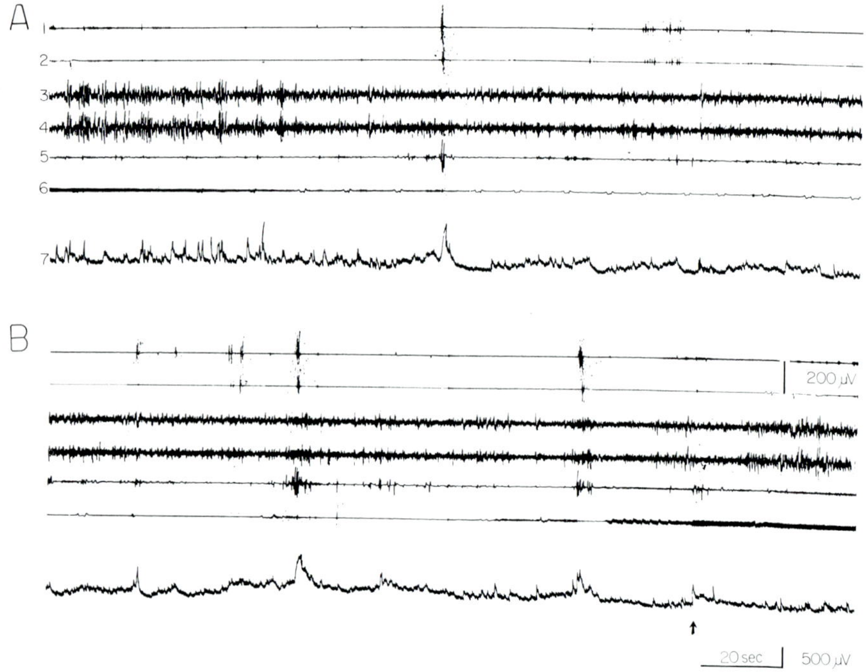

Fig. 1. Muscular twitches and phasic increases in the pyramidal activity during the bursts of REM occurring in desynchronized sleep. Unrestrained, unanesthetized cat. Experiment made 2 days after the operation. Bipolar records. 1: left tibialis anterior (EMG); 2: right tibialis anterior (EMG); 3: left parieto-occipital (EEG); 4: right parieto-occipital (EEG); 5: electro-oculogram (EOG); 6: posterior cervical muscles (EMG); 7: pyramidal integrated record. Upper voltage calibration applies to channels 1 and 2, lower voltage calibration applies to channels 3–6. Continuous episode of desynchronized sleep. The most striking increases in the pyramidal activity occur during the bursts of REM, associated with myoclonic twitches. Note in B a phasic abolition of the residual neck muscular activity which appears during the last burst of REM, together with an increase in pyramidal activity and myoclonic twitches. The arrow indicates arousal produced by acoustic stimulation (whistle) (MARCHIAFAVA and POMPEIANO, 1964b)

lary reticular formation (MAGOUN and RHINES, 1947). This activity is triggered by the same pontine mechanisms which are assumed to be responsible for the appearance of the tonic events during desynchronized sleep (cf. JOUVET, 1962, 1967).

In reference to the process of *phasic* inhibition of the spontaneous postural activity, which occurs synchronously with the REM bursts (Fig. 1B), it is worthwhile to anticipate here what will be mentioned later, namely that it is due to supraspinal descending volleys exerting presynaptic inhibition on the primary afferents (MORRISON and POMPEIANO, 1965c, d, 1966c).

A second phasic phenomenon that occurs during desynchronized sleep is represented by the rapid muscle contractions or twitches which appear at the time of the REM (cf. GASSEL et al., 1964c). The pattern and organization of these muscular contractions have been studied in unrestrained cats by recording simultaneously the activity from flexor and extensor muscles of proximal and distal parts of both hindlimbs and from the posterior neck muscles, both before and after section of spinal tracts and roots (GASSEL et al., 1964c). As pointed out previously, the muscular contractions appear predominantly during the episodes of REM (Fig. 1), *i.e.*, paradoxically just when a phasic increase of the inhibitory influences is present. This coincidence was particularly evident when the tonic EMG activity of the muscle was only partially depressed. The twitches usually occurred when the tonic muscle activity disappeared during the bursts of REM. The relationship between the depression of spontaneous muscle activity during REM and the simultaneous occurrence of muscular contractions may be of some importance for elucidating the nature of the influences acting on the motoneurons during sleep.

These large twitches are more likely to occur in association with the most intense and prolonged bursts of REM. However, some REM bursts may not be accompanied by muscular contractions, and when isolated ocular movements occur, no phasic change in muscular activity can be detected. Moreover muscle twitches, occurring independently of the outbursts of REM, may also be observed. Muscular contractions have been found in all hindlimb muscles tested. They are generally more prominent in flexor than extensor muscles and more frequent in distal than in proximal ones. In addition, twitches affect both red and white muscles.

Although some γ-fusimotor neurons can fire synchronously with REM (KUBOTA and TANAKA, 1966), the twitches are basically due to phasic excitatory influences acting directly upon the α-motoneurons. In fact section of the dorsal roots influences neither the frequency nor the pattern of the myoclonic jerks (GASSEL et al., 1964c).

Bilateral section of the ventral funicle and of the ventral half of the lateral funicle, where the descending efferent projections from the vestibular nuclei are located, does not result in any distinct alteration in muscular twitches occurring during desynchronized sleep (GASSEL et al., 1964c). However, a striking reduction of the twitches after ipsilateral section of the dorsolateral funicle indicates that some effective pathways are interrupted. It is of interest that all the supraspinal descending pathways running along the dorsolateral funicle do not affect motoneurons monosynaptically but through spinal interneurons (cf. LUND and POMPEIANO, 1965, 1968). The important descending tracts located in this region are the corticospinal, rubrospinal and reticulospinal tracts.

B. Activity of the Pyramidal Tract Neurons and the Red Nucleus

In the cat the corticospinal tract influences mainly the flexor motoneurons, this effect being mediated through the same interneurons of the flexion reflex pathway (LUNDBERG et al., 1962; LUNDBERG and VOORHOEVE, 1962). It has also been shown that the motor response to electrical stimulation of the red nucleus is specifically flexor in type (POMPEIANO, 1956, 1957, 1966b, 1967a). Recent investigation of the influence of the rubrospinal tract on the interneuronal pathway (HONGO et al., 1965) resulted in the hypothesis that phasic outbursts descending along these tracts are responsible for, or at least contribute to, the myoclonic twitches.

EVARTS (1964, 1965, 1967) recorded the discharge of single pyramidal tract neurons in the precentral gyrus of unanesthetized monkeys during natural sleep and wakefulness. He observed a similarity between the average unit activities in pyramidal tract neurons during wakefulness and during desynchronized sleep (cf. also ARDUINI et al., 1963). He found, however, striking differences in the temporal patterns of discharge during the two experimental conditions. While relaxed wakefulness was associated with a regular discharge, bursts of activity alternating with periods of silence appeared during synchronized sleep (cf. ADRIAN and MORUZZI, 1939); these bursts became much more intense and were separated by long intervals of complete inactivity during the desynchronized phase. Similar findings were also obtained by recording the unit activity in the red nucleus of the cat during physiological sleep (GASSEL et al., 1965c). Further analysis of the integrated activity of the pyramidal (MARCHIAFAVA and POMPEIANO, 1964a, b, 1966a) and extrapyramidal (rubral) discharges (GASSEL et al., 1965b, c) during desynchronized sleep has shown that the striking increase in the activity of the pyramidal tract originating from the precentral motor cortex and the red nucleus is related in time with the outbursts of REM (Fig. 1).[1] The muscular contractions, therefore, appear to be associated not only with the REM, as stated previously, but also with outbursts of pyramidal and rubral discharges. Ablation experiments indicate, however, that neither the pyramidal tract (MARCHIAFAVA and POMPEIANO, 1964a, b, 1966a) nor the rubrospinal tract (GASSEL et al., 1965b, c) is essential for the appearance of the muscular twitches.

This negative result would be understood if we knew the degree of effectiveness of the pyramidal volleys impinging upon the spinal motoneurons during the REM of desynchronized sleep. Observations by MARCHIAFAVA and POMPEIANO (1964a, b, 1966a), later confirmed (BALDISSERA and MANCIA, 1966; IWAMA and KAWAMOTO, 1966), showed that the motor effects produced by pyramidal (MARCHIAFAVA and POMPEIANO, 1964a, b, 1966a; BALDISSERA and MANCIA, 1966) and cortical stimulation (BALDISSERA and MANCIA, 1966; IWAMA and KAWAMOTO, 1966) are blocked during desynchronized sleep. Even the crossed flexor responses elicited by stimulation of the red nucleus (POMPEIANO, 1956, 1957) are tonically depressed during this phase of sleep (GASSEL et al., 1965b, c). Depression of the motoneuronal response to pyramidal and rubrospinal volleys is due to tonic postsynaptic inhibition of the α-motoneurons characteristic of desynchronized sleep (POMPEIANO, 1965, 1966a, 1967b).

When the pyramidal tract is repeatedly stimulated during the bursts of REM, it is unable to produce motor discharges, nor it is able to prolong the duration and the amplitude of the muscular twitches, when these contractions occurred spontaneously (MARCHIAFAVA and POMPEIANO, 1964a, b; 1966a). On the other hand, the response recorded in the contralateral sciatic nerve to repetitive stimulation

1 It is of interest that even the excitability of the motor cortex, as detected by recording the cortical response to pyramidal tract stimulation (ROSSI et al., 1965) or by recording from the pyramidal tract the efferent discharges of the corticospinal neurons elicited by single shock stimulation of the motor cortex, is modified during desynchronized sleep (DAGNINO et al., 1965d; FAVALE et al., 1965; IWAMA and KAWAMOTO, 1966). A specific result is that cortical responsiveness is phasically increased during the bursts of REM (DAGNINO et al., 1965d; FAVALE et al., 1965).

of the motor cortex, which is markedly reduced or abolished during desynchronized sleep, reappears during the bursts of REM (BALDISSERA et al., 1966c). This finding may be due, at least in part, to an increase in the excitability of cortical neurons occurring synchronously with the REM (DAGNINO et al., 1965d; FAVALE et al., 1965). Hence the phasic increase of pyramidal (and possibly also of the rubral) discharges cannot explain, exclusively at least, the appearance of muscular twitches during REM. The possibility must be considered that other supraspinal pathways are responsible for these muscular contractions. This possibility is only indirectly supported by the observation that the activity of single units recorded from the brain stem reticular formation increases phasically during the bursts of REM (HUTTENLOCHER, 1961; BIZZI et al., 1964c).

Summing up, the muscular contractions which occasionally appear during desynchronized sleep represent the phasic response of motoneurons to volleys descending from supraspinal structures, which become suddenly and transiently active mainly in correspondence with the outbursts of REM. The twitches occur whenever the excitatory volley is powerful enough to overwhelm the inhibitory barrage that characterizes the desynchronized phase of sleep.

III. Transmission of Sensory Input through Spinal Reflex Pathways during REM

A. Depression of the Mono- and Polysynaptic Reflexes

In an initial group of experiments (GIAQUINTO et al., 1963a, b, 1964a) we reported that the electrically-induced heteronymous monosynaptic reflexes of both extensor and flexor muscles as well as the polysynaptic reflexes produced by repetitive electrical stimulation of muscular afferents are strongly depressed throughout the desynchronized phase of sleep. These effects are due to inhibitory volleys arising from supraspinal structures and impinging upon the spinal segments (GIAQUINTO et al., 1963c, d, 1964b). In these experiments no phasic enhancement of inhibition could be demonstrated because the heteronymous monosynaptic reflexes were completely abolished.

It has been found, however, that other spinal reflexes are only partially depressed when the animal enters the desynchronized phase of sleep. This happens with the homonymous monosynaptic reflex elicited by single shock stimulation of group I afferents of the nerve supplying the muscle whose action potentials are being recorded. Also the polysynaptic reflexes are not entirely blocked by the desynchronized sleep when single shock stimulation excites a large number of group II and III afferents (GASSEL et al., 1964d, e). The demonstration that these spinal reflexes are only tonically depressed, but never abolished, has led to the observation that a further phasic depression occurs synchronously with the outbursts of REM (Fig. 2A–C) (GASSEL et al., 1964d, e; LENZI et al., 1968a, b).

Experiments carried out in free-moving, unanesthetized cats (KUBOTA et al., 1964, 1965; BALDISSERA et al., 1964b, c; TOKIZANE, 1966) and in man (HODES and DEMENT, 1964; HISHIKAWA and KANEKO, 1965; HISHIKAWA et al., 1965; SHIMIZU et al., 1966) have confirmed the tonic depression of both the monosynaptic (KUBOTA et al., 1964, 1965; BALDISSERA et al., 1964b, c; HODES and DEMENT,

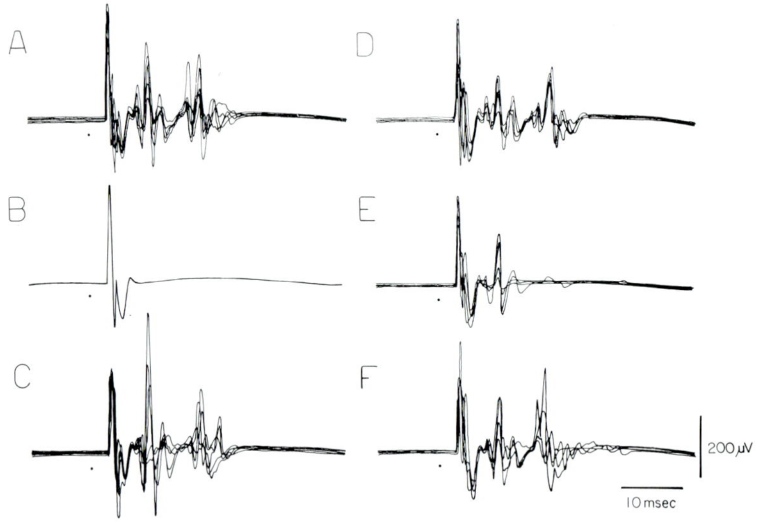

Fig. 2. Phasic inhibition of spinal reflexes during bursts of REM. Experiment made in the unrestrained, unanesthetized cat, 4 days after the permanent implantation of the electrodes. Stimulation of the left tibial nerve with rectangular pulses (0.07 msec duration, 1.25 times the threshold for the direct motor response) elicited an early monosynaptic reflex followed by a late polysynaptic response. The two reflexes, which follow the direct motor action potential, were recorded electromyographically from the left plantar muscles, before (A, D), during (B, E) and after (C, F) two bursts of REM. Both the monosynaptic and the polysynaptic reflexes are completely abolished during a large burst of REM (B). Note in E the abolition of the polysynaptic reflex but not of the monosynaptic reflex during a small burst of REM (LENZI et al., 1958a)

1964; HISHIKAWA and KANEKO, 1965; HISHIKAWA et al., 1965; SHIMIZU et al., 1966; TOKIZANE, 1966) and polysynaptic (BALDISSERA et al., 1964b, c; TOKIZANE, 1966) spinal reflexes. Even the phasic enhancement of the inhibitory influences in correspondence with the REM has been confirmed both in the animal experiments (BALDISSERA et al., 1964a, 1966a) and in man (HODES and DEMENT, 1964; STUART et al., 1965; SHIMIZU et al., 1966).

One may recall that the depression of spinal reflexes is particularly striking when the bursts of REM are not accompanied by twitches. The simultaneous occurrence of muscular contractions in the same muscle reduces the extent of the reflex depression brought about during the bursts of REM. Indeed the reflex response may be enhanced when strong twitches occur during lulls between the bursts of REM.

Thus, both the monosynaptic and the polysynaptic reflexes, which are tonically depressed during desynchronized sleep, show a further phasic depression during the bursts of REM, characteristic of this phase of sleep. When muscular contractions appear during the outbursts of REM, the monosynaptic reflexes simultaneously induced in the homonymous muscle are only moderately depressed but not completely abolished.

B. Presynaptic Inhibition of the Group I Muscular Afferents

Experiments summarized in previous reports (POMPEIANO, 1966a, 1967b) have shown that the excitability of the motoneurons to antidromic (GASSEL et al., 1964f, 1965a) and direct stimulation (MORRISON and POMPEIANO, 1965a, b, 1966b) is tonically depressed during the desynchronized phase of sleep, *i.e.*, during the tonic depression of the spinal reflexes. For reasons which have been discussed in the full papers (loc. cit.), it is concluded that this effect is due to postsynaptic inhibition of the α-motoneurons.

The phasic depression of monosynaptic and polysynaptic reflexes that occurs during REM, at least in the absence of muscular twitches, cannot be explained by a mechanism of postsynaptic inhibition, since no phasic enhancement in the depression of the response of the α-motoneurons to their antidromic or direct stimulation could be detected. It has been suggested therefore that these phasic phenomena are due to presynaptic inhibition of the primary afferents.

Experiments in which the excitability of the spinal endings of group I muscle afferents was tested according to WALL's method (1958) support the presynaptic hypothesis (MORRISON and POMPEIANO, 1965c, d, 1966c). The experiments were performed on unrestrained, unanesthetized cats following complete deafferentation of the hindleg of one side. The excitability of group I primary afferent fibers was tested by recording the antidromic responses to single shocks applied unipolarly to the ventral horns through a stainless steel microelectrode (100 KΩ–600 KΩ) chronically implanted and completely insulated. The tibial and the deep peroneal nerves were dissected and mounted on chronically implanted bipolar electrodes so that the antidromic response to ventral horn stimulation could be recorded in either the extensor (tibial) or flexor (deep peroneal) muscle afferents.

Rectangular pulses (0.05 msec at 1.5–2/sec) were used at a strength of 1.2–1.8 times the threshold for the antidromic response. Because the ventral roots had been cut (de-efferentation), the spike potential recorded from the muscle nerves could only be due to impulses propagating, antidromically, along afferent fibers. Measurements of conduction velocity indicated that group I afferent fibers (120–80 m/sec) were involved in the antidromic response. The size of the spike potential was taken as a measure of the number of group I fibers excited by the stimulus.

There was no significant change in the mean amplitude and standard deviation of the group I antidromic volley during transition from quiet waking to drowsiness or to synchronized sleep, nor was there any significant change in these values found during desynchronized sleep in the absence of REM. The main change in excitability of the central terminals of group I afferent fibers occurred during desynchronized sleep, where a phasic increase of the antidromic volley appeared at the time of the large bursts of REM (Fig. 3). The more intense the REM burst, the greater was the enhancement. The antidromic response of the group I afferent fibers was then increased up to 110–140% of the mean value observed during synchronized sleep, both in tibial and deep peroneal nerves. The increase in excitability of the group I muscle afferent fibers during REM can be referred to presynaptic depolarization of the central endings of the primary afferents due to

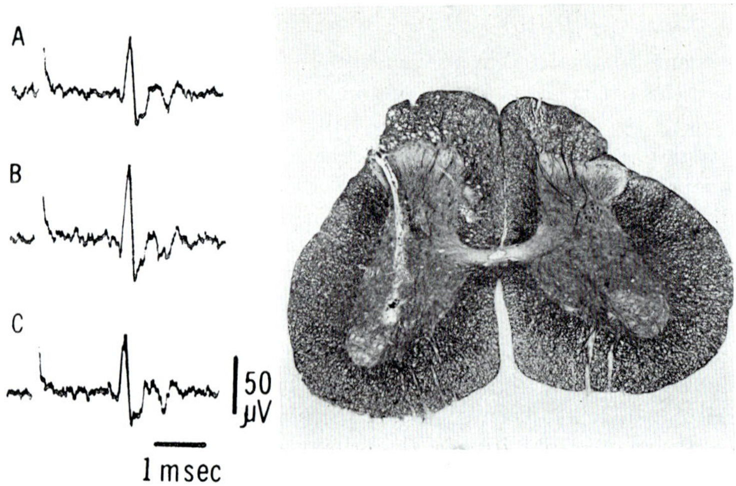

Fig. 3. Increase in amplitude of the antidromic group I volley during a REM period of desynchronized sleep in the unrestrained, unanesthetized cat. Experiment made 2 days after implantation of the electrodes and section of the left ventral roots (L5–S2). A stainless steel microelectrode (600 KΩ) was permanently inserted into the motoneuronal pool supplying the left tibial nerve. Rectangular pulses were used (0.05 msec duration, 1.62 times the threshold for the antidromic group I volley recorded from the left tibial nerve). The records show the antidromic potential recorded from group I afferent fibers of left tibial nerve following stimulation of ventral horn terminals before (A), during (B) and after (C) a burst of REM. The electrolytic lesion in the ventral horn of lower L7 indicates the position of the stimulating spinal cord electrode (MORRISON and POMPEIANO, 1965d)

supraspinal descending volleys. This effect would lead to a reduced postsynaptic efficacy of the orthodromic volley, *i.e.*, to presynaptic inhibition (ECCLES, 1964).

BALDISSERA et al. (1965a) were unable to find any increase in the antidromic group I volley during desynchronized sleep. However, after publication of our reports showing that an increase in the excitability of the group I primary afferents occurred during the bursts of REM (MORRISON and POMPEIANO, 1965c, d), the last group of investigators confirmed our finding (BALDISSERA et al., 1965b, 1966b).

In summary, during desynchronized sleep supraspinal descending volleys exert a depolarizing action on the central terminals of group I primary afferents. This influence is phasic in nature and is related in time only with the large bursts of REM. This terminal depolarization is known to be responsible for presynaptic inhibition, which in turn would account for the striking depression of the homonymous monosynaptic reflex that occurs during the bursts of REM.

C. Presynaptic Inhibition of the Flexion Reflex Afferents

The phasic depression of the polysynaptic reflex that occurs synchronously with the bursts of REM can be due either to presynaptic inhibition of the primary afferents responsible for the flexion reflex [flexion reflex afferents (FRA): ECCLES and LUNDBERG, 1959] or to postsynaptic effects on the interneurons responsible for the flexion reflex. The experiments reported here provide only indirect evidence in support of the first hypothesis (MORRISON and POMPEIANO, 1965e, f).

Experiments reported above showed that the increase in the pyramidal discharge that occurs during desynchronized sleep (EVARTS, 1964, 1965, 1967) appears to be synchronous with the bursts of REM (MARCHIAFAVA and POMPEIANO, 1964a, b, 1966a). This effect is due in part to corticospinal volleys arising from the motor cortex, since it can still be observed after bilateral ablation of the sensory cortical areas SI and SII (MARCHIAFAVA and POMPEIANO, 1964a, b, 1966a).

The corticospinal fibers, however, are not exclusively involved in the transmission to α-motoneurons of volleys arising from the motor cortex. Electrical stimulation of the sensorimotor cortex of the cat is followed in fact by depolarization of the primary afferent endings of both cutaneous and high threshold muscle afferents (ANDERSEN et al., 1962, 1964e; CARPENTER et al., 1962b, 1963). Although this effect is produced by electrical stimulation not only of the sensory areas SI and SII but also of the motor (precruciate) cortex, experimental evidence indicates that the precruciate cortex depolarizes the primary afferents not directly, *i.e.*, through its own projection pathway, but indirectly, through synaptic activation of neurons in the postcruciate cortex. Observations made by MORRISON and POMPEIANO (1965e, f) indicate that after ablation of the precruciate area there is still a phasic increase in the corticofugal discharge during desynchronized sleep which originates from the somatosensory areas of the cortex (SI and SII). Acute experiments performed in these animals after decerebration showed that stimulation of the pyramidal tract up to 49 days after ablation of the precruciate area (*i.e.*, when the corticofugal fibers originating from the motor cortex were partially

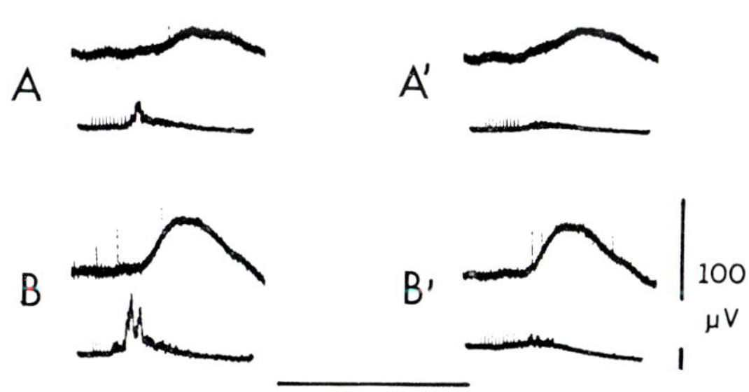

Fig. 4. Dorsal root potentials and ventral root discharges evoked by pyramidal stimulation. The upper traces were recorded from a dorsal root filament (upper L7), on the right side. The filament was cut 15 mm from the dorsal root entry zone and placed on two electrodes, one close to the entry zone and the other on the cut end. Upwards deflection denotes negativity of the central electrode. The lower traces were recorded from ventral roots L7–S1, on the right side. A, B: control records taken from a cat with sensorimotor cortex intact. A′, B′: records taken from another experiment, after ablation of the left motor cortex. Experiment made forty-nine days after cortical topectomy. A, B and A′, B′: effects of repetitive stimulation of the left pyramid at the medullary level above the *decussatio* with a train of 10 shocks at 500/sec, 1.0 msec in duration, and at intensities 1.5 (*A*, *A′*), and 2.5 (*B*, B′) times the threshold for dorsal root potentials. The cats were anesthetized with Nembutal, paralyzed with Flaxedil, and artificially respired (MORRISON and POMPEIANO, 1965f)

or completely degenerated) produced a ventral root discharge which was strikingly reduced or even abolished, as compared to results from intact animals used as controls. However the dorsal root potentials elicited by this pyramidal stimulation were about the same in both size and shape in the experimental and the control animals (Fig. 4).

Since the dorsal root potentials elicited by pyramidal volleys are attributed to presynaptic depolarization of the FRA (Andersen et al., 1962, 1964e; Carpenter et al., 1962b, 1963) one can conclude that the pyramidal mechanisms responsible for this effect are operative during the REM of desynchronized sleep. They may at least contribute to the phasic depression of the polysynaptic reflexes synchronous with the bursts of REM (Gassel et al., 1964d, e). It should be pointed out, however, that a phasic depression of the polysynaptic reflex during REM can still be observed after bilateral ablation of the sensorimotor cortex.

Summing up, the pyramidal discharge originating from the somatosensory cortex increases phasically during desynchronized sleep particularly at the time of the bursts of REM. These volleys might contribute, through a mechanism of presynaptic inhibition, to the phasic depression of the polysynaptic reflex that occurs during the bursts of REM.

D. Postsynaptic Effects on the Interneurons of the Polysynaptic Reflex Pathway

It has been reported elsewhere that the amount of the depression of spinal reflexes during desynchronized sleep may vary according to the different motoneuronal population tested (Gassel and Pompeiano, 1965a, b). If one could, however, submit the *same* motoneuronal pool to reflex excitation through both the monosynaptic and the polysynaptic reflex pathways during desynchronized sleep, then one would know whether there is a difference in the amount of depression of the polysynaptic as compared to the monosynaptic reflex during the *same* bursts of REM. We found recently (Pompeiano, 1968b) that when a single shock is applied to the tibial nerve, it is possible to record from the intrinsic plantar muscles not only a monosynaptic reflex, but also a late response, which is polysynaptic in nature since it occurs at a latency of about 20 msec.

An analysis of the modulation during sleep of the mono- and polysynaptic reflexes involving the *same* motoneuronal population (Lenzi et al., 1968a, b) has shown that both these reflexes are phasically depressed at the time of the REM (Fig. 2). However the amount of the depression is generally greater for the polysynaptic than for the monosynaptic reflex. This occurs in spite of the fact that any reduction in amplitude of the monosynaptic reflex would allow a larger fraction of the motoneuronal pool to be available for the late polysynaptic excitation. The greater depression of the polysynaptic as compared to the monosynaptic reflex involving the *same* motoneuronal population during the *same* bursts of REM could be referred to postsynaptic effects on the interneurons of the polysynaptic reflex pathway (inhibition, occlusion). Summing up, evidence is presented suggesting that the interneurons of the polysynaptic reflex pathway are influenced by supraspinal descending volleys, thus contributing to the phasic depression of the polysynaptic reflex that occurs during the REM of desynchronized sleep.

IV. Transmission of Sensory Input through the Cuneate Nucleus during REM

A. Depression of the Orthodromic Lemniscal Response

It might be asked whether the depressed transmission of somatic afferent volleys through spinal reflex pathways occurring during the REM periods of desynchronized sleep is also associated with a reduced transmission of somatic afferent volleys through spinal ascending systems.

Carli et al. (1966a, 1967a) found that the orthodromic lemniscal response elicited in the unrestrained, unanesthetized cat by single shock stimulation of the superficial radial nerve did not show any significant change in amplitude during transition from quiet waking to synchronized sleep. Nor did they find a significant

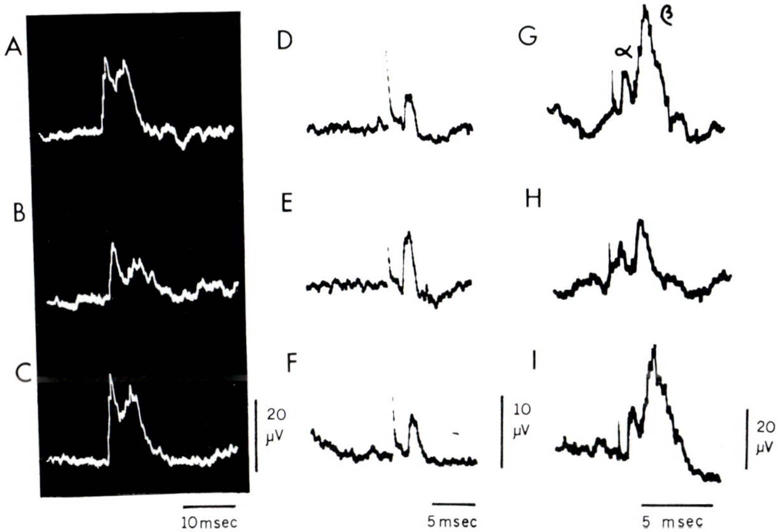

Fig. 5. Synaptic transmission of somatic afferent volleys through the cuneate nucleus during bursts of REM in unrestrained, unanesthetized cats. A–C: Phasic depression of the orthodromic lemniscal response during a burst of REM. Experiment performed 2 days after permanent implantation of the electrodes. Stimulation of the left superficial radial nerve with 0.05 msec rectangular pulses, 3 times the threshold for the orthodromic lemniscal responses recorded from the right medial lemniscus. The records illustrate the orthodromic lemniscal response recorded before (A), during (B) and after (C) a burst of REM. D–F: Phasic increase in amplitude of the antidromic group II cutaneous volley during a REM period. Experiment made 2 days after implantation of the electrodes. Stimulation of the left cuneate nucleus with 0.02 msec rectangular pulses, 2 times the threshold for the antidromic response of group II cutaneous fibers of the left superficial radial nerve. The records illustrate the antidromic response recorded before (D), during (E) and after (F) a burst of REM. G–I: Phasic depressions of the lemniscal responses to direct stimulation of the cuneate nucleus during a burst of REM. Experiment made 5 days after implantation of the electrodes. Stimulation of the left cuneate nucleus with 0.05 msec rectangular pulses, 2.15 times the threshold for the direct responses recorded from the right medial lemniscus. The response consists of an initial α-spike followed by a much more prolonged β potential. The records indicate the response recorded before (G), during (H) and after (I) a burst of REM (Carli et al., 1967a, b)

difference in the amplitude of the evoked potentials observed during desynchronized sleep as compared with those during the synchronized phase. This finding is different from that which occurs in the spinal cord, where both the monosynaptic and the polysynaptic reflexes are tonically depressed during this phase of sleep. However, similarly to the responses involving the spinal reflexes even the orthodromic lemniscal responses were phasically depressed during the large bursts of REM (Fig. 5A–C). This effect is still present after section of the ipsilateral dorsolateral funicle, performed at high cervical level. With this section the spinocervical (Morin's) pathway is interrupted. It is concluded that the modulation during sleep of the orthodromic lemniscal response is due mainly to reduced transmission of somatic afferent volleys through the dorsal column pathway.

The phasic depression of the lemniscal response is not due to interaction between the electrically induced ingoing volley and the proprioceptive afferent volleys related to the appearance of muscular twitches, since it is still present after bilateral section of the dorsal half of the lateral funicles, performed at high cervical level (CARLI et al., 1967a). This lesion prevents the normal occurrence of the muscular contractions during intense outbursts of REM (GASSEL et al., 1964c).

Summing up, a phasic depression of the orthodromic lemniscal response occurs during the bursts of REM. This effect is still present after interruption of the spinocervical (Morin's) pathway, thus indicating that somatic afferent transmission through the cuneate nucleus is phasically depressed during desynchronized sleep.

B. Presynaptic Inhibition of the Group II Cutaneous and the Group I Muscular Afferents to the Cuneate Nucleus

Experiments have been performed to determine whether mechanisms of presynaptic and postsynaptic inhibition (cf. ANDERSEN et al., 1964a–d) could be responsible for the changes in the synaptic transmission occurring at the level of the dorsal column nuclei during desynchronized sleep, particularly at the time of the REM (CARLI et al., 1966b–d, 1967b). In particular the presynaptic hypothesis was tested by studying the sleep-produced excitability changes of the cutaneous and muscular afferents to the cuneate nucleus, close to their synaptic terminals. The experiments were performed in unrestrained, unanesthetized cats. The excitability of the primary afferents was tested using WALL's method (1958), by recording from the superficial and the deep radial nerves the antidromic responses to single shocks applied unipolarly to the cuneate nucleus through a stainless steel microelectrode (300 KΩ–1 MΩ) completely insulated except at the tip.

There were no significant changes in the mean amplitude and standard deviation of the antidromic group II cutaneous or group I muscular volleys recorded respectively from the superficial or the deep radial nerve during quiet wakefulness, synchronized sleep or desynchronized sleep in the absence of REM. An enhancement of the antidromic volleys occurred only during the REM characteristics of desynchronized sleep (Fig. 5 D–F). The higher the repetition rate of the ocular movements within the REM burst, the greater was the increase of the antidromic response.

Summing up, the antidromic group II cutaneous volley and the antidromic group I muscular volley recorded from the superficial and the deep radial nerves respectively are phasically enhanced during the bursts of REM. This increased excitability of the central endings of the cuneate tract fibers is considered an indication of the presynaptic depolarization of the terminals of the primary afferents within the cuneate nucleus, an effect which is considered the cause of presynaptic inhibition on synaptic transmission through the cuneate nucleus.

C. Postsynaptic Inhibition of the Cuneothalamic Relay Neurons

Andersen et al. (1964a) showed that when a brief current pulse is applied through a microelectrode in the cuneate nucleus, an initial brief positive spike (α-spike), followed by a much more prolonged and complex positive potential (β-spike), can be recorded from the lemniscal tract. Similar potentials were recorded in our experiments (Carli et al., 1966b–d, 1967b) where single shock stimulation of the cuneate nucleus was performed in unrestrained, unanesthetized cat through a chronically implanted microelectrode, while the evoked potential was recorded from the contralateral medial lemniscus with a bipolar electrode.

In agreement with the findings of Andersen et al. (1964a), the latency of the initial spike (α-spike) was so short (0.7–0.8 msec) that it must be due to impulses generated by direct stimulation of cuneate neurons or their axons. The secondary or β-spike had a latency that was 0.7–0.8 msec longer than the α-spike and so was just long enough for one synaptic delay; hence it can be attributed to direct excitation of presynaptic fibers and consequent synaptic excitation of cuneate neurons.

There was no tonic change of cuneate cell excitability during relaxed wakefulness, synchronized sleep or desynchronized sleep. Only during the large bursts of REM was there a phasic depression of both the α- and β-spikes. However the degree of depression was greater for the β-spike than for the α-spike (Fig. 5G–I).

It has been clearly shown that the test for α-spike depression provides a direct assessement of postsynaptic inhibition of cuneothalamic relay neurons (Andersen et al., 1964a). Therefore the depression of the α-excitability during the desynchronized phase of sleep indicates that hyperpolarization, possibly due to postsynaptic inhibition, affects the cuneothalamic relay neurons during REM. The depression of the β-spike during REM is more difficult to interpret. We have shown that the presynaptic depolarization of the primary afferents to the cuneate nucleus produced by REM results in a large increase in the number of presynaptic fibers being excited. The resulting increase in the number of presynaptic fibers excited by the test stimulus would tend to increase the size of the β-spike. This increase has to be weighed against i) the depression of synaptic excitation that results from presynaptic depolarization, *i.e.*, presynaptic inhibition, and ii) the depression that results from the postsynaptic hyperpolarization, *i.e.*, postsynaptic inhibition. In summary, both mechanisms of presynaptic and postsynaptic inhibition occur during the bursts of REM.

Summing up, the excitability of the cuneate neurons was tested during sleep and wakefulness. A depression of the direct excitability of the cuneothalamic relay neurons occurs particularly during REM, an effect which is attributed to postsynaptic inhibitory action. This postsynaptic inhibitory mechanism of synaptic transmission in the cuneate nucleus, together with the presynaptic mechanism documented in the previous section, contributes to the phasic depression of transmission of somatic afferent volleys through the cuneate nucleus, which also occurs during desynchronized sleep at the time of REM.

V. Transmission of Sensory Input through the Lateral Geniculate Nucleus during REM

A. Activity Recorded from the Lateral Geniculate Nucleus

Monophasic potentials 100–300 μV in amplitude, about 100 msec in duration, appear during desynchronized sleep in the pontine reticular formation (JOUVET et al., 1959; JOUVET, 1962) and also in the lateral geniculate nucleus (LGN) (MIKITEN et al., 1961; JOUVET, 1962; BIZZI and BROOKS, 1963; BROOKS and BIZZI, 1963; HENDLEY, 1963; MOURET et al., 1963; MICHEL et al., 1964a, b; MOURET, 1964; JEANNEROD, 1965; BROOKS, 1967a, b). As described by BIZZI and BROOKS (1963), they occur synchronously in both these structures, and they are related in time with the ocular movements (cf. BROOKS and BIZZI, 1963).

The observations that i) geniculate responses, having the same temporal behavior of the spontaneous potentials, can be evoked by single shock stimulation of pontine structures during desynchronized sleep (BIZZI and BROOKS, 1963), and ii) that they can be abolished by certain brain-stem lesions (HOBSON, 1965), indicate the existence of an extraretinal input upon the LGN during this phase of sleep, originating from the pontine reticular formation (BROOKS and BIZZI, 1963; JEANNEROD, 1965).

The activity of single geniculate neurons during desynchronized sleep has been recently recorded in the intact cat. If both unit and mass discharges were recorded from the LGN simultaneously, it was found that the ongoing unit activity was temporarily suppressed during the geniculate waves, but following its subsidence, the units fired in burst temporarily (SAKAKURA and IWAMA, 1966). A detailed analysis of this pattern of discharge (BIZZI, 1966b) indicated that in most of the geniculate cells a silent period of about 15–20 msec corresponding to the rising phase of the geniculate waves was followed by a burst of discharge. Each burst began at the peak of the wave or immediately after it and continued on the descending phase of the wave for about 100 msec. Bursts of discharges were also recorded during desynchronized sleep from optic radiations (GARDNER-MEDWIN, 1967).

The phasic increase in the discharge of geniculate neurons cannot be the result of a modulation of tonic retinofugal discharge (BENOIT, 1964a), nor can it be attributed to afferent discharge from eye muscle proprioceptors, because similar effects were also obtained following enucleation of eyes and extraocular muscles (BIZZI, 1966b). One can hypothesize that the phasic discharges of lateral geniculate neurons are the result of the activity of oculomotor centers located in the brain stem.

The simplest way to interpret these findings is that this premotor center controlling the oculomotor activity during desynchronized sleep sends excitatory volleys on the LGN neurons, particularly at the time of REM.

Summing up, most of the lateral geniculate neurons show bursts of high frequency discharge which are related in time with the monophasic geniculate potentials and the ocular movements characteristic of the desynchronized phase of sleep.

B. Orthodromic Transmission through the Lateral Geniculate Nucleus

It has been clearly shown that the orthodromic response of the lateral geniculate neurons to electrical stimulation of the primary optic fibers, which is minimum during synchronized sleep, increased during wakefulness and even more so in desynchronized sleep. These results were obtained by recording the postsynaptic response of the lateral geniculate neurons from the LGN (SAKAKURA and IWAMA, 1965; BIZZI, 1966a; IWAMA and KASAMATSU, 1966; IWAMA et al., 1966; KASAMATSU and IWAMA, 1966), the geniculocortical radiation (FAVALE et al., 1964; DAGNINO et al., 1967) and the visual cortex (BENOIT, 1964b; CORDEAU et al., 1965; DAGNINO et al., 1965c). The conclusion of these experiments is that the responsiveness of the lateral geniculate nucleus to orthodromic stimulation is larger during desynchronized sleep than in wakefulness, while it is reduced during synchronized sleep (OKUMA and FUJIMORI, 1963; CORDEAU et al., 1965; DAGNINO et al., 1965c; WALSH and CORDEAU, 1965; PALESTINI et al., 1965, 1967).[2] All of the preceding effects persisted throughout the episodes of desynchronized sleep. It should be mentioned here that the responses elicited by flashes at the level of the retina and of the optic nerve do not show any change during this phase of sleep (MOURET et al., 1963; PALESTINI et al., 1967).

One may now ask whether transmission through the lateral geniculate nucleus is modified during the phasic events of desynchronized sleep. Unfortunately the evidence on this subject is contradictory. It appears in fact that transmission of impulses through the LGN elicited by electrical shock stimulation of the optic tract increases phasically during the REM and also during the lateral geniculate waves occurring either spontaneously (DAGNINO et al., 1965b; IWAMA and SAKAKURA, 1965; IWAMA et al., 1966; IWAMA and KASAMATSU, 1966; SAKAKURA and IWAMA, 1966; cf. BIZZI, 1966a) or induced by stimulation of the pontine reticular formation (DAGNINO et al., 1966b).[3] On the other hand, the LGN postsynaptic responses to a flash of light are apparently reduced in amplitude during the lateral geniculate waves (JEANNEROD, 1965; BIZZI, 1966a).

The discrepancy between responses elicited by electrical and photic stimulation has been found not only at the geniculate but also at the cortical level. It is of interest that while the amplitude of both the presynaptic and the postsynaptic

2 It is of interest that even the responsiveness of the LGN to direct stimulation of the geniculate structure (ROSSI et al., 1965; WALSH and CORDEAU, 1965; DAGNINO et al., 1965c; PALESTINI et al., 1967) or to antidromic stimulation of the optic radiation (IWAMA and KASAMATSU, 1966) is larger during desynchronized sleep than during wakefulness. On the contrary it is reduced in amplitude during synchronized sleep.

3 Similarly the responsiveness of the LGN to antidromic stimulation of the optic radiation increases in amplitude at the peak of the lateral geniculate wave. This facilitation of the antidromic response has been ascribed to phasic depolarization of the cell bodies of the lateral geniculate neurons (IWAMA and KASAMATSU, 1966).

components of the cortical-evoked potentials elicited in the visual areas by electrical stimulation of the optic tract or chiasma increases phasically during the REM as well as during the monophasic lateral geniculate waves (Dagnino et al., 1965a, 1966a, 1967), the responses evoked by flashes diminish in amplitude or disappear at this time (Mouret et al., 1963). The latter finding, however, has not been confirmed by Jeanneron (1965). All these findings will be discussed later. We can simply anticipate here that during the ocular movements of desynchronized sleep, the postsynaptic excitation of the lateral geniculate neurons is associated with presynaptic depolarization of the primary optic tract endings.

Summing up, the orthodromic transmission through the lateral geniculate nucleus of volleys running along the primary optic fibers increases tonically throughout the desynchronized sleep. During the geniculate potentials associated with the ocular movements typical of this phase of sleep, orthodromic transmission can either be facilitated or depressed.

C. Presynaptic Inhibition of the Primary Optic Fibers

Recent observations performed in unrestrained, unanesthetized animals (Sakakura and Iwama, 1965; Bizzi, 1966a; Iwama and Kasamatsu, 1966; Iwama et al., 1966; Kasamatsu and Iwama, 1966) have shown that i) the presynaptic spike in the LGN following orthodromic electrical stimulation of the optic tract is reduced during geniculate waves and ii) the excitability of the intrageniculate endings of optic fibers is enhanced during the LGN waves, particularly related in time with the REM. The reduction of the presynaptic spike in the LGN following orthodromic stimulation as well as the increase of optic tract antidromic response during REM indicates a depolarization of optic nerve terminals. A positive Wall's test (1958) is generally regarded as major evidence in favor of presynaptic inhibition.

Summing up, during desynchronized sleep there is a presynaptic depolarization of the central endings of the primary optic fibers to the LGN. This effect occurs only during the geniculate potentials associated with the ocular movements typical of desynchronized sleep.

VI. Transmission of Sensory Volleys through the Thalamic Nuclei during REM

Accumulated evidence indicates that during desynchronized sleep the transmission of somatic centripetal impulses elicited either by peripheral stimulation (Favale et al., 1963c, 1965; Albe-Fessard et al., 1964; Guilband and Yamaguchi, 1964; Guilband and Kummer, 1965) or by central lemniscal (Favale et al., 1963b, c, 1965; Allison, 1965; Dagnino et al., 1967) or thalamic (Pisano et al., 1962; Favale et al., 1963b, c, 1965; Rossi et al., 1965; Allison, 1965) stimulations is constantly facilitated at the level of the nucleus ventralis posterolateralis (VPL) of the thalamus (cf. also Dagnino et al., 1965c). This facilitation lasts throughout the episode of desynchronized sleep. There is also a constant parallelism between the facilitation of the thalamic responses and that of the cortical ones (cf. also Favale et al., 1963a). Moreover a further increase in the lemniscocortical (ALLISON, 1965; DAGNINO et al., 1965a, 1967) and thalamocortical responses (ALLISON, 1965) has been found to occur synchronously with the REM. It has been mentioned previously that the neurons of the somatosensory cortex show bursts of high frequency discharge (EVARTS, 1964, 1965, 1967) that are related in time with the trains of REM (MARCHIAFAVA and POMPEIANO, 1964a, b, 1966a; MORRISON and POMPEIANO, 1965e, f).

A certain parallelism can be found between transmission of somatic afferent volleys through the VPL nucleus of the thalamus and transmission of the optic nerve volleys through the thalamic (geniculate) station of the visual pathways. It was shown in the previous section that transmission through the LGN is tonically facilitated during desynchronized sleep, while a further phasic facilitation may occur during the bursts of REM.

Similarly an increase in cortical responsiveness in the visual areas was found during desynchronized sleep which persisted throughout this phase of sleep (BENOIT, 1964b; FAVALE et al., 1964; CORDEAU et al., 1965; WALSH and CORDEAU, 1965; Rossi et al., 1965; DAGNINO et al., 1965c; PALESTINI et al., 1967). Moreover, superimposed on these tonic changes, phasic increases in cortical responsiveness were also found to occur at irregular intervals of the desynchronized episodes. This further increase appeared during the monophasic lateral geniculate waves as well as during the bursts of REM (DAGNINO et al., 1965a, 1966a, 1967). The latter finding is of particular interest since during desynchronized sleep monophasic waves appear not only in the pontogeniculate system, but also in the visual cortex (MOURET et al., 1963; MICHEL et al., 1964a; JEANNEROD, 1965; JEANNEROD et al., 1965a; BROOKS, 1967b). They are probably correlated with the bursts of high frequency discharge recorded from single units in the visual cortex during the REM periods of desynchronized sleep (EVARTS, 1962, 1965; VALLEALA, 1967).

Summing up, the responses evoked in the specific cortical (somatosensory and visual) areas during stimuli applied at the prethalamic level (medial lemniscus, optic tract) increase tonically during desynchronized sleep and phasically at the time of the REM. These observations are attributed to phenomena of thalamic and probably also of cortical facilitation.

VII. Central Mechanisms Responsible for the Motor Activities during REM

A. Vestibular Influences on the Oculomotor Nuclei

Experiments were performed in order to localize the structures responsible for the REM and the related phasic contractions affecting the skeletal muscles. We concentrated our attention on the vestibular complex, because the second-order vestibular neurons connect directly with the oculomotor nuclei and control their activity (cf. BRODAL et al., 1962). It was then assumed that the vestibular nuclei which control eye movements were involved during the outbursts of REM of desynchronized sleep. A microelectrode analysis of the spontaneous activity of the vestibular nuclei performed in the unrestrained, unanesthetized cat during natural sleep and wakefulness has shown that most of the neurons localized in the medial and descending vestibular nuclei but not in the lateral vestibular nuclei increase their activity during desynchronized sleep (BIZZI et al., 1964a–c). In particular the pattern of discharge consists of bursts of rapid firing (80 to 160 spikes per second) which are invariably associated with the ocular movements typical of this phase of sleep (Fig. 6).

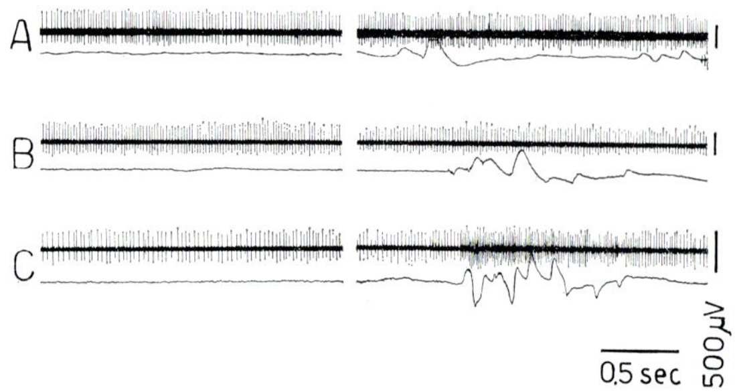

Fig. 6. Activity of vestibular neurons during sleep. Spontaneous discharge of single units recorded in unrestrained, unanesthetized cat from lateral (A), superior (B), and medial (C) vestibular nucleus during synchronized sleep (left column) and during the episodes of rapid eye movements occurring in desynchronized sleep (right column). Upper records show the unit activity; lower records show the eye movements recorded from electrodes placed above the orbit. Voltage calibrations apply to the units (BIZZI et al., 1964c)

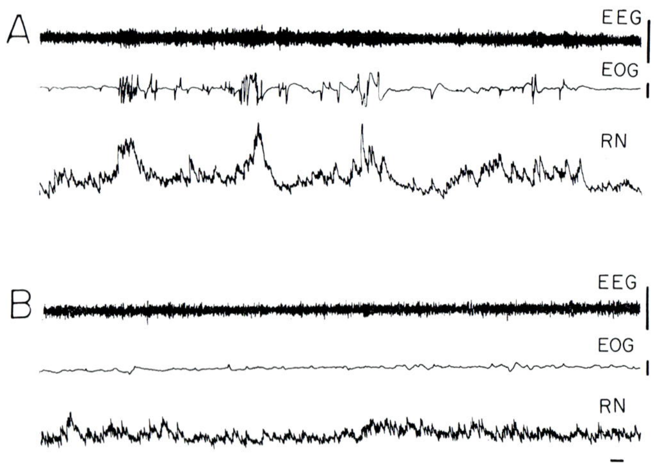

Fig. 7. Phasic increase in the rubral activity during the REM of desynchronized sleep, and its abolition following vestibular lesion. Unrestrained, unanesthetized cat. Bipolar records. EEG: electroencephalogram (left parieto-occipital); EOG: electro-oculogram; RN: integrated red nucleus activity. Time calibration: 1 sec. Voltage calibration: 0.5 mV. A. Experiment made 3 days after permanent implantation of the electrodes. During desynchronized sleep there are large phasic increases in the rubral discharge which are strikingly related in time with the bursts of REM. B. Same animal as in A. Experiment made 7 days after permanent implantation of the electrodes and 2 days after bilateral lesion of the medial and descending vestibular nuclei. Absence during desynchronized sleep of the large bursts of REM and related phasic enhancements of rubral discharge (POMPEIANO and SATOH, 1967)

The increased activity of the units localized in the medial and descending vestibular nuclei indicates that these structures are in some way related to the REM occurring during desynchronized sleep. The crucial proof was provided by lesions of the vestibular nuclei (Pompeiano and Morrison, 1965a, b, 1966b). The most impressive finding of these experiments is the demonstration that after well-defined vestibular lesions, the episodes of desynchronized sleep are still characterized by typical low voltage, fast activity in the EEG and by complete electrical silence of the cervical antigravity muscles. However the typical bursts of REM are abolished (Fig. 7). The abolition of these bursts of REM lasted throughout the survival of the animal, *i.e.*, up to 36 days after the lesion. Histologic controls indicated that a complete and persistent abolition of the REM occurs only when the lesion affects completely the medial and descending vestibular nuclei on both sides in their entire rostrocaudal extent. Bilateral and symmetrical lesions of either the superior or the lateral vestibular (Deiters') nucleus do not prevent the appearance of the bursts of REM.

The abolition of the REM is due neither to interruption of primary vestibular fibers nor to lesion of cerebellofugal fibers which cross the area of the vestibular regions before reaching the brain stem (Walberg et al., 1962a, b). A regular occurrence of REM could still be observed after bilateral chronic section of the vestibular nerves or complete cerebellectomy (Pompeiano and Morrison, 1965a, b, 1966b; cf. Jouvet, 1962). The conclusion was drawn that the vestibular nuclei represent a necessary link in the causal chain of events leading to the activation of the oculomotor nuclei, which is responsible for the outbursts of REM.

B. Vestibular Influences on the Pyramidal Tract Neurons and the Red Nucleus

After the demonstration that the vestibular nuclei are responsible for the oculomotor activity during the REM bursts, an attempt was made to determine i) whether the increase in the pyramidal and rubral discharge related in time with the REM depends upon the integrity of the vestibular nuclei, and ii) whether the destruction of these nuclei also prevents the appearance of the muscular twitches (Morrison and Pompeiano, 1965h, 1966a).

Bilateral destruction of the medial and descending vestibular nuclei did not abolish the modulation of the integrated pyramidal discharge during synchronized sleep. Only the phasic enhancement of the integrated pyramidal activity related in time with the large bursts of REM disappeared. Even the phasic increases in rubral activity related in time with the large bursts of REM depend upon ascending vestibular volleys, since they disappeared following vestibular lesion (Fig. 7) (Pompeiano and Satoh, 1967). This effect, however, did not require the presence of the sensorimotor cortex, since it could still be observed after ablation of this cortical region, from which the corticorubral projection originates.

It is of interest that even the large muscular contractions which occurred synchronously with the REM were abolished by the vestibular lesions (Morrison and Pompeiano, 1965h, 1966a).

Summing up, a complete, bilateral lesion of the medial and descending vestibular nuclei abolishes the typical bursts of REM. In this experimental condition the episodes of desynchronized sleep are simply characterized by the typical low-voltage, fast activity in the EEG and by complete abolition of neck muscular activity. The integrity of the medial and descending vestibular nuclei is necessary not only for the occurrence of the bursts of REM during desynchronized sleep, but also for the appearance of the phasic increases in the pyramidal and rubral discharge and of the related muscular contractions.

VIII. Central Mechanisms Responsible for Inhibition of Sensory Transmission during REM

A. Vestibular Control of Somatic Afferent Transmission in the Spinal Cord

Analysis of spontaneous and reflex muscular activity during desynchronized sleep indicates that supraspinal inhibitory influences, namely those presynaptic in nature, impinge upon the spinal reflex pathways during the typical outbursts of REM (Morrison and Pompeiano, 1965c, d, 1966c). It will be shown here that the phasic inhibitory influences are selectively abolished by the vestibular lesions (Pompeiano and Morrison, 1965c, 1966a).

The homonymous monosynaptic reflex was elicited in the flexor digitorum brevis by single shock stimulation of group I afferents of the tibial nerve. Both tonic and phasic depression of the monosynaptic reflex could still be detected in the unrestrained, unanesthetized cat after bilateral ablation of the sensorimotor cortex. Following a bilateral lesion of all vestibular nuclei, or after a bilateral lesion limited to the medial and descending vestibular nuclei, the tonic depression of the monosynaptic reflex could still be observed throughout desynchronized sleep. The most remarkable change, however, was the abolition of the phasic depression of the monosynaptic reflex. It was possible, therefore, to dissociate tonic from phasic inhibitory events.

Summing up, the medial and descending vestibular nuclei are the structures which are critically important not only for the occurrence of the bursts of REM, but also for the appearance of the phasic depression of the monosynaptic reflexes. Since this depression is due to a mechanism of presynaptic inhibition (Morrison and Pompeiano, 1965c, d, 1966c) it can be concluded that the supraspinal inhibitory volleys which depolarize the group I primary afferents during the REM periods of desynchronized sleep originate from or are triggered by the vestibular discharge.

B. Vestibular Control of Somatic Afferent Transmission in the Dorsal Column Nuclei

It has been shown that during REM there is a phasic depression of the orthodromic lemniscal response (Carli et al., 1966a, 1967a) which is due to mechanisms of both presynaptic and postsynaptic inhibition (Carli et al., 1966b–d, 1967b). In experiments performed to localize the structures which are responsible for the inhibitory control of synaptic transmission in the cuneate nucleus during desynchronized sleep (Carli et al., 1966e, 1967c), attention was devoted to the vestibular nuclei. These were found to be responsible not only for REM (Pompeiano and Morrison, 1965a, b, 1966b), but also for the phasic enhancement of the pyramidal discharge, related in time with the REM (Morrison and Pompeiano, 1965b, 1966a).

Since stimulation of the sensorimotor cortex, performed in acute experiments, inhibits the transmission of cutaneous afferent volleys through the cuneate nucleus by mechanisms of both presynaptic and postsynaptic inhibition (cf. Andersen et al., 1964a), the possibility exists that excitation of the pyramidal neurons elicited by ascending vestibular volleys during the REM periods of desynchronized sleep is responsible for the inhibition of synaptic transmission in the cuneate nucleus which occurs at the time of the REM.

We have shown that bilateral destruction of the medial and descending vestibular nuclei abolishes not only REM but also the related phasic depression of the orthodromic lemniscal response evoked by single shock stimulation of the superficial radial nerve. The absence of any modulation of the lemniscal response during sleep, following vestibular lesion, is also duplicated in experiments of bilateral ablation of the sensorimotor cortex. Bilateral ablation, however, does not prevent the appearance of the typical bursts of ocular movements.

Summing up, the depression of the orthodromic lemniscal response elicited by single shock stimulation of the superficial radial nerve during the bursts of REM is abolished by bilateral lesion of the vestibular nuclei, or by complete ablation of the sensorimotor cortex. It appears, therefore, that during REM the vestibular nuclei depress the synaptic transmission at the level of the dorsal column nuclei through the roundabout way of the sensorimotor cortex and the pyramidal tract.

C. Vestibular Control of Afferent Transmission in the Lateral Geniculate Nucleus

Experiments were performed to determine i) whether the geniculate potentials recorded during the REM periods of desynchronized sleep were due, at least in part, to bursts of high frequency discharge originating from the second-order vestibular neurons and running along their ascending pathways (Morrison and Pompeiano, 1966d; Pompeiano and Morrison, 1966c, d) and ii) whether the vestibular system controls presynaptically the transmission of visual impulses at the LGN during the REM (Marchiafava and Pompeiano, 1966b, c).

In the first group of experiments performed in unrestrained, unanesthetized cats, the integrated activity of the LGN was recorded during desynchronized sleep, both before (Fig. 8A) and after bilateral electrolytic lesion of the medial and descending vestibular nuclei (Fig. 8B). All data were recorded in complete darkness (Morrison and Pompeiano, 1966d; Pompeiano and Morrison, 1966c, d).

The integrated activity of all-or-none events in the LGN is smaller during synchronized sleep, but increases during wakefulness and even more so during desynchronized sleep (cf. also Benoit, 1964a). Using this technique, two kinds of geniculate activity can be differentiated during desynchronized sleep (Fig. 8A). The first type is represented by brief rhythmic enhancements which precede by 10–90 sec the onset of the desynchronized EEG and the disappearance of the EMG activity in the cervical muscles. These waves, which have been called "type I

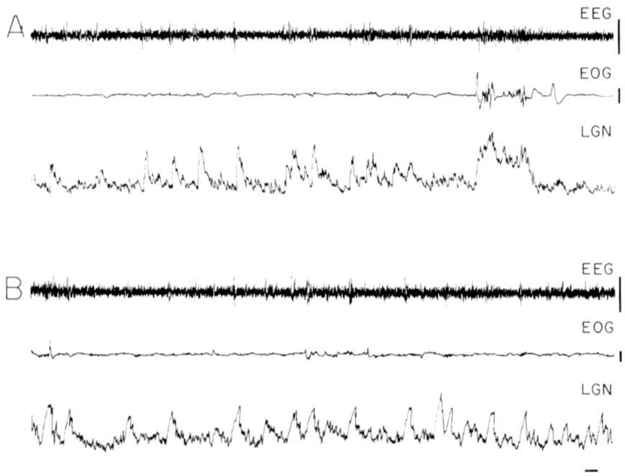

Fig. 8. Phasic increase in the lateral geniculate activity during REM of desynchronized sleep, and its abolition following vestibular lesion. Unrestrained, unanesthetized cat. Bipolar records. EEG: electroencephalogram (left parieto-occipital); EOG: electro-oculogram; LGN: integrated geniculate activity. Time calibration: 1 sec. Voltage calibration: 0.2 mV. A: Experiment made 4 days after permanent implantation of the electrodes. Two kinds of activity are recorded from the lateral geniculate nucleus during desynchronized sleep. The first is made by regular, rhythmic enhancements, which are sometimes associated with isolated ocular movements. The second type of activity is characterized by a phasic increase in the integrated geniculate discharge, larger in amplitude and longer in duration than those described above, which is strikingly related in time with a large burst of REM. B: Same animal as in A. Experiment made 6 days after permanent implantation of the electrodes and 2 days after complete bilateral lesion of the medial and descending vestibular nuclei. Persistence during desynchronized sleep of the first type of rhythmic activity and abolition of the large bursts of REM and related phasic enhancements of geniculate discharge (POMPEIANO and MORRISON, 1966d)

LGN waves", were sometimes but not always related with single ocular jerks or isolated twitches of the limb musculature. The second type of geniculate activity was characterized by phasic increases, 1.5 to 2.0 times larger in amplitude and 2 to 6 times longer in duration than those described above. Only the latter type of wave, designated as "type II LGN waves", appeared to be strictly related in time with the large bursts of REM.

The most prominent changes in geniculate activity produced by vestibular lesion include the abolition of the second group of large amplitude deflections and of the related bursts of REM. The rhythmic geniculate activity which started several seconds before the occurrence of the other signs of desynchronized sleep, and which was apparently unrelated to the large bursts of REM, however, persisted throughout the episode of desynchronized sleep (Fig. 8B).

These results suggest that two extraretinal inputs influence the LGN during desynchronized sleep: i) a vestibular input, originating from the medial and descending vestibular nuclei, which impinges upon the geniculate nucleus at the time of the large bursts of REM, and ii) an extravestibular input, probably localized in the pontine reticular formation, which affects rhythmically the geniculate activity throughout the episode of desynchronized sleep.

These experiments indicate that mechanisms of optovestibular integration may occur not only at the level of the visual cortex (JUNG et al., 1963; KORNHUBER and DA FONSECA, 1964), but also at the level of the lateral geniculate nucleus.

The second group of experiments, performed to determine whether vestibular volleys enhance the excitability of the intrageniculate optic fiber endings, possibly leading to presynaptic inhibition (MARCHIAFAVA and POMPEIANO, 1966b, c), was performed on cats under light Nembutal anesthesia. The excitability changes of the central endings of the optic nerve fibers induced by conditioning stimulation of the VIIIth nerve or of the vestibular nuclei were investigated using WALL's method (1958). It was found in particular that brief conditioning stimulation (20–50 msec) of the left VIIIth nerve or of the medial and descending vestibular nuclei, with rectangular pulses at 300–500/sec, 0.2–1.0 msec pulse duration, increases the amplitude of the antidromic response elicited in the contralateral optic nerve on single shock stimulation of the LGN of either side. This effect starts soon after the end of the conditioning stimulation, reaches a maximum 30–80 msec later and disappears within 300 msec (Fig. 9).

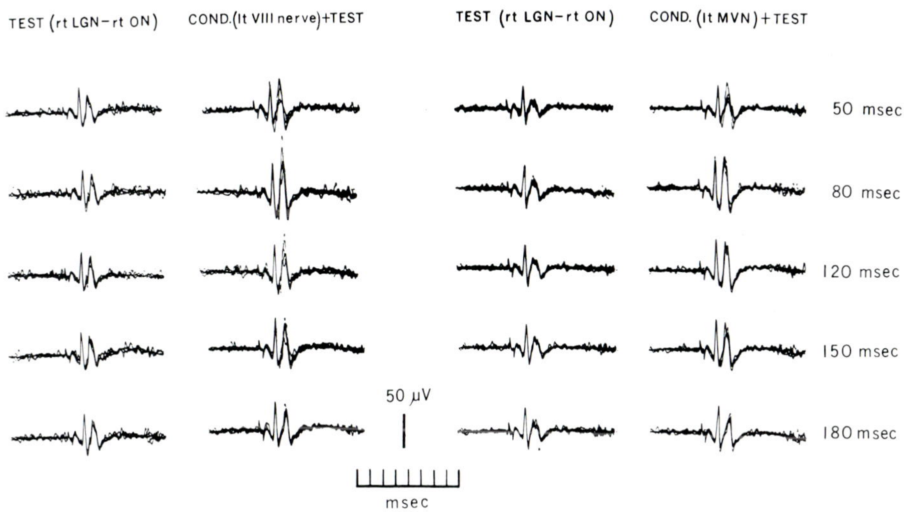

Fig. 9. Changes in the antidromic response of the optic nerve fibers to intrageniculate shocks following electrical stimulation of the vestibular system. The terminals of the primary optic afferents are excited through an electrode inserted in the right lateral geniculate nucleus (rt LGN) while the antidromic discharge is recorded peripherally in the right optic nerve (rt ON). Conditioning stimulation of the left VIII nerve or of the left medial vestibular nucleus (lt MVN) was made with 1 msec rectangular pulses at 330/sec, for 20 msec. The lateral geniculate nucleus was stimulated with a testing shock, 0.5 msec in duration, of such a strength that the amplitude of the test responses illustrated on the left and right sides of the figure corresponded to 41% of the maximum amplitude of the antidromic volleys. The times in msec indicate the intervals between the beginning of the conditioning stimulation and the testing shock. Each record represents a series of 5 superimposed sweeps taken at the repetition rate of 1 every 4 sec (MARCHIAFAVA and POMPEIANO, 1966c)

The increase in excitability of the optic nerve endings produced by repetitive stimulation of the vestibular nuclei and the VIII nerve is due to presynaptic depolarization of the intrageniculate terminals of the optic fibers, possibly leading to inhibition of transmission through the LGN. Further experiments, however, are required to ascertain the postsynaptic effects that the ascending vestibular volleys might exert on LGN. It can be concluded that the phasic increase in unit activity recorded from the medial and descending vestibular nuclei during desynchronized sleep (Bizzi et al., 1964a–c) is likely to be responsible for presynaptic depolarization of the optic tract fibers which occurs during desynchronized sleep at the time of the large bursts of REM (Sasakura and Iwama, 1965; Bizzi, 1966a; Iwama and Kasamatsu, 1966; Iwama et al., 1966; Kasamatsu and Iwama, 1966). This effect may not be a direct one, but may be mediated by the reticular formation (cf. Angel et al., 1965).

The differing amounts of presynaptic inhibition and postsynaptic facilitation occurring within the LGN during "type I" and "type II" geniculate waves may partially explain the discrepancy in the results obtained so far on the orthodromic transmission through the LGN during the phasic events of desynchronized sleep.

Summing up, two extraretinal inputs influence the LGN during desynchronized sleep: i) a vestibular input, originating from the medial and descending vestibular nuclei, which impinge upon the geniculate nucleus at the time of the large bursts of REM and ii) an extravestibular input, probably localized in the pontine reticular formation, which affects rhythmically the geniculate activity throughout the episode of desynchronized sleep. Both these inputs can alter the orthodromic transmission of afferent volleys through the LGN by the mechanisms of presynaptic inhibition and postsynaptic excitation.

D. Vestibular Control of Vegetative Functions

Tonic changes in pupillary diameter and blood pressure occur during desynchronized sleep. The autonomic nervous system is also clearly affected, phasically, during the outbursts of REM. In particular, phasic changes have been described in the regulation of the pupillary diameter and of the neural control of circulation. Whenever an outburst of REM occurs, one observes; i) pupillary dilation (Berlucchi et al., 1964; Hodes, 1964; Jeannerod et al., 1965b) and ii) a slight increase in the heart rate and blood pressure followed by a marked slowing of the heart rhythm and fall of arterial pressure (Gassel et al., 1964a, b). The most striking effect of a vestibular lesion was the abolition of the brief, and occasionally quite pronounced, pupillary dilations which in the intact animal are correlated with the ocular outbursts. Also, the phasic changes in heart rate were completely abolished following vestibular lesion (Fig. 10) (Morrison and Pompeiano, 1965g, 1970).

The critical region, the destruction of which is responsible for the effects described above, includes the medial and descending vestibular nuclei. The lesion must be bilateral and affect these vestibular nuclei in their entire rostrocaudal extent. The conclusion is that the medial in descending vestibular nuclei are critically involved also in the phasic autonomic changes which appear simultaneously with the REM periods of desynchronized sleep.

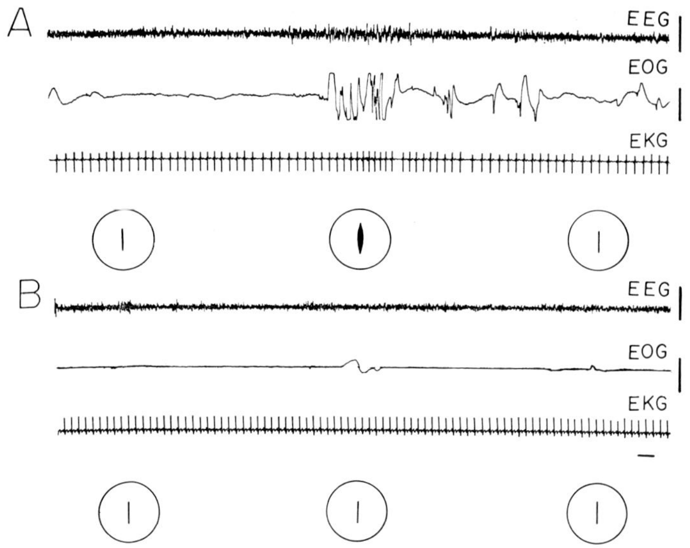

Fig. 10. Effects of vestibular lesions on the vegetative changes characteristic of the desynchronized phase of sleep. Unrestrained unanesthetized cat. Bipolar records. EEG: Electroencephalogram (right parieto-occipital); EOG: electro-oculogram; EKG: electrocardiogram. Time calibration: 1 sec. Voltage calibration: 0.2 mV (EEG) and 0.5 mV (EOG). The pupillary changes are indicated by the diagrams. A: Intact animal showing a pupillary dilation and a phasic increase followed by a reduction in heart rate synchronously with a REM burst of desynchronized sleep. B: Cat 3 days after bilateral lesion of the medial and descending vestibular nuclei. During desynchronized sleep the large bursts of REM are abolished, as well as the related changes in pupillary diameter and heart rate. Note the regularity of the heart rate throughout the episode of desynchronized sleep (Morrison and Pompeiano, 1965g)

IX. Conclusion

An analysis of the central mechanisms responsible for the motor events occurring during desynchronized sleep, made both by microelectrode recording of single vestibular neurons in unrestrained, unanesthetized animals (Bizzi et al., 1964a–c) and also by lesion experiments, clearly shows that the medial and descending vestibular nuclei represent the triggering mechanism responsible not only for the REM (Pompeiano and Morrison, 1965a, b, 1966b) but also for the phasic excitation of the spinal motoneurons (Morrison and Pompeiano, 1965h, 1966a). However, the efferent projections from these vestibular nuclei to the spinal cord do not seem to be of critical importance for the appearance of the muscular twitches, since they are not apparently modified by lesions of the ventral funicles, which condition interrupts all the vestibulospinal projections (Gassel et al., 1964c). The descending volleys responsible for the phasic excitation of the α-motoneurons run mainly along the dorsolateral funiculi, where corticospinal, rubrospinal and reticulospinal pathways are located. Although selective lesion of the pyramidal tract (Marchiafava and Pompeiano, 1964a, b, 1966a) and of the red nucleus (Gassel et al., 1965b, c) produces only a transitory depression of the twitches, thus suggesting that other pathways contribute to their appearance, it is of interest that: i) during desynchronized sleep a phasic increase in the pyramidal and rubral discharges occurs during the REM, and ii) the abolition of the muscular twitches following lesion of the vestibular nuclei is always associated with the abolition of the pyramidal (Morrison and Pompeiano, 1965h, 1966a) and rubral activity (Pompeiano and Satoh, 1967, 1968) that occurs synchronously with the bursts of REM.

The demonstration that during sleep vestibular efferent volleys impinge upon the sensorimotor cortex is supported by the observation that in acute experiments labyrinthine volleys are able to alter the pattern of discharge of some neurons localized in this cortical area (Kornhuber and Aschoff, 1963, 1964; Jung et al., 1963). A discharge of impulses can actually be recorded from the bulbar pyramid on single shock stimulation of the vestibular nerves (Megirian and Troth, 1964).

In summary, a motor pattern is performed during desynchronized sleep due to increased activity of the vestibular neurons. It consists not only of REM, due to direct excitation of the oculomotor neurons, but also of muscular contractions related in time with the REM. These phasic events are associated with reflex excitation of corticospinal and rubrospinal neurons due to ascending vestibular volleys impinging upon the motor cortex. Other structures, however, also triggered by the ascending vestibular system, contribute to the phenomenon. For sake of simplicity they have not been considered in the present report.

Parallel to this phasic excitation of the extrinsic ocular and spinal motoneurons, occurring during desynchronized sleep, phasic inhibitory events affect the transmission of sensory inputs along several sensory pathways. The result is that, in terms of the specific sensory inputs, the animal is functionally deafferented during REM every time the oculomotor and spinal motoneurons are phasically excited. Experimental evidence clearly indicates that mechanisms of presynaptic and/or postsynaptic inhibition are responsible for the inhibitory control of the somatic sensory input during the bursts of REM. In particular the striking depression of the monosynaptic reflex that occurs during bursts of REM (Gassel et al., 1964d, e) is due to presynaptic depolarization of the group I primary afferents from muscle spindles, thus leading to presynaptic inhibition (Morrison and Pompeiano, 1965c, d, 1966c). The phasic depression of the polysynaptic reflex during REM has been attributed to presynaptic inhibition of the flexion reflex afferents (Morrison and Pompeiano, 1965e, f) and/or to reduced transmission through the interneurons of the polysynaptic reflex pathway (Lenzi et al., 1968a, b). Finally, the phasic depression of the orthodromic lemniscal response during REM is shown to be related to mechanisms of both presynaptic and postsynaptic inhibition occurring within the cuneate nucleus (Carli et al., 1966a–d, 1967a b).

An analysis of the central structures responsible for the phasic depression of the spinal reflexes during REM shows that this effect can still be detected even after bilateral ablation of the sensorimotor cortex. On the other hand, electrolytic lesions localized in the medial and descending vestibular nuclei on both sides abolish not only the bursts of REM, but also the phasic depression of the spinal reflexes that occurs synchronously with the ocular phenomena (Pompeiano and Morrison, 1965c, 1966a).

The conclusion can be drawn, therefore, that the supraspinal descending inhibitory influences which bring about presynaptic depolarization of the primary afferents to the spinal motoneurons during the bursts of REM originate from or are triggered by the medial and descending vestibular nuclei. Similar effects can also be obtained by electrical stimulation of the VIIIth nerve (COOK et al., 1968a, b), the vestibular nuclei and the medial longitudinal fascicle (CARPENTER et al., 1962a, 1966; COOK et al., 1968a, b) in the decerebrate cat.

It has been pointed out previously that the increase in the activity of the vestibular nuclei, occurring during the bursts of REM, is capable of exciting cortical and probably also subcortical structures, which exert descending excitatory influences on the α-motoneurons. This effect would occur when the proprioceptive afferent volleys running along the group I pathway as well as along the FRA pathway are filtered at the presynaptic level by descending volleys originating from or triggered by the same vestibular nuclei.

It is of interest that just at the time when descending excitatory influences impinge on the α-motoneurons, thus initiating movements, there is a presynaptic block of peripheral afferent impulses which otherwise would reach the discharging motoneurons along the primary sensory fibers. In other words, at the moment when the motoneurons are being stimulated to discharge by supraspinal descending volleys, the segmental control of the same neurons by the primary afferents is depressed due to a mechanism of presynaptic inhibition.

It should be mentioned that during desynchronized sleep the α-motoneurons are tonically hyperpolarized (GASSEL et al., 1964f, 1965a; MORRISON and POMPEIANO, 1965a, b) and that the depression of somatic afferent transmission occurs during REM sleep in the absence of muscle twitches. When supraspinal descending volleys depolarize the α-motoneurons, particularly during the large bursts of REM, the monosynaptic reflex, far from being depressed, is actually enhanced (GASSEL et al., 1964d, e). At this time the reduced postsynaptic efficacy of the orthodromic volley, due to presynaptic inhibition, has to be weighed against an increased excitability of discharging motoneurons.

Even in the decerebrate cat the presynaptic inhibitory effect exerted on primary afferents by electrical stimulation of the VIIIth nerve (COOK et al., 1968a, b) is counteracted by an increased excitability of motoneurons. The result is that the motoneurons are not completely uncoupled from their segmental afferents as shown by an enhancement of the spinal reflexes. These observations may explain why, for instance, a facilitation of the monosynaptic reflex occurs during increased gravity in the unrestrained, unanesthetized cat (HUERTAS et al., 1966).

The effects described above do not represent the only events elicited by the vestibular volleys, which control the transmission of somatosensory information during desynchronized sleep.

The excitatory influences exerted by the vestibular nuclei on the cerebral cortex during the bursts of REM involve not only the pyramidal neurons originating from the motor cortex but also those originating from the somatosensory cortex (MORRISON and POMPEIANO, 1965e, f). While the pyramidal volleys originating from the motor cortex act mainly on flexor motoneurons through the interneurons of the flexion reflex pathway (LUNDBERG and VOORHOEVE, 1962; LUNDBERG et al., 1962), the pyramidal discharge originating from the somatosensory cortex exerts presynaptic inhibitory influences on the central endings of both cutaneous and high threshold muscular afferents, which are known to be related to the polysynaptic spinal reflex (Andersen et al., 1962, 1964e; Carpenter et al., 1962b, 1963). Furthermore our findings indicate that the ascending volleys originating from the vestibular nuclei at the time of the REM influence also those pyramidal neurons whose fibers are directed to the cuneate and gracilis nuclei in the cat (Carli et al., 1966e, 1967c). Bilateral destruction of this cortical structure duplicates in fact the effects of the vestibular lesion on somatic afferent transmission in the dorsal column system during desynchronized sleep, while the appearance of the bursts of REM is not prevented by the cortical ablation. As a result of both of these lesions, the phasic depression of somatic afferent transmission through the lemniscal pathway during the REM is abolished. These observations suggest that volleys ascending from the vestibular nuclei affect neurons of the somatosensory cortex, whose efferent discharge is finally responsible for the depressed transmission at dorsal column level. It has been pointed out previously that the phasic depression of transmission of somatic afferent volleys through the cuneate nucleus during bursts of REM is due to mechanisms of presynaptic and postsynaptic inhibition (Carli et al., 1966b–d, 1967b) and that both of these mechanisms occurring during physiological sleep in unrestrained animals can also be elicited in acute experiments on repetitive stimulation of the sensorimotor cortex, as described by Andersen et al. (1964a–d).

These observations lead to the conclusion that the vestibular activity occurring during REM periods of desynchronized sleep is able to block the transmission of somatic afferent volleys to the polysynaptic spinal reflex pathway not only directly, but also through the roundabout way of the sensorimotor cortex. The same mechanism is also responsible for the parallel depression in transmission of somatic afferent volleys to the ascending lemniscal pathway.

It is surprising that, contrary to the depressed transmission of somatic afferent volleys at dorsal column level, the transmission of somatic volleys through the VPL is greatly facilitated during REM (Allison, 1965; Dagnino et al., 1965a, 1967).

It has been assumed by several authors that the sensory feedback dependent upon active movement plays an important role in motor coordination (Held, 1965; Held and Freedman, 1963). It is interesting that while during the movements associated with REM the somatic sensory volleys are partially inhibited at spinal cord level or at medullary level, a postsynaptic facilitation occurs simultaneously within the specific thalamic nuclei. We can postulate therefore that some part of the efferent vestibular activity giving rise to contraction of the limb musculature is fed into the somatosensory system, particularly the nucleus ventralis posterolateralis, where it interacts with the incoming somatic information filtered at dorsal column level. The result is that external stimulation due to sensory feedback is partially substituted by internal stimulation which is incorporated at thalamic level and elaborated by the somatosensory cortex.

This mechanism of sensorimotor integration which affects the transmission of somatosensory volleys through the dorsal column-medial lemniscal system during the hypnic contractions of the limb musculature is paralleled by similar findings involving visual transmission through the LGN during the rapid eye movements.

It has been recently shown that during the REM phase of sleep there is an increase of the optic tract antidromic response, which indicates the occurrence of presynaptic inhibition during these ocular movements. Depolarization of optic tract terminals at the time of the REM might decrease the amount of retinal activity impinging upon geniculate neurons (Bizzi, 1966a). Evidence suggesting inhibition in the transmission of visual impulses during eye movements has been reviewed recently (cf. Pompeiano, 1968a).

It appears now that during desynchronized sleep the vestibular afferent volleys impinge upon the lateral geniculate nucleus (Pompeiano and Morrison, 1966c, d; Morrison and Pompeiano, 1966d). Though evidence for vestibular influence on the postsynaptic activity recorded from the lateral geniculate neurons is still lacking, enhancement in the excitability of the intrageniculate optic tract endings is clearly elicited by stimulating electrically the VIIIth nerve as well as the medial and descending vestibular nuclei (Marchiafava and Pompeiano, 1966b, c), *i.e.*, those structures which contribute to the appearance of ocular movements during desynchronized sleep.

The extraretinal inputs, originating from the oculomotor centers in the brain stem (particularly localized in the pontine reticular formation and the vestibular nuclei) may lead not only to presynaptic depolarization of the primary optic fibers during REM, but also to postsynaptic excitation of the lateral geniculate units (Bizzi, 1966b; Sakakura and Iwama, 1966). This effect is comparable to the process of postsynaptic facilitation involving the specific thalamic nuclei of the somatosensory pathway mentioned previously. It appears therefore that a central discharge originating from the oculomotor centers in the brain stem reaches the geniculate neurons simultaneously with the efferent discharge which gives rise to the eye movements. The existence of such "corollary" central discharges, *i.e.*, discharges from motor to sensory structures, has been postulated in order to account for the perceptual constancy of the environment during eye movements (Sperry, 1950; Teuber, 1964).

One may propose that also during the somatic and ocular movements elicited by natural labyrinthine stimulation in the awake animal, vestibular volleys interact with proprioceptive afferent and visual impulses at different relay stations of both the somatosensory and visual pathways, thus leading to proper perception during body and eye movements.

References

Adrian, E.D., Moruzzi, G.: Impulses in the pyramidal tract. J. Physiol. (Lond.) **97**, 153–199 (1939).

Albe-Fessard, D., Massion, J., Hall, R., Rosenblith, W.: Modifications au cours de la veille et du sommeil des valeurs moyennes de réponses nerveuses centrales induites par des stimulations somatique chez le chat libre. C. R. Acad. Sci. (Paris) **258**, 353–356 (1964).

Allison, T.: Cortical and subcortical evoked responses to central stimuli during wakefulness and sleep. E.E.G. clin. Neurophysiol. **18**, 131–139 (1965).

Andersen, P., Eccles, J.C., Oshima, T., Schmidt, R.F.: Mechanisms of synaptic transmission in the cuneate nucleus. J. Neurophysiol. **27**, 1096–1116 (1964a).

Andersen, P., Eccles, J.C., Schmidt, R.F., Yokota, T.: Slow potential waves produced in the cuneate nucleus by cutaneous volleys and by cortical stimulation. J. Neurophysiol. **27**, 78–91 (1964b).

Andersen, P., Eccles, J.C., Schmidt, R.F., Yokota, T.: Depolarization of presynaptic fibers in the cuneate nucleus. J. Neurophysiol. **27**, 92–106 (1964c).

Andersen, P., Eccles, J.C., Schmidt, R.F., Yokota, T.: Identification of relay cells and interneurons in the cuneate nucleus. J. Neurophysiol. **27**, 1080–1095 (1964d).

Andersen, P., Eccles, J.C., Sears, T.A.: Presynaptic inhibitory action of cerebral cortex on the spinal cord. Nature (Lond.) **194**, 740–741 (1962).

Andersen, P., Eccles, J.C., Sears, T.A.: Cortically evoked depolarization of primary afferent fibers in the spinal cord. J. Neurophysiol. **27**, 63–77 (1964e).

Angel, A., Magni, F., Strata, P.: Excitability of intrageniculate optic tract fibres after reticular stimulation in the mid-pontine pretrigeminal preparation. Arch. ital. Biol. **103**, 668–693 (1965).

Arduini, A., Berlucchi, G., Strata, P.: Pyramidal activity during sleep and wakefulness. Arch. ital. Biol. **101**, 530–544 (1963).

Aserinsky, E., Kleitman, N.: Regularly occurring periods of eye motility and concomitant phenomena, during sleep. Science **118**, 273–274 (1953).

Aserinsky, E., Kleitman, N.: Two types of ocular motility occurring in sleep. J. appl. Physiol. **8**, 1–10 (1955).

Baldissera, F., Broggi, G., Mancia, M.: Analisi dei riflessi spinali durante la veglia e il sonno. Boll. Soc. ital. Biol. sper. **40**, 1868–1871 (1964a).

Baldissera, F., Broggi, G., Mancia, M.: Spinal reflexes in normal unrestrained cats during sleep and wakefulness. Experientia (Basel) **20**, 577–579 (1964b).

Baldissera, F., Broggi, G., Mancia, M.: Modificazioni del riflesso spinale monosinaptico e polisinaptico nel gatto normale non anestetizzato durante le varie fasi del sonno e della veglia. Rend. Accad. naz. Lincei, Cl. Sci. fis., mat. nat., Serie VIII, **36**, 539–542 (1964c).

Baldissera, F., Broggi, G., Mancia, M.: Monosynaptic and polysynaptic spinal reflexes during physiological sleep and wakefulness. Arch. ital. Biol. **104**, 112–133 (1966a).

Baldissera, F., Cesa-Bianchi, M.G., Mancia, M.: Studio della depolarizzazione delle fibre afferenti primarie al midollo spinale durante le fasi naturali del sonno e della veglia. Boll. Soc. ital. Biol. sper. **41**, fasc. 20 bis, n. 3 (1965a).

Baldissera, F., Cesa-Bianchi, M.G., Mancia, M.: Eventi fasici nel midollo spinale quali prove di inibizione presinaptica durante il sonno desincronizzato. Rend. Accad. naz. Lincei, Cl. Sci. fis., mat. nat., Serie VIII, **39**, 321–324 (1965b).

Baldissera, F., Cesa-Bianchi, M.G., Mancia, M.: Phasic events indicating presynaptic inhibition of primary afferents to the spinal cord during desynchronized sleep. J. Neurophysiol. **29**, 871–887 (1966b).

Baldissera, F., Ettore, G., Infuso, L., Mancia, M., Pagni, C.A.: Comparative study of peripheral responses evoked by cortico-spinal stimulation during wakefulness and sleep in cat and man. E.E.G. clin. Neurophysiol. **21**, 512 (1966c).

Baldissera, F., Mancia, M.: Sciatic nerve activity evoked by sensory-motor cortex stimulation during paradoxical sleep. Nature (Lond.) **209**, 1030 (1966).

Benoit, O.: Activité unitaire du nerf optique, du corps genouillé latéral de la formation réticulaire durant des différents stades de sommeil. J. Physiol. (Paris) **56**, 259–262 (1964a).

Benoit, O.: Variations avec l'état de vigilance et au cours du sommeil des réponses électrocorticales obtenues par stimulation des voies visuelles. C.R. Acad. Sci. (Paris) **258**, 1076–1079 (1964b).

Berlucchi, G., Moruzzi, G., Salvi, G., Strata, P.: Pupil behavior and ocular movements during synchronized and desynchronized sleep. Arch. ital. Biol. **102**, 230–244 (1964).

Bizzi, E.: Changes in the orthodromic and antidromic response of optic tract during the eye movements of sleep. J. Neurophysiol. **24**, 861–870 (1966a).

Bizzi, E.: Discharge patterns of single geniculate neurons during the rapid eye movements of sleep. J. Neurophysiol. **29**, 1087–1095 (1966b).

Bizzi, E., Brooks, D.C.: Functional connections between pontine reticular formation and lateral geniculate nucleus during deep sleep. Arch. ital. Biol. **101**, 666–680 (1963).

Bizzi, E., Pompeiano, O., Somogyi, I.: Attività spontanea di singole unità registrate dai nuclei vestibolari nei gatti integri non anestetizzati nel corso del sonno e della veglia. Boll. Soc. ital. Biol. sper. **40**, 138–141 (1964a).

BIZZI, E., POMPEIANO, O., SOMOGYI, I.: Vestibular nuclei: activity of single neurons during natural sleep and wakefulness. Science **145**, 414–415 (1964b).

BIZZI, E., POMPEIANO, O., SOMOGYI, I.: Spontaneous activity of single vestibular neurons of unrestrained cats during sleep and wakefulness. Arch. ital. Biol. **102**, 308–330 (1964c).

BRODAL, A., POMPEIANO, O., WALBERG, F.: The vestibular nuclei and their connections. Anatomy and functional correlations. Edinburgh: Oliver and Boyd 1962.

BROOKS, D.C.: Localization of the lateral geniculate nucleus monophasic waves associated with paradoxical sleep in the cat. E.E.G. clin. Neurophysiol. **23**, 123–133 (1967a).

BROOKS, D.C.: Effect of bilateral optic nerve section on visual system monophasic wave activity in the cat. E.E.G. clin. Neurophysiol. **23**, 134–141 (1967b).

BROOKS, D.C., BIZZI, E.: Brain stem electrical activity during deep sleep. Arch. ital. Biol. **101**, 648–665 (1963).

CARLI, G., DIETE-SPIFF, K., POMPEIANO, O.: Modulazione ipnica della risposta lemniscale alla stimolazione elettrica di afferenze cutanee. Boll. Soc. ital. Biol. sper. **42**, 638–639 (1966a).

CARLI, G., DIETE-SPIFF, K., POMPEIANO, O.: Inibizione presinaptica e postsinaptica nel nucleo cuneato durante il sonno. Boll. Soc. ital. Biol. sper. **42**, 640–641 (1966b).

CARLI, G., DIETE-SPIFF, K., POMPEIANO, O.: The transfer of sensory information through the lemniscal pathway during sleep. J. Physiol. (Lond.) **184**, 19–21P (1966c).

CARLI, G., DIETE-SPIFF, K., POMPEIANO, O.: Presynaptic and postsynaptic inhibition on transmission of cutaneous afferent volleys through the cuneate nucleus during sleep. Experientia (Basel) **22**, 239–240 (1966d).

CARLI, G., DIETE-SPIFF, K., POMPEIANO, O.: Influenze vestibolari sulla trasmissione d'impulsi somatici lungo la via lemniscale. Rend. Accad. Naz. Lincei, Cl. Sci. fis., mat. nat. **40**, 113–115 (1966e).

CARLI, G., DIETE-SPIFF, K., POMPEIANO, O.: Transmission of sensory information through the lemniscal pathway during sleep. Arch. ital. Biol. **105**, 31–51 (1967a).

CARLI, G., DIETE-SPIFF, K., POMPEIANO, O.: Presynaptic and postsynaptic inhibition on transmission of somatic afferent volleys through the cuneate nucleus during sleep. Arch. ital. Biol. **105**, 52–82 (1967b).

CARLI, G., DIETE-SPIFF, K., POMPEIANO, O.: Vestibular influences during sleep. V. Vestibular control on somatic afferent transmission in the cuneate nucleus during desynchronized sleep. Arch. ital. Biol. **105**, 83–103 (1967c).

CARPENTER, D., ENGBERG, I., LUNDBERG, A.: Presynaptic inhibition in the lumbar cord evoked from the brain stem. Experientia (Basel) **18**, 450–451 (1962a).

CARPENTER, D., ENGBERG, I., LUNDBERG, A.: Primary afferent depolarization evoked from the brain stem and the cerebellum. Arch. ital. Biol. **104**, 73–85 (1966).

CARPENTER, D., LUNDBERG, A., NORRSELL, U.: Effects from the pyramidal tract on primary afferents and on spinal reflex actions to primary afferents. Experientia (Basel) **18**, 337–338 (1962b).

CARPENTER, D., LUNDBERG, A., NORRSELL, U.: Primary afferent depolarization evoked from the sensorimotor cortex. Acta physiol. scand. **59**, 126–142 (1963).

COOK, W.A., JR., CANGIANO, A., POMPEIANO, O.: Vestibular influences on primary afferents in the spinal cord. Pflügers Arch. ges. Physiol. **299**, 334–338 (1968a).

COOK, W.A., JR., CANGIANO, A., POMPEIANO, O.: Vestibular evoked primary afferent depolarization in the lumbar spinal cord. Proc. XXIV int. Congr. physiol. Sci., Washington, D.C. **7**, 272 (1968b).

CORDEAU, J.P., WALSH, J., MAHUT, H.: Variations dans la transmission des messages sensoriels en fonction des différents états d'éveil et de sommeil. In: Aspects anatomo-fonctionnels de la physiologie du sommeil. Paris: Éditions du Centre National de la Recherche Scientifique 1965.

DAGNINO, N., FAVALE, E., LOEB, C., MANFREDI, M.: Trasmissione talamica e movimenti oculari durante il sonno profondo. Boll. Soc. ital. Biol. sper. **41**, 1269–1271 (1965a).

DAGNINO, N., FAVALE, E., LOEB, C., MANFREDI, M.: Thalamic transmission changes during the rapid eye movements of deep sleep. Arch. int. Physiol. **73**, 858–861 (1965b).

DAGNINO, N., FAVALE, E., LOEB, C., MANFREDI, M.: Sensory transmission in the geniculostriate system of the cat during natural sleep and arousal. J. Neurophysiol. **28**, 443–456 (1965c).

Dagnino, N., Favale, E., Loeb, C., Manfredi, M., Massazza, G., Seitun, A.: Afferenze oculari (retiniche e propriocettive) e variazioni fasiche della trasmissione talamica durante il sonno profondo. Boll. Soc. ital. Biol. sper. **42**, 1775–1777 (1966a).

Dagnino, N., Favale, E., Loeb, C., Manfredi, M., Seitun, A.: Variazioni fasiche della trasmissione sinaptica nel nucleo geniculato laterale durante le "deep sleep waves" spontanee ed evocate. Boll. Soc. ital. Biol. sper. **42**, 1777–1779 (1966b).

Dagnino, N., Favale, E., Loeb, C., Manfredi, M., Seitun, A.: Accelerated synaptic transmission in nucleus ventralis-postero-lateralis during deep sleep. Experientia (Basel) **22**, 329–330 (1966c).

Dagnino, N., Favale, E., Loeb, C., Manfredi, M., Seitun, A.: Nervous mechanisms underlying phasic changes in thalamic transmission during deep sleep. E.E.G. clin. Neurophysiol., Suppl. **26**, 156–163 (1967).

Dagnino, N., Favale, E., Manfredi, M.: Le risposte cortico-piramidali durante il ciclo sonno-veglia. Boll. Soc. ital. Biol. sper. **41**, 1271–1274 (1965d).

Dement, W.: The occurrance of low voltage, fast electroencephalogram patterns during behavioral sleep in the cat. E.E.G. clin. Neurophysiol. **10**, 291–296 (1958).

Dement, W.C.: Eye movements during sleep. In: M.B. Bender, Ed. The oculomotor system. New York: Hoeber Medical Division, Harper and Row 1964.

Dement, W.C., Kleitman, N.: The relation of eye movements during sleep to dream activity: an objective method for the study of dreaming. J. exp. Psychol. **53**, 339–346 (1957a).

Dement, W.C., Kleitman, N.: Cyclic variations in EEG during sleep and their relation to eye movements, body motility and dreaming. E.E.G. clin. Neurophysiol. **9**, 673–690 (1957b).

Eccles, J.C.: The physiology of synapses. Berlin-Göttingen-Heidelberg-New York: Springer 1964.

Eccles, R.M., Lundberg, A.: Synaptic actions in motoneurones by afferents which may evoke the flexion reflex. Arch. ital. Biol. **97**, 199–221 (1959).

Evarts, E.V.: Activity of neurons in visual cortex of the cat during sleep with low voltage fast EEG activity. J. Neurophysiol. **25**, 812–816 (1962).

Evarts, E.V.: Temporal patterns of discharge of pyramidal tract neurons during sleep and waking in the monkey. J. Neurophysiol. **27**, 152–171 (1964).

Evarts, E.V.: Neuronal activity in visual and motor cortex during sleep and waking. In: Aspects anatomo-fonctionnels de la physiologie du sommeil. Paris: Éditions du Centre National de la Recherche Scientifique 1965.

Evarts, E.V.: Activity of individual cerebral neurons during sleep and arousal. In: S.S. Kety, E.V. Evarts and H.L. Williams, Eds. Sleep and altered states of consciousness. Res. Publ. Ass. nerv. ment. Dis. **45**, 319–337 (1967).

Favale, E., Loeb, C., Manfredi, M.: Le risposte corticali somatiche durante il sonno profondo: particolare comportamento delle risposte radiato-corticali. Boll. Soc. ital. Biol. sper. **39**, 430–432 (1963a).

Favale, E., Loeb, C., Manfredi, M.: Somatic responses evoked by central stimulation during natural sleep and during arousal. Arch. int. Physiol. **71**, 229–235 (1963b).

Favale, E., Loeb, C., Manfredi, M.: Somatic evoked responses in cats during natural sleep. Experientia (Basel) **19**, 189–192 (1963c).

Favale, E., Loeb, C., Manfredi, M.: Cortical responses evoked by stimulation of the optic pathways during natural sleep and during arousal. Arch. int. Physiol. **72**, 221–228 (1964).

Favale, E., Loeb, C., Manfredi, M., Sacco, G.: Somatic afferent transmission and cortical responsiveness during natural sleep and arousal in the cat. E.E.G. clin. Neurophysiol. **18**, 354–368 (1965).

Gardner-Medwin, A.R.: Is there activity in geniculo-striate fibres during rapid eye movement sleep? J. Physiol. (Lond.) **191**, 41–42P (1967).

Gassel, M.M., Ghelarducci, B., Marchiafava, P.L., Pompeiano, O.: Modificazioni fasiche della pressione arteriosa e della frequenza cardiaca durante i movimenti rapidi oculari caratteristici della fase desincronizzata di sonno. Rend. Accad. naz. Lincei, Cl. Sci. fis., mat. nat., Serie VIII, **36**, 550–551 (1964a).

GASSEL, M.M., GHELARDUCCI, B., MARCHIAFAVA, P.L., POMPEIANO, O.: Phasic changes in blood pressure and heart rate during the rapid eye movement episodes of desynchronized sleep in unrestrained cats. Arch. ital. Biol. **102**, 530–544 (1964b).

GASSEL, M.M., MARCHIAFAVA, P.L., POMPEIANO, O.: Phasic changes in muscular activity during desynchronized sleep in unrestrained cats. An analysis of the pattern and organization of myoclonic twitches. Arch. ital. Biol. **102**, 449–470 (1964c).

GASSEL, M.M., MARCHIAFAVA, P.L., POMPEIANO, O.: Depressione tonica e fasica dei riflessi spinali monosinaptici omonimi e polisinaptici durante il sonno desincronizzato. Rend. Accad. naz. Lincei, Cl. Sci. fis., mat. nat., Serie VIII, **36**, 543–546 (1964d).

GASSEL, M.M., MARCHIAFAVA, P.L., POMPEIANO, O.: Tonic and phasic inhibition of spinal reflexes during deep, desynchronized sleep in unrestrained cats. Arch. ital. Biol. **102**, 471–499 (1964e).

GASSEL, M.M., MARCHIAFAVA, P.L., POMPEIANO, O.: Modulazione ipnica della scarica ricorrente dei motoneuroni spinali nel gatto. Boll. Soc. ital. Biol. sper. **40**, 1937–1939 (1964f).

GASSEL, M.M., MARCHIAFAVA, P.L., POMPEIANO, O.: An analysis of the supraspinal influences acting on motoneurons during sleep in the unrestrained cat. Modification of the recurrent discharge of the alpha motoneurons during sleep. Arch. ital. Biol. **103**, 25–44 (1965a).

GASSEL, M.M., MARCHIAFAVA, P.L., POMPEIANO, O.: Rubrospinal influences during desynchronized sleep. Nature (Lond.) **209**, 1218–1220 (1965b).

GASSEL, M.M., MARCHIAFAVA, P.L., POMPEIANO, O.: Activity of the red nucleus during deep, desynchronized sleep in unrestrained cats. Arch. ital. Biol. **103**, 369–396 (1965c).

GASSEL, M.M., POMPEIANO, O.: Modulazione ipnica dell'attività motoria fusale. Rend. Accad. naz. Lincei, Cl. Sci. fis., mat. nat., Serie VIII, **38**, 561–564 (1965a).

GASSEL, M.M., POMPEIANO, O.: Fusimotor function during sleep in unrestrained cats. An account of the modulation of the mechanically and electrically evoked monosynaptic reflexes. Arch. ital. Biol. **103**, 347–368 (1965b).

GIAQUINTO, S., POMPEIANO, O., SOMOGYI, I.: Modificazioni nel sonno dei riflessi spinali mono- e polisinaptici prodotti dalla stimolazione graduata di afferenze propriocettive. Rend. Accad. naz. Lincei, Cl. Sci. fis., mat. nat., Serie VIII, **34**, 317–319 (1963a).

GIAQUINTO, S., POMPEIANO, O., SOMOGYI, I.: Reflex activity of extensor and flexor muscles following muscular afferent excitation during sleep and wakefulness. Experientia (Basel) **19**, 481–482 (1963b).

GIAQUINTO, S., POMPEIANO, O., SOMOGYI, I.: Meccanismi responsabili delle modificazioni dei riflessi propriocettivi nel sonno. Boll. Soc. ital. Biol. sper. **39**, 1261–1264 (1963c).

GIAQUINTO, S., POMPEIANO, O., SOMOGYI, I.: Supraspinal inhibitory control of spinal reflexes during natural sleep. Experientia (Basel) **19**, 652–653 (1963d).

GIAQUINTO, S., POMPEIANO, O., SOMOGYI, I.: Supraspinal modulation of monosynaptic and polysynaptic spinal reflexes during natural sleep and wakefulness. Arch. ital. Biol. **102**, 245–281 (1964a).

GIAQUINTO, S., POMPEIANO, O., SOMOGYI, I.: Descending inhibitory influences on spinal reflexes during natural sleep. Arch. ital. Biol. **102**, 282–307 (1964b).

GUILBAND, G., KUMMER, J.L.: Comparaison de l'évolution au cours du sommeil, des activités évoquées par stimulation somatique dans le noyaux ventral postérieur et ventral latéral du thalamus et au niveau du cortex moteur chez le Chat. J. Physiol. (Paris) **57**, 617–618 (1965).

GUILBAND, G., YAMAGUCHI, Y.: Évolution au cours des diverses phases du sommeil des activités évoquées de différentes régions du cortex somato-moteur du Chat. J. Physiol. (Paris) **56**, 370–371 (1964).

HELD, R.: Plasticity in sensory-motor systems. Sci. Amer. **213**, 84–94 (1965).

HELD, R., FREEDMAN, S.J.: Plasticity in human sensorimotor control. Science **142**, 455–462 (1963).

HENDLEY, C.D.: Sharp waves in lateral geniculate of cat with eye movements during low-voltage sleep. Fed. Proc. **22**, 637 (1963).

HISHIKAWA, Y., KANEKO, Z.: Electroencephalographic study on narcolepsy. E.E.G. clin. Neurophysiol. **18**, 249–259 (1965).

HISHIKAWA, Y., SUMITSUJI, N., MATSUMOTO, K., KANEKO, Z.: H-reflex and EMG of the mental and hyoid muscles during sleep, with special reference to narcolepsy. E.E.G. clin. Neurophysiol. **18**, 487–492 (1965).

Hobson, J.A.: The effects of chronic brain-stem lesions on cortical and muscular activity during sleep and waking in the cat. E.E.G. clin. Neurophysiol. **19**, 41–62 (1965).

Hodes, R.: Ocular phenomena in the two stages of sleep in the cat. Exp. Neurol. **9**, 34–42 (1964).

Hodes, R., Dement, W.C.: Depression of electrically induced reflexes ("H-reflexes") in man during low voltage EEG sleep. E.E.G. clin. Neurophysiol. **17**, 617–629 (1964).

Hongo, T., Jankowska, E., Lundberg, A.: Effects evoked from the rubrospinal tract in cats. Experientia (Basel) **21**, 525–526 (1965).

Huertas, J., Bracchi, F., Epstein, B.: Spinal reflexes during increased gravity. In: Second symposium on the role of the vestibular organs in space exploration. NASA SP-**115**, 151–158 (1966).

Huttenlocher, P.R.: Evoked and spontaneous activity of single units of medial brain stem during natural sleep and waking. J. Neurophysiol. **24**, 451–468 (1961).

Iwama, K., Kasamatsu, T.: Effects of sleep and wakefulness upon antidromic responsiveness of the lateral geniculate body. Tohoku J. exp. Med. **90**, 269–276 (1966).

Iwama, K., Kawamoto, T.: Responsiveness of cat motor cortex to electrical stimulation in sleep and wakefulness. In: T. Tokizane and J.P. Schadé, Eds. Progress in Brain Research. Vol. 21B: Correlative Neurosciences. Part B. Clinical Studies. Amsterdam: Elsevier Publ. Co. 1966.

Iwama, K., Kawamoto, T., Sakakura, H., Kasamatsu, T.: Responsiveness of cat lateral geniculate at pre- and postsynaptic levels during natural sleep. Physiol. Behav. **1**, 45–53 (1966).

Iwama, K., Sakakura, M.: Impulse transmission in cat lateral geniculate and so-called deep sleep wave. Proc. Jap. Acad. **41**, 499–502 (1965).

Jeannerod, M.: Organisation de l'activité électrique phasique du sommeil paradoxal. Lyon: Imprimerie L.M.D. 1965.

Jeannerod, M., Mouret, J., Jouvet, M.: Effects secondaires de la dé-afférentation visuelle sur l'activité électrique phasique ponto-géniculo-occipitale du sommeil paradoxal. J. Physiol. (Paris) **57**, 255–256 (1965a).

Jeannerod, M., Mouret, J., Jouvet, M.: Étude de la motricité oculaire au cours de la phase paradoxale du sommeil chez le chat. E.E.G. clin. Neurophysiol. **18**, 554 (1965b).

Jouvet, M.: Recherches sur les structures nerveuses et les mécanismes responsables des differentes phases du sommeil physiologique. Arch. ital. Biol. **100**, 125–206 (1962).

Jouvet, M.: Neurophysiology of the states of sleep. Physiol. Rev. **47**, 117–177 (1967).

Jouvet, M., Michel, F., Courjon, J.: Sur un stade d'activité électrique cérébrale rapide au cours du sommeil physiologique. C. R. Soc. Biol. (Paris) **153**, 1024–1028 (1959).

Jung, R., Kornhuber, H.H., Fonseca, J.S. da: Multisensory convergence on cortical neurons. Neuronal effects of visual, acoustic and vestibular stimuli in the superior convolutions of the cat's cortex. In: G. Moruzzi, A. Fessard and H.H. Jasper, Eds. Progress in Brain Research. Vol. 1: Brain Mechanisms. Amsterdam: Elsevier Publ. Co. 1963.

Kasamatsu, T., Iwama, K.: Two types of light sleep and central visual function in cats. Tohoku J. exp. Med. **88**, 289–303 (1966).

Kornhuber, H.H., Aschoff, J.C.: Somatisch-vestibuläre Konvergenz und Interaktion an Neuronen des motorischen und des somatosensiblen Cortex der Katze. Pflügers Arch. ges. Physiol. **278**, 72–73 (1963).

Kornhuber, H.H., Aschoff, J.C.: Somatisch-vestibuläre Integration an Neuronen des motorischen Cortex. Naturwissenschaften **51**, 62–63 (1964).

Kornhuber, H.H., Fonseca, J.S. da: Optovestibular integration in the cat's cortex: a study of sensory convergence on cortical neurons. In: M.B. Bender, Ed. The oculomotor system. New York: Hoeber Medical Division 1964.

Kubota, K., Iwamura, Y., Niimi, Y.: Monosynaptic reflex and sleep. Experientia (Basel) **20**, 316–317 (1964).

Kubota, K., Iwamura, Y., Niimi, Y.: Monosynaptic reflex and natural sleep in the cat. J. Neurophysiol. **28**, 125–138 (1965).

Kubota, K., Tanaka, R.: The fusimotor activity and natural sleep in the cat. Brain Res. **3**, 198–201 (1966).

LENZI, G.L., POMPEIANO, O., RABIN, B.: Supraspinal control of transmission in the polysynaptic reflex pathway to motoneurones during sleep. Pflügers Arch. ges. Physiol. **301**, 311–319 (1968a).

LENZI, G.L., POMPEIANO, O., RABIN, B.: Transmission of somatic afferent volleys through the flexion reflex pathway during sleep. Proc. XXIV int. Congr. physiol. Sci., Washington, D.C. **7**, 780 (1968b).

LUND, S., POMPEIANO, O.: Descending pathways with monosynaptic action on motoneurones. Experientia (Basel) **21**, 602–603 (1965).

LUND, S., POMPEIANO, O.: Monosynaptic excitation of alpha motoneurones from supraspinal structures in the cat. Acta physiol. scand. **73**, 1–21 (1968).

LUNDBERG, A., NORRSELL, U., VOORHOEVE, P.: Pyramidal effects on lumbo-sacral interneurones activated by somatic afferents. Acta physiol. scand. **56**, 220–229 (1962).

LUNDBERG, A., VOORHOEVE, P.: Effects from the pyramidal tract on spinal reflex arcs. Acta physiol. scand. **56**, 201–219 (1962).

MAGHERINI, P.C., POMPEIANO, O., THODEN, U.: Cholinergic mechanisms related to REM sleep. I. Rhythmic activity of the vestibulo-oculomotor system induced by an anticholinesterase in the decerebrate cat. Arch. ital. Biol. **110**, 234–259 (1972).

MAGOUN, H.W., RHINES, R.: Spasticity. The stretch-reflex and extrapyramidal systems. Springfield, Ill.: C.C. Thomas 1947.

MARCHIAFAVA, P.L., POMPEIANO, O.: Scariche cortico-spinali e inibizione di risposte motorie a stimolazione piramidale nel sonno desincronizzato. Rend. Accad. naz. Lincei, Cl. Sci. fis., mat. nat., Serie VIII, **36**, 547–549 (1964a).

MARCHIAFAVA, P.L., POMPEIANO, O.: Pyramidal influences on spinal cord during desynchronized sleep. Arch. ital. Biol. **102**, 500–529 (1964b).

MARCHIAFAVA, P.L., POMPEIANO, O.: Attività piramidale durante il sonno desincronizzato. Riv. Neurol. **32**, 118–129 (1966a).

MARCHIAFAVA, P.L., POMPEIANO, O.: Excitability changes of the intrageniculate optic tract fibres produced by electrical stimulation of the vestibular system. Pflügers Arch. ges. Physiol. **290**, 275–278 (1966b).

MARCHIAFAVA, P.L., POMPEIANO, O.: Enhanced excitability of intra-geniculate optic tract endings produced by vestibular volleys. Arch. ital. Biol. **104**, 459–479 (1966c).

MEGIRIAN, D., TROTH, R.: Vestibular and muscle nerve connections to pyramidal tract neurons of cat. J. Neurophysiol. **27**, 481–492 (1964).

MICHEL, F., JEANNEROD, M., MOURET, J., RECHTSCHAFFEN, A., JOUVET, M.: Sur les mécanismes de l'activité de pointes au niveau du système visuel au cours de la phase paradoxal du sommeil. C. R. Soc. Biol. (Paris) **158**, 103–106 (1964a).

MICHEL, F., RECHTSCHAFFEN, A., VIMONT, P.: Activité électrique des muscles oculaires extrinsèques au cours du cycle veille-sommeil. C. R. Soc. Biol. (Paris) **158**, 106–109 (1964b).

MIKITEN, T.H., NIEBYL, P.H., HENDLEY, C.D.: EEG desynchronization during behavioral sleep associated with spike discharges from the thalamus of the cat. Fed. Proc. **20**, 327 (1961).

MORRISON, A.R., POMPEIANO, O.: Risposta degli α-motoneuroni alla stimolazione elettrica diretta durante il sonno desincronizzato. Rend. Accad. naz. Lincei, Cl. Sci. fis., mat. nat., Serie VIII, **39**, 329–331 (1965a).

MORRISON, A.R., POMPEIANO, O.: An analysis of the supraspinal influences acting on motoneurons during sleep in the unrestrained cat. Responses of the alpha motoneurons to direct electrical stimulation during sleep. Arch. ital. Biol. **103**, 467–516 (1965b).

MORRISON, A.R., POMPEIANO, O.: Inibizione presinaptica della via riflessa spinale monosinaptica nel sonno fisiologico. Boll. Soc. ital. Biol. sper. **41**, 631–633 (1965c).

MORRISON, A.R., POMPEIANO, O.: Central depolarization of group Ia afferent fibers during desynchronized sleep. Arch. ital. Biol. **103**, 517–537 (1965d).

MORRISON, A.R., POMPEIANO, O.: Corticospinal influences on primary afferents during sleep and wakefulness. Experientia (Basel) **21**, 660–661 (1965e).

MORRISON, A.R., POMPEIANO, O.: Pyramidal discharge from somatosensory cortex and cortical control of primary afferents during sleep. Arch. ital. Biol. **103**, 538–568 (1965f).

MORRISON, A.R., POMPEIANO, O.: Vestibular influences on vegetative functions during the rapid eye movement periods of desynchronized sleep. Experientia (Basel) **21**, 667–668 (1965g).

Morrison, A.R., Pompeiano, O.: Influenze vestibolari sull'attività piramidale durante i movimenti rapidi oculari nel sonno desincronizzato. Boll. Soc. ital. Biol. sper. **41**, 937–939 (1965h).

Morrison, A.R., Pompeiano, O.: Vestibular influences during sleep. II. Effects of vestibular lesions on the pyramidal discharge during desynchronized sleep. Arch. ital. Biol. **104**, 214–230 (1966a).

Morrison, A.R., Pompeiano, O.: Response of alpha motoneurones to direct electrical stimulation during desynchronized sleep. Nature (Lond.) **211**, 636–637 (1966b).

Morrison, A.R., Pompeiano, O.: Depolarization of central terminals of group Ia muscle afferent fibres during desynchronized sleep. Nature (Lond.) **210**, 201–202 (1966c).

Morrison, A.R., Pompeiano, O.: Vestibular influences during sleep. IV. Functional relations between vestibular nuclei and lateral geniculate nucleus during desynchronized sleep. Arch. ital. Biol. **104**, 425–458 (1966d).

Morrison, A.R., Pompeiano, O.: Vestibular influences during sleep. VI. Vestibular control of autonomic functions during the rapid eye movements of desynchronized sleep. Arch. ital. Biol. **108**, 154–180 (1970).

Moruzzi, G.: Active processes in the brain stem during sleep. Harvey Lect. **58**, 233–297 (1963).

Mouret, J.: Les mouvements oculaires au cours du sommeil paradoxal. Recherches sur leur nature et leurs méchanismes chez le chat et chez l'homme. Lyon: Imprimerie des Beaux-Arts 1964.

Mouret, U., Jeannerod, M., Jouvet, M.: L'activité éléctrique du système visuel au cours de la phase paradoxale du sommeil chez le chat. J. Physiol. (Paris) **55**, 305–306 (1963).

Okuma, T., Fujimori, M.: Electrographic and evoked potential studies during sleep in the cat. I. The study on sleep. Folia psychiat. neurol. jap. **17**, 25–50 (1963).

Palestini, M., Pisano, M., Rosadini, G., Rossi, G.F.: Excitability cycle of the visual cortex during sleep and wakefulness. E.E.G. clin. Neurophysiol. **19**, 276–283 (1965).

Palestini, M., Pisano, M., Rosadini, G., Rossi, G.F.: Visual cortical responses evoked by stimulating lateral geniculate body and optic radiations in awake and sleeping cats. Exp. Neurol. **9**, 17–30 (1967).

Pisano, M., Rosadini, G., Rossi, G.F.: Risposte corticali evocate da stimoli dromici e antidromici durante il sonno e la veglia. Riv. Neurobiol. **8**, 414–426 (1962).

Pompeiano, O.: Sulle risposte posturali alla stimolazione elettrica del nucleo rosso nel gatto decerebrato. Boll. Soc. ital. Biol. sper. **32**, 1450–1451 (1956).

Pompeiano, O.: Analisi degli effetti della stimolazione elettrica del nucleo rosso nel gatto decerebrato. Rend. Accad. naz. Lincei, Cl. Sci. fis., mat. nat., Serie VIII, **22**, 100–103 (1957).

Pompeiano, O.: Ascending and descending influences of somatic afferent volleys in unrestrained cats: supraspinal inhibitory control of spinal reflexes during natural and reflexly induced sleep. In: Aspects anatomo-fonctionnels de la physiologie du sommeil. Paris: Éditions du Centre National de la Recherche Scientifique 1965.

Pompeiano, O.: Muscular afferents and motor control during sleep. In: R. Granit, Ed. Nobel Symposium I. Muscular afferents and motor control. Stockholm: Almqvist and Wiksell 1966a.

Pompeiano, O.: Sui rapporti anatomo-funzionali tra cervelletto e midollo spinale. Riv. Pat. nerv. ment. 33–164 (1966b).

Pompeiano, O.: Functional organization of the cerebellar projections to the spinal cord. In: C.A. Fox and R.S. Snider, Eds. Progress in Brain Research. Vol. 25. The cerebellum. Amsterdam: Elsevier Publ. Co. 1967a.

Pompeiano, O.: The neurophysiological mechanisms of the postural and motor events during desynchronized sleep. In: S.S. Kety, E.V. Evarts and H.L. Williams, Eds. Sleep and altered states of consciousness. Res. Publ. Ass. nerv. ment. Dis. **45**, 351–423 (1967b).

Pompeiano, O.: Sensory inhibition during motor activity in sleep. In: M.D. Yahr and D.P. Purpura, Eds. Neurophysiological basis of normal and abnormal motor activities. Hewlett, N.Y.: Raven Press 1967c.

Pompeiano, O.: Mechanisms of sensory-motor integration during sleep. In: E. Stellar and J.M. Sprague, Eds. Progress in Physiological Psychology. New York: Academic Press **3**, 1–179 (1968a).

Pompeiano, O.: Monosynaptic and polysynaptic reflex excitation of motoneurones to plantar muscles in the unrestrained cat. Brain Res. **10**, 252–256 (1968b).

Pompeiano, O.: Sleep mechanisms. In: M.M. Jasper, A.A. Ward and A. Pope, Eds. Basic mechanisms of the epilepsies. Boston: Little, Brown & Co. 1969.

Pompeiano, O.: Interaction between vestibular and nonvestibular sensory inputs. In: Fourth symposium on the role of the vestibular organs in space exploration. NASA-SP **187**, 209–236 (1970).

Pompeiano, O.: Reticular control of the vestibular nuclei: physiology and pharmacology. In: A. Brodal and O. Pompeiano, Eds. Progress in Brain Research. Vol. 37. Basic aspects of central vestibular mechanisms. Amsterdam: Elsevier Publ. Co. 1972.

Pompeiano, O.: A neuronal model of REM sleep. In: W.P. Koella and P. Levin, Eds. Sleep. Basel: S. Karger AG 1973.

Pompeiano, O., Morrison, A.R.: Abolizione dei movimenti rapidi oculari nel sonno desincronizzato prodotta da lesioni vestibolari. Boll. Soc. ital. Biol. sper. **41**, 935–937 (1965a).

Pompeiano, O., Morrison, A.R.: Vestibular influences during sleep. I. Abolition of the rapid eye movements during desynchronized sleep following vestibular lesions. Arch. ital. Biol. **103**, 569–595 (1965b).

Pompeiano, O., Morrison, A.R.: Origine vestibolare della depressione fasica dei riflessi spinali durante i movimenti rapidi oculari nel sonno desincronizzato. Boll. Soc. ital. Biol. sper. **41**, 939–941 (1965c).

Pompeiano, O., Morrison, A.R.: Vestibular influences during sleep. III. Dissociation of the tonic and phasic inhibition of spinal reflexes during desynchronized sleep following vestibular lesions. Arch. ital. Biol. **104**, 231–246 (1966a).

Pompeiano, O., Morrison, A.R.: Vestibular origin of the rapid eye movements during desynchronized sleep. Experientia (Basel) **22**, 60–61 (1966b).

Pompeiano, O., Morrison, A.R.: Influenze vestibolari sull'attività del nucleo genicolato laterale nel sonno desincronizzato. Rend. Accad. naz. Lincei, Cl. Sci. fis., mat. nat., Serie VIII, **40**, 116–118 (1966c).

Pompeiano, O., Morrison, A.R.: Vestibular input to the lateral geniculate nucleus during desynchronized sleep. Pflügers Arch. ges. Physiol. **290**, 272–274 (1966d).

Pompeiano, O., Satoh, T.: Vestibular influences on the red nucleus during sleep. Pflügers Arch. ges. Physiol. **298**, 159–162 (1967).

Pompeiano, O., Swett, J.E.: EEG and behavioral manifestations of sleep induced by cutaneous nerve stimulation in normal cats. Arch. ital. Biol. **100**, 311–342 (1962).

Rossi, G.F., Palestini, M., Pisano, M., Rosadini, G.: An experimental study of the cortical reactivity during sleep and wakefulness. In: Aspects anatomo-fonctionnels de la physiologie du sommeil. Paris: Éditions du Centre National de la Recherche Scientifique 1965.

Sakakura, H., Iwama, K.: Presynaptic inhibition and postsynaptic facilitation in lateral geniculate body and so-called deep sleep wave activity. Tohoku J. exp. Med. **87**, 40–51 (1965).

Sakakura, H., Iwama, K.: Unitary recording from cat lateral geniculate during natural sleep. Proc. Jap. Acad. **42**, 418–423 (1966).

Seguin, J.J., Magherini, P.C., Pompeiano, O.: Cholinergic mechanisms related to REM sleep. III. Tonic and phasic inhibition of monosynaptic reflexes induced by an anticholinesterase in the decerebrate cat. Arch. ital. Biol. **111**, 1–28 (1973).

Shimizu, A., Yamada, Y., Yamamoto, J., Fujiki, A., Kaneko, Z.: Pathways of descending influence on H reflex during sleep. E.E.G. clin. Neurophysiol. **20**, 337–347 (1966).

Sperry, R.W.: Neural basis of the spontaneous optokinetic response produced by visual inversion. J. comp. physiol. Psychol. **43**, 482–489 (1950).

Stuart, D., Ishikawa, K., Bors, E., Porter, R.W.: The H-reflex in spinal and normal man. Physiologist **8**, 282 (1965).

Teuber, H.L.: The riddle of frontal lobe function in man. In: J.M. Warren and K. Akert, Eds. The frontal granular cortex and behavior. New York: McGraw Hill 1964.

Thoden, U., Magherini, P.C., Pompeiano, O.: Cholinergic mechanisms related to REM sleep. II. Effects of an anticholinesterase on the discharge of central vestibular neurons in the decerebrate cat. Arch. ital. Biol. **110**, 260–283 (1972).

Tokizane, T.: Studies on the paradoxical phase of sleep in the cat. In: T. Tokizane and J.P. Schadé, Eds. Progress in Brain Research. Vol. 21B. Correlative Neurosciences. Part B. Clinical Studies. Amsterdam: Elsevier Publ. Co. 1966.

Valleala, P.: The temporal relation of unit discharge in visual cortex and activity of the extraocular muscles during sleep. Arch. ital. Biol. **105**, 1–14 (1967).

Walberg, F., Pompeiano, O., Brodal, A., Jansen, J.: The fastigio-vestibular projection in the cat. An experimental study with silver impregnation methods. J. comp. Neurol. **118**, 49–75 (1962a).

Walberg, F., Pompeiano, O., Westrum, L.E., Hauglie-Hanssen, E.: Fastigioreticular fibers in the cat. An experimental study with silver methods. J. comp. Neurol. **119**, 187–199 (1962b).

Wall, P.D.: Excitability changes in afferent fibre terminations and their relation to slow potentials. J. Physiol. (Lond.) **142**, 1–21 (1958).

Walsh, J.T., Cordeau, J.P.: Responsiveness in the visual system during various phases of sleep and waking. Exp. Neurol. **11**, 80–103 (1965).

Author Index

Page numbers in *italics* refer to the bibliography

Subject Index